Springer

*Berlin*
*Heidelberg*
*New York*
*Barcelona*
*Hong Kong*
*London*
*Milan*
*Paris*
*Singapore*
*Tokyo*

Z. Petrovich · L. Baert · L.W. Brady (Eds.)

# Carcinoma of the Kidney and Testis, and Rare Urologic Malignancies

## Innovations in Management

With Contributions by

J. A. L. L. Baert · L. Baert · M. Bamberg · A. Belldegrun · G. A. Bogaert · R. Bouillon
L.W. Brady · C. Catton · J. Classen · F. A. Corso · P. Dal Cin · D. J. M. K. De Ridder
H. Dumez · M. Dzeda · R. A. Figlin · A. J. Figueroa · S. C. Formenti · B. E. Henderson
S. Horenblas · G. Jozsef · B. A. Kogan · J. E. Lahaniatis · R. Lavey · B. K. Lee · B. Micaily
J. M. Michalski · A. Mohrbacher · P. W. Nichols · R. J. M. Nijman · R. H. Oyen
H. Ozer · A. Pawinski · C. L. Pearce · Z. Petrovich · H. Raat · M. Roach III · T. Roskams
R. K. Ross · C. E. Salem · D. G. Skinner · E. C. Skinner · J. P. Stein · L. Stockx
O. E. Streeter · S. J. Tucker · B. Van Damme · H. Van den Berghe · A. Van den Bruel
A. Van Oosterom · H. P. Van Poppel · L. Vanuytsel · B. M. Verbist · G. A. Verswijvel
W. Wynendaele · M. C. Yu · J.-M. Yuan · C.-S. Zee

Foreword by

L.W. Brady and H.-P. Heilmann

Preface by

Z. Petrovich · L. Baert · L.W. Brady

With 189 Figures in 266 Separate Illustrations, Some in Color and 92 Tables

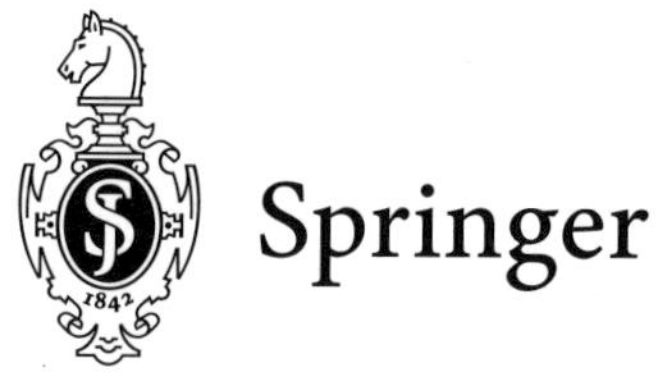

Springer

Zbigniew Petrovich, MD, FACR
Professor of Radiation Oncology and Urology
Chairman, Department of Radiation Oncology
University of Southern California School of Medicine
Kenneth Norris Jr. Cancer Hospital and Research Institute
1441 Eastlake Avenue
Los Angeles, CA 90033-004
USA

Luc Baert, MD, PhD
Professor and Chairman, Department of Urology
Catholic University of Leuven, University Hospitals Gasthuisberg
49, Herestraat
B-3000 Leuven
Belgium

Luther W. Brady, MD
Hylda Cohn/American Cancer Society
Professor of Clinical Oncology, and
Professor, Department of Radiation Oncology
Allegheny University of the Health Sciences
Allegheny University Hospitals, Hahnemann
Broad & Vine Sts., Mail Stop 200,
Philadelphia, PA 19102-1192
USA

---

MEDICAL RADIOLOGY · Diagnostic Imaging and Radiation Oncology

Continuation of
Handbuch der medizinischen Radiologie
Encyclopedia of Medical Radiology

---

ISSN 0942-5373
ISBN 3-540-63215-8 Springer-Verlag Berlin Heidelberg New York

Library of Congress Cataloging-in-Publication Data. Carcinoma of the kidney and testis, and rare urologic malignancies: innovations in management / Z. Petrovich, L. Baert, L.W. Brady (eds.) ; with contributions by J.A.L.L. Baert... [et al.] ; foreword by L. W. Brady and H.-P. Heilmann.   p.   cm. -- (Medical radiology)   Includes bibliographical references and index. ISBN 3-540-63215-8 (alk. paper)   1. Genitourinary organs--Cancer. 2. Kidneys--Cancer. 3. Testis--Cancer. I. Petrovich, Zbigniew.   II. Baert, L. (Luc)   III. Brady, Luther W., 1925- . IV.   Series   [DNLM: 1. Urogenital Neoplasms--therapy. WJ 160 C265 1999]   RC280.G4C37   1999   616.99'46--dc21   DNLM/DLC   for Library of Congress   98-21388   CIP



Printed in Germany



Typesetting: Best-set Typesetter Ltd., Hong Kong

SPIN: 10546236          21/3135 – 5 4 3 2 1 0 – Printed on acid-free paper

This book is dedicated to

*Zofia Petrovich, MD and Mrs. Bea Baert*

# Foreword

In the United States in 1997, 28 800 new cases of malignant tumors of the kidney and renal pelvis were diagnosed along with 2100 new cases of malignant tumors of the ureter and other urinary organs, 7200 primary malignant tumors of the testis, and 1300 primary malignant tumors of the penis and other genital organs. In large measure, surgery is the treatment of choice for these tumors, but radiation therapy is increasingly recognized as having significant and important curative and palliative benefits in each of these tumor sites. Surgery is the standard form of treatment for nonmetastatic renal cell carcinomas as well as for malignancies of the renal pelvis and ureter, with radical nephrectomy and radical uretectomy being employed. However, postoperative radiation therapy is of value for those patients who demonstrate evidence of residual tumor following surgery, transection of tumor during surgery, or positive regional lymph node drainage. As regards the rare tumors that involve the female urethra, surgical resection is appropriate for those that are limited and local in character and amenable to partial ureterectomy. With tumors that are more advanced in character, however, local recurrence and lymphatic dissemination are significant problems, and treatment by radiation therapy programs alone yield satisfactory control rates as well as limited recurrences and long-term survivors.

For primary tumors involving the testis, the major approach to nonseminomatous tumors is surgical resection with postsurgical systemic chemotherapy. On the other hand, seminomas are best managed by surgical resection with orchiectomy and high cord ligation along with postoperative radiation therapy in the appropriate circumstances; this strategy produces significant survival figures in patients with seminomas.

Tumors that involve the penis and the male urethra are difficult problems to tackle because of both the location and the pattern of local tumor spread. Generally, surgical management is the appropriate approach to the problem but when there is evidence of regional lymph node involvement, radiation therapy can be used with good results; certainly radiation therapy has the primary advantage of preserving the phallus intact.

The current volume, *Carcinoma of the Kidney and Testis, and Rare Urologic Malignancies. Innovation in Management*, compiles all of the pertinent data with regard to epidemiology, workup, and treatment for these tumor types, presenting results relative to management; it also discusses basic research and clinical research into appropriate treatment regimens for each of these tumor sites. The authors of this volume stress the need for careful selection of cases for each treatment regimen, careful follow-up, and carefully carried out treatment programs.

<table>
<tr><td>Philadelphia</td><td style="text-align:right">LUTHER W. BRADY</td></tr>
<tr><td>Hamburg</td><td style="text-align:right">HANS-PETER HEILMANN</td></tr>
</table>

# Preface

During the past decade, major advances have taken place in the diagnosis and management of patients with carcinoma of the kidney and testicle. At the same time quality of life issues have reached a level of importance nearly equal to that of patient survival rates. It appears appropriate and relevant to summarize these important advances in the present volume.

Renal cell carcinoma (RCC) is the predominant primary tumor of the kidney. It is an important and relatively common tumor. In the past decade in the United States there has been an approximate 20% increase in the incidence of RCC with a simultaneous major improvement in patient survival. This improvement in survival has primarily been, due to major progress in the imaging modalities and better understanding of the natural history of this disease, permitting early diagnosis and timely application of appropriate surgical therapy. Radical nephrectomy remains the only effective therapy in the management of primary RCC, with newer surgical techniques such as partial nephrectomy becoming an important  and widely recognized treatment in properly selected patients. RCC patients presenting with or relapsing with metastatic disease remain a major challenge to uro-oncology in spite of recent developments in immunotherapy and a possibility of applying gene therapy. Contemporary radiotherapy has become an important palliative treatment in many RCC patients with metastasis.

Testicular tumors are relatively small in number but important malignancies with an estimated 7600 patients expected to be diagnosed in the United States in 1998. In the past decade these tumors have shown a nearly 30% increase in incidence, which is most apparent  in white males. The management of testicular tumors has become a success story through the use of surgery in combination with systemic chemotherapy. In the early 1960s in the United States, the 5-year survival of patients with testicular carcinoma was less than 63% but it had increased to more than 95% by the early 1990s. This increase in survival was largely due to advances in chemotherapy. Current efforts in therapy for testicular tumors are directed towards improvement in quality of life of the treated patients who are expected to have survival rates similar to those of a matched group of males in the general population. The importance of these quality of life issues is reflected in the four chapters dedicated to this topic in this volume.

The management of uncommon tumors of the genitourinary tract presents a special problem. Due to their rarity only major medical centers acquire the experience needed for the frequently complex management of these tumors. In view of the above the authors believe that patients with rare urologic malignancies should be referred for treatment to centers specializing in the management of genitourinary tumors.

This work, together with the previously published two volumes including carcinoma of the prostate and bladder, attempts to present the state-of-the-art in the diagnosis and management of patients with genitourinary tumors. It is apparent that successful management of these tumors depends on the presence and frequent interaction of a multidisciplinary team of specialists dedicated to genitourinary carcinoma. This team of specialists should include: urologists, medical oncologists, radiation oncologists, diagnostic radiologists, pathologists, epidemiologists, geneticists, immunologists, molecular biologists, highly skilled technologists, and nursing staff.

<br>

| | |
|---|---|
| Los Angeles | Z. Petrovich |
| Leuven | L. Baert |
| Philadelphia | L.W. Brady |

# Contents

# Renal Cell Carcinoma

# 1 Epidemiology of Renal Cell Carcinoma

M.C. Yu, J.-M. Yuan, and R.K. Ross

CONTENTS



## 1.1
## Introduction

Kidney cancer is a relatively rare malignancy. In the United States, there are roughly 30 000 new cases of kidney cancer each year, accounting for approximately 2% of all incident cancer cases diagnosed annually (Parker et al. 1996).

Renal cell carcinoma accounts for 80%–85% of all kidney cancers occurring in the United States (Devesa et al. 1990). The remaining 15%–20% of kidney cancers are mostly cancers of the renal pelvis, which are anatomically and histologically distinct from renal cell carcinoma. The following description of international variations of renal cell carcinoma incidence is based on data given for kidney cancer as a whole since these two distinct types of renal cancer are not reported separately in international comparisons.

M.C. Yu, PhD, Professor of Preventive Medicine, Department of Preventive Medicine, University of Southern California, Norris Comprehensive Cancer Center, 1441 Eastlake Avenue, Los Angeles, CA 90033-0800, USA
J.-M. Yuan, MD, PhD, Department of Preventive Medicine, University of Southern California, Norris Comprehensive Cancer Center, 1441 Eastlake Avenue, Los Angeles, CA 90033-0800, USA
R.K. Ross, MD, Department of Preventive Medicine, University of Southern California, Norris Comprehensive Cancer Center, 1441 Eastlake Avenue, Los Angeles, CA 90033-0800, USA

## 1.2
## Demographic Pattern

### 1.2.1
### International Variation

There is an approximately sixfold difference in incidence of kidney cancer between high- and low-risk countries on a worldwide basis. Highest rates are found among Western Europeans and Scandinavians with age-standardized incidence rates of 10–13/100 000 in men and 5–7/100 000 in women, respectively. Lowest rates are found in Asian countries such as India and China, where age-standardized incidence rates in men and women are 1–2/100 000 and 0.5–1/100 000, respectively (Parkin et al. 1997).

### 1.2.2
### U.S. Incidence

Similar to many other cancers, renal cell carcinoma shows variation in incidence among the major racial-ethnic groups constituting the U.S. population. Highest rates are observed among Hispanics, followed by African-Americans and non-Hispanic whites. Rates in Hispanics tend to be about 3%–7% higher than in African-Americans (depending on gender) whereas larger differences of about 10%–20% are noted between African-Americans and non-Hispanic whites. Rates are substantially lower among Asians (including Chinese, Japanese, Filipinos, and Koreans), being roughly half the rates in non-Asians (Table 1.1). Alaskan Natives and Native-Americans have been reported to have particularly high rates of renal cell carcinoma (Nutting et al. 1993). The Native-Americans' high risk with respect to renal cell carcinoma may have contributed to

**Table 1.1.** Age-adjusted incidence rates (per 100 000) for men and women by major racial-ethic groups, Los Angeles County, California, 1972–1995[a]

| Race-Ethnicity | Males | | Females | |
|---|---|---|---|---|
| | Rate | No. | Rate | No. |
| African-Americans | 9.3 | 722 | 4.4 | 457 |
| Chinese | 3.8 | 57 | 1.6 | 27 |
| Japanese | 3.6 | 55 | 1.5 | 29 |
| Filipinos | 4.9 | 65 | 2.2 | 32 |
| Koreans | 4.0 | 29 | 2.2 | 19 |
| Non-Hispanic Whites | 8.6 | 4789 | 3.7 | 2651 |
| Hispanics | 9.5 | 981 | 4.7 | 618 |

[a] Based on data from the Los Angeles County Cancer Surveillance Program/Surveillance Epidemiology and End Results (SEER) Cancer Ragistry; age adjustment according to the 1970 U.S. population.

the observed high rates in Hispanics, many of whom have Mexican origins with Native-American admixture.

### 1.2.3
### Sex and Age

Renal cell carcinoma is a disease with a strong male dominance, which is present across all populations. Among U.S. populations, there is generally at least a twofold excess incidence in men relative to women (Table 1.1).

Similar to most epithelial cancers, renal cell carcinoma is strongly related to age. There is a linear relationship between age and renal cell carcinoma incidence when both variables are expressed in logarithmic units (Fig. 1.1). The magnitude of the slope of this logarithmic age-incidence curve is approximately 4.5, which is relatively low compared to the steep slopes (magnitude of 9–10 or greater) associated with cancers such as prostate cancer. The age-incidence pattern is similar across racial-ethnic groups and in both sexes.

### 1.2.4
### Time Trends

Renal cell carcinoma rates have increased in the United States over the past 25 years. Data from one large population-based cancer registry (the Los Angeles County Cancer Surveillance Program) active during this entire period are shown in Fig. 1.2. Rates

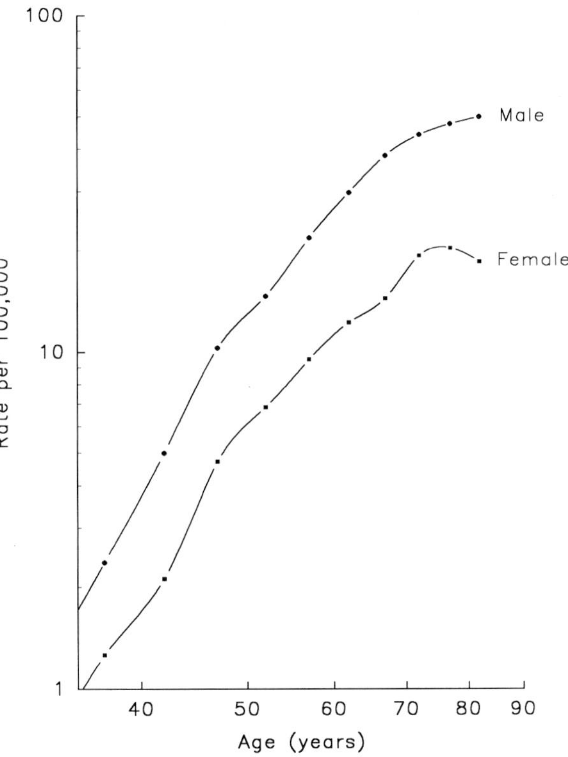


**Fig. 1.1.** Annual age-specific incidence rates of renal cell carcinoma in non-Hispanic whites in Los Angeles County, 1972–1995

increased by approximately 30%–40% from the early 1970s through the mid- to late 1980s in non-Hispanic whites and more substantially in African-Americans in Los Angeles. These increases occurred in both men and women. This rate of increase has slowed and in non-Hispanic white males at least, may even have reversed in the past few years.

### 1.2.5
### Social Class

Some population-based cancer registries in the United States classify cases according to social class characteristics. This is achieved on a group rather than individual basis. Typically, census information on income and/or educational levels of residents in the neighborhoods where cancer patients reside is used to rank cancer cases into one of four or five social class groupings. In Los Angeles, for men there is no clear association between social class and risk of renal cell carcinoma. Men in the highest quintile have approximately the same risk as men in the lowest quintile. For women, there is a weak inverse

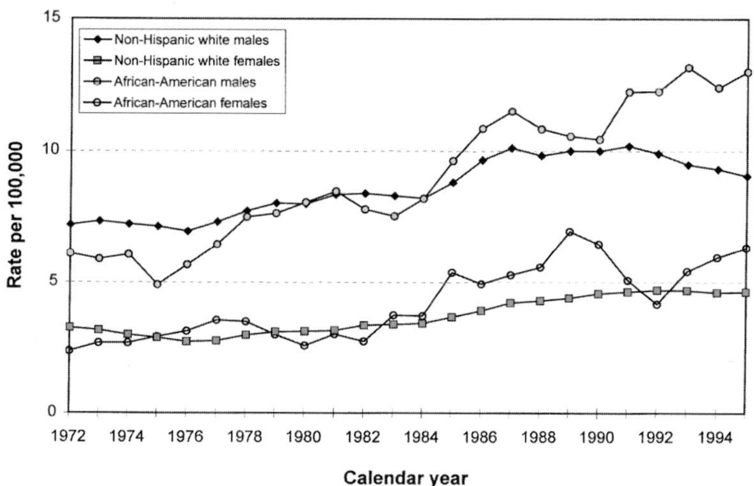



**Fig. 1.2.** Secular trend in incidence rates of renal cell carcinoma in non-Hispanic whites and African-Americans in Los Angeles County, 1972–1995

**Table 1.2.** Age-adjusted incidence rates (per 100000) in non-Hispanic white males and females by socioeconomic status (SES) groupings, Los Angeles County, California, 1972–1995[a]

| SES grouping | Males | Females |
| --- | --- | --- |
| 1 (High) | 8.4 | 3.1 |
| 2 | 8.6 | 3.8 |
| 3 | 8.2 | 3.7 |
| 4 | 8.2 | 3.7 |
| 5 (Low) | 8.4 | 3.8 |

[a] Based on data from the Los Angeles County Cancer Surveillance Program/Surveillance Epidemiology and End Results (SEER) Cancer Registry; age adjustment according to the 1970 U.S. population.

relationship (i.e., rates are slightly higher in the lower than in the upper quintiles) (Table 1.2). Since the best-studied major risk factors for renal cell carcinoma, including obesity, hypertension, and cigarette smoking (see below), tend to be negatively related to social class, these data suggest that in men at least, other important, as yet unidentified risk factors for renal cell carcinoma must exist to explain these social class gradients.

## 1.2.6
## Comparison with Bladder Cancer

It is of some interest to compare the epidemiology of renal cell carcinoma with that of bladder cancer, since both sites share common exposure to the same urinary carcinogens. The etiology of bladder cancer is relatively well understood; cigarette smoking and occupational exposure to a class of chemical carcinogens known as arylamines are believed to account for as many as 60% of all bladder cancer cases diagnosed in the United States (YU and Ross 1998). Bladder cancer is also a disease with a male predominance, with men having a threefold or greater risk than women in all major racial-ethnic groups in the United States. However, the racial-ethnic pattern of bladder cancer incidence in the United States is dramatically different from that of renal cell carcinoma. Non-Hispanic whites have the highest risk of bladder cancer (almost twice that of any other group), and African-Americans have slightly higher rates than Hispanics. As with renal cell carcinoma, Asians have the lowest risk of bladder cancer among all racial-ethnic groups in the United States (YU and Ross 1998).

## 1.3
## Environmental Risk Factors

### 1.3.1
### Cigarette Smoking

Cigarette smoking in relation to renal cell carcinoma risk has been investigated in multiple case-control and cohort studies. All study results are consistent with a modest association between cigarette use and renal cell carcinoma risk (DOLL 1996). The overall evidence strongly supports cigarette smoking as a cause of renal cell carcinoma.

**Table 1.3.** Cigarette smoking in relation to risk of renal cell carcinoma (adapted from YUAN et al. 1998a)

| | Total | | Males | | Females | |
|---|---|---|---|---|---|---|
| | Ca/Co | OR (95% Cl) | Ca/Co | OR (95% Cl) | Ca/Co | OR (95% Cl) |
| Never | 404/491 | 1.00 | 223/288 | 1.00 | 181/203 | 1.00 |
| Ever | 800/713 | 1.35 (1.14, 1.60) | 558/493 | 1.42 (1.14, 1.77) | 242/220 | 1.23 (0.93, 1.64) |
|   Former smokers | 463/450 | 1.24 (1.02, 1.50) | 350/331 | 1.34 (1.05, 1.70) | 113/119 | 1.07 (0.77, 1.49) |
|   No. of years since quitting | | | | | | |
|     20 | 169/177 | 1.15 (0.89, 1.50) | 135/145 | 1.18 (0.86, 1.61) | 34/32 | 1.19 (0.70, 2.02) |
|     10–19 | 135/135 | 1.25 (0.94, 1.64) | 98/99 | 1.26 (0.90, 1.76) | 37/36 | 1.23 (0.74, 2.04) |
|     1–9 | 159/138 | 1.33 (1.02, 1.74) | 117/87 | 1.64 (1.17, 2.29) | 42/51 | 0.88 (0.56, 1.40) |
|   Current smokers | 337/262 | 1.53 (1.23, 1.90) | 208/162 | 1.58 (1.20, 2.08) | 129/100 | 1.46 (1.03, 2.08) |
|   No. of cigarettes/day | | | | | | |
|     1–19 | 87/73 | 1.48 (1.04, 2.12) | 45/38 | 1.58 (0.96, 2.58) | 42/35 | 1.39 (0.83, 2.32) |
|     20–39 | 183/146 | 1.45 (1.11, 1.88) | 114/92 | 1.46 (1.05, 2.03) | 69/54 | 1.41 (0.91, 2.22) |
|     40 | 67/43 | 1.90 (1.25, 2.90) | 49/32 | 1.92 (1.17, 3.17) | 18/11 | 1.93 (0.88, 4.23) |
|   Total no. of cigarettes smoked over lifetime (×1000) | | | | | | |
|     <117 | 239/237 | 1.22 (0.97, 1.53) | 154/152 | 1.28 (0.96, 1.71) | 85/85 | 1.13 (0.79, 1.62) |
|     117–<283 | 244/236 | 1.25 (0.99, 1.58) | 172/171 | 1.27 (0.96, 1.69) | 72/65 | 1.22 (0.82, 1.83) |
|     283 | 316/239 | 1.60 (1.28, 2.01) | 231/170 | 1.69 (1.29, 2.22) | 85/69 | 1.43 (0.93, 2.18) |

Ca/Co, Number of cases/number of controls; OR, odds ratio; Cl, confidence interval.

Results of a large-scale, population-based case-control study conducted in Los Angeles serve to illustrate selected details of the smoking/renal cell carcinoma relationship (YUAN et al. 1998a). Overall, ever smokers have a 35% increased risk relative to lifelong nonsmokers (Table 1.3). Cigarette smokers who quit the habit experience a reduced risk of renal cell carcinoma relative to current smokers, with increasing magnitude in risk reduction as time interval since smoking cessation increases. The average number of cigarettes smoked per day is proportional to risk, with an approximate twofold risk of renal cell carcinoma in 2 or more packs per day current smokers relative to lifelong nonsmokers. Use of filtered (as opposed to nonfiltered) cigarettes and pattern of inhalation do not seem to influence risk of renal cell carcinoma. There is little evidence that use of other tobacco products (such as cigar, pipe, chew tobacco, and snuff) elevates an individual's risk for renal cell carcinoma. For any given level of smoking, risks of renal cell carcinoma in men and women are remarkably similar. It is estimated that in Los Angeles, 17% (21% in men and 11% in women) of renal cell carcinoma cases can be attributed to cigarette smoking (YUAN et al. 1998a).

The mechanism by which cigarette smoking causes renal cell carcinoma is still unclear. Nonetheless, it is known that cigarette smokers excrete mutagenic urine while nonsmokers do not (YAMASAKI and AMES 1977). Also, $N$-nitrosodimethylamine, a renal carcinogen in a number of animal species, is detected in cigarette smoke (International Agency for Research on Cancer 1986).

It is of interest that the magnitude of increased risk for renal cell carcinoma associated with a given level of cigarette smoking is considerably less than that observed for cancer of the renal pelvis and ureter (Ross et al. 1989; MCLAUGHLIN et al. 1992). The transitional cell urothelium of the renal pelvis and ureter is exposed to the same potential carcinogens in urine as the renal tubular cells which give rise to renal cell carcinoma. It appears that either the tubular cells are less sensitive to the tobacco carcinogens in urine or the exposure level of the target cells to these compounds is higher for the renal pelvis.

### 1.3.2
### Iatrogenic Factors

#### 1.3.2.1
#### Diuretics

In 1986, YU et al. first reported that use of diuretics might be related to risk of renal cell carcinoma, independent of history of hypertension. A number of subsequent case-control studies have noted similar findings (MCLAUGHLIN et al. 1988; FINKLE et al. 1993; KREIGER et al. 1993; HIATT et al. 1994; WEINMANN et al. 1994). However, these earlier studies all possess one or more major design flaws that can impact on the validity of study findings, including crude assessment of medication history, inclusion of proxy interviews, small sample size, and limited analysis to separate treatment effects from their indications.

Two recent studies specifically designed to circumvent the methodological limitations of earlier studies have failed to confirm a role for diuretics in renal cell carcinoma development that is independent of the medical condition (i.e., hypertension) for which the drugs are prescribed. In a multicenter study involving 1732 cases of renal cell carcinoma and 2309 population controls, McLaughlin et al. (1995) noted no association between diuretic use and cancer risk after adjustment for history of hypertension and other confounding factors. In Los Angeles, Yuan et al. (1998b) conducted a population-based study involving 1204 patients with renal cell carcinoma and an equal number of individually matched (by age, sex, and race) neighborhood controls. The investigators reported that: (1) among the relatively small number of individuals who had used diuretics for purposes other than treatment for hypertension, there was no increased cancer risk even for those with high lifetime cumulative doses; (2) among hypertensive subjects, cancer risk was unrelated to cumulative lifetime dose of diuretics; and (3) hypertensive subjects treated with diuretics and/or other antihypertensives exhibited risk levels for renal cell carcinoma quite comparable to those who had never been medically treated. Yuan et al. (1998b) concluded that hypertension per se, rather than its treatment, is the principal determinant of risk for renal cell carcinoma.

### 1.3.2.2
### Nondiuretic Antihypertensives

There is no a priori reason to suspect that nondiuretic antihypertensives (beta-blockers, central antiadrenergic agents, neuronal depleting agents, angiotensin-converting enzyme inhibitors, and vasodilators) are renal carcinogens. However, McLaughlin et al. (1995) reported that long-term use (5 or more years) of these drugs was associated with a significant increase in risk of renal cell carcinoma independent of a history of hypertension, although no dose-response relationship was observed with cumulative dosage of any of the major classes of antihypertensives. Heath et al. (1997) showed that use of antihypertensives was associated with a statistically significant increase in risk of death from renal cell carcinoma among female participants of the

American Cancer Society Cohort Study. But the effects of antihypertensives and history of hypertension could not be disentangled in this latter study and there was no dose-response relationship between cancer risk and either dosage or duration of use. In their recent case-control study of renal cell carcinoma in Los Angeles in which all commonly prescribed brand names of antihypertensives in the United States since the 1950s were explicitly asked about during the in-person interviews conducted with study subjects, Yuan et al. (1998b) detected no association between regular use of such drugs and renal cell carcinoma risk after adjustment for hypertension status. Therefore, the overall evidence does not support an etiologic link between antihypertensive use and renal cell carcinoma development.

### 1.3.2.3
### Analgesics

Chronic use of analgesics was first linked to the development of kidney cancer through a series of case reports which documented cancer of the renal pelvis occurring in heavy users of phenacetin (Hultengren et al. 1965; Bengtsson et al. 1968; Mahony et al. 1977). These uncontrolled observations were later confirmed by a number of case-control studies conducted in diverse populations (McCredie et al. 1982, 1986; McLaughlin et al. 1985; Jensen et al. 1989; Ross et al. 1989). Phenacetin has been absent from all drugs manufactured in the United States since 1987.

A possible link between heavy use of analgesics and renal cell carcinoma was first suggested by Armstrong and co-workers in 1976 (Armstrong et al. 1976). In that study, subjects reporting daily use of analgesics had a tenfold increase in risk of renal cell carcinoma relative to nonusers. A number of subsequent studies have substantiated that finding, implicating chronic use of phenacetin (McLaughlin et al. 1985, 1992; McCredie et al. 1986, 1988, 1995; Kreiger et al. 1993; Mellemgaard et al. 1994a), acetaminophen (McCredie et al. 1993, 1995; Derby and Jick, 1996) and aspirin (Asal et al. 1988; Paganini-Hill et al. 1989; Mellemgaard et al. 1994a) as risk factors for renal cell carcinoma, although the exposure-risk associations were much more modest.

The recently completed population-based case-control study in Los Angeles provides the most definitive results to date on the analgesic–renal cell carcinoma relationship (GAGO-DOMINGUEZ et al., unpublished work). This study involved 1204 incident cases of renal cell carcinoma and an equal number of age-, sex-, and race-matched population controls. During in-person interviews, subjects were asked explicitly about use of common over-the-counter and prescription brand name analgesics marketed in the United States since the 1950s. A picture album of the listed drugs was available to the respondents to aid in their recalls. For every prescription analgesic named by the respondent, every attempt was made to validate its use from the prescribing physician. Results of this validation effort indicate comparable degrees of recall accuracy between cancer cases and controls. GAGO-DOMINGUEZ et al. (unpublished work) reported an overall 60% increase in risk of renal cell carcinoma among regular users of analgesics, with increasing risk as level of intake increased. Each of the four major classes of analgesics – aspirin, nonsteroidal anti-inflammatory agents other than aspirin, acetaminophen, and phenacetin – was clearly shown to be independently related to risk of renal cell carcinoma. Interestingly, risks per unit of intake (in grams) were comparable across these four classes of formulations. There was no evidence of an increase in risk of renal cell carcinoma among subjects who ingested one regular-strength (i.e., 325 mg) aspirin or less a day for cardiovascular health, a finding with obvious public health implications.

There are experimental data in support of analgesics as renal carcinogens. Phenacetin is known to induce renal cell carcinoma in rodents (JOHANSSON 1981; NAKANISHI et al. 1982). Acetaminophen, a major metabolite of phenacetin in humans, can induce renal proximal tubular necrosis in rodents (NEWTON et al. 1983; HART et al. 1991) and increase the incidence of renal cell carcinomas in rodents previously treated with a known renal carcinogen (TSUDA et al. 1984; KURATA et al. 1987). Aspirin and other non-steroidal anti-inflammatory agents are known to induce tubular necrosis (PLUMMER et al. 1975; KARI et al. 1995) and renal cell carcinoma in rodents (KARI et al. 1995).

### 1.3.2.4
### Amphetamines

In 1986, YU et al. first suggested that use of diet pills might be a risk factor for renal cell carcinoma. This association was recently confirmed in a large-scale case-control study in Los Angeles in which all prescription and nonprescription diet pills commonly used in the United States since the 1950s were listed in the structured questionnaire administered in-person to all study subjects. The investigators noted that the increased risk for renal cell carcinoma among users of diet pills was confined to those taking amphetamine-containing diet pills. There was an overall twofold risk in regular users of amphetamines relative to nonusers. This increase in risk of renal cell carcinoma was amphetamine dose-dependent, and regardless of the reason for use (Table 1.4). However, only a small fraction (no more than 5%) of renal cell carcinoma cases in Los Angeles

**Table 1.4.** Use of diet pills in relation to risk of renal cell carcinoma (adapted from YUAN et al. 1998b)

|  | Cases | Controls | OR (95%Cl) |
|---|---|---|---|
| Regular use of any diet pill |  |  |  |
| No | 1028 | 1094 | 1.0 |
| Yes | 176 | 110 | 1.6 (1.2, 2.1) |
| Amphetamines only | 89 | 47 | 2.0 (1.3, 2.9) |
| Nonamphetamines only | 57 | 49 | 1.1 (0.7, 1.7) |
| Combined use | 30 | 14 | 2.0 (0.96, 4.0) |
| Regular use of amphetamine-containing diet pills |  |  |  |
| No | 1085 | 1143 | 1.0 |
| Yes | 119 | 61 | 2.0 (1.4, 2.8) |
| Maximum weekly dose of amphetamine (mg) |  |  |  |
| 1–37.5 | 25 | 18 | 1.5 (0.7, 2.9) |
| 37.6–75.0 | 33 | 22 | 1.9 (1.04, 3.4) |
| ≥75.1 | 55 | 18 | 2.6 (1.5, 4.6) |
| Reason for use |  |  |  |
| Weight reduction | 68 | 31 | 2.1 (1.3, 3.3) |
| Other | 45 | 28 | 1.8 (1.1, 3.0) |

OR, odds ratio; Cl, confidence interval.

County are possibly related to this putative renal carcinogen (YUAN et al. 1998b).

In a multicenter study, MELLEMGAARD et al. (1995) also reported a statistically significant increase in risk of renal cell carcinoma among amphetamine users, but with no evidence of increasing risk with increasing cumulative dose or duration of use. This lack of association with exposure indices involving duration of use is not surprising. The usage pattern of diet pills typically is sporadic and intermittent; thus, self-reported duration of use is likely to be inaccurate.

## 1.3.3
### Obesity and Hypertension

Multiple studies have noted that obese individuals are at a high risk of renal cell carcinoma (YU et al. 1986; MELLEMGAARD et al. 1995; CHOW et al. 1996; YUAN et al. 1998b). Numerous case-control and cohort studies also have reported that individuals with a history of hypertension experienced an increased risk of renal cell carcinoma (RAYNOR et al. 1981;

GROVE et al. 1991; KREIGER et al. 1993; HEATH et al. 1997; YUAN et al. 1998b).

Details of the relationships between obesity, hypertension, and renal cell carcinoma have been published recently, based on a large-scale, population-based case-control study in Los Angeles (YUAN et al. 1998b). Results of that study indicate comparable risk levels between men and women for any given level of exposure. There is increasing risk of renal cell carcinoma with increasing body mass index (defined as weight in kilograms divided by height in meters squared), a marker of obesity. Individuals whose usual body mass index is 30 or higher are over 4 times as likely to develop renal cell carcinoma as compared to those whose body mass index is below 22 (Table 1.5). A history of hypertension confers a twofold risk of renal cell carcinoma. This elevation in risk is independent of the time interval between the diagnoses of hypertension and renal cell carcinoma, thus dispelling the possibility that hypertension results from advanced renal disease. Risk of renal cell carcinoma in hypertensives who have received medical treatments is only modestly elevated compared with never-treated hypertensives (Table 1.6). Obesity

**Table 1.5.** Relative body weight in relation to risk of renal cell carcinoma (adapted from YUAN et al. 1998b)

| Usual body mass index (kg/m$^2$) | Total | | | Males | | | Females | | |
|---|---|---|---|---|---|---|---|---|---|
| | Cases | Controls | OR (95% Cl) | Cases | Controls | OR (95% Cl) | Cases | Controls | OR (95% Cl) |
| <22 | 188 | 289 | 1.0 | 62 | 112 | 1.0 | 126 | 177 | 1.0 |
| 22–<24 | 247 | 269 | 1.6 (1.3, 2.2) | 152 | 179 | 1.7 (1.1, 2.5) | 95 | 90 | 1.7 (1.1, 2.5) |
| 24–<26 | 266 | 294 | 1.5 (1.2, 2.0) | 200 | 229 | 1.6 (1.1, 2.4) | 66 | 65 | 1.5 (0.96, 2.3) |
| 26–<28 | 164 | 170 | 1.7 (1.3, 2.4) | 129 | 128 | 2.0 (1.3, 3.1) | 35 | 42 | 1.3 (0.7, 2.2) |
| 28–<30 | 139 | 96 | 2.5 (1.8, 3.5) | 107 | 76 | 2.7 (1.7, 4.3) | 32 | 20 | 2.3 (1.2, 4.2) |
| ≥30 | 200 | 86 | 4.3 (3.0, 6.1) | 131 | 57 | 4.6 (2.9, 7.5) | 69 | 29 | 4.0 (2.3, 7.0) |

OR, odds ratio; Cl, confidence interval.

**Table 1.6.** History of hypertension in relation to risk of renal cell carcinoma (adapted from YUAN et al. 1998b)

| | Cases | Controls | OR (95% Cl) |
|---|---|---|---|
| No | 669 | 875 | 1.0 |
| Yes | 535 | 329 | 2.2 (1.8, 2.6) |
| Number of years since first diagnosis | | | |
| <5 | 55 | 40 | 2.1 (1.3, 3.2) |
| 5–9 | 122 | 85 | 1.8 (1.4, 2.5) |
| 10–19 | 188 | 96 | 2.6 (2.0, 3.4) |
| 20–29 | 97 | 62 | 2.2 (1.6, 3.2) |
| ≥30 | 63 | 40 | 2.0 (1.3, 3.1) |
| Unknown | 10 | 6 | 1.8 (0.7, 5.2) |
| Ever medically treated (by diuretics or antihypertensive drugs) | | | |
| No | 98 | 74 | 1.7 (1.2, 2.3) |
| Yes | 437 | 255 | 2.3 (1.9, 2.9) |

OR, odds ratio; Cl, confidence interval.

**Table 1.7.** Relative body weight and history of hypertension in relation to risk of renal cell carcinoma (adapted from YUAN et al. 1998b)

| Usual body mass index (kg/m$^2$) | No hypertension | | | Hypertension | | |
|---|---|---|---|---|---|---|
| | Cases | Controls | OR (95% Cl) | Cases | Controls | OR (95% Cl) |
| <22 | 135 | 236 | 1.0 | 53 | 53 | 1.8 (1.1, 2.8) |
| 22–<24 | 157 | 211 | 1.5 (1.1, 2.1) | 90 | 58 | 3.4 (2.2, 5.2) |
| 24–<26 | 165 | 212 | 1.5 (1.1, 2.1) | 101 | 82 | 2.3 (1.6, 3.4) |
| 26–<28 | 72 | 104 | 1.5 (0.98, 2.2) | 92 | 66 | 2.8 (1.9, 4.3) |
| 28–<30 | 60 | 63 | 1.8 (1.2, 2.9) | 79 | 33 | 4.6 (2.9, 7.5) |
| ≥30 | 80 | 49 | 3.2 (2.0, 5.2) | 120 | 37 | 7.0 (4.4, 11.3) |

OR, odds ratio; Cl, confidence interval.

and hypertension are independently related to risk of renal cell carcinoma. Regardless of hypertension status, cancer risk increases with increasing usual body mass index. Similarly, irrespective of level of usual body mass index, individuals with a history of hypertension experience a twofold risk for renal cell carcinoma (Table 1.7).

Diabetes and stroke have been reported to be positively related to renal cell carcinoma risk. The evidence indicates that these are indirect, noncausal associations, due to the close relations between the two medical conditions and obesity/hypertension (YUAN et al. 1998b).

Experimental work in rodents has demonstrated that obesity and hypertension can lead to renal glomerulosclerosis and tubulointerstitial cell proliferation (KEANE et al. 1993; MAI et al. 1993; O'DONNELL et al. 1993; ENG et al. 1994). None of these rodent models included tumor development as an outcome measurement. At the present, the relevance of these animal findings to human renal carcinogenesis is unclear.

### 1.3.4
### Dietary Factors

Relatively few epidemiologic studies have examined the role of diet in the development of renal cell carcinoma. Nonetheless, there is suggestive evidence that a "Western" diet high in meat and low in vegetables and fruit promotes renal cell carcinoma development (McLAUGHLIN et al. 1984, 1992; FRASER et al. 1990; TALAMINI et al. 1990; KREIGER et al. 1993; WOLK et al. 1996; YUAN et al. 1998c). In Los Angeles, YUAN et al. (1998c) found a strong inverse association between intake of cruciferous vegetables and risk of renal cell carcinoma. In terms of nutrients, there were significant inverse associations of renal cell carcinoma risk with consumption of a variety of carotenoids including alpha-carotene, beta-carotene, beta-cryptoxanthin, and lutein. Interestingly, the investigators still observed a significant residual effect of cruciferous vegetables on renal cell carcinoma risk after adjustment for carotenoid intake, suggesting that other compounds present in cruciferous vegetables may protect against renal cell carcinoma.

Experimental data have implicated cured meats as a possible risk factor for renal cell carcinoma in humans. Cured meats are potential sources of nitrosamines, which are known renal carcinogens in rodents (HAMILTON 1975). YUAN et al. (1998c) specifically tested this hypothesis in the Los Angeles-based case-control study described above. No association was observed between cured meat intake and renal cell carcinoma risk.

A fair number of epidemiologic studies have investigated the relationships between intakes of coffee, tea, and alcoholic beverages and renal cell carcinoma risk (WYNDER et al. 1974; ARMSTRONG et al. 1976; McLAUGHLIN et al. 1984; YU et al. 1986; KREIGER et al. 1993; WOLK et al. 1996; YUAN et al. 1998c). The overall evidence indicates a lack of association between intake of these beverages and the development of renal cell carcinoma.

### 1.4
### Genetic Factors

Several case-control studies have found that patients with renal cell carcinoma were more likely than control subjects to report having one or more first-degree relatives with the same malignancy. Individuals with a family history of renal cell carcinoma are more than twice as likely to develop renal cell carcinoma than those without such a family history (MᶜLᴀᴜɢʜʟɪɴ et al. 1984; Mᴇʟʟᴇᴍɢᴀᴀʀᴅ et al. 1994b; Sᴄʜʟᴇʜᴏғᴇʀ et al. 1996).

von Hippel-Lindau disease is a hereditary cancer syndrome associated with germline mutations of the von Hippel-Lindau tumor suppressor gene that is located on the short arm of chromosome 3 (Lᴀᴛɪғ et al. 1993). The disease is characterized by a high frequency of tumor development in affected individuals, including renal cell carcinoma, pheochromocytomas, and hemangioblastomas of the retina and central nervous system (Mᴇʟᴍᴏɴ and Rᴏsᴇɴ 1964; Lᴀᴍɪᴇʟʟ et al. 1989). The incidence of von Hippel-Lindau disease is rare, occurring in about one per 36 000 live births in England (Mᴀʜᴇʀ et al. 1991). Affected individuals carry an extremely high risk of developing renal cell carcinoma in their lifetimes, approaching 70% by age 60 years (Mᴀʜᴇʀ et al. 1990). Somatic mutations of the von Hippel-Lindau gene also have been detected in sporadic cases of renal cell carcinoma (Fᴏsᴛᴇʀ et al. 1994; Gɴᴀʀʀʀᴀ et al. 1994; Sʜᴜɪɴ et al. 1994).

Zʙᴀʀ et al. (1994) reported on another class of hereditary renal cell carcinoma. Nine members over three generations of this high-risk family developed papillary renal cell carcinoma, a histologic type of renal cell carcinoma that is found in only 10% of sporadic cases of renal cell carcinoma. Results of linkage analysis using multiple polymorphic markers on chromosome 3p were negative, and no 3p allele loss was detected in tumor tissues.

# References


Armstrong B, Garrod A, Doll R (1976) A retrospective study of renal cancer with special reference to coffee and animal protein consumption. Br J Cancer 33:127–136

Asal NR, Lee ET, Geyer JR, Kadamani S, Risser DR, Cherng N (1988) Risk factors in renal cell carcinoma. II. Medical history, occupation, multivariate analysis, and conclusions. Cancer Detect Prev 13:263–279

Bengtsson U, Angerval L, Ekman H, Lehmann L (1968) Transitional cell tumors of the renal pelvis in analgesic abusers. Scand J Urol Nephrol 2:145–150

Chow WH, McLaughlin JK, Mandel JS, Wacholder S, Niwa S, Fraumeni JF (1996) Obesity and risk of renal cell cancer. Cancer Epidemiol Biomarkers Prev 5:17–21

Derby LE, Jick H (1996) Acetaminophen and renal and bladder cancer. Epidemiology 7:358–362

Devesa SS, Silverman DT, McLaughlin JK, Brown CC, Connelly RR, Fraumeni JF (1990) Comparison of the descriptive epidemiology of urinary tract cancers. Cancer Caus Contr 1:133–141

Doll R (1996) Cancers weakly related to smoking. Br Med Bull 52:35–49

Eng E, Veniant M, Floege J, et al. (1994) Renal proliferative and phenotypic changes in rats with two-kidney, one-clip Goldblatt hypertension. Am J Hypertens 7:177–185

Finkle WD, McLaughlin JK, Rasgon SA, Yeoh HH, Low JE (1993) Increased risk of renal cell cancer among women using diuretics in the United States. Cancer Caus Contr 4:555–558

Foster K, Prowse A, van de Berg A, et al. (1994) Somatic mutations of the von Hippel-Lindau disease tumor suppressor gene in non-familial clear cell renal carcinoma. Human Mol Genet 3:2169–2173

Fraser GE, Phillips RL, Beeson WL (1990) Hypertension, antihypertensive medication and risk of renal carcinoma in California Seventh-Day Adventists. Int J Epidemiol 19:832–838

Gnarra JR, Tory K, Weng Y, et al. (1994) Mutations of the *VHL* tumour suppressor gene in renal carcinoma. Nature Genet 7:85–90

Grove JS, Nomura A, Severson RK, Stemmermann GN (1991) The association of blood pressure with cancer incidence in a prospective study. Am J Epidemiol 134:942–947

Hamilton JM (1975) Renal carcinogenesis. Adv Cancer Res 22:1–56

Hart SGE, Beierschmitt WP, Bartolone JB, Wyand DS, Khairallah EA, Cohen SD (1991) Evidence against deacetylation and for cytochrome P450-mediated activation in acetaminophen-induced nephrotoxicity in the CD-1 mouse. Toxicol Appl Pharmacol 107:1–15

Heath CW, Lally CA, Calle EE, McLaughlin JK, Thun MJ (1997) Hypertension, diuretics, and antihypertensive medications as possible risk factors for renal cell cancer. Am J Epidemiol 145:607–613

Hiatt RA, Tolan K, Quesenberry CP (1994) Renal cell carcinoma and thiazide use: a historical, case-control study (California, USA). Cancer Caus Contr 5:319–325

Hultengren N, Lagergren C, Ljungqvist A (1965) Carcinoma of the renal pelvis in renal papillary necrosis. Acta Chir Scand 130:314–320

International Agency for Research on Cancer (1986) IARC monographs on the evaluation of carcinogenic risks to humans, vol. 28. Tobacco smoking. International Agency for Research on Cancer, Lyon

Jensen OM, Knudsen JB, Tomasson H, Sorensen BL (1989) The Copenhagen case-control study of renal pelvis and ureter cancer: role of analgesics. Int J Cancer 44:965–968

Johansson SL (1981) Carcinogenicity of analgesics: long-term treatment of Sprague-Dawley rats with phenacetin, phenazone, caffeine and paracetamol (acetaminophen). Int J Cancer 27:521–529

Kari F, Bucher J, Haseman J, Eustis S, Huff J (1995) Long-term exposure to the anti-inflammatory agent phenylbutazone induces kidney tumors in rats and liver tumors in mice. Jpn J Cancer Res 86:252–263

Keane WF, Kasiske BL, O'Donnell MP, Kim Y (1993) Hypertension, hyperlipidemia, and renal damage. Am J Kidney Dis 21:43–50

Kovacs G, Erlandsson R, Boldog F, Ingvarsson S, Muller-Brechlin R, Klein G, Sumegi J (1988) Consistent chromosome 3p deletion and loss of heterozygosity in renal cell carcinoma. Proc Natl Acad Sci USA 85:1571–1575

Kreiger N, Marret LD, Dodds L, Hilditch S, Darlington GA (1993) Risk factors for renal cell carcinoma: results of a population-based case-control study. Cancer Caus Contr 4:101–110

Kurata Y, Tsuda H, Sakata T, Yamashita T, Ito N (1987) Reciprocal modifying effects of isomeric forms of aminophenol on induction of neoplastic lesions in rat liver and kidney initiated by *N*-ethyl-*n*-hydroxyethylnitrosamine. Carcinogenesis 8:1281–1285

Lamiell JM, Salazar FG, Hsia YE (1989) von Hippel-Lindau disease affecting 43 members of a single kindred. Medicine (Baltimore) 68:1–29

Latif F, Tory K, Gnarra J, et al. (1993) Identification of the von Hippel-Lindau tumor suppressor gene. Science 260:1317–1320

Maher ER, Yates JRW, Harris R, Benjamin C, Harris R, Moore AT, Ferguson-Smith MA (1990) Clinical features and natural history of von Hippel-Lindau disease. Q J Med 77:1151–1163

Maher ER, Iselius L, Yates JRW, et al. (1991) von Hippel-Lindau disease: a genetic study. J Med Genet 28:443–447

Mahony JF, Stoney BG, Ibanez RC, Stewart JH (1977) Analgesic abuse, renal parenchymal disease and carcinoma of the kidney or ureter. Aust NZ J Surg 7:463–469

Mai M, Geiger H, Hilgers KF, Veelken R, Mann JFE, Dammrish J, Luft FC (1993) Early interstitial changes in hypertension-induced renal injury. Hypertension 22:754–765

McCredie M, Ford JM, Taylor JS, Stewart JH (1982) Analgesics and cancer of the renal pelvis in New South Wales. Cancer 49:2617–2625

McCredie M, Stewart JH, Carter JJ, Turner J, Mahony JF (1986) Phenacetin and papillary necrosis: independent risk factors for renal pelvic cancer. Kidney Int 30:81–84

McCredie M, Ford JM, Stewart JM (1988) Risk factors for cancer of the renal parenchyma. Int J Cancer 42:13–16

McCredie M, Stewart JH, Day NE (1993) Different roles for phenacetin and paracetamol in cancer of the kidney and renal pelvis. Int J Cancer 53:245–249

McCredie M, Pommer W, McLaughlin JK, et al. (1995) International renal cell cancer study. II. Analgesics. Int J Cancer 60:345–349

McLaughlin JK, Mandel JS, Blot WJ, Schuman LM, Mehl ES, Fraumeni JF (1984) A population-based case-control study of renal cell carcinoma. J Natl Cancer Inst 72:275–284

McLaughlin JK, Blot WJ, Mehl ES, Fraumeni JF (1985) Relation of analgesic use to renal cancer: population-based findings. Natl Cancer Inst Monogr 69:217–222

McLaughlin JK, Blot WJ, Fraumeni JF (1988) Diuretics and renal cell cancer. J Natl Cancer Inst 80:378

McLaughlin JK, Silverman DT, Hsing AW, et al. (1992) Cigarette smoking and cancers of the renal pelvis and ureter. Cancer Res 52:254–257

McLaughlin JK, Chow WH, Mandel JS, et al. (1995) International renal cell cancer study. VIII. Role of diuretics, other anti-hypertensive medictions and hypertension. Int J Cancer 63:216–221

Mellemgaard A, Niwa S, Mehl ES, Engholm G, McLaughlin J, Olsen JH (1994a) Risk factors for renal cell carcinoma in Denmark. II. Role of medication and medical history. Int J Epidemiol 23:923–930

Mellemgaard A, Engholm G, McLaughlin JK, Olsen JH (1994b) Risk factors for renal cell carcinoma in Denmark. I. Role of socioeconomic status, tobacco use, beverages, and family history. Cancer Causes Control 5:105–113

Mellemgaard A, Lindblad P, Schlehofer B, et al. (1995) International renal-cell cancer study. III. Role of weight, height, physical activity, and use of amphetamines. Int J Cancer 60:350–354

Melmon KL, Rosen SW (1964) Lindau's disease: review of the literature and study of a large kindred. Am J Med 36:595–617

Nakanishi K, Kurata Y, Oshima M, Fukushima S, Ito N (1982) Carcinogenicity of phenacetin: long-term feeding study on B6C3F mice. Int J Cancer 29:434–444

Newton JF, Yoshimoto M, Bernstein J, Rush GF, Hook JB (1983) Acetaminophen nephrotoxicity in the rat. I. Strain differences in nephrotoxicity and metabolism. Toxicol Appl Pharmacol 69:291–306

Nutting PA, Freeman WL, Risser DR, et al. (1993) Cancer incidence among American Indians and Alaska Natives, 1980 through 1987. Am J Public Health 83:1589–1598

O'Donnell MP, Kasiske BL, Kim Y, Schmitz PG, Keane WF (1993) Lovastatin retards the progression of established glomerular disease in obese Zucker rats. Am J Kidney Dis 22:83–89

Paganini-Hill A, Chao A, Ross RK, Henderson BE (1989) Aspirin use and chronic diseases: a cohort study of the elderly. BMJ 299:1247–1250

Parker SL, Tong T, Bolden S, Wingo PA (1996) Cancer statistics, 1996. CA Cancer J Clin 46:5–27

Parkin DM, Whelan SL, Ferlay J, Raymond L, Young J (1997) Cancer incidence in five continents, vol VII. IARC Scientific Publications No. 143, International Agency for Research on Cancer, Lyon

Plummer DT, Leatherwood PD, Blake ME (1975) Urinary enzymes and kidney damage by aspirin and phenacetin. Chem Biol Interact 10:277–284

Raynor WJ, Shekelle RB, Rossof AH, Maliza C, Paul O (1981) High blood pressure and 17-year cancer mortality in the Western Electric Health Study. Am J Epidemiol 113:371–377

Ross RK, Paganini-Hill A, Landolph J, Gerkins V, Henderson BE (1989) Analgesics, cigarette smoking, and other risk factors for cancer of the renal pelvis and ureter. Cancer Res 49:1045–1048

Schlehofer B, Pommer W, Mellemgaard A, et al. (1996) International renal-cell-cancer study. VI. The role of medical and family history. Int J Cancer 66:723–726

Shuin T, Kondo K, Torigoe S, et al. (1994) Frequent somatic mutations and loss of heterozygosity of the von Hippel-Lindau tumor suppressor gene in primary human renal cell carcinoma. Cancer Res 54:2852–2855

Talamini R, Baron AE, Barra S, et al. (1990) A case-control study of risk factor for renal cell cancer in northern Italy. Cancer Caus Contr 1:125–131

Tsuda H, Sakata T, Masui T, Imaida K, Ito N (1984) Modifying effects of butylated hydroxyanisole, ethoxyquin and acetaminophen on induction of neoplastic lesions in rat liver and kidney initiated by *N*-ethyl-*n*-hydroxyethylnitrosamine. Carcinogenesis 5:525–531

Weinmann S, Glass AG, Weiss NS, Psaty BM, Siscovick DS, White E (1994) Use of diuretics and other antihypertensive medications in relation to the risk of renal cell cancer. Am J Epidemiol 140:792–804

Wolk A, Gridley G, Niwa S, et al. (1996) International renal cell cancer study. VII. Role of diet. Int J Cancer 65:67–73

Wynder EL, Mabuchi K, Whitmore WF (1974) Epidemiology of adenocarcinoma of the kidney. J Natl Cancer Inst 53:1619–1634

Yamasaki E, Ames BN (1977) Concentration of mutagens from urine by adsorption with the nonpolar resin XAD-2: cigarette smokers have mutagenic urine. Proc Natl Acad Sci USA 74:3555–3559

Yu MC, Mack TM, Hanisch R, Cicioni C, Henderson BE (1986) Cigarette smoking, obesity, diuretic use, and coffee consumption as risk factors for renal cell carcinoma. J Natl Cancer Inst 77:351–356

Yu MC, Ross RK (1998) Epidemiology of bladder cancer. In: Petrovich Z, Baert L, Brady LW (eds) Carcinoma of the bladder, innovations in management. Springer, Berlin Heidelberg, New York, pp 1–13

Yuan J-M, Castelao JE, Gago-Dominguez M, Yu MC, Ross RK (1998a) Tobacco use in relation to renal cell carcinoma. Cancer Epidemiol Biomarkers Prev 7:429–433, 1998

Yuan J-M, Castelao JE, Gago-Dominguez M, Ross RK, Yu MC (1998b) Hypertension, obesity and their medications in relation to renal cell carcinoma. Br J Cancer 77:1508–1513, 1998

Yuan J-M, Gago-Dominguez M, Castelao E, Hankin JH, Ross RK, Yu MC (1998c) Cruciferous vegetables in relation to renal cell carcinoma. Int J Cancer 77:211–216, 1998

Zbar B, Tory K, Merino M, et al. (1994) Hereditary papillary renal cell carcinoma. J Urol 151:561–566

**Table 2.1.** Classification of renal cell tumors in relation to the nephron and its cell types

|  | Proximal tubule |  | Distal tubule | Connecting tubule |  | Cortical medullary collecting duct |
|---|---|---|---|---|---|---|
| Basic types | Clear cell RCC | Chromophil RCC |  | Chromophobe RCC | Oncocytoma | Bellini duct ca. |
| Eosinophilic variants | Clear cell RCC | Chromophil RCC |  | Chromophobe RCC |  | Bellini duct ca. |
| Sarcomatoid variants | Clear cell RCC | Chromophil RCC |  | Chromophobe RCC |  | Bellinic duct ca. |

**Table 2.2.** Overview of different types of RCC and differential diagnostic criteria

|  | Clear cell RCC | Chromophil RCC | Chromophobe RCC | Bellini duct ca. | Oncocytoma |
|---|---|---|---|---|---|
| Gross pathology | Yellow | Tan or brown | Light brown | White or gray | Tan-brown |
|  | Well circumscribed | Well circumscribed | Well circumscribed | Irregular extensions | Central stellate scar |
|  | Necrosis, hemorrhage | Necrosis, hemorrhage |  | Necrosis | Hemorrhage |
|  | Cysts | Multifocal, bilateral | Solitary | Centered in medulla | Necrosis is rare |
| Growth pattern | Compact | Papillary | Compact | Tubular | Compact or insular |
|  | Tubulocystic | Tubulopapillary | (tubular) | (Papillary) | Tubules often present |
|  | Delicate fibrovascular septa |  |  | Abundant loose or desmoplastic stroma | Edematous stroma |
| Cell type | Clear (empty) cells (Eosinophilic granular cells) | Small cells with scanty pale cytoplasm | Pale, reticular cytoplasm Eosinophilic cytoplasm | Hobnail cells | Eosinophilic cytoplasm |
|  | (Spindle cells) | Large cells with abundant eosinophilic cytoplasm | Prominent cell membranes Perinuclear halo |  |  |
| Immunohistochemical features | Cytokeratin + Vimentin + (partly) *Ulex europaeus* − Coll. iron droplike + | Cytokeratin + Vimentin + (partly) *Ulex Europaeus* − Coll. iron droplike + | Cytokeratin + Vimentin − *Ulex Europaeus* − Colloidal iron ++ (reticular) | *Ulex europaeus* + | Cytokeratin + Vimentin − Coll. iron weakly + |
| Ultrastructural features |  |  | Vesicles Plus Numerous mitochondria in eosinophilic variant |  | Numerous mitochondria |

morphological criteria, subsequent genetic studies have confirmed its validity by showing characteristic genetic abnormalities in each subtype; other genetic changes have been related to tumor progression (Kovacs 1993; van den Berg et al. 1993).

After a discussion on the controversial diagnosis "adenoma," the following sections discuss each of the currently recognized subtypes of RCC (for an overview see Table 2.2).

## 2.2
## Renal Adenoma

The differential diagnosis between renal cell adenomas and carcinomas has been a matter of con-troversy for decades. Discovery of small cortical lesions at autopsy might suggest that these lesions lack the capacity to develop into clinical cancer. However, small examples of each of the currently recognized subtypes of RCC are found in surgical and autopsy specimens (Eble and Warfel 1991). Conversely, no histological pattern found among the small cortical tumors has no counterpart in clinical cancer. For a long time, Bell's rule (1950) was followed: a lesion <3 cm was regarded as adenoma, a lesion >3 cm as carcinoma (Bell 1950). Since incidental discovery of small renal tumors by ultrasonography and computed tomography conducted for other disorders is increasing, a definition of renal adenoma based on the size of the tumor is unreliable (Dal Bianco et al. 1988). The new WHO classification proposed the following rules: (1) adenoma: nuclear grade 1 tumor <1 cm diameter; (2) carcinoma: grade 1 tumor >3 cm diameter and every grade 2, 3, or 4 tumor; (3) grade 1 tumors of 1–3 cm diameter are considered of dubious malignancy (Murphy et al. 1994). Presently, there are no studies showing that tumors <1 cm in diameter can be safely left in place and that they will not progress and grow, particularly if they are of the clear cell type. So caution has to be taken and it seems appropriate to follow patients with incidentally found small tumors very closely or to perform a local resection.

## 2.3
## Clear Cell Renal Cell Carcinoma

Clear cell RCC is the most common type of RCC, accounting for 70% of the cases in surgical series.

### 2.3.1
### Gross Pathology

The typical macroscopic appearance of clear cell RCC is a solid, yellow-light orange tumor, often lobulated and bulging above the cut surface. Usually these neoplasms are surrounded by a pseudocapsule, but sometimes they diffusely infiltrate and replace the kidney. Pale areas of necrosis and darker areas of hemorrhage are frequently seen, giving the tumor a mottled aspect. Sarcomatoid (dedifferentiated) areas are pale and firm. Cysts are common and rarely the tumor is nearly completely cystic (Hartman et al. 1986; Murad et al. 1991). The cysts usually have a smooth surface. Occasionally, clear cell RCC arises in a preexisting simple cyst. A cystic appearance can also be the result of necrosis and degeneration. Multicentric tumors in the same kidney appear in approximately 13% of cases of clear cell RCC (Cheng et al. 1991), particularly in association with von Hippel-Lindau disease (Seizinger et al. 1988) and with acquired cystic disease in chronically dialyzed patients (Hughson et al. 1980). Bilateral clear cell RCC is rarely seen, usually occurring in association with von Hippel-Lindau disease (Seizinger et al. 1988).

### 2.3.2
### Microscopic Pathology

As already stated in the introduction, clear cell RCCs originate from the proximal tubule. This was first

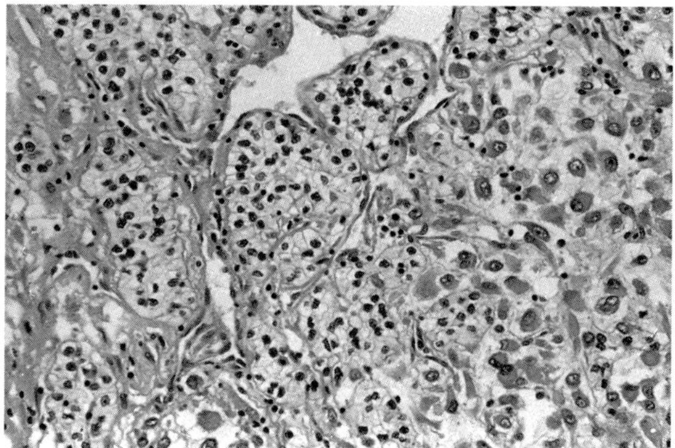

**Fig. 2.1.** Clear cell RCC composed of clear (empty) cells (*left*) and eosinophilic granular cells (*right*), organized in broad trabeculae, separated by delicate fibrovascular septa (solid pattern). Hematoxylin-eosin, original magnification ×200

indicated in 1960 by the findings of Oberling et al. that these tumors exhibit apical brush borders of microvilli, pinocytotic vesicles, and a glycocalyx-like matrix. Subsequent immunohistochemical studies have supported the proximal tubule origin (Thoenes et al. 1990): clear cell RCCs typically express cytokeratin and vimentin, which are also present in the normal proximal tubule.

Clear cell RCC is composed of cells with abundant clear cytoplasm due to lipid (visualized with oil red O stain on frozen sections) and/or glycogen (visualized on PAS stain) storage. Although this feature has given the tumor its name, it is common for tumor cells to exhibit a more eosinophilic, granular cytoplasm, especially in areas of necrosis or bleeding. Sometimes, tumor areas consist almost entirely of eosinophilic granular cells, which by no means contradicts the diagnosis of the clear cell variant of RCC. The eosinophilic appearance of the cytoplasm is due to the presence of a large number of mitochondria.

Clear cell RCC can have several architectural patterns, which commonly occur in combination. Most often, the tumor cells are organized in broad sheets and trabeculae, separated by delicate fibrovascular septa (compact, solid, or alveolar pattern) (Fig. 2.1). The pattern of thin-walled blood vessels is striking and diagnostically valuable. Tumor cells can also be arranged in more or less dilated tubular structures, merging with the cystic pattern. Small tubular structures are usually empty, while larger dilated tubules or cysts often contain eosinophilic fluid or blood. In poorly differentiated tumors, sarcomatoid areas can be seen, in which the tumor cells become spindled and have a more or less bundled growth pattern. If a tumor seems entirely sarcomatoid, extensive sam-

**Table 2.3.** Fuhrman nuclear grading system

| Grade | Characteristics |
| --- | --- |
| Grade 1 | Round, uniform nuclei; ±10 µm in diameter with minute or absent nucleoli |
| Grade 2 | Slightly irregular nuclear contours; ±15 µm in diameter; nucleoli visible at 400 × |
| Grade 3 | Moderately to markedly irregular nuclear contours; ±20 µm in diameter; large nucleoli, visible at 100 × |
| Grade 4 | Nuclei similar to those of grade 3, but also multilobular or multiple nuclei or bizarre nuclei and heavy clumps of chromatin |

pling should be carried out in the search for epithelial areas.

Degenerative changes – necrosis, hemorrhage, edema, fibrosis, hemosiderin, cholesterol clefts, and calcification – are common in tumors of any architectural pattern.

In cases of clear cell RCC the nuclei are usually spherical and centrally located, ranging from small and hyperchromatic without visible nucleoli to large and pleomorphic with prominent nucleoli. Based on the size and contour of the nuclei and on the conspicuousness of the nucleoli, the FUHRMAN nuclear grading system has been developed (FUHRMAN et al. 1982) (Table 2.3) and has been shown to correlate well with survival (MEDEIROS et al. 1988).

## 2.4
## Chromophil Renal Cell Carcinoma

The second most common carcinoma arising from the renal tubular epithelium is chromophil RCC, also called papillary RCC because of the predominant papillary growth pattern. Chromophil RCC accounts for 10%–15% of RCCs in large clinical series (EBLE 1996).

There is considerable immunohistochemical evidence that chromophil RCCs originate in the proximal tubules (STORKEL 1993; STORKEL and JACOBI 1989). However, other studies have shown that papillary RCCs express markers of both proximal and distal tubular epithelium (HUGHSON et al. 1993). A recent study in a series of 105 chromophil RCCs showed a variable expression of cytokeratin 7 (DELAHUNT and EBLE 1997), which is also present in normal renal distal tubule and collecting duct epithelium, but not in the proximal tubule (GATALICA

et al. 1995), and vimentin, which is present in the normal proximal tubule, but not in the distal tubule.

### 2.4.1
### Gross Pathology

Chromophil RCC is well circumscribed, with frequent cystic change, hemorrhage, and necrosis. Hemorrhage and necrosis may be extensive, causing the tumor to appear hypovascular on angiography (MANCILLA-JIMENEZ et al. 1976). Size is highly variable and many tumors are large. Calcifications and psammoma bodies are more often seen in chromophil RCC than in other subtypes. Multifocality and bilaterality are also prominent features in chromophil RCCs (AMIN et al. 1997; KOVACS and KOVACS 1993).

### 2.4.2
### Microscopic Pathology

The large majority of chromophil RCCs have a papillary or tubulopapillary architecture (AMIN et al. 1997; DELAHUNT and EBLE 1997; THOENES et al. 1990) (Fig. 2.2). The remainder have a "compact" or "trabecular" pattern. In our experience and also that of others (AMIN et al. 1997), a compact pattern is mostly the result of tight packing of papillae, while a trabecular pattern results from long parallel arrays of papillae; if one pays special attention, the fibrovascular cores of the papillae can still be recognized in these "other" growth patterns. Papillary cores can be extended by edema, giving a false impression of cysts on low magnification (DELAHUNT and EBLE 1997).

There are three variants of chromophil RCC: (1) basophilic (Fig. 2.2a), (2) eosinophilic (Fig. 2.2b), and (3) intermediate. The *basophilic* variant consists of papillae with a fibrovascular core, covered with a single layer of small epithelial cells with scanty pale or clear cytoplasm. The basophilic appearance is due to the small volume of the cytoplasm and, accordingly, the relatively high nuclear/cytoplasmic ratio. The nuclei show a low to medium degree of pleomorphism and usually inconspicuous nucleoli (Furhman grades I and II; grade III is rare). Accumulations of foamy macrophages that fill and extend the papillary cores are common in the basophilic variant (DELAHUNT and EBLE 1997). If tubules are present, they are lined by similar cells and often result from cross-sectioning of papillae. The *eosinophilic* variant

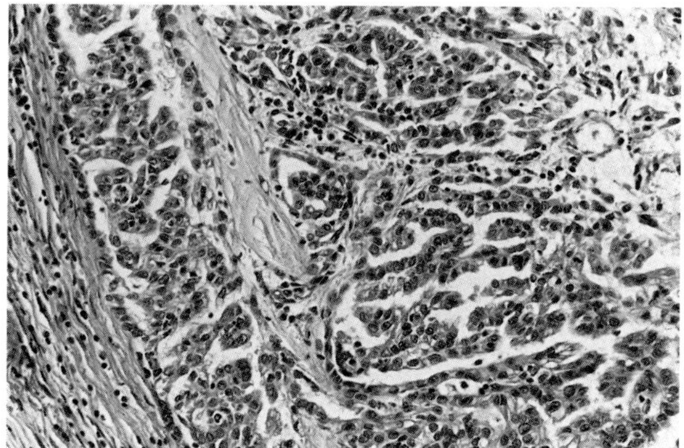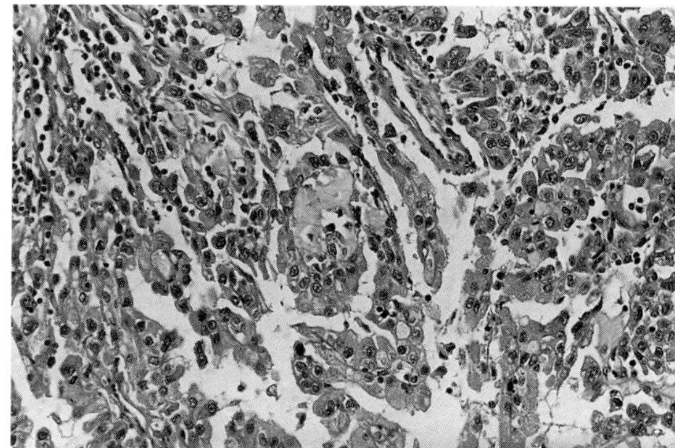

**Fig. 2.2 a,b.** Chromophil RRC. **a** Basophilic variant. Papillary structures are lined by a single layer of small epithelial cells. The nuclei show a low degree of pleomorphism. **b** Eosinophilic variant. Papillae are covered by large cells with abundant eosinophilic cytoplasm. Nuclear pleomorphism is more prominent. In the *center* of the figure, foamy macrophages are present in the core of the papillary structures. Hematoxylineosin, original magnification ×200

is composed of papillae, covered by epithelial cells with abundant eosinophilic cytoplasm, arranged in a pseudostratified or irregularly stratified manner. Areas with clear cells may be prominent (AMIN et al. 1997). Nuclei show predominantly medium- to high-grade nuclear pleomorphism (Fuhrman grades II, III, and IV; grade I is rare). Foamy macrophages in the papillary cores are rarely seen in the eosinophilic variant (DELAHUNT and EBLE 1997). Mitotic figures are rare in both variants, while tumor-related inflammation is a prominent feature. Sarcomatoid dedifferentiation occurs occasionally, at a rate not much different from that of other types of RCC (DELAHUNT and EBLE 1997).

## 2.5
## Chromophobe Renal Cell Carcinoma

Chromophobe RCC was discovered by BANNASCH in experimentally induced tumors in rats in 1974 (BANNASCH et al. 1974); THOENES et al. described the first cases in humans in 1985 (THOENES et al. 1985). This tumor represents approximately 4%–5% of neoplasms of the renal tubular epithelium in surgical series (CROTTY et al. 1995; DELONG et al. 1996; DURHAM et al. 1996; THOENES et al. 1986). The tumor cells are characterized by numerous cytoplasmic vesicles on electron microscopic examination: these vesicles are characteristic and define the entity (BONSIB and LAGER 1990; THOENES et al. 1988). The vesicles resemble vesicles seen in the intercalated cells of the collecting duct (BONSIB and LAGER 1990; STORKEL et al. 1989; THOENES et al. 1988).

### 2.5.1
### Gross Pathology

Chromophobe RCCs vary in size from less than 2 cm to more than 20 cm. The tumors are typically solitary, circumscribed, globular, and solid. The cut surface is characteristically beige to light brown, but may be yellow or gray-white. Foci of hemorrhage or necrosis are rare.

### 2.5.2
### Microscopic Pathology

Most tumors have a solid growth pattern, but tubular areas may be present. The nuclei are central or slightly eccentric, and may be either low or high grade. Mitotic figures are rare, but can be detected in the majority of cases. Two histological variants are recognized: typical and eosinophilic. In the *typical* variant, the cells have a voluminous, pale (but not clear) reticular cytoplasm (Fig. 2.3). The cytoplasm is condensed at the periphery of the cell, accentuating the cell boundaries. The typical variant may be mistaken for clear cell RCC. In clear cell RCC, however, the transparency of the cytoplasm is due to dissolution of glycogen and lipid from the cells during tissue processing. The transparency of cytoplasm in chromophobe cell carcinoma is chiefly due to the accumulation of membranous microvesicles (THOENES et al. 1988). In the *eosinophilic* variant, the cytoplasm is markedly eosinophilic and finely granular. The cytoplasm surrounding the nucleus may be pale, creating a halo. Ultrastructurally, nu-

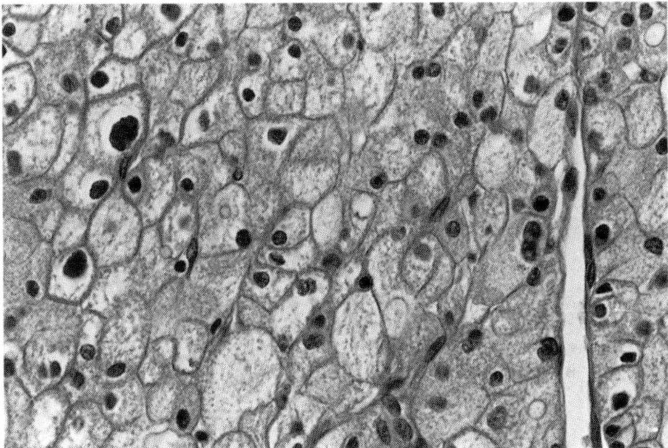

**Fig. 2.3.** Chromophobe RCC. Solid growth pattern. Cells with voluminous pale, reticular cytoplasm and prominent cell borders are intermingled with smaller cells with eosinophilic cytoplasm. A perinuclear halo can also be recognized (*upper left corner*). Hematoxylin-eosin, original magnification ×400

merous mitochondria are mixed with the cytoplasmic vesicles. Mixtures of the two cell types are not uncommon. The tumor cells are arranged in trabeculae, with the pale cells often showing an affinity for the periphery, where they are juxtaposed to the vascular septa. The cells in the center of the trabeculae have more granularity with perinuclear clearing. It is imperative to pay attention to the diffuse growth pattern with a variable yet often unique interplay of the two distinct cell types (Durham et al. 1996).

The eosinophilic variant may be difficult to distinguish from eosinophilic chromophil RCC and oncocytoma (Bonsib and Lager 1990; Thoenes et al. 1986; Thoenes et al. 1988). This differential diagnosis is highly significant given the different implications for the expected clinical course of the disease (benign versus malignant). Some authors suggest that most (if not all) published cases of "malignant" oncocytoma of the kidney actually represent misdiagnosed chromophobe RCC (Bonsib and Lager 1990; Kovacs 1993; Thoenes et al. 1986).

Hale's colloidal iron stain is diagnostically most helpful and stains the cytoplasm of chromophobe cells a vivid blue with a reticular pattern (DeLong et al. 1996). Also PAS staining reveals strong positivity in a reticular pattern; staining is abolished by diastase predigestion (DeLong et al. 1996). Some degree of Hale's colloidal iron reactivity can be seen in other types of tumors, although the pattern of reactivity is distinctly different (DeLong et al. 1996). In oncocytoma, there is faint, diffuse positivity without the reticular pattern. In clear cell and eosinophilic chromophil RCCs, reactivity is scattered and droplike, frequently corresponding to hemosiderin

deposits. A reticular pattern is not observed. Immunohistochemically, chromophobe RCCs cannot be distinguished from other tumors. Chromophobe RCCs are typically positive for cytokeratin and epithelial membrane antigen and negative for vimentin (DeLong et al. 1996; Storkel et al. 1989). Interestingly, chromophobe RCC shows an unusual reactivity pattern for cytokeratin, with scattered strongly positive cells among negative cells (DeLong et al. 1996; Storkel et al. 1989). This pattern is not seen in the other types of RCC. Vimentin immunoreactivity is helpful in the differential diagnosis with clear cell RCC, since all chromophobe RCCs are negative and some clear cell RCCs are positive. Oncocytoma is also typically negative for vimentin. The most characteristic feature of chromophobe RCCs is the presence of abundant cytoplasmic microvesicles (150–300 nm) on ultrastructural examination. In the eosinophilic variant, these vesicles are admixed with large numbers of mitochondria, which can again lead to confusion with oncocytoma (Bonsib and Lager 1990; DeLong et al. 1996; Thoenes et al. 1985, 1988). Bonsib and Lager (1990) have shown that the vesicles disintegrate in routine processing for paraffin embedding, so it is crucial that tissue for electron microscopy be primarily fixed in glutaraldehyde.

## 2.6
## Collecting Duct Carcinoma (Bellini Duct Carcinoma)

The collecting ducts begin in the renal cortex and descend through the medulla to the renal papillae. The short segments just above the papillary orifices are called Bellini's ducts. There is evidence that the intercalated cells of the collecting duct may be the origin of chromophobe RCC (Storkel et al. 1989) and renal oncocytoma (Storkel et al. 1988). In addition, a heterogeneous group of tumors with a presumed collecting duct origin has been described (Aizawa et al. 1987; Fleming and Lewi 1986; Kennedy et al. 1990; Rumpelt et al. 1991), representing about 2% of renal neoplasms.

### 2.6.1
### Gross Pathology

The tumor mass is usually localized in the renal medulla, often with irregular extensions into the adjacent renal cortex and hilar structures and with distortion of the pelvicalyceal system (FLEMING and LEWI 1986; KENNEDY et al. 1990). The tumors are generally firm and white or gray.

## 2.6.2
## Microscopic Pathology

Collecting duct carcinoma has features of both adenocarcinoma and urothelial carcinoma (EBLE 1990; RUMPELT et al. 1991). The tumors consist of anastomosing tubules, cords, and nests in an abundant, loose, or desmoplastic stroma (Fig. 2.4). The cells have small or moderate amounts of cytoplasm and often pleomorphic nuclei, oriented towards the lumen of tubules. This "hobnail" appearance is a useful feature since it is rarely found in other types of RCC and is not found in urothelial carcinoma. In some reported cases, a papillary architecture predominates, giving rise to a differential diagnostic problem with chromophil RCC (AIZAWA et al. 1987; KENNEDY et al. 1990). Occasionally, atypical cells are found in adjacent distal tubules or collecting ducts, providing a clue to the collecting duct origin of the tumor (KENNEDY et al. 1990). Sarcomatoid dedifferentiation has been reported (BAER et al. 1993).

*Ulex europaeus* lectin is the best marker for collecting duct carcinoma: all presently reported cases are strongly immunoreactive, while other types of RCC are consistently negative (DELAHUNT and EBLE 1997; RUMPELT et al. 1991). The majority of cases are immunoreactive for vimentin (KENNEDY et al. 1990).

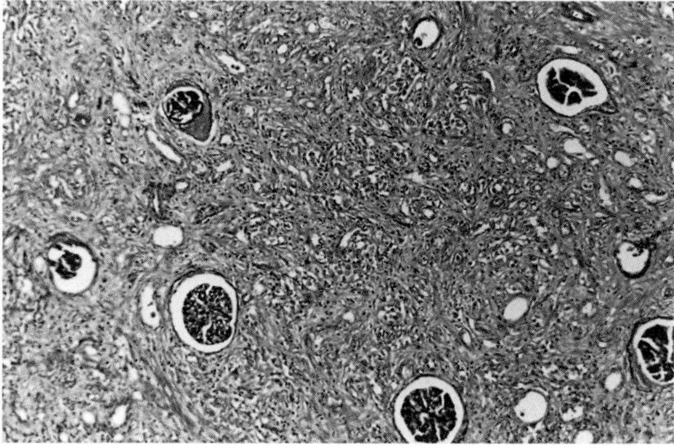

**Fig. 2.4.** Collecting duct carcinoma (Bellini duct carcinoma) consisting of irregular tubular structures, lined by atypical cells with pleomorphic nuclei (hobnail cells). The tumor infiltrates the cortex, in between preexisting glomeruli. PAS after α-amylase digestion, original magnification ×100

Intraluminal mucin production staining positive on PAS and mucicarmine stain is also a feature of collecting duct carcinoma.

## 2.7
## Renal Oncocytoma

In 1976 KLEIN and VALENSI drew attention to renal oncocytoma as a renal tumor previously classified as granular cell RCC, but having a benign course (KLEIN and VALENSI 1976). Renal oncocytoma accounts for approximately 5% of renal neoplasms. There is evidence that they originate from intercalated cells of the collecting duct (STORKEL et al. 1988).

## 2.7.1
## Gross Pathology

Renal oncocytomas are usually well circumscribed, solid, and tan-brown. Larger tumors tend to have a central stellate scar. Foci of hemorrhage are frequent, but necrosis is unusual and often related to concurrent conditions such as vasculitis, sickle cell anemia, or sepsis (DAVIS et al. 1991). Bilaterality or multicentricity occurs. Rarely, large numbers of small oncocytomas are present in the cortices of both kidneys, a condition referred to as oncocytomatosis (WARFEL and EBLE 1982).

## 2.7.2
## Microscopic Pathology

The tumor consists of cells with abundant granular eosinophilic cytoplasm; cells with clear cytoplasm are not present. The nuclei are generally low grade (nuclear grade I or II) and uniform, but focal areas may have marked nuclear atypia. However, the presence of nuclei with features of nuclear grade IV in an apparent oncocytoma strongly suggests that the tumor is a carcinoma. Mitotic activity is not seen, and foci of necrosis are uncommon. The cells are usually arranged either in diffuse sheets or as cellular islands in a background of loose edematous connective tissue (archipelagic architecture) (Fig. 2.5). Tubules, often mildly dilated, are also common. Ultrastructurally, the cytoplasm is filled with mitochondria rich in cristae, and other organelles are scant. Microvilli are sparse and completely formed brush borders are usually absent (EBLE and HULL 1984).

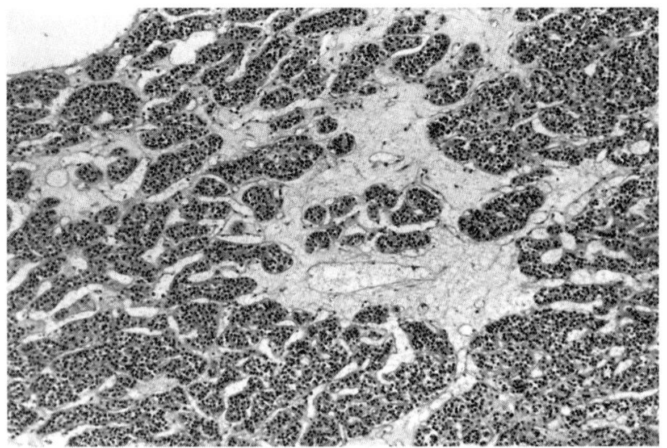

**Fig. 2.5.** Renal oncocytoma. Islands of cells with eosinophilic cytoplasm in a background of loose edematous connective tissue. Hematoxylin-eosin, original magnification ×100

Microscopic vascular invasion and microscopic extension into perirenal fat is seen in 5%–10% of cases and appears to have no adverse effect (DAVIS et al. 1991); however, more cases need to be studied to confirm this. Features that are impermissible in (benign) renal oncocytoma and which imply the diagnosis of (malignant) carcinoma are gross vascular invasion or gross extension into perirenal fat, presence of clear cells or spindle cells, papillary architecture, and presence of mitotic figures. The main differential diagnostic problem is the eosinophilic variant of chromophobic RCC: in the latter, a colloidal iron stain is positive and the typical chromophobe-type vesicles are seen by electron microscopy.

## 2.8
## Neuroendocrine Tumors of the Kidney

Neuroendocrine tumors of the kidney range from carcinoid tumors to small cell carcinomas and are extremely rare (EBLE 1990).

### 2.8.1
### Gross Pathology

Carcinoid tumors are often well circumscribed and consist of red or tan-colored tissue with areas of necrosis and hemorrhage. Small cell carcinomas are large and often show invasion of local structures (EBLE 1990).

### 2.8.2
### Microscopic Pathology

The histological appearance of both carcinoid and small cell carcinoma is identical to that of their counterparts in other organs. Ultrastructurally, neurosecretory granules are present and immunohistochemically, they are immunoreactive for cytokeratin, chromogranin, neuron-specific enolase, and other neuroendocrine markers.

## References

Aizawa S, Kikuchi Y, Suzuki M, et al. (1987) Renal cell carcinoma of lower nephron origin. Acta Pathol Jpn 37:567–574

Amin M, Corless C, Renshaw A, Tickoo S, Kubus J, Schultz D (1997) Papillary (chromophil) renal cell carcinoma: histomorphologic characteristics and evaluation of conventional pathologic prognostic parameters in 62 cases. Am J Surg Pathol 21:621–635

Baer S, Ro J, Ordonez N, Maiese R, Loose J, Grignon D, Ayala A (1993) Sarcomatoid collecting duct carcinoma: a clinicopathologic and immunohistochemical study of five cases. Hum Pathol 24:1017–1022

Bannasch P, Zerban H (1990) Animal models and renal carcinogenesis. In: Eble J (ed) Tumors and tumor-like conditions of the kidneys and ureters. Churchill Livingstone, New York, pp 1–34

Bannasch P, Schacht U, Storch E (1974) Morphogenese und Mikromorphologie epithelialer Nierentumoren bei Nitrosomorpholin-vergifteten Ratten. I. Induktion und Histologie der Tumoren. Z Krebsforsch 81:311–331

Bell E (1950) Renal diseases, 2nd edn. Lea and Febiger, Philadelphia

Bonsib S, Lager DJ (1990) Chromophobe cell carcinoma: analysis of five cases. Am J Surg Pathol 14:260–267

Cheng W, Farrow G, Zincke H (1991) The incidence of multicentricity in renal cell carcinoma. J Urol 146:1221–1223

Crotty T, Farrow G, Lieber M (1995) Chromophobe renal cell carcinoma: clinicopathologic features of 50 cases. J Urol 154:964–967

Dal Bianco M, Artibani W, Bassi P, et al. (1988) Prognostic factors in renal cell carcinoma. Eur Urol 15:73–76

Davis CJ, Mostofi F, Sesterhenn I, et al. (1991) Renal oncocytoma, clinicopathological study of 166 patients. J Urogenital Pathol 1:41–52

Delahunt B, Eble J (1997) Papillary renal cell carcinoma: a clinicopathologic and immunohistochemical study of 105 tumors. Mod Pathol 10:537–544

DeLong W, Sakr W, Grignon D (1996) Chromophobe renal cell carcinoma: a comparative histochemical and immunohistochemical study. J Urol Pathol 4:1–8

Durham J, Keohane M, Amin M (1996) Chromophobe renal cell carcinoma. Adv Anat Pathol 5:336–342

Eble J (1990) Unusual renal tumors and tumor-like conditions. In: Eble J (ed) Tumors and tumor-like conditions of the kidneys and ureters. Churchill Livingstone, New York

Eble J (1996) Neoplasms of the kidney. In: Bostwick D, Eble J (eds) Urologic surgical pathology. Mosby, St. Louis, pp 82–147

Eble J, Hull M (1984) Morphologic features of renal oncocytoma: a light and electron microscopic study. Hum Pathol 15:1054–1061

Eble J, Warfel K (1991) Early human renal cortical epithelial neoplasia. Mod Pathol 4:45A

Fleming S (1993) The impact of genetics on the classification of renal carcinoma. Histopathology 22:89–92

Fleming S, Lewi H (1986) Collecting duct carcinoma of the kidney. Histopathology 10:1131–1141

Fuhrman S, Lasky L, Limas C (1982) Prognostic significance of morphologic parameters in renal cell carcinoma. Am J Surg Pathol 6:655–663

Gatalica Z, Kovatich A, Miettinen M (1995) Consistent expression of cytokeratin 7 in papillary renal-cell carcinoma. An immunohistochemical study in formalin-fixed, paraffin-embedded tissues. J Urol Pathol 3:205–211

Grawitz P (1883) Die sogenannten Lipomen der Nieren. Virchows Arch A 93:39–45

Hartman D, Davis CJ, Johns T, et al. (1986) Cystic renal cell carcinoma. Urology 28:145–153

Hughson M, Hennigar G, McManus J (1980) Atypical cysts, acquired renal cystic disease and renal cell tumors in end stage dialysis kidneys. Lab Invest 42:475–480

Hughson M, Johnson L, Silva F, Kovacs G (1993) Nonpapillary and papillary renal cell carcinoma: a cytogenetic and phenotypic study. Mod Pathol 6:449–456

Kennedy S, Merino M, Linehan W, Roberts J, Robertson C (1990) Collecting duct carcinoma of the kidney. Hum Pathol 21:449–456

Klein M, Valensi Q (1976) Proximal tubular adenomas of kidney with so-called oncocytic features, a clinicopathologic study of 13 cases of a rarely reported neoplasm. Cancer 38:9096–9104

Kovacs G (1993) Molecular differential pathology of renal cell tumours. Histopathology 22:1–8

Kovacs G, Kovacs A (1993) Parenchymal abnormalities associated with papillary renal cell tumors: a morphologic study. J Urol Pathol 1:301–312

Mancilla-Jimenez R, Stanley R, Blath R (1976) Papillary renal cell carcinoma, a clinical, radiologic, and pathologic study of 34 cases. Cancer 38:2469–2480

Medeiros L, Gelb A, Weiss L (1988) Renal cell carcinoma: prognostic significance of morphologic parameters in 121 cases. Cancer 61:1639–1651

Murad T, Komaiko W, Oyasu T, et al. (1991) Multilocular cystic renal cell carcinoma. Am J Clin Pathol 95:633–637

Murphy W, Beckwith J, Farrow K (1994) Tumors of the kidney, bladder, and related urinary structures. Armed Forces Institute of Pathology, Washington, DC

Oberling C, Riviere M, Hagueneau F (1960) Ultrastructure of the clear cells in renal carcinomas and its importance for the demonstration of their renal origin. Nature 186:402–403

Rumpelt H, Storkel S, Moll R, Scharfe T, Thoenes W (1991) Bellini duct carcinoma: further evidence for this rare variant of renal cell carcinoma. Histopathology 18:115–122

Seizinger B, Rouleau G, Ozelius L, et al. (1988) Von Hippel-Lindau disease maps to the region of chromosome 3 associated with renal cell carcinoma. Nature 332:268–269

Storkel S (1993) Karzinome und Onkozytome der Niere. Gustav Fischer, Stuttgart

Storkel S, Jacobi G (1989) Systematik, Histogenese und Prognose der Nierenzellkarzinome und des renalen Onkozytoms. Verh Dtsch Ges Pathol 73:321–513

Storkel S, van den Berg E (1995) Morphological classification of cancer. World J Urol 13:153–158

Storkel S, Pannen B, Thoenes W, et al. (1988) Intercalated cells as a probable source for the development of renal oncocytoma. Virchows Arch B Cell Pathol 56:185–189

Storkel S, Steart P, Drenckhahn D, Thoenes W (1989) The human chromophobe cell renal carcinoma: its probable relation to intercalated cells of the collecting duct. Virchows Arch B Cell Pathol 56:237–245

Thoenes W, Storkel S, Rumpelt H-J (1985) Human chromophobe cell renal carcinoma. Virchows Arch B Cell Pathol 48:207–217

Thoenes W, Storkel S, Rumpelt H (1986) Histopathology and classification of renal cell tumors (adenomas, oncocytomas and carcinomas). The basic cytological and histopathological elements and their use for diagnostics. Pathol Res Pract 181:125–143

Thoenes W, Storkel S, Rumpelt H-J, et al. (1988) Chromophobe cell renal carcinoma and its variants: a report on 32 cases. J Pathol 155:277–287

Thoenes W, Storkel S, Rumpelt H, Moll R (1990) Cytomorphological typing of renal cell carcinoma: a new approach. Eur Urol 18 (Suppl):6–9

van den Berg E, van der Hout A, Oosterhuis J, et al. (1993) Cytogenetic analysis of epithelial renal cell tumors: relationship with a new histopathological classification. Int J Cancer 55:223–227

van der Hout A, van den Berg E, van der Vlies P, et al. (1993) Loss of heterozygosity at the short arm of chromosome-3 in renal cell cancer correlates with the cytological tumour type. Int J Cancer 53:353–357

Warfel K, Eble J (1982) Renal oncocytomatosis. J Urol 127:1179–1180

# 3 Genetics of Renal Cell Carcinoma

P. Dal Cin and H. Van Den Berghe

CONTENTS



## 3.1
## Introduction

The classification of renal cell carcinomas is still a matter of debate. The World Health Organization (WHO) nomenclature subdivided renal tumors into adenomas, carcinomas (with and without papillary growth pattern), and others (Murphy et al. 1994). A new refined classification of renal cell tumors was suggested by Thoenes et al. (1986), based not on the growth pattern but on the cell type from which they are derived in different parts of the tubules. Five basic tumor cell types can thus be distinguished: clear and chromophilic cells derived from the proximal tubules; chromophobe and oncocytic cells derived from the cortical connecting tubules and Bellini duct cells derived from the medullary connecting duct. Variants can be assigned to all


P. Dal Cin, PhD, Center for Human Genetics, University Hospitals Gasthuisberg, Catholic University of Leuven, Herestraat 49, B-3000 Leuven, Belgium
H. Van Den Berghe, PhD, Professor and Chairman, Center for Human Genetics, University Hospitals Gasthuisberg, Catholic University of Leuven, Herestraat 49, B-3000 Leuven, Belgium


these basic cells, resulting from an accumulation of mitochondria (eosinophilic variants). An ultimate form of dedifferentiation may occur when spindle cells (sarcomatoid transformation) are present in a smaller or greater part of a tumor together with any of the basic cell subtypes (carcinomatous area). In 1995, two new subtypes were introduced, neuroendocrine renal cell carcinoma and metanephric adenomas (Storkel and van den Berg 1995).

Specific genomic changes mark the majority of each morphological subtype, and other changes have been related to tumor progression (Kovacs 1993; van den Berg et al. 1993).

## 3.2
## Renal Cell Carcinoma
## of the Clear Cell Type

### 3.2.1
### Cytogenetics

A pivotal finding leading to the recognition of the target region 3p, important in the histogenesis of clear cell renal cell carcinoma (RCC), has been the identification of families carrying a constitutional translocation involving the 3p region, i.e., t(3;8)(p14.2;q24.1) and t(3;6)(p13;q25), in which an unusual number of members have developed a clear cell RCC (Cohen et al. 1979; Kovacs et al. 1989).

Since the first observation of involvement of chromosome 3 in RCC in a series of cell lines as well as in primary renal tumors, reported by Wang et al. (1983), loss of the short arm (p) of chromosome 3 has frequently been observed in sporadic clear cell type/nonpapillary RCC, mostly as the sole chromosome change. This partial monosomy 3p can occur via at least three different mechanisms: (1) as a deletion, terminal or interstitial; (2) as an unbalanced translocation between the 3p region and another chromosome, the long arm (q) of chromosome 5 being a preferential partner; (3) as a result of loss of

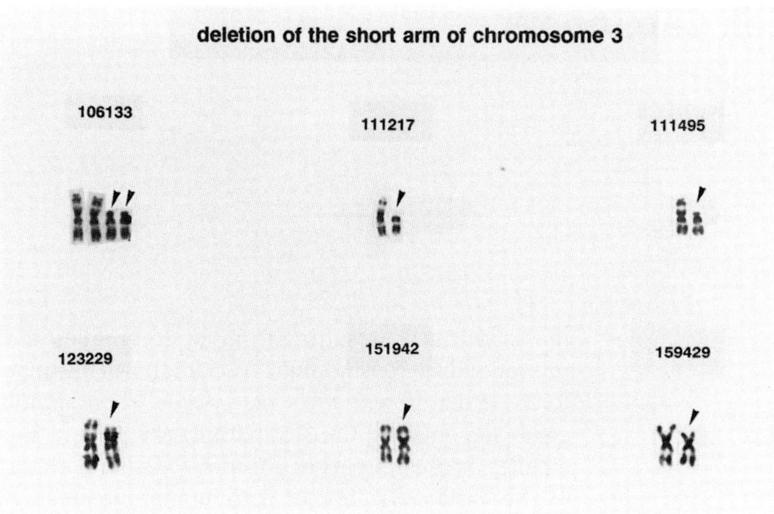


**Fig. 3.1.** Partial karyotypes from six different clear cell RCCs, showing different deletions of the short arm of chromosome 3 (*arrowheads*)

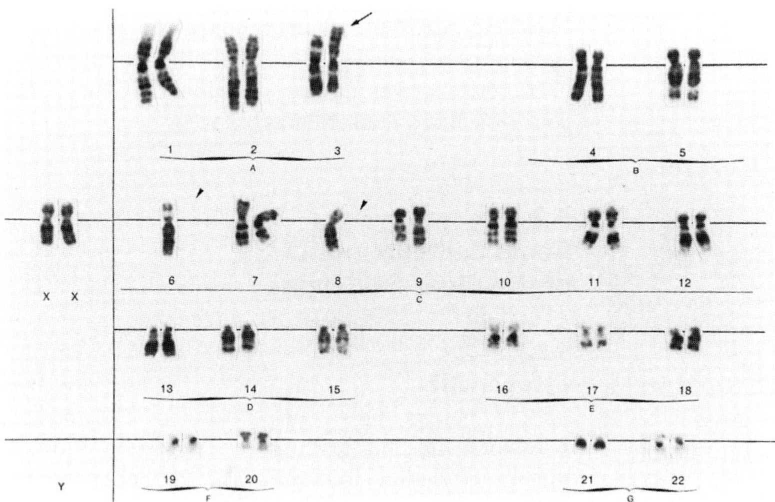


**Fig. 3.2.** G-banded karyotype of a clear cell RCC showing loss of 3p by unbalanced translocation t(2;3)(p11;p11) (*arrow*). *Arrowheads* point to secondary chromosome abnormalities

one chromosome 3 material, 3pter 3q11–12 or 3pter 3q21 being deleted with a concomitant translocation of the remaining part of the long arm of chromosome 3 (Figs. 3.1–3.3).

The region of chromosome 3p most frequently lost varies from p11.2 to pter with a clustering of breakpoints at 3p14.2, which is the locus of fragile site FRA 3B (SUTHERLAND and HECHT 1985).

Besides a 3p abnormality, other recurrent chromosome aberrations can be observed in clear cell RCC, which seem to be associated with tumor progression. Among the numerical changes, monosomies of chromosomes 8, 9, 13, and 14 and trisomies of chromosomes 12 and 20 are the most frequent anomalies observed. Also nonrandom structural changes involving 5q, 6q, 8p, 10q and 14q have been described (KÄLBLE and KOVACS 1994).

Most of the bilateral solitary RCCs are of the clear cell type, and cytogenetic investigations have shown that the abnormal karyotype of the tumor of one kidney is usually different from that of the other (DAL CIN et al. 1996).

## 3.2.2
## Molecular Aspects

From the findings in two families with hereditary clear cell RCC exhibiting a constitutional translocation involving 3p, i.e., t(3;8) and t(3;6) (COHEN et al. 1979; KOVACS et al. 1989), it has been suggested that the translocation inactivated a tumor suppressor gene on chromosome 3. Further molecular studies on these families have shown that, as different chro-

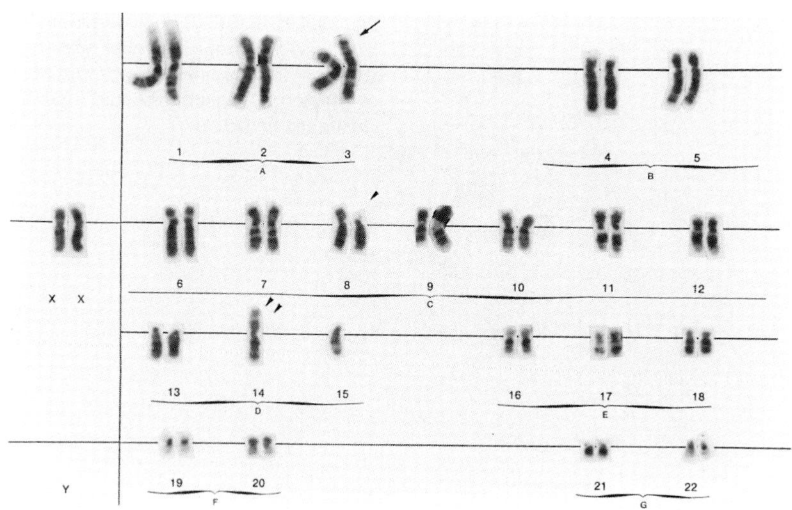

**Fig. 3.3.** G-banded karyotype showing a der(3)t(3;5)(p13;q22) (*arrow*) leading to loss of 3p and partial trisomy 5q22 qter. *Arrowheads* point to secondary chromosome abnormalities

mosomal sites are affected by the translocations, it is unlikely that they would disrupt the same tumor suppressor gene, consequently implying the presence of two different tumor suppressor genes in the 3p12–p14 region (VAN DEN BERG et al. 1995b). The von Hippel-Lindau (VHL) gene located at 3p25 (LATIF et al. 1993) was found to be involved not only in the hereditary cancer syndrome but also in the development of sporadic clear cell RCCs. The VHL gene therefore was suggested to be the RCC gene (GNARRA et al. 1994). Recently another gene on chromosome 3, FHIT, has been found to be disrupted in hereditary RCC with a (3;8) constitutional translocation (OTHA et al. 1995). Its causative role in RCC, however, is very much debated (LUAN et al. 1997; VAN DEN BERG et al. 1997).

Furthermore, loss of heterozygosity has been demonstrated with high frequency in clear cell/nonpapillary RCC in several regions of 3p, i.e., 3p12–p14, 3p21 and 3p25 (for review see VAN DEN BERG et al. 1996). The true nature of the apparently complex genomic changes that may occur in the 3p11.2–p14.1 large breakpoint region, however, is far from being established (BUGERT et al. 1996).

Finally, loss of heterozygosity at chromosomes 8p, 9p, and 14q is probably more related to tumor evolution as it has been described mainly in advanced stages of nonpapillary RCC and potentially represent a good prognostic marker for these tumors (SCHULLERUS et al. 1997).

## 3.3
## Renal Cell Adenoma/Carcinoma of the Chromophilic Type

### 3.3.1
### Cytogenetics

Renal cell adenomas/carcinomas of the chromophilic type are generally referred to as papillary renal cell tumors. Two subgroups of papillary/chromphilic renal tumors may be distinguished on the basis of karyotypic changes. The combination of sex chromosome loss with trisomy or tetrasomy 7 and trisomy 17 is a unique combination of numerical changes found as the only karyotypic alteration in some papillary tumors. Such tumors do not display invasive and metastatic growth; therefore they must be considered benign and should be referred to as papillary adenoma (DAL CIN et al. 1989; KOVACS et al. 1991) (Fig. 3.4). When, however, additional trisomies 12, 16, and 20 appear, they are associated with a more aggressive behavior and with progression to the carcinoma stage, papillary RCC. In these cases trisomy 3/+3q is also frequently found (Fig. 3.5).

In a recent study BROWN and co-workers (1997) argued that simultaneous chromosome 7 and 17 gain with or without sex chromosome loss also characterizes a newly identified entity, metanephric adenoma, suggesting that these tumors may be related to the common papillary tumors.

Bilateral multifocal RCCs are always of the papillary/chromophilic type and the karyotypes show more or less the same numerical anomalies with trisomies in different combinations in the same kidney

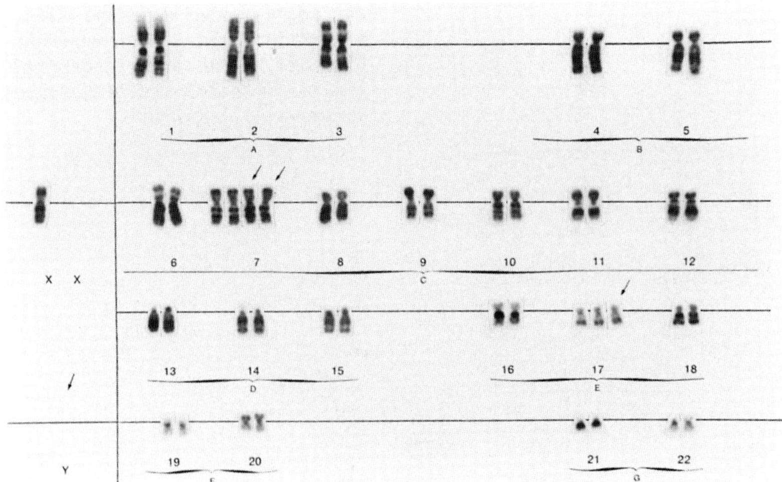

**Fig. 3.4.** G-banded karyotype of a papillary/chromophilic renal adenoma showing the characteristic combination of tetrasomy 7, trisomy 17, and loss of Y chromosome (*arrow*)

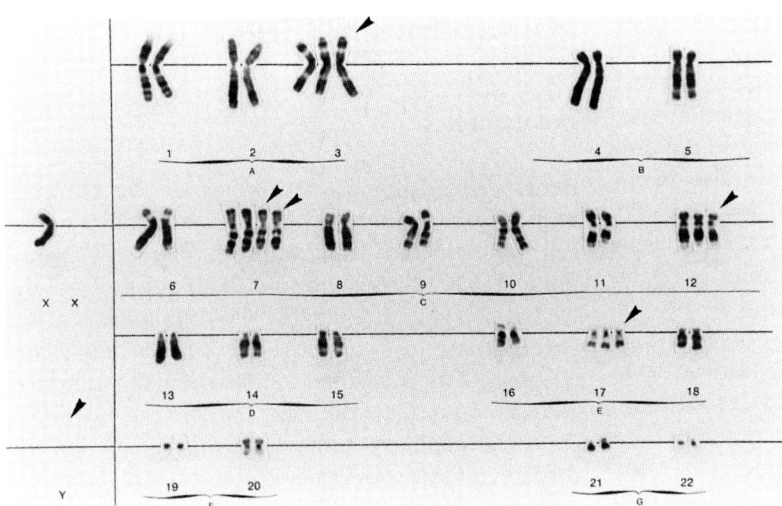

**Fig. 3.5.** G-banded karyotype of a papillary/chromophilic RCC showing the presence of additional trisomies of chromosomes 3 and 12 (*arrowheads*)

as well as in both kidneys (Kovacs et al. 1991; Henn et al. 1993).

### 3.3.2
### Molecular Aspects

Little is known about molecular lesions in chromophilic tumors. Missense mutations in the tyrosine kinase domain of the MET proto-oncogene, located at 7q31, have recently been described in the germline of affected members of hereditary papillary renal carcinoma families and in a subset of sporadic papillary RCCs (Schmidt et al. 1997).

### 3.3.3
### Chromophilic Renal Cell Carcinomas
### with Aberration of Xp11.2

Fifteen RCCs have been reported with X; autosome translocations (for review see Dal Cin et al. 1998). The most frequently reported translocation partner of the Xp11.2 band has been the 1q21 band, followed by another chromosome 1 band, 1p34 (Fig. 3.6). The three remaining RCCs exhibited a t(X;17)(p11.2;q25), a t(X;10)(p11.2;q23), and a del(X)(p11). Interestingly, the age distribution of these cases is strikingly different from that of kidney tumors in general, more than 50% of the patients

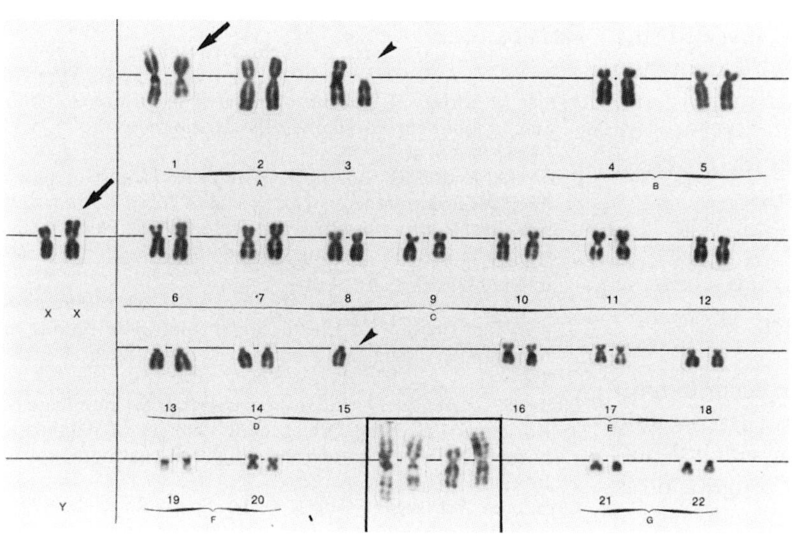

**Fig. 3.6.** G-banded karyotype showing a der(X)t(X;1)(p11.2;q21), which is a characteristic chromosome abnormality in some chromophilic RCCs

being younger than 45 years. There is also a marked predominance of males (ratio 4:1), whereas in the general population a ratio of 1.5:1 is found.

Histologically, most of the cases have revealed a chromophilic/papillary growth pattern, with some clear cell-like features due to the deposition of fat and glycogen, which results in a possible misdiagnosis of clear cell RCC. There are no data on the prognosis of this subset of chromophilic RCCs. The finding of metastases 31 years after nephrectomy (DAL CIN et al. 1998) could be a truly exceptional event, but could also indicate a more indolent course of the disease.

The genes involved in the t(X;1) have recently been identified. The translocation results in a fusion of the transcription factor TFE3 gene on the X chromosome to a novel gene, designated PRCC, on chromosome 1 (WETERMAN et al. 1996).

## 3.4
## Bellini Duct Carcinoma

Data concerning the cytogenetic abnormalities of Bellini duct carcinoma are limited to seven cases (FÜZESI et al. 1992; GREGORI-ROMERO et al. 1996; CAVAZZANA et al. 1996). Conflicting findings have been reported, with monosomies on the one hand (FÜZESI et al. 1992) and trisomies on the other (CAVAZZANA et al. 1996; GREGORI-ROMERO et al. 1996).

Molecular studies in this particular type of kidney tumor have suggested frequent loss of heterozygosity of 8p and 13q, and no loss of material of the short arm of chromosome 3 (SCHOENBERG et al. 1995; POLASCIK et al. 1996).

## 3.5
## Renal Cell Carcinoma of the Chromophobic Cell Type

Cytogenetics, comparative genomic hybridization, and microsatellite and DNA cytometric analysis have suggested that a combination of monosomies of chromosomes 1, 2, 6, 10, 13, 17, and 21 characterizes this type of RCC (BUGERT et al. 1997; SCHWERDTLE et al. 1996; SHUIN et al. 1996; SPEICHER et al. 1994).

Chromophobic RCCs do not grow very well in vitro, but correct genetic characterization is not trivial since the two variants, the typical one and the eosinophilic one, may be misdiagnosed as clear cell RCC and oncocytoma, respectively. However, the latter two renal tumors exhibit different chromosomal patterns: loss of 3p material in clear cell RCCs, and at least two different cytogenetic subgroups in oncocytomas, i.e., those with coincident loss of chromosomes Y and 1, and those with involvement of 11q13 (NEUHAUS et al. 1997).

## 3.6
## Other Types of Renal Cell Carcinoma

There are no cytogenetic data on RCCs of the transitional cell type. Investigations of only two cases of neuroendocrine type RCC have been reported. In one case cytogenetic investigation revealed the presence of two different abnormal karyotypes, both involving chromosome 13, i.e., trisomy 13 and t(13;14)(q31;q11.2) (VAN DEN BERG et 1995a); by contrast loss of heterozygosity on 3p21 was observed by EL-NAGGAR and co-workers (1995).

## 3.7
## Sarcomatoid Renal Cell Cancers

Sarcomatoid transformation seems to occur in most of the RCC subtypes. The appearance of sarcomatoid features, such as a spindle cell pattern with little differentiation, may be an indication of progression in RCC rather than of the existence of a specific type of tumor.

To our knowledge, a few sarcomatoid RCCs have been cytogenetically investigated (EL-NAGGAR and PATHAK 1992; GRAMMATICO et al. 1993; AKTHAR et al. 1996; DIJKHUIZEN et al. 1997). Cytogenetic findings on two presumed papillary sarcomatoid RCCs did not confirm the papillary nature of the tumor since the changes characteristic of papillary tumors were not found (EL-NAGGAR and PATHAK 1992; GRAMMATICO et al. 1993). On the other hand, a low chromosome number usually characterizing chromophobic RCC was found in both chromophobe and sarcomatous components of a case described by AKTHAR and co-workers (1996). Loss of 3p sequences, p53 mutation and complex karyotype pointed to a clear cell rather than to a chromophilic origin in the case investigated by DIJKHUIZEN et al. (1997). Interesting, ODA and co-workers (1995) described an association between p53 and the sarcomatoid transformation in RCC.

## 3.8
## Renal Cell Carcinoma in Children

Little is known about the cytogenetics of RCC in the pediatric age group. Three cases have been reported with a single chromosome change: a t(X;1)(p11.2;q21.2) in a trabecular carcinoma composed of large clear cells (DE JONG et al. 1986), a t(X;17)(p11.2;q25) in a clear cell RCC (TOMLINSON et al. 1991), and a t(6;17)(p21;q24–25) in a clear cell RCC (DAL CIN et al. 1991).

## References

Akthar M, Kfoury H, Kardar A, Linjafwi T, Kovacs G (1996) Sarcomatoid chromophobe cell carcinoma of the kidney. J Urol Pathol 4:155–166

Brown JA, Anderl KL, Borell TJ, Qian J, Bostwick DG, Jenkins RB (1997) Simultaneous chromosome 7 and 17 gain and sex chromosome loss provide evidence that renal metanephric adenoma is related to papillary renal cell carcinoma. J Urol 158:370–374

Bugert P, Kenck C, Wilhelm M, Kovacs G (1996) Refining a proximal breakpoint cluster at chromosome 3p11.2 in non-papillary renal cell carcinomas. Int J Cancer 68:723–726

Bugert P, Gaul C, Weber K, Herbers J, Akhtar M, Ljungberg B, Kovacs G (1997) Specific genetic changes of diagnostic importance in chromophobe renal cell carcinomas. Lab Invest 76:203–208

Cavazzana AO, Prayer-Galetti T, Tirabosco R, et al. (1996) Bellini duct carcinoma. A clinical and in vitro study. Eur Urol 30:340–344

Cohen AJK, Li FP, Berg S, Marchetto DJ, Tsai S, Jacobs SC, Brown RS (1979) Hereditary renal-cell carcinoma associated with a chromosomal translocation. N Eng J Med 301:592–595

Dal Cin P, Gaeta J, Huben R, Li FP, Prout GR JR, Sandberg AA (1989) Renal cortical tumors: cytogenetic characterization. Am J Clin Pathol 92:408–414

Dal Cin P, Van Gool S, Brock P, et al. (1991) Renal cell carcinoma in a child. Cancer Genet Cytogenet 53:137–138

Dal Cin P, Van Poppel H, Van Damme B, Baert L, Van Den Berghe H (1996) Cytogenetic investigation of synchronous bilateral renal tumors. Cancer Genet Cytogenet 89:57–60

Dal Cin P, Stas M, Sciot R, De Wever I, Van Damme B, Van den Berghe H (1998) Translocation X;1 reveals metastasis after 31 years of renal cell carcinoma. Cancer Genet Cytogenet, in press

de Jong B, Molenaar IM, Leeuw JA, Idebburg VJS, Oosterhuis JW (1986) Cytogenetics of a renal cell carcinoma in a 2-year-old child. Cancer Genet Cytogenet 21:165–169

Dijkhuizen T, van den Berg E, van den Berg A, et al. (1997) Genetics as a diagnostic tool in sarcomatoid renal-cell cancer. Int J Cancer 72:265–269

El-Naggar AK, Pathak S (1992) Cytogenetic and corresponding flow cytometric DNA analysis of renal cell neoplasms. Anticancer Res 12:1491–1500

El-Naggar AK, Troncoso P, Ordonez NG (1995) Primary renal carcinoid tumor with molecular abnormality characteristic of conventional renal cell neoplasms. Diagn Mol Pathol 1:41–53

Füzesi L, Cober M, Mittermayer C (1992) Collecting duct carcinoma: cytogenetic characterization. Histopathology 21:155–160

Gnarra JR, Tory K, Weng Y, et al. (1994) Mutations of the *VHL* tumour suppressor gene in renal carcinoma. Nature Genet 7:85–90

Grammatico P, Cianciulli AM, Grammatico B, Di Rosa C, Del Porto G (1993) The first cytogenetic study of a sarcomatoid renal cell carcinoma. J Exp Clin Cancer Res 12:19–21

Gregori-Romero MA, Morell-Quadreny L, Llombart-Bosch A (1996) Cytogenetic analysis of three primary Bellini duct carcinomas. Genes Chromosom Cancer 15:170–172

Henn W, Zwergel T, Wullich B, Thonnes M, Zang KD (1993) Bilateral multicentric papillary renal tumors with heteroclonal origin based on tissue-specific karyotype instability. Cancer 72:1315–1318

Kälble T, Kovacs G (1994) Molecular genetics in the diagnosis and prognosis of renal cancer. Klin Lab 40: 1209–1234

Kovacs G (1993) Molecular differential pathology of renal cell tumours. Histopathology 22:1–8

Kovacs G, Brusa, De Riese W (1989) Tissue-specific expression of a constitutional 3;6 translocation: development of multiple bilateral renal-cell carcinomas. Int J Cancer 43: 422–427

Kovacs G, Fuzesi L, Emanuel A, Kung HF (1991) Cytogenetics of papillary renal cell tumors. Genes Chromosom Cancer 134:27–34

Latif F, Tory K, Gnarra J, et al. (1993) Identification of the von Hippel-Lindau disease tumor suppressor gene. Science 260: 1317–1320

Luan X, Shi G, Zohouri M, Paradee W, Smith DI, Decker HJ, Cannizzaro LA (1997) The FHIT gene is alternatively spliced in normal kidney and renal cell carcinoma. Oncogene 15:79–86

Murphy WM, Beckwith JB, Farrow KGM (1994) Tumors of the kidney, bladder, and related urinary structures. Armed Forces Institute of Pathology, Washington, D.C.

Neuhaus C, Dijkhuizen T, van den Berg E, et al. (1997) Involvement of the chromosomal region 11q13 in renal oncocytoma: case report and literature review. Cancer Genet Cytogenet 94:95–98

Oda H, Nakatsura Y, Ishikawa T (1995) Mutations of p53 gene and p53 protein expression are associated with sarcomatoid transformation in renal cell carcinoma. Cancer Res 55:658–662

Otha M, Inoue H, Cotticelli MG, et al. (1995) The *FHIT* gene, spanning the chromosome 3p14.2 fragile site and renal carcinoma-associated t(3;8) breakpoint, is abnormal in digestive tract cancers. Cell 84:587–597

Polascik TJ, Cairns P, Epstein JI, et al. (1996) Distal nephron renal tumors: micro-satellite allelotype. Cancer Res 56:1892–1895

Schmidt L, Duh F-M, Chen F, et al. (1997) Germline and somatic mutations in the tyrosine kinase domain of the *MET* proto-oncogene in papillary renal carcinomas. Nature Genet 16: 68–73

Schoenberg M, Cairns P, Brooks DB, Marshall FF, Epstein JI, Isaacs WB, Sidransky D (1995) Frequent loss of chromosome arms 8p and 13p in collecting duct carcinoma of kidney. Genes Chromosom Cancer 12:76–80

Schullerus D, Herbers J, Chudek J, Kanamaru H, Kovacs G (1997) Loss of heterozygosity at chromosomes 8p, 9p, and 14q is associated with stage and grade of non-papillary renal cell carcinomas. J Pathol 183:151–155

Schwerdtle RF, Störkel S, Neuhaus C, et al. (1996) Allelic losses at chromosomes 1p, 2p, 6p, 10p, 13q, 17p, and 21q significantly correlate with the chromophobe subtype of renal cell carcinoma. Cancer Res 56:2927–2930

Shuin T, Kondo K, Sakai N, et al. (1996) A case of chromophobe renal cell carcinoma associated with low chromosome number and microsatellite instability. Cancer Genet Cytogenet 86:69–71

Speicher MR, Schoell B, du Manoir S, et al. (1994) Specific loss of chromosomes 1, 2, 6, 10, 13, 17, and 21 in chromophobe renal cell carcinomas revealed by comparative genomic hybridization. Am J Pathol 145:356–364

Storkel S, van den Berg E (1995) Morphological classification of cancer. World J Urol 13:153–158

Sutherland GR, Hecht F (1985) Fragile sites on human chromosomes. Oxford University Press, New York

Thoenes W, Storkel S, Rumplet HJ (1986) Histopathology and classification of renal cell tumors (adenomas, oncocytomas, and carcinomas). The basic cytological and histopathological elements and their use for diagnostics. Pathol Res Pract 181:125–143

Tomlinson GE, Nisen PD, Timmons CF, Schneider NR (1991) Cytogenetics of renal cell carcinoma in a 17-month-old child: evidence for Xp11.2 as a recurring breakpoint. Cancer Genet Cytogenet 57:11–17

van den Berg E, van der Hout AH, Oosterhuis JW, et al. (1993) Cytogenetic analysis of epithelial renal-cell tumors: relationship with a new histopathological classification. Int J Cancer 55:223–227

van den Berg E, Gauw ASH, Oosterhuis JWK, Störkel S, Dijkhkuizen T, Mensink HJA, de Jong B (1995a) Carcinoid in a horseshoe kidney. Morphology, immunohistochemistry, and cytogenetics. Cancer Genet Cytogenet 84:95–98

van den Berg A, van der Veen AYK, Hulsbeen MMF, Kovacs G, Gemmill RM, Drabkin HA, Buys CHCM (1995b) Defining the position of the breakpoint of the constitutional t(3;6) occurring in a family with renal cell carcinoma. Genes Chromosom Cancer 12:224–228

van den Berg A, Hulsbeek MMF, de Jong D, Kok K, Veldhuis PMJF, Roch J, Buys CHCM (1996) Major role for a 3p21 region and lack of involvement of the t(3;8) breakpoint region in the development of renal cell carcinoma suggested by loss of heterozygosity analysis. Genes Chromosom Cancer 15:64–72

van den Berg A, Draaijers TG, Kok K, et al. (1997) Normal *FHIT* transcripts in renal cell cancer- and lung cancer-derived cell lines, including a cell line with a homozygous deletion in the FRA3B region. Genes Chromosom Cancer 19:220–227

Wang N, Soldat L, Fan S, Figemshau S, Clayman R, Fraley E (1983) The consistent involvement of chromosome 3 and 6 aberrations in renal cell carcinoma (abstract). Am J Hum Genet 35:73A

Weterman MAJ, Wilbrink M, Geurts van Kessel A (1996) Fusion of the transcription factor *TFE3* gene to a novel gene, *PRCC* in t(X;1)(p11;q21)positive papillary renal cell carcinomas. Proc Natl Acad Sci USA 93:15294–15298

# 4 Imaging of Renal Parenchymal Tumors

R.H. OYEN and G.A. VERSWIJVEL

CONTENTS



## 4.1
## Introduction

The detection of renal masses by ultrasonography (US), computed tomography (CT), and magnetic resonance imaging (MRI) relies on high-quality examinations. Therefore, optimization of the imaging techniques is a continuous challenge for radiologists. Once a renal mass is detected, the radiologist is faced with two additional tasks: (1) to determine whether it is a simple renal cyst/benign lesion or a malignant tumor, or more simply, whether or not it is renal cancer; and (2) in cases of suspected malignancy, to ascertain the stage, or, ultimately, whether the case is operable. Therefore, imaging strategies must be directed towards appropriate differentiation and staging of any renal mass lesion.

R.H. OYEN, MD, PhD, Adjunct Clinic Head, Department of Radiology, University Hospitals Gasthuisberg, Catholic University of Leuven, Herestraat 49, B-3000 Leuven, Belgium
G.A. VERSWIJVEL, MD, Department of Radiology, University Hospitals Gasthuisberg, Catholic University of Leuven, Herestraat 49, B-3000 Leuven, Belgium

## 4.2
## Imaging Techniques

### 4.2.1
### Ultrasonography

Ultrasonography is now widely accepted for the detection and noninvasive evaluation of renal masses. Its major advantage is the ability to reliably differentiate simple renal cysts and solid renal masses (which in general require surgery). In selected cases, US can be an excellent adjunct for the evaluation of complex cyst-like lesions detected with CT or MRI (in general such lesions require further investigation or follow-up).

Gray-scale US remains the modality of choice for routine assessment of the renal parenchyma and renal mass lesions. Color-Doppler and duplex-Doppler US may be helpful for further lesion characterization in selected cases. TAKASE et al. (1994) showed that US angiography has a possible role in the detection of small nodules in patients with chronic renal failure. In TAKASE et al.'s study, US was useful for the detection of nodules but did not allow differentiation of malignant from benign lesions. US is less accurate than CT or MRI in tumor staging. Failure to visualize adequately the central retroperitoneal region, renal vessels, and infrahepatic vena cava may occur in more than 50% of patients, usually because of overlying intestinal gas (WEBB et al. 1987).

A few reports have been published on the advantages of intraoperative US for visualizing renal masses, major renal vessels, and the inferior vena cava (LONG et al. 1993; HARRIS et al. 1994; POLASCIK et al. 1995).

### 4.2.2
### Computed Tomography

At the outset, it should be clearly stated that the imaging diagnosis of a renal mass depends on high-quality imaging studies (BOSNIAK 1997). An experienced observer is an additional and essential prerequisite to improve the diagnostic accuracy of CT. Indeed, many lesions are "indeterminate," not so much because of the character of the lesion but because of suboptimal imaging studies and because of lack of confidence of the observer.

Detection of tumor vascularity remains the single most important discriminator of solid lesions from renal cysts (BOSNIAK 1991). Therefore it is necessary to perform scans prior to and after the intravenous administration of iodinated contrast material (ZEMAN et al. 1988). Thus, in general, the quality of a CT scan to a great extent depends on the quality of the equipment and the care given in study performance. A high-quality CT scan includes the following:

1. Performance with modern equipment.
2. Performance before and after i.v. contrast; in small lesions (or in small suspect areas of a large lesion), thin sections must be obtained.
3. Rapid injection (mechanical if possible) of an adequate amount of contrast medium (30–40 g of iodine in patients with normal renal function) so that a high blood concentration of contrast is present at the time of scanning.
4. Accuracy of the numbers when measurement of Hounsfield units (HU) is important in diagnosis (BOSNIAK 1991).

The same technical parameters employed to obtain the precontrast scan should be used to acquire the postcontrast scan, and it must be ensured that artefacts are not affecting the measurements. Multiple measurements are needed in cases in which the enhancement is minimal. With well-calibrated equipment, increase of at least 20 HU is considered to be sufficient for the diagnosis of a solid mass. Nowadays, the sensitivity of incremental CT has been markedly improved by spiral (helical) CT. Spiral CT eliminates respiratory misregistration and allows examination of the entire kidney in virtually the same phase after injection of iodinated contrast material (SILVERMAN et al. 1994). Some studies have illustrated the superiority of scanning in the nephrographic phase compared with the earlier corticomedullary phase (COHAN et al. 1995; SZOLAR et al. 1997). Scanning in the nephrographic phase is certainly more efficient in visualizing small lesions originating in or near the renal medulla. Therefore, spiral CT scanning is preferably initiated 35–40 s after injection and repeated after 70–80 s. A total amount of 120–150 ml contrast containing 40–45 g iodine is administered at a rate of 1.5–3 ml/s. A collimation of 5 mm and a pitch (ratio of table speed to collimation) of 1 is used. Furthermore, this technique permits the evaluation of the liver parenchyma prior to the equilibrium phase.

Lesion detection is significantly improved with CT compared to US and excretory urography (WARSHAUER et al, 1988). With appropriate CT technique a diagnostic accuracy exceeding 95% can be achieved (LEVINE 1995).

### 4.2.3
### Magnetic Resonance Imaging

Magnetic resonance imaging is gaining in status for the diagnosis, characterization, and staging of renal masses. MRI should include T1- and T2-weighted images in the axial plane. Both coronal and sagittal planes are helpful in selected cases. Fat-suppressed T1-weighted spin-echo images before and after intravenous gadolinium (0.1 mmol/kg) enhancement are also useful in evaluating renal masses. As with CT, the diagnosis of a renal mass relies on the demonstration of vascularity. Renal cell carcinoma (RCC) is the most frequent solid renal mass; since most RCCs have areas of hemorrhage or necrosis, they can be easily demonstrated on heavily T2-weighted images (HASTE) and without administration of gadolinium. In practice, though, tumors smaller than 3 cm in diameter are isointense to normal renal parenchyma on both T1- and T2-weighted images and are therefore detected in only 63% of unenhanced sequences (HRICAK et al. 1988). Therefore, contrast administration for lesion detection and characterization is required in most cases (HRICAK et al. 1988; ROMINGER et al. 1992; NARUMI et al. 1997). On gadolinium-enhanced gradient-echo images there is a marked increase in contrast between tumor and normal renal parenchyma, and RCCs usually show heterogeneous enhancement less than that of normal renal parenchyma. Others have likewise observed superior lesion detection and characterization with gadolinium-enhanced spin-echo sequences with fat saturation compared with unenhanced MRI (EILENBERG et al. 1990; SEMELKA et al. 1991, 1992, 1993). Especially in a patient with renal insufficiency or allergy to iodinated contrast material, contrast-enhanced dynamic MRI is a useful technique for the diagnosis of small RCC (ROFSKY et al. 1991; YAMASHITA et al. 1995). A disadvantage of MRI is that tumor calcification is difficult to appreciate on almost all MR pulse sequences; tumor calcification can occasionally be helpful in the differential diagnosis of renal masses.

New technical developments allow for the simultaneous evaluation of the renal arteries (MR angiography; both arteries and veins are visible), the renal parenchyma, and the collecting system (MR urography) in a single examination after injection of a small amount of contrast medium. This is very promising, since MRI now seems to be applicable in virtually all patients, irrespective of their age and their ability to cooperate. MR angiography provides useful additional information and is considered a complementary technique to the spin-echo sequences for the evaluation of thrombotic conditions and venous anomalies, and in the study of the relationship of the renal artery and renal neoplasms with aortic aneurysms (CARRIERO et al. 1994). Finally, CHOYKE et al. (1997) have shown that dual-phase MR angiography of the kidney may be a useful technique in depicting renal vessels before nephrectomy.

With current techniques, MRI is of equal value to CT in the overall detection and differential diagnosis of renal masses (SEMELKA et al. 1992; KREFT et al. 1997). MRI is particularly helpful for further differential diagnosis of lesions which are equivocal on CT (especially in the differentiation between complicated cysts and cystic or hypovascular RCC) and enhancement of tumor thrombus and adenopathy.

## 4.2.4
## Angiography

Angiography has an extremely limited role in the diagnosis of renal masses, even though it may have a role in the management of RCC and angiomyolipoma (MAURO et al. 1982). Angiography can be used to evaluate the renal blood vessels if this information is needed in the planning of a surgical procedure. This information can also be abtained with MR angiography (CHOYKE et al. 1997). Occasionally, angiography is used for the therapeutic embolization of renal neoplasms to decrease vascularity, to stop bleeding, or to cure postoperative complications (BARBARIC 1996). Likewise, embolization may be indicated in angiomyolipoma to control bleeding (DE WEVER et al. 1996).

## 4.2.5
## Needle Aspiration or Biopsy

Needle aspiration puncture or biopsy has a limited role in the evaluation of renal masses in the CT/MRI era and has been abandoned as a routine procedure (IMAIDE and SAITOH 1995). The procedure has occasional value in the evaluation of the cystic indeterminate mass, but its success in these cases is limited because clear fluid, even with negative cytology, does not rule out neoplasm, and hemorrhagic fluid does not necessarily indicate malignancy (HAYAKAWA et al. 1996). Also, in complex multiloculated lesions, multiple needle passes would be necessary. In the occasional case in which a lesion is highly suspicious for neoplasm in a patient who is a very poor surgical risk, the technique could be performed to help establish a diagnosis and determine the treatment approach.

On the other hand, there are a number of occasions on which needle aspiration or biopsy is definitely indicated. These include the following: (1) differentiation of a chronic abscess from a cystic carcinoma; (2) differentiation of a simple cyst from an infected cyst; (3) differentiation of a primary renal neoplasm from metastasis in a patient who has had a previous primary tumor in another organ; and (4) differentiation of a primary renal neoplasm from renal lymphoma in a patient with lymphoma, particularly when the lesion does not regress with treatment whereas the rest of the lymphomatous disease does (BARBARIC 1996). Even in these cases, it should be known that at least 50% of renal masses will turn out to be primary renal epithelial neoplasms rather than metastases or lymphoma.

## 4.3
## Renal Masses

There has been a great increase in the detection and earlier diagnosis of renal tumors because of the wider application of US and CT. While this has tended to improve the cure rate of malignant renal parenchymal tumors because of earlier and more accurate diagnosis, these new techniques have also increased the detection of all types of renal masses, including those that require surgery. In practice, any nonfatty renal mass that enhances with intravenous contrast should be considered a RCC until proved otherwise. On the other hand, not all renal masses that enhance are malignant renal tumors. The goal of imaging is essentially to separate the carcinomas from all other renal masses that finally do not require surgery. This means that simple and complicated benign renal cysts, abscesses, hematomas, infarcts, localized inflammatory pseudotumors, angiomyolipomas, lymphoma, and metastatic cancer should be identified and differentiated from other primary malignant renal neoplasms, if possible. The combination of clinical history, CT findings, MRI, and needle aspiration (in highly selected cases only) enables the distinction between these lesions in the majority of cases.

This overview almost exclusively deals with the most frequent renal mass lesions in adults, including simple renal cysts. RCC accounts for almost 90% of primary malignant renal epithelial neoplasms in the adult age group (median age at diagnosis about 57 years) and approximately 3% of adult malignancies. The tumor occurs about twice as commonly in men as in women. Most RCCs occur sporadically. The tumor occurs in about 36% of patients with von Hippel-Lindau disease, and the incidence is greater among long-term dialysis patients (LEVINE 1995). Since so-called complicated cysts and angiomyolipomas may cause problems in differential diagnosis, they will be taken into consideration as well.

### 4.3.1
### Cysts and Cyst-like Lesions

#### 4.3.1.1
#### Simple Renal Cysts

The imaging criteria of simple renal cysts are well established. The US diagnosis of a simple cyst is based on four criteria: a well-marginated (rounded) fluid collection, without a discernible wall, without internal echoes, and with good sound through-transmission producing acoustic enhancement. In selected cases color-Doppler US is helpful to differentiate solid lesions from cysts (DENYS et al. 1991). On CT, a cyst has a rounded shape, with attenuation numbers of water (0–20 HU), and without enhancement after intravenous contrast administration. On T1-weighted MR images, simple cysts are hypointense with no internal architecture or debris, while on predominantly T2-weighted images the content exhibits high signal intenstities. The cyst wall is thin and almost imperceptible with both pulse sequences. There is no enhancement of any portion of the cyst after administration of gadolinium.

Solid protrusions inside the confines of a cystic lesion exclude the radiological diagnosis of benignity: such lesions must be considered as a carcinoma and require surgery.

#### 4.3.1.2
#### "Complex" Cysts

When a "complicated" cystic lesion is encountered in an imaging study, determination of its benignity or malignancy is based on the evaluation of the thickness and contour of the wall of the lesion; the number, contour, and thickness of any septa; the amount, character, and location of any calcifications; the density of fluid in the lesion; and the margination of the lesion and the presence of solid components (BOSNIAK 1986, 1997; DAVIDSON et al. 1997). Any partially or entirely calcified lesion detected at US must always be investigated with CT or MRI because of the possibility that it is an RCC (WEYMAN et al. 1982; BOSNIAK 1986, 1997; VANDEPUTTE et al. 1996). Cystic RCCs may have large cystic components, but also have some solid protrusions and irregular shaggy margins, which allow a definitive diagnosis of malignancy, especially when there is enhancement of the protrusions after contrast medium administration (SIEGEL et al. 1997).

Minimally complicated cysts are benign lesions that give rise to some radiological findings that cause concern but can be appreciated as benign. This category includes septated (thickness ≤ 1 mm), minimally calcified, and infected cysts and some high-density cysts (Figs. 4.1, 4.2). Some of these lesions require follow-up, i.e., those that, although "most likely benign are somewhat suspicious." In these lesions, a nonoperative approach is appropri-

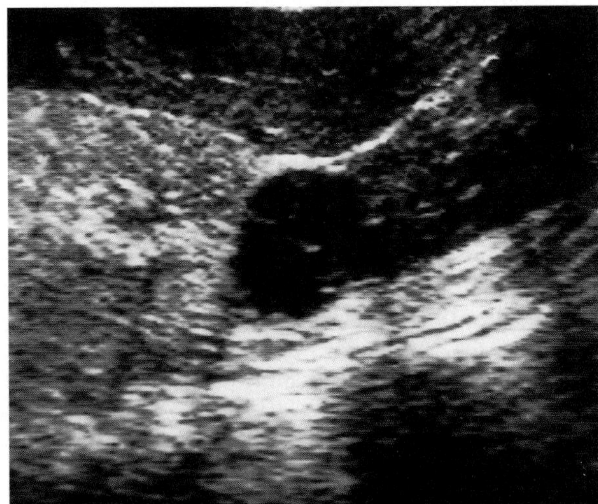

Fig. 4.1. US; benign septated cyst. Cystic lesion in the lower pole of the kidney with thin internal septations. There is no border, no internal reflections, and no internal protrusions: this lesion was considered to be a benign cyst. The septations were probably due to an old intracystic hemorrhage

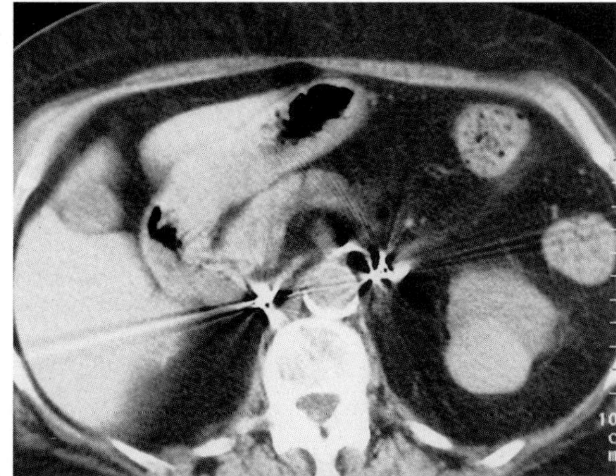

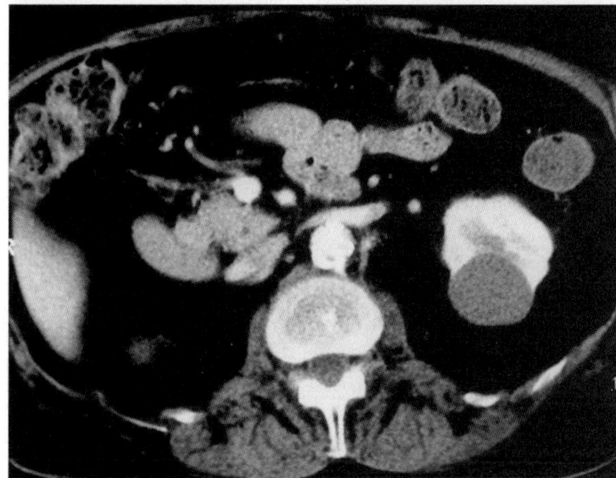

**Fig. 4.2 a,b.** CT; hyperdense cyst. Precontrast scan (**a**) showing a hyperdense lesion at the posterior aspect of the upper pole of the left kidney (52 HU), not enhancing after intravenous administration of contrast medium (**b**) (61 HU)

ate, but follow-up is needed to prove that the lesion is benign. Follow-up scans will be able to show that the lesion is not growing or changing. These studies could be performed after 3 months, then 6 months, then 1 year. Examples of such lesions are some hyperdense cysts, some lesions with more calcium in the wall, or slightly more complicated lesions. Some lesions have features seen in malignancies and cannot be clearly distinguished from malignancies by any imaging study. In most instances, these lesions must be surgically explored and are basically "indeterminate." Some of them will be found to be benign, such as hemorrhagic, complex septated, and multiloculated cysts, multiloculated cystic nephromas, and densely calcified cysts, whereas others will prove to be malignant cystic tumors (BOSNIAK 1986; DAVIDSON et al. 1997). When just one of these abnormalities is present, generally, the

lesion can be considered as a benign, nontumor cyst. The MR appearance of complicated cysts can overlap that of cystic or necrotic RCCs and documentation of contrast enhancement, as with CT, is crucial in distinguishing these two entities (ROMINGER et al. 1992). Because complicated cysts can be hyperintense on T1-weighted images, signal intensities before and after contrast material administration should be compared and fat suppression techniques should be used to exclude the possibility of fat-containing lesions.

One of the more difficult problems in the diagnosis of cystic lesions remains the evaluation of the hyperdense cyst at CT (COLEMAN et al. 1984; SUSSMAN et al. 1984; BOSNIAK 1986). These benign lesions contain old, degenerated blood, clotted blood, or coagulation of old blood, milk of calcium, a high-protein content, or rarely contrast medium, and therefore the attenuation of their contents is increased (Fig. 4.2). These high-density cysts are difficult to evaluate radiologically because the criteria that one usually applies to diagnose a cyst are not available for study. That is, the thickness of the wall and the internal structure of the lesion cannot be evaluated. US may not be helpful, as only approximately 50% of these hyperdense lesions show characteristics of a typical cyst. The principal criterion to evaluate these lesions is whether the lesion enhances with contrast. Therefore, extremely high-quality scans are required (BOSNIAK 1986, 1997). Thin sections before and after contrast are needed. Multiple measurements should be obtained in all lesions, at comparable portions (Fig. 4.3). If this type of detailed examination is available and the following criteria are fulfilled, a diagnosis of benign hyperdense cyst can be made, and surgical approach can be avoided: (1) the lesion is ≤ 3.0 cm; (2) the lesion extends outside the kidney (at least approximately one-quarter of its circumference) so that the smoothness of a portion of the wall can be evaluated; (3) the lesion is round and sharply marginated and is examined with narrow window settings to be certain it is homogeneous in attenuation; and (4) most important of all, the lesion does not enhance with contrast medium (BOSNIAK 1986). Lesions that fulfil the above criteria but are more than 3 cm in size or are totally intrarenal may be benign hyperdense cysts as well, but the diagnosis cannot be made with total confidence, and the patient will have to be managed by surgical exploration or follow-up, depending on other clinical aspects. Follow-up studies could also be performed for lesions that appear solid on US, especially if there is any question as to whether

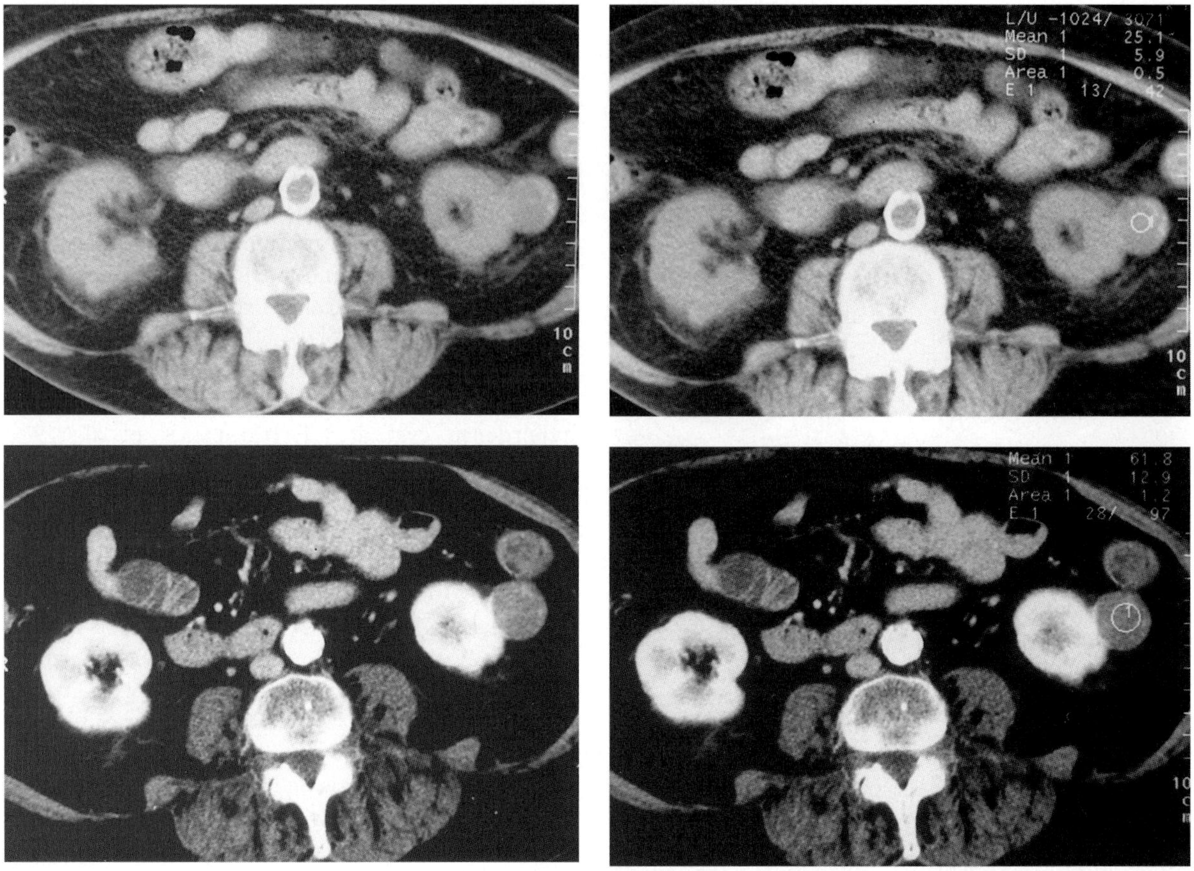

**Fig. 4.3 a–d.** CT; chromophobe carcinoma. CT before (**a,b**) and after (**c,d**) intravenous injection of contrast medium. **a,b** Peripherally calcified isodense nodule at the lateral aspect of the left lower pole (attenuation number 25.1 HU). The attenu- ation number increased to 61.8 HU (**c,d**). This indicates a solid, hypovascular mass, consistent with a carcinoma, proven at partial nephrectomy

enhancement has occurred. Lesions that enhance with contrast must be considered RCCs and should be treated generally by removal, possibly by partial nephrectomy (Figs. 4.3, 4.4). While the surgeon has the ultimate responsibility for selecting the type of operation that will be performed, the appearance of the lesion can provide a clue as to whether it is more likely to be benign or malignant. This is considered to be a major task for the radiologist. Along with other clinical aspects, the size of the lesion and its position in the kidney will help to determine the surgical approach.

### 4.3.1.3
### *Benign Cystic Nephroma*

The multilocular cystic nephroma (adult Wilms' tumor) is a benign lesion consisting of multiple

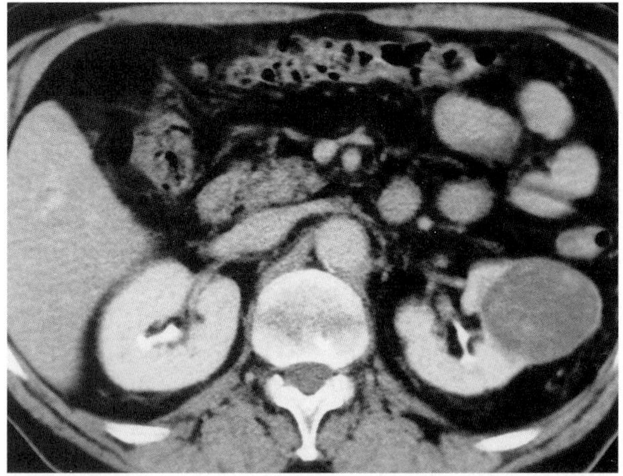

**Fig. 4.4.** CT; cystic renal cell carcinoma. Cyst-like lesion with thick wall and internal protrusions, enhancing after intrave- nous injection of contrast medium. These protrusions basi- cally exclude the diagnosis of a benign cyst. This was surgically proved cystic RCC

noncommunicating cystic anechoic areas separated by rather thick echogenic septations, sometimes with focal thickening (CASTILLO et al. 1991; YAMASHITA et al. 1994). Sometimes the cysts are very tiny and numerous in parts of the lesion, which then appear as hyperechoic, solid-like portions. Color-Doppler is helpful neither for further histological diagnosis nor for discrimination from cystic RCC.

On CT, multilocular cystic nephroma consits of multiple noncommunicating low-density cysts of varying size and contrast-enhancing septations of varying thickness. Many of these tumors typically protrude into the collecting system, which may jeopardize partial nephrectomy.

The MR features are multiple hyperintense spaces on T2-weighted images separated by thick septations.

Whatever imaging modality is used, it remains impossible to distinguish this lesion from septated ("multicystic") RCC based on imaging criteria, because RCC may have the same features.

### 4.3.2
### Angiomyolipoma/Hamartoma

#### 4.3.2.1
#### The Typical Case

The benign tumor known as angiomyolipoma (AML) or hamartoma occurs in the kidney in a number of clinical settings: (1) in association with tuberous sclerosis, in which case the lesions usually are multiple and bilateral; (2) in association with lymphangiomyomatosis; (3) not in association with other diseases, rather being discovered because of clinical symptomatology resulting from bleeding (usually a single lesion, most often in women aged 35–60 years); and (4) in asymptomatic patients, in whom the tumor is found incidentally by US or CT. The tumor might be small (less than 1 cm) or as large as 10–15 cm, but most are 3–5 cm in size. The term AML describes their tissue make-up, but they may contain only two tissue elements such as angiolipoma, angiomyoma, or myolipoma (JINZAKI et al. 1997). AMLs grow with time; multiple AMLs show more growth than solitary AMLs (LEMAITRE et al. 1995). This observation necessitates clinical and radiological follow-up in all cases of AML at regular intervals since the chance of hemorrhage increases with size.

An AML presents as a highly echogenic nodular mass at US, comparable to the echogenicity of fat

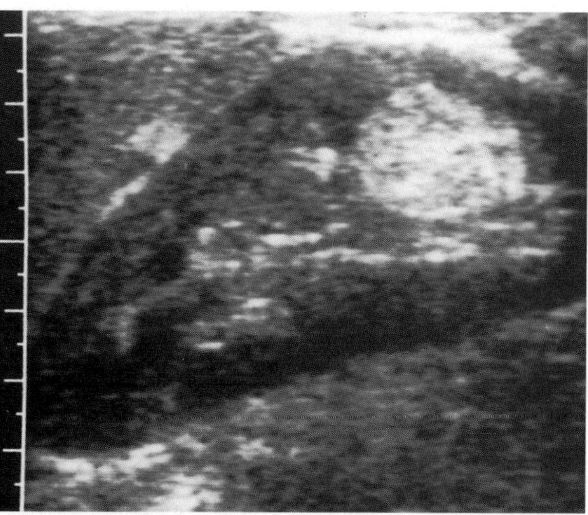

**Fig. 4.5.** US; angiomyolipoma. Hyperechoic lesion in the lower pole of the kidney. There is no halo and there are no intratumoral cystic areas. The lesion characteristics are typical for an angiomyolipoma

(Fig. 4.5). Sometimes, the mass is lobulated and smaller satellite nodules can be seen adjacent to the largest lesion. The size of the lesion may be underestimated when the AML extends into the perirenal fat or into the renal hilum. AMLs can be diagnosed at CT based on the presence of fat (DAVIDSON et al. 1997) (Fig. 4.6). Thin-section CT is required, as the detection of fat is difficult if lesions are small, or if there is only a limited amount of fat. AMLs have high signal intensities on both T1- and T2-weighted MR images (Fig. 4.7). Complicated cysts can be hyperintense on T1-weighted images. Therefore, signal intensities before and after contrast material administration should be compared and fat suppression techniques employed to exclude the possibility of fat-containing lesions. The key to diagnosis is precise demonstration that the lesion contains fat. This can be done by showing either persistence of high signal intensity on images obtained with water suppression or loss of signal intensity on images obtained with fat suppression.

#### 4.3.2.2
#### Problems in Differential Diagnosis

##### 4.3.2.2.1
HYPERECHOIC RENAL CELL CARCINOMA
The problem with a hyperechoic mass in practice is that approximately one-third of RCCs smaller than 3 cm in diameter are hyperechoic too (FORMAN et al.

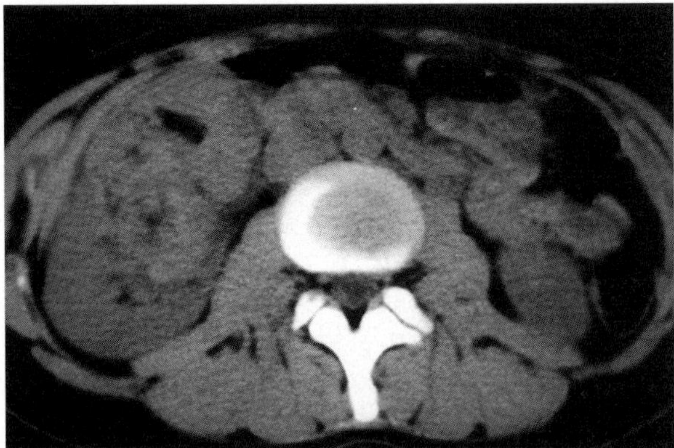

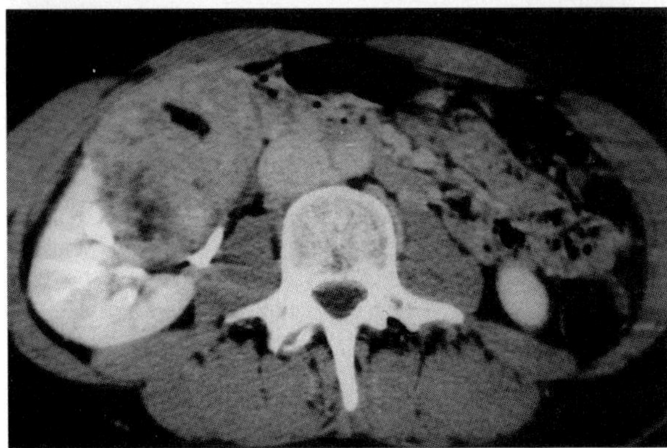

**Fig. 4.6 a,b.** CT; angiomyolipoma. Slightly hyperattenuating mass at the anterior aspect of the right kidney with low-density areas (−102 HU) consistent with fat on the precontrast scan (**a**). On the contrast-enhanced images (excretory phase, **b**) the lesion enhances heterogeneously; the fatty areas are clearly visible

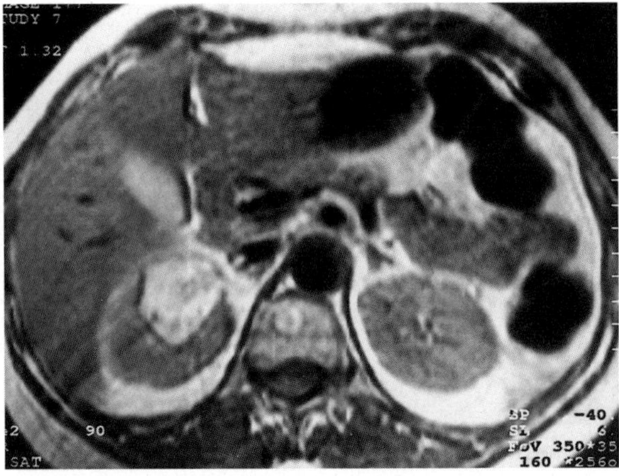

**Fig. 4.7.** MRI; angiomyolipoma. Hyperintense lesion in the upper pole of the right kidney on this T1-weighted image, consistent with an angiomyolipoma

1993). Small cystic areas inside the lesion and a hypoechoic halo surrounding the lesion are more likely to be present in (hyperechoic) RCCs (YAMASHITA et al. 1993) (Fig. 4.5). However, in the individual patient such criteria may not be useful for reliable discrimination between AML and RCC. Because CT can establish the presence of fat with great accuracy, the diagnosis of this tumor can be made in virtually every case except on the rare occasions when there is no mature fat in the tumor, such as in those hamartomas that are in fact angiomyomas (BOSNIAK et al. 1988). MRI may prove to be useful in further lesion discrimination.

### 4.3.2.2.2
#### ANGIOMYOLIPOMA "WITHOUT" FAT
MRI may be helpful in these cases: angiomyomas tend to be hypointense on both T1- and T2-weighted images (RUECKFORTH et al. 1995; JINZAKI et al. 1997).

### 4.3.2.2.3
#### RENAL CELL CARCINOMA CONTAINING FAT
Fat-containing RCC has been reported (HELENON et al. 1993a, 1997; OUTWATER et al. 1997). Malignant fat-containing RCC, however, tends to be heterogeneous with coarse calcifications that are unlikely to be present in AML.

### 4.3.2.2.4
#### ANGIOMYOLIPOMA WITH AGGRESSIVE BEHAVIOR
Sometimes AMLs has an "aggressive" appearance with thrombosis of the renal vein and/or the inferior vena cava, and extension into the perirenal space and eventually adjacent organs (BAERT et al. 1995; CITTADINI et al. 1996).

### 4.3.3
### Primary Renal Epithelial Neoplasms

The differentiation between benign and malignant lesions is a challenge for many radiologists. RCCs are the most frequent solid renal parenchymal tumor (90%). It is felt by nonradiologists and (inexperienced) radiologists that there are no useful radiological characteristics that permit a histological diagnosis. This is not entirely true: experienced uroradiologists will be able to characterize many solid renal masses on the basis of objective CT and/or MRI criteria.

Renal epithelial neoplasms include RCC (clear cell/granular cell type), oncocytoma, chromophobic carcinoma, papillary carcinoma, collecting duct carcinoma, and neuroendocrine tumors (WEISS et al. 1995; KOVACS et al. 1992).

### 4.3.3.1
### Renal Cell Carcinoma: "Classic Type"

The classic RCC (clear cell or granular cell) is the most common malignant renal epithelial tumor (80%). Well-differentiated lesions have a homogeneous echo texture and are isoechoic, slightly hypoechoic, or even hyperechoic compared with the normal renal parenchyma (FORMAN et al. 1993) (Fig. 4.8). As nuclear grade increases, RCCs are more likely to be of higher stage and greater size at presentation, and appear more heterogeneous (hemorrhage, necrosis, or fibrosis) and less marginated (BIRNBAUM et al. 1994). Necrosis or hemorrhage is usually located eccentrically (in contrast to scarring in oncocytoma, which is located near the center of the mass in the majority of cases). Necrosis and hemorrhage explain the heterogeneity on imaging studies. According to the study of YAMASHITA et al. (1992), histologically homogeneous tumors of solid architecture are hypoechoic on US and hypervascular on contrast-enhanced CT (Figs. 4.9, 4.10). Tumors of papillary, tubular, and multilocular cystic architecture are hyperechoic on US and hypovascular on contrast-enhanced CT. In selected cases color-Doppler US is helpful to differentiate

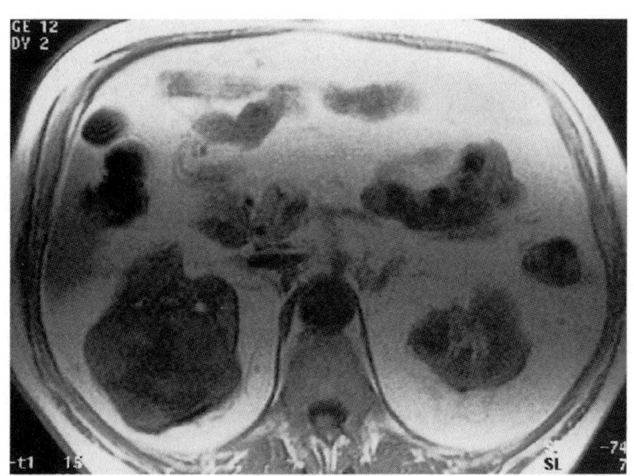
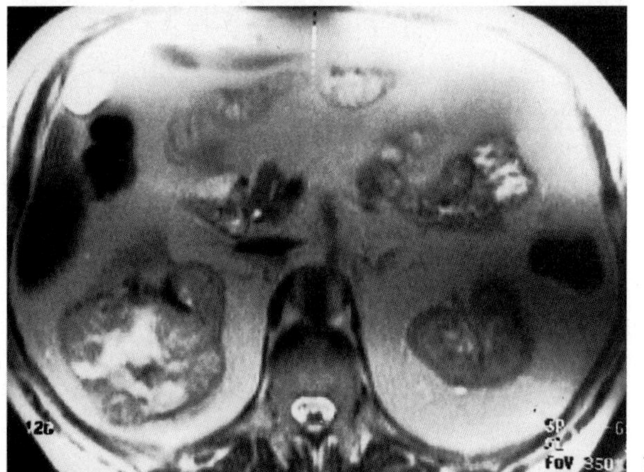
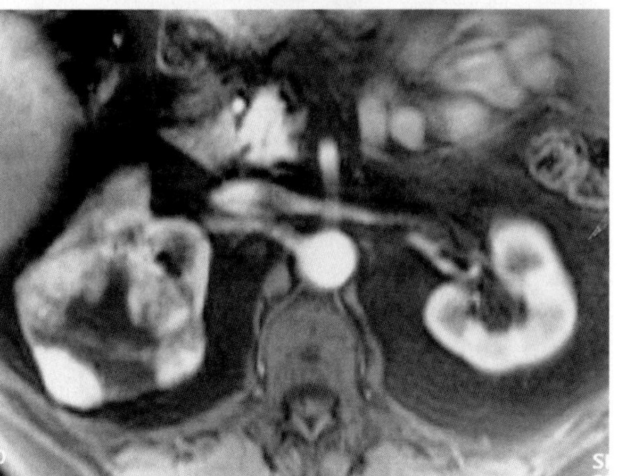

Fig. 4.9 a–c. MRI; RCC. Nearly isointense mass at the posterior aspect of the right kidney on the T1-weighted image (a). The tumor is heteregeneous on T2-weighted images, with extensive areas of necrosis exhibiting high signal intensities (b). After intravenous injection of gadolinium, the peripheral viable tissue clearly enhances; a large eccentric area of necrosis is present (c)

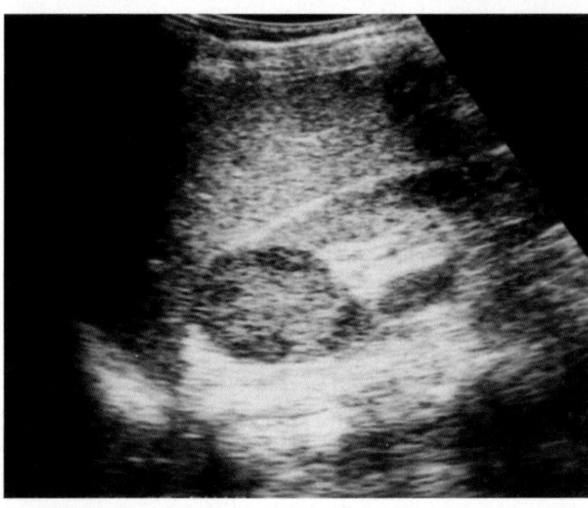

Fig. 4.8. US; RCC. Heterogeneous rounded soft tissue mass at the upper pole of the right kidney in a 22-year-old male who was referred to the hospital with flank pain and fever. Histologically proved RCC

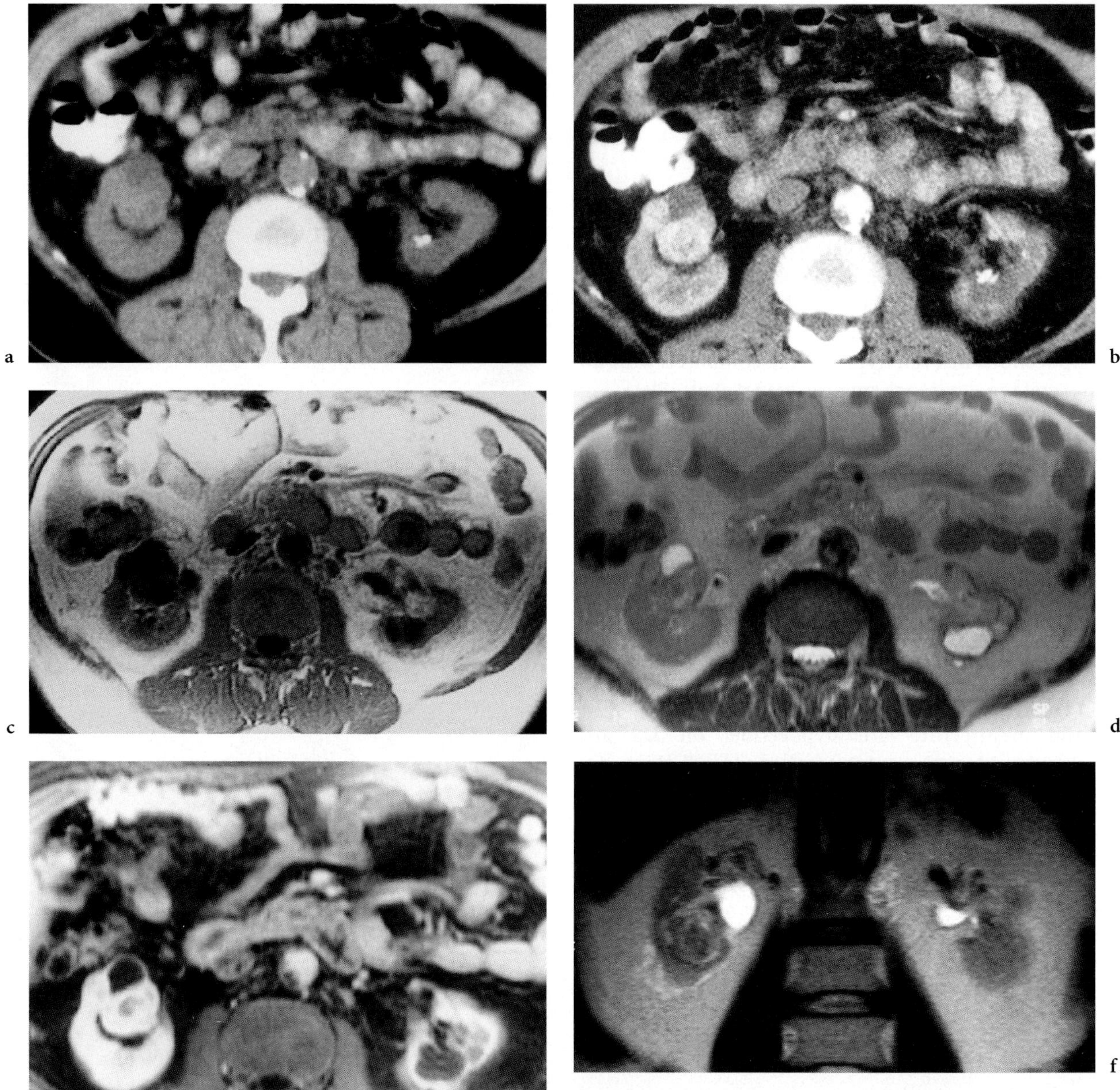

**Fig. 4.10 a–f.** CT and MRI; RCC. Heterogeneous nodular lesion at the anterior aspect of the right kidney on precontrast CT scan (**a**). After contrast administration, two nodular well-vascularized lesions are in fact recognizable, anteriorly separated by a fluid-filled lesion (**b**). The masses are isointense on T1-weighted MR images (**c**). On the HASTE sequence the larg- est lesion exhibits heterogeneous signal intensities with hyperintense areas due to necrosis (**d**). After intravenous administration of gadolinium, the heterogeneous lesions again are easily seen (**e**). On the coronal images (**f**), the position of the lesions relative to the renal hilum and to the collecting system is more easily assessed

solid lesions from cysts (DENYS et al. 1991). The MR appearance of RCC is variable, depending on the histological differentiation of the tumor and the presence of necrosis and cystic change (Fig. 4.9).

Most RCCs show eccentric areas of necrosis or hemorrhage, appearing as hypodense areas within a hyperattenuating mass after intravenous injection of contrast medium (Figs. 4.9, 4.10). Some RCCs are hypovascular. In such cases, differential diagnosis with other lesions is needed, such as chromophobic carcinoma, papillary carcinoma, lymphoma, and metastasis. As already mentioned above, RCCs rarely contain areas of fat (HELENON et al. 1993a, 1997; STROTZER et al. 1993). The presence of fat is considered characteristic for angiomyolipoma. Malignancy should be suspected based on the following criteria: (1) presence of intratumoral calcifications; (2) large, irregular tumor invading the perirenal or sinus fat; (3) large necrotic tumor with small foci of fat; and (4) association with nonfatty lymph nodes or venous invasion (HELENON et al. 1997). On opposed-phase images, some clear cell carcinomas show relative focal or diffuse of signal intensity. In renal masses, this signal intensity loss, which is consistent with lipid, does not necessarily indicate AML (OUTWATER et al. 1997).

Cystic RCCs can be classified into four distinct histopathological growth patterns: (1) multilocular, (2) unilocular, (3) cystic necrosis, and (4) tumors originating in the wall of a simple cyst (YAMASHITA et al. 1994). The appearance on CT varies from cystic with mural nodules to a multiloculated mass with irregular architecture. Neovascularity is expected in the periphery of the lesion (YAMASHITA et al. 1994) (Fig. 4.4). Rarely cystic RCC has CT findings simulating a benign hyperdense cyst (HARTMAN et al. 1992).

According to JAMIS-DOW et al. (1996), a substantial proportion of lesions under 1 cm are not detected with US or CT in patients with von Hippel-Lindau disease. Neither CT nor US proved to be superior in the characterization of lesions of 3 cm or less. Therefore, CT and particularly US screening studies in patients with von Hippel-Lindau disease should be interpreted cautiously because missed or mischaracterized small renal lesions are a frequent problem in these patients. There is nothing specific about the US features. The tumors can be small (<3 cm diameter) and are either completely isoechoic, slightly hypoechoic, or hyperechoic (PRESS et al. 1984).

Occasionally anatomical variants (junctional parenchyma, postoperative), inflammatory masses, or unexpected masses have a pseudotumoral appearance (GRIETEN et al. 1992) (Fig. 4.11).

#### 4.3.3.2
#### Renal Oncocytoma

Renal oncocytoma is a benign renal parenchymal neoplasm which in fact is indistinguishable from RCC. Oncocytoma may be bilateral (SANCHEZ-CHAPADO et al. 1995). Only 10%–20% of oncocytomas are correctly diagnosed before surgery

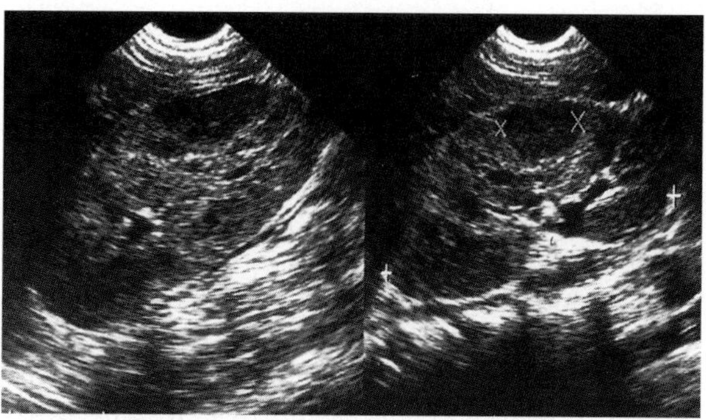

**Fig. 4.11.** US; acute pyelonephritis. Wig-shaped to rounded hypoechoic lesion in the right kidney in a patient with acute pyelonephritis. At times it can be difficult to distinguish the lesion from lymphoma or RCC

(TIKKAKOSKI et al. 1991). Most reported oncocytomas have behaved in a benign manner, but local or distant metastases may occur (LIEBER et al. 1987; AMIN et al. 1997). However, it is now felt that most, if not all, malignant oncocytomas described in the literature are in fact nonpapillary, papillary, or chromophobe RCCs with eosinophilic granular cytoplasm which would have been expected to have displayed a deletion of 3p or trisomy 17 or mitochondrial alterations had genetic analysis been undertaken (KOVACS et al. 1992).

Renal oncocytoma may appear isoechoic, hyperechoic, or hypoechoic on US (TIKKAKOSKI et al. 1991). Some oncocytomas have a "characteristic" appearance with sharp margination and homogeneity on CT, often with a central scar, but this appearance can be mimicked by some cases of RCC, so that imaging diagnosis is not sufficiently specific for treatment to be based on these findings. It is not fully clear why this central scar occurs so frequently in oncocytoma. One manifestation of ischemia is the pattern of growth of oncocytomas in which cells accumulate in more or less rounded, solid cell nests that become smaller, fewer, and farther apart toward the center of the tumor. Eventually these ischemic tumor cells are replaced by fibroblasts that give rise to the classic gross pathological and radiological finding of a central scar (DAVIS et al. 1992). The same evolutionary changes of ischemia and fibrosis also occur in regions other than the center of an oncocytoma. This is the most likely explanation for the observations of heterogeneity in the enhancement pattern of oncocytomas.

DAVIDSON et al. (1993) studied the hypothesis that oncocytoma and RCC of the kidney can be differentiated with CT criteria and that differences will become more apparent as tumors enlarge. On contrast-enhanced scans, homogeneous attenuation throughout the tumor and a central, sharply marginated stellate area of low attenuation were considered predictors of oncocytoma. Any area of decreased attenuation in the tumor except for a stellate, central area was used as a predictor of RCC. Among oncocytomas larger than 3 cm in diameter, 67% exhibited criteria for oncocytoma and 33% met the criterion for RCC; among smaller oncocytomas, the respective results were 82% and 18%. Among RCCs larger than 3 cm in diameter, 84% fulfilled the criterion for malignancy and 16% were incorrectly predicted to be oncocytomas; among smaller RCCs, the respective results were 58% and 42%. The authors conclude that the CT criteria used are poor predictors of the diagnosis of oncocytoma or RCC regardless of tumor size. A low-intensity homogeneous mass on T1-weighted images which appears with increased intensity on T2-weighted images, the presence of a capsule, a central scar or stellate pattern, and the absence or either hemorrhage or necrosis suggest oncocytoma (SASAKI et al. 1995; HARMON et al. 1996).

A pseudocapsule seems to be present in RCC and oncocytoma only; in the study of YAMASHITA et al. (1992, 1996), in 66%–69% of RCCs of 4 cm in diameter or smaller a pseudocapsule was seen. T2-weighted MRI was the most sensitive technique for exhibiting this feature. In general, encapsulated RCCs are likely to have a more favorable pathological stage (SOYER et al. 1997).

Only very rarely may calcifications be seen in an oncocytoma (HADDAD and MUFARRIJ 1992). Very rarely, oncocytomas contain fat, thus mimicking AML (CURRY et al. 1990).

### 4.3.3.3
### Renal Chromophobe Cell Carcinoma

Chromophobe carcinomas have only been described since 1985 and are usually detected at lower stages. Their prognosis seems to be more favorable than that of the classic RCC (AKHTAR et al. 1995; CROTTY et al. 1995).

There is nothing specific about the US appearance of this histological subtype. They tend to be at low stages at the time of detection and are either nearly isoechoic or slightly hyperechoic compared with the renal parenchyma. They are hypovascular on color-Doppler US. Chromophobe carcinomas tend to be homogeneously hypovascular on contrast-enhanced

CT/MRI. They are predominately hypointense on T2-weighted MR images (Fig. 4.3).

### 4.3.3.4
### Renal Papillary Carcinoma

There are two variants of papillary carcinomas: one where a single bulky tumor develops, sometimes largely cystic, and with distant metastases; the other where multifocal tumors occur (often <3 cm in diameter) in one kidney or in both; many of them are of microscopic size only and therefore not detectable by any radiological method (DELAHUNT and EBLE 1997; ROBERTS et al. 1997). Papillary tumors with high nuclear grade are more likely to behave in an aggressive fashion (LAGER et al. 1995).

There is nothing specific about the US features. The tumors can be small (<3 cm diameter) and are either completely isoechoic, slightly hypoechoic, or hyperechoic (PRESS et al. 1984). Therefore, and since papillary carcinomas tend to be multiple, many lesions are missed at US. When papillary carcinoma is suspected, careful examination of the entire kidney, preferably by contrast-enhanced spiral CT, is necessary (PRESS et al. 1984). These tumors are hypovascular and differential diagnosis from renal lymphoma or renal metastases can only be achieved with needle biopsy. Similar results can be expected from MRI examinations. Rarely, papillary carcinomas are large, partially or almost completely cystic tumors, with a solid appearance on US, or with internal wall proliferations and heterogeneous on CT and MRI (ROBERTS et al. 1997) (Fig. 4.12).

### 4.3.3.5
### Collecting Duct (Bellini Duct) Carcinoma

Renal collecting duct carcinoma (Bellini duct carcinoma) arises from collecting duct epithelium. These tumors contain the higher molecular weight keratin characteristic of the collecting ducts rather than the low molecular weight keratins of renal tubular epithelium (FLEMING and LEWI 1986; FLEMING 1993; FÜZESI et al. 1992). They represent approximately 1% of renal neoplasms. Hematuria is the most common symptom. The mean age of patients at presentation has been about 55 years, although several cases have occurred in the 2nd and 3rd decades of life. Their clinical behavior is not well defined, but they appear to be aggressive, often with metastatic disease

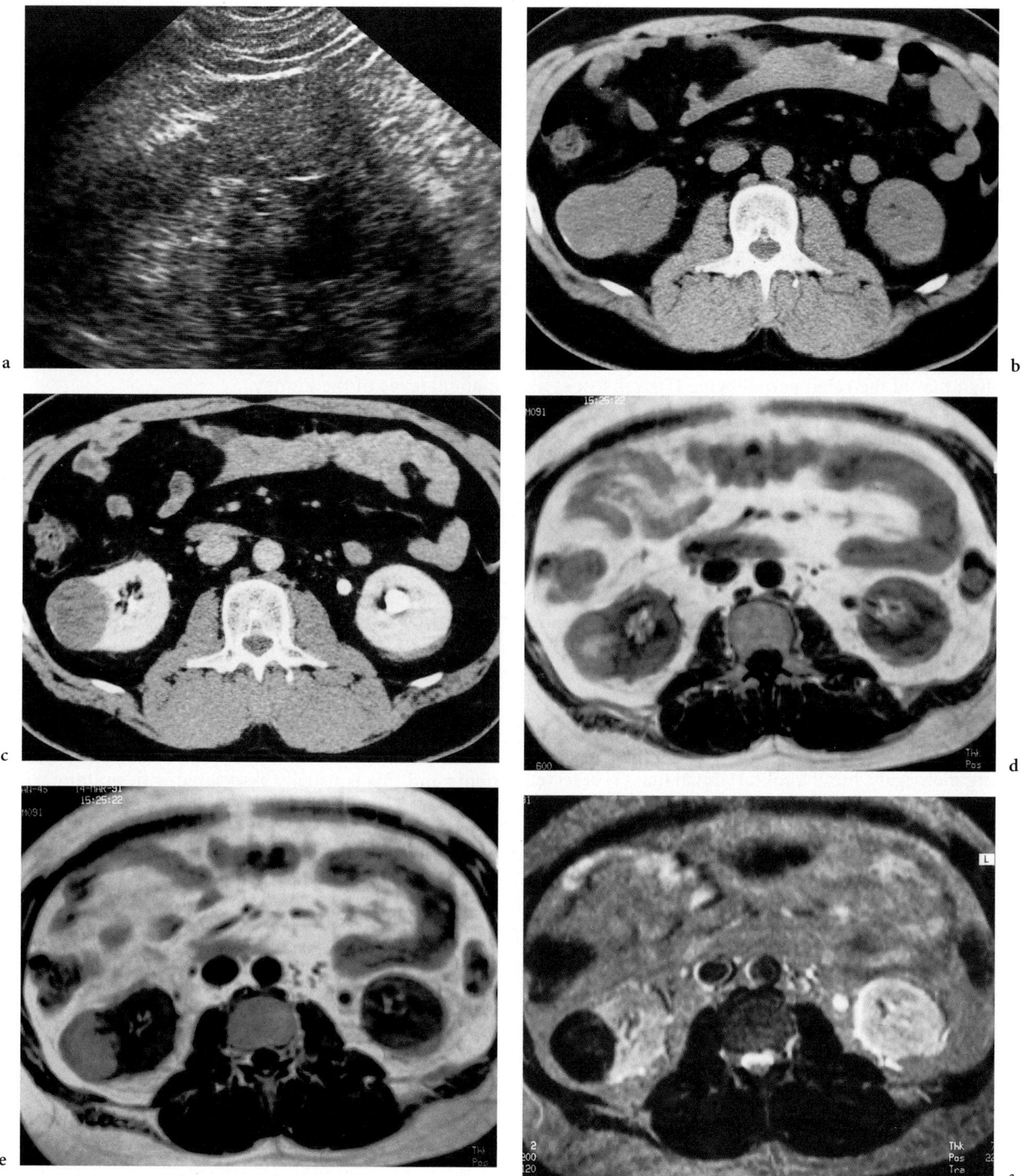

**Fig. 4.12 a–f.** US, CT, and MRI; papillary carcinoma. Slightly hyperechoic rounded mass lesion at the lower pole of the right kidney with egg-shell peripheral calcifications (**a**). On CT, the mass was isodense to the renal parenchyma (42 HU, **b**) and there was no enhancement after intravenous contrast administration (52 HU, **c**). On T1-weighted MR images (**d,e**), the lesions exhibited heterogeneous signal characteristics, with nodular irregularities at the inplantation border. On T2-weighted images, the lesion was heterogeneously hypointense (**f**); there was no enhancement after gadolinium. This was proven to be an RCC at surgery. Note: slight dilation of the left ureter due to a stone. The tumor in the right kidney was an incidental finding at the time of the diagnosis of the ureteral calculus

at manifestation and rapid progression despite surgery (MacLennan et al. 1997).

The tumor is usually localized to the renal medulla, with distortion of the pelvicaliceal system and often with irregular extensions into the adjacent renal cortex. The tumors are generally firm and white or gray, which is probably due to an accompanying desmoplasmatic reaction. Some are cystic with endophytic papillary projections. Unlike RCCs, they are not yellow and do not usually show necrosis or hemorrhage (Gohji et al. 1994).

In many cases, the affected kidney preserves its normal outer margins and the mass protrudes into the sinus. The contrast enhancement at CT is less than that of the renal parenchyma (Davidson et al. 1995; Fukuya et al. 1996). Collecting duct carcinoma may be multifocal (Kutta et al. 1993).

### 4.3.4
### Renal Lymphoma

Rarely a lymphomatous mass can cause a problem in differentiation from primary parenchymal tumor, because almost all cases of renal lymphoma occur in patients with systemic lymphoma and because renal lymphoma has a CT pattern of involvement quite different from RCC. Most often, renal lymphoma presents with multiple lymph nodes and organomegaly, but if a solitary renal mass is detected in a patient with lymphoma, in the overwhelming majority of cases it will represent renal lymphoma. Lymphomatous tissue is usually homogeneous and often shows an invasive character. The tissue enhances 10–25 HU after contrast administration, and usually is isoechoic to hypoechoic on US. Analysis of the margins, architecture, and effects of the collecting system and renal sinus by the mass are helpful in the diagnosis of lymphoma and other diseases that characteristically infiltrate the kidney (Hartman et al. 1988). If the lesion responds to therapy as the rest of the patient's lymphomatous disease does, no further evaluation is necessary. If the renal lesion persists or grows, then needle biopsy is indicated.

### 4.3.5
### Renal Metastases

Metastases to the kidneys from primaries in other sites are not uncommon; although not often symptomatic, they have been seen with greater frequency because of the widespread use of CT for tumor staging. By far the most common tumor that metastasises to the kidney is carcinoma of the lung. Most metastases to the kidneys are multiple and bilateral and are associated with metastases to other organs. Therefore, in the proper clinical setting, the diagnosis is obvious. Occasionally, a single large metastatic focus occurs, and differentiation from a primary renal neoplasm is not clear. In such cases, if there is a history of a primary neoplasm, renal biopsy should be performed to determine the histologic nature and etiology of the tumor so that correct therapy can be instituted. More than 50% of solitary renal masses detected in patients with a history of malignancy and with no other metastases will turn out to be primary malignancies of the kidney.

## 4.4
## Staging

Renal cell carcinoma spreads by direct growth with eventual breaching of the renal capsule and spread into the perirenal area. Later, adjacent organs and the abdominal wall may be invaded. Involvement of the renal vein may be expected in approximately one-quarter of patients with RCC (Parks and Kellett 1994). Metastases may occur in the lymph node around the renal vessels and the aorta. Spread to the mediastinal nodes is seen in 8%–10% of patients and this is usually associated with pulmonary metastases.

Tumor stage at diagnosis has an important bearing on the ultimate prognosis. While incidental detection of RCC has become more frequent in recent years, it appears to have impacted minimally on the discovery of earlier stage tumors than those with presenting clinical symptoms (Smith et al. 1989). In contrast to prior reports, Mevorach et al. (1992) showed that the natural history of RCC is not significantly altered by the incidental detection of tumor.

It must be emphasized that pathological stage remains the most important prognostic factor. Therefore, imaging essentially provides information regarding the operability of renal masses.

Renal cell carcinomas customarily have been removed with radical nephrectomy regardless of size to establish a conclusive pathological diagnosis. Management strategies for solid renal masses other than traditional radical nephrectomy are often required in patients with compromised renal function, in those with multiple and/or bilateral tumors or a solitary kidney, and in patients with adverse surgical risk factors. In addition, the application of kidney-sparing surgery by means of segmental resection of a tumor would be enhanced if a confident preoperative prediction of a benign tumor could be made, an approach made more urgent by the increasing number of renal tumors now being discovered in asymptomatic patients (ZINCKE et al. 1985; SMITH et al. 1989).

## 4.4.1
## T-Staging

Computed tomography is an important tool for staging. Most experienced radiologists are convinced that similar or even better results can be expected from MRI.

### 4.4.1.1
### Single or Multifocal Neoplasms

In view of the above evolution towards nephron-sparing surgery, detection or exclusion of multi-focality is very important. Indeed, it is becoming clear that complete local excision of a small serendipitously discovered renal tumor is feasible and reasonable in the patient with an otherwise normal opposite kidney (VAN POPPEL and BAERT 1992; HERR 1994). Involvement of the contralateral kidney is seen in 11% of patients at autopsy. Multifocality is more likely in papillary carcinoma. Whenever a small (≤3 cm diameter) hypovascular neoplasm is detected, the possibility of a multifocal papillary carcinoma, and thus multifocality, should be taken into account. Other histological subtypes (clear cell carcinoma, oncocytoma, Bellini duct carcinoma) may be multifocal as well (Figs. 4.13, 4.14).

The great advantage of spiral CT is that the entire renal parenchyma can be examined in the same corticomedullary and/or nephrographic phase (Fig. 4.13). This enables the detection of multifocal neoplams in virtually all cases, at least if the lesions are larger than 1 cm in diameter. Contrast-enhanced MRI provides similar accuracy for tumor detection.

### 4.4.1.2
### Tumor Delineation

Tumor extension beyond the capsule causes blurring of the tumor margins, thickening of the renal capsule, or obliteration of the perirenal fat. Perinephric soft tissue stranding, however, is an unreliable indi-cator of tumor extension because it may also result from a resolving perinephric hematoma, fat necrosis, dilated collateral blood vessels, or edema of connective tissue septa (Fig. 4.15). The inability to determine accurately the presence or absence of small amounts of extracapsular, perinephric tumor extension accounts for over half of CT staging errors (JOHNSON et al. 1987). At times, invasion of adjacent organs (e.g., liver, spleen, pancreas, colon) is difficult to assess on axial images. Loss of fat planes between the tumor and adjacent structures such as the liver or psoas muscle is not necessarily a sign of tumor invasion (JOHNSON et al. 1987). Multiplanar reformatted CT images (coronal, sagittal, parasagittal) can be helpful to define tumor margins more accurately (Figs. 4.16, 4.17). US is often helpful in determining whether the tumor is merely adjacent to or has invaded a structure such as the liver or psoas muscle (LEVINE 1995). Perhaps MRI has some advantages over CT concerning the evaluation of involvement of neighboring organs because of direct multiplanar imaging and good tissue differentiation.

Intraoperative US is a useful adjunct for the dynamic evaluation of renal tumors in the surrounding environment of cysts, the collecting system, and the renal vasculature (POLASCIK et al. 1995). It is particularly beneficial in defining preoperative indeterminate lesions and in evaluating extrarenal structures for tumor involvement, such as the renal vein, inferior vena cava, adrenal gland, and liver. At some centers, intraoperative US turns out to be most useful during partial nephrectomy because it may improve tumor-free surgical margins.

### 4.4.1.3
### Venous Involvement

There is probably no preoperative staging decision more important than that concerning venous propagation and its cephalad extension, followed by regional lymph node metastases (BARBARIC 1996).

Involvement of the renal vein with tumor thrombus occurs in 21%–35% of patients, while vena caval involvement is seen in 5%–10% of patients, and is more common in patients with a right-sided tumor (GONCHARENKO et al. 1979). In 20% of patients with caval involvement extension of the thrombus is seen into the right side of the heart and the pulmonary artery (MADAYAG et al. 1979; PARKS and KELLETT 1994).

Since the introduction of spiral CT, image acquisition can be obtained within one breath hold. This

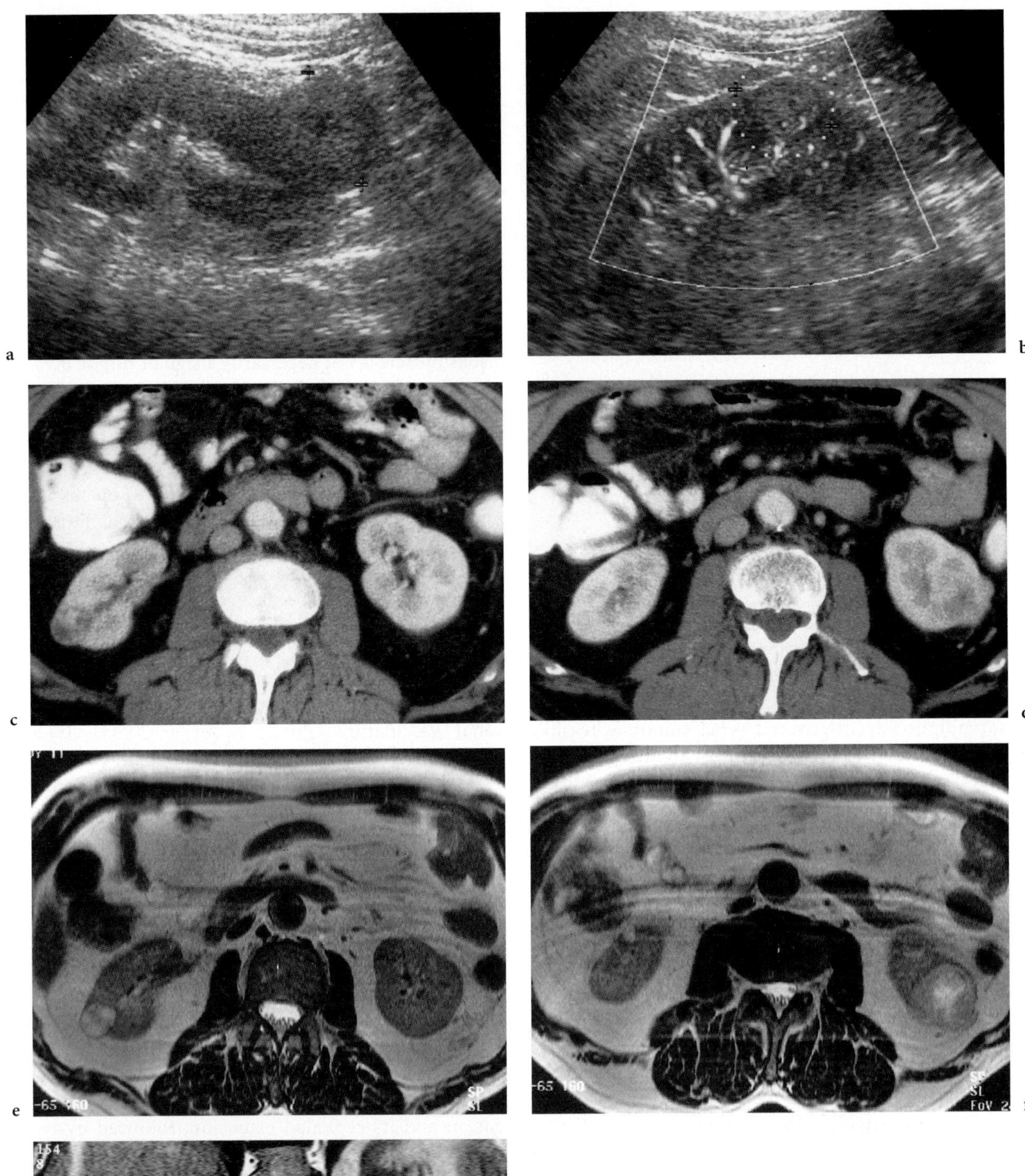

**Fig. 4.13 a–g.** US, CT, and MRI; bilateral RCC. On US, both lesions are slightly hyperechoic compared with the renal parenchyma (right kidney, **a**; left kidney, **b**). The central hypoechoic area in the left lesion is due to necrosis. Note that vascularity is only exhibited at the implantatoin base of the small lesion in **a**. Based on color-Doppler such a lesion could be erroneously misinterpreted as a complicated cyst. The contrast-enhanced CT scan shows both lesions, heterogeneously enhancing at the periphery and with areas of necrosis or hemorrhage (**c,d**). T2-weighted MR images (axial, **e,f**; coronal, **g**) likewise show the necrotic carcinomas in both kidneys. The lesion in the right kidney is predominately hyperintense with subtle low-intensity areas representing viable tumor tissue

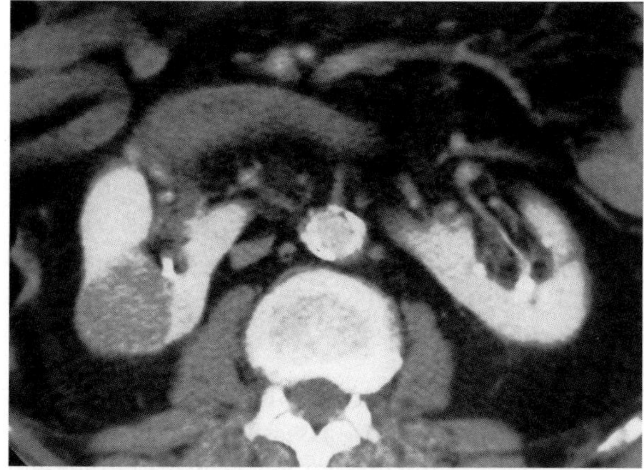

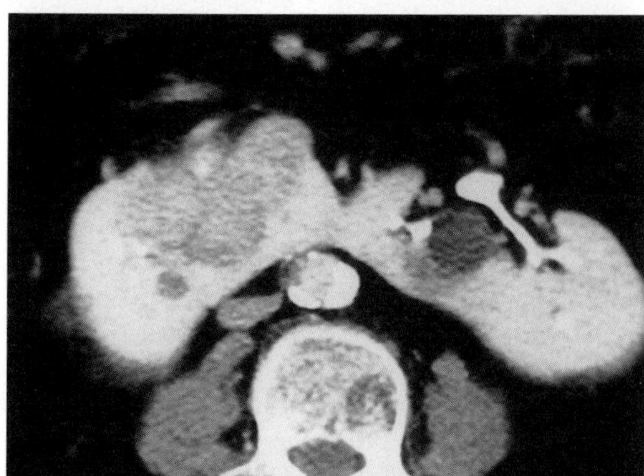

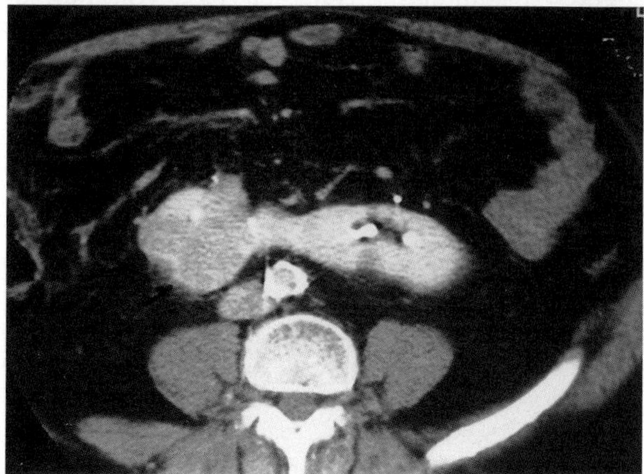

Fig. 4.14 a–c. CT; RCC. Horse-shoe kidney with multifocal RCCs, clear cell type. There are multiple hypovascular tumors in the right kidney and a cluster of tumors is present in the isthmus. Heminephrectomy was performed

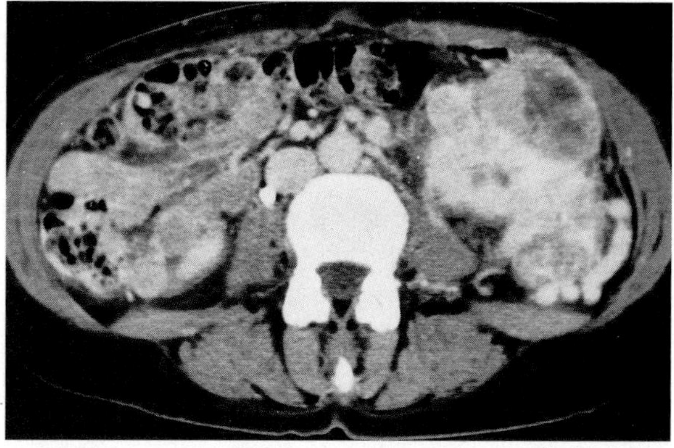

Fig. 4.15. CT; RCC. Malignant tumor extending from the lower pole of the left kidney indiscernible from the anterior abdominal wall, from the intestines, and from the psoas muscle. However, it is difficult to discriminate between invasion of these structures and compression

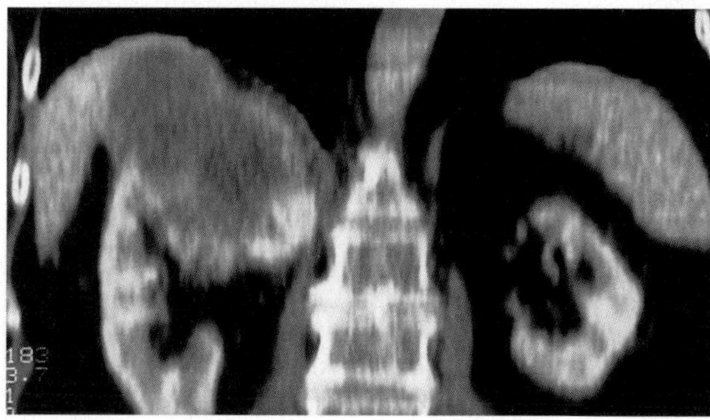

Fig. 4.16. CT; RCC. Malignant tumor at the upper pole of the right kidney, indiscernible from the liver and the diaphragm. At surgery, there was invasion of the liver, but not of the diaphragm. Partial hepatectomy had to be performed

increases the ability to identify a venous tumor thrombus and also allows computer-generated reconstruction in a different plane or use of a three-dimensional reconstruction technique, such as maximum intensity projection (MIP). The accuracy of the CT diagnosis of tumoral involvement of the main renal vein and the inferior vena cava reaches 78%–93%. Axial imaging is usually sufficient for the diagnosis and evaluation of the extension of venous involvement. Reformatted imaging to visualize the course of the veins in the coronal or sagittal spatial plane can be attractive for surgeons who are used to angiograms (Fig. 4.18).

The study of SEMELKA et al. (1993) suggested that MRI is moderately better than CT for the detection and staging of renal cancer, especially for detecton of tumor thrombi. This was confirmed by other studies (HELENON et al. 1993b; ROUBIDOUX et al. 1992; KALLMAN et al. 1992). MRI allows for differentiation between a native thrombus and a tumor thrombus based on signal characteristics and demonstration of patchy flow within the thrombus (NGUYEN et al. 1996). Tumor thrombus in the renal vein and infe-

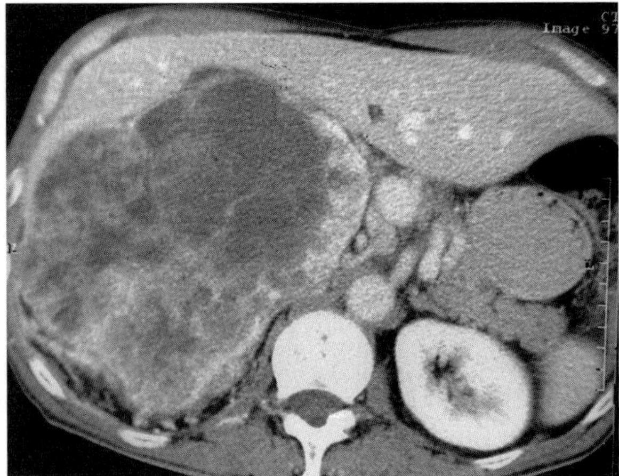

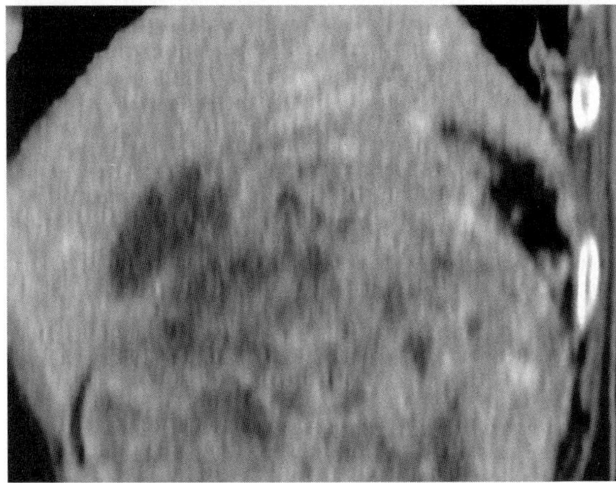

**Fig. 4.17 a,b.** CT; RCC. Bulky mass originating in the right kidney and displacing the liver. It is not clear whether there is invasion of the liver on axial images (**a**). Reformatted imaging (sagittal plane, **b**) is not always helpful in further discrimination between compression and invasion. At surgery, the tumor could be easily dissected from the liver capsule

rior vena cava may be suspected on T1-weighted SE pulse sequences if the signal void of flowing blood is replaced by relatively high signal because of tumor thrombus. Tumor thrombi emit signal with an intensity similar to that of the primary neoplasm on different pulse sequences. MRI using sagittal and coronal planes is particularly helpful in evaluating the superior extent of caval tumor thrombus relative to the diaphragm, hepatic veins, and right atrium. Furthermore, MRI has the potential to detect venal wall invasion.

In patients with RCC, color-Doppler US appears to be fairly accurate in assessing tumor extension into renal veins, the inferior vena cava, and the right side of the heart (Kallman et al. 1992) (Fig. 4.19). Although CT and MRI are the imaging techniques of choice for staging RCC, color-Doppler US may be used as a complementary technique for assessing venous extension in patients with equivocal results (Habboub et al. 1997).

Occasionally, the results of preoperative staging will be called into question intraoperatively. Then, intraoperative US can be used to clarify the presence or extent of thrombus (Long et al. 1993; Harris et al. 1994).

The ability of CT and MRI to detect microscopic tumor extension into the renal capsule or perinephric fat is limited, but standard radical therapy techniques include en bloc resection of Gerota's fascia. Although this is an important prognosticator (Van Poppel et al. 1997), this cannot be considered a serious limitation of either imaging technique in terms of impact on standard surgical

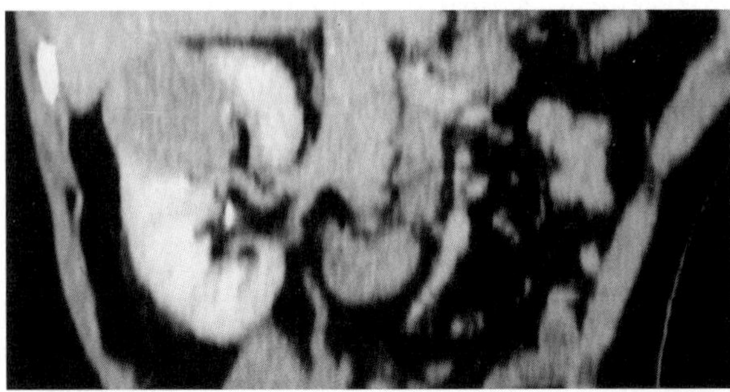

**Fig. 4.18.** CT; chromophobe carcinoma. Parasagittal reformatted image showing the hypovascular tumor in the upper pole of the right kidney in relation to the renal veins and inferior vena cava

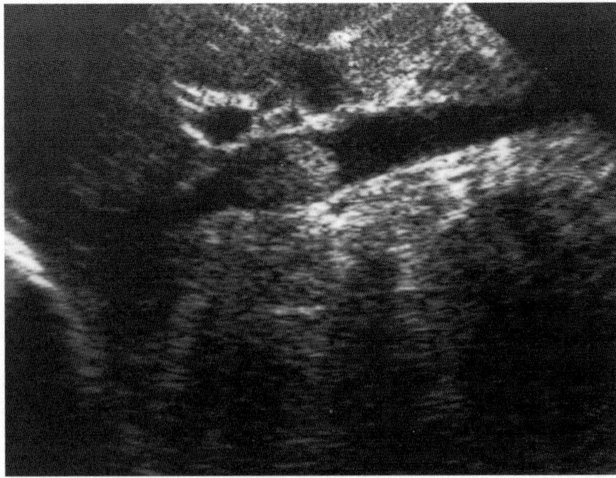

**Fig. 4.19.** US; thrombus in the inferior vena cava. Sagittal scan of the inferior vena cava showing an intraluminal thrombus from an RCC of the right kidney

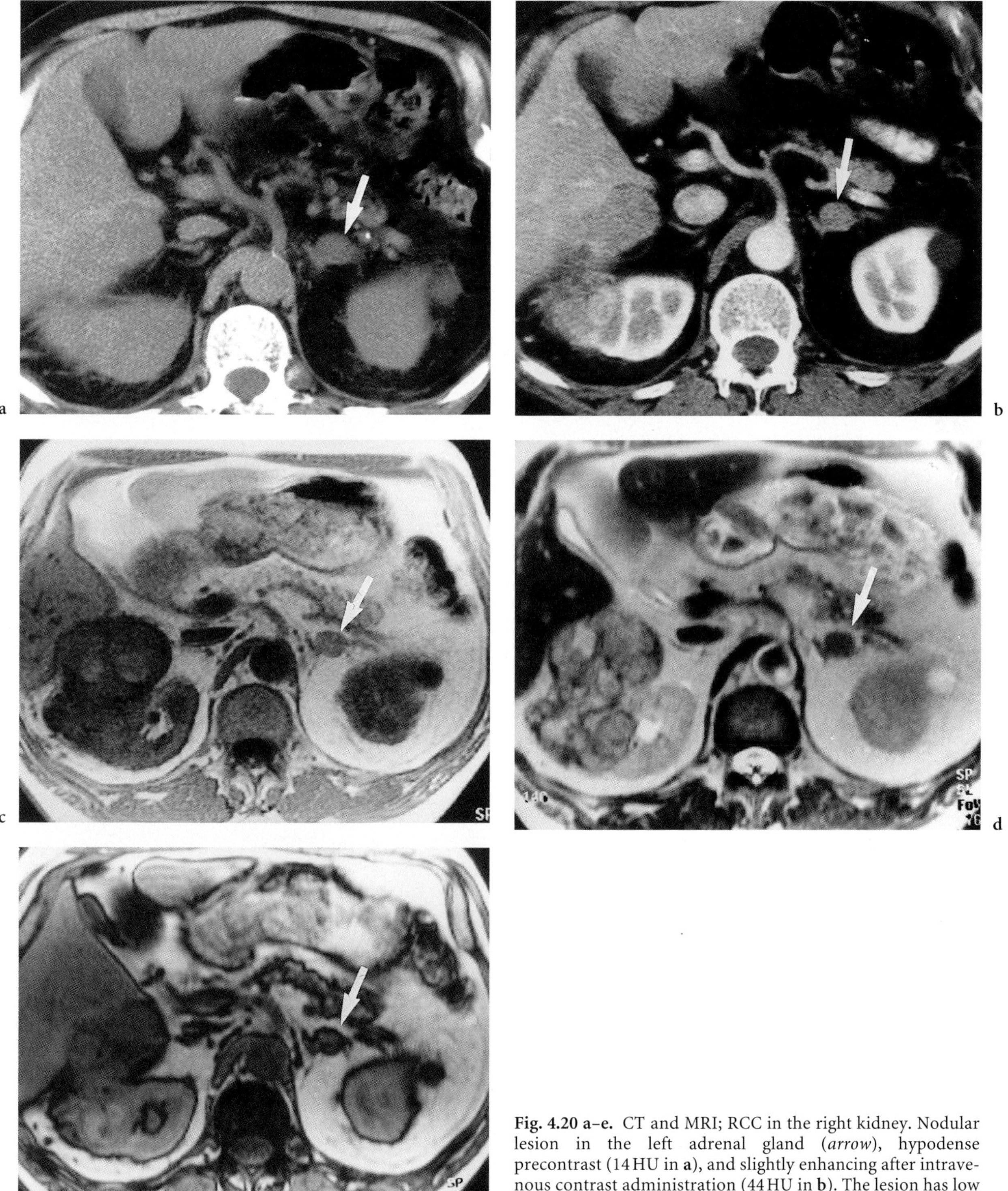

**Fig. 4.20 a–e.** CT and MRI; RCC in the right kidney. Nodular lesion in the left adrenal gland (*arrow*), hypodense precontrast (14 HU in **a**), and slightly enhancing after intravenous contrast administration (44 HU in **b**). The lesion has low signal characteristics on both T1- and T2-weighted images (**c,d**), and is isointense to the liver on the out-phase images (**e**)

technique (Fig. 4.15). The accuracy rate for the detection of visceral invasion has been reported to be 97%–100%.

Reports in the literature have recorded an 80%–96% accuracy for staging renal tumors, and it seems that MRI is at least as accurate as CT for staging purposes (FEIN et al. 1987; HRICAK et al. 1988; KABALA et al. 1990). MRI appears to be the best technique for detecting venous tumor involvement (HRICAK et al. 1985; ROUBIDOUX et al. 1992). One hundred percent accuracy has been reported for inferior vena cava thrombus diangosis and 80% accuracy for right atrial thrombus (PARKS and KELLETT 1994).

### 4.4.2
### N-Staging

Lymph nodes can be detected with a reasonably high degree of accuracy. Size, however, is not a reliable criterion to differentiate benign (reactive) from malignant lymph nodes. Significant lymph node enlargement frequently may be caused by inflammatory changes, especially in the presence of tumor necrosis (STUDER et al. 1990). Enlarged hyperplastic or reactive lymph nodes may be present in more than 50% of patients with renal carcinoma (STUDER et al. 1990). Furthermore, micrometastases may be present in lymph nodes of normal size.

The sensitivity of CT lymph node staging is reported to be 83%–89% (JOHNSON et al. 1987; LONDON et al. 1989). MRI appears to be as accurate as CT for the detection of lymph node involvement (PARKS and KELLETT 1994). US is less accurate than CT or MRI in tumor staging. Failure to visualize adequately the central retroperitoneal region, renal vessels, and infrahepatic vena cava may occur in more than 50% of patients, usually because of overlying intestinal gas (WEBB et al. 1987).

The reported sensitivity and specificity for stages T1, T3, and T4 range from 90% to 100% (JOHNSON et al. 1987; ZEMAN et al. 1988). The sensitivity and specificity for stage T2 disease are 44% and 91% respectively. Understaging is more frequent than overstaging (DINNEY et al. 1992).

### 4.4.3
### M-Staging

Bone, liver, and adrenal glands are also common sites for secondary deposits. Involvement of the

adrenals can be easily assessed by MRI, and differentiation between adenoma and metastasis is feasible with great accuracy (PEPPERCORN and REZNEK 1997) (Fig. 4.20). Normal size and normal attenuation numbers of the adrenals virtually exclude the presence of metastases from a primary tumor in the kidneys.

The lung is the most common site for secondary deposits, and these are seen in 55% of patients at autopsy (PARKS and KELLETT 1994). Accurate staging of lung disease is of great importance as complete surgical resection of a solitary metastasis has been shown to increase the 5-year survival rate from 32% to 58.3% (PARKS and KELLETT 1994). For the most

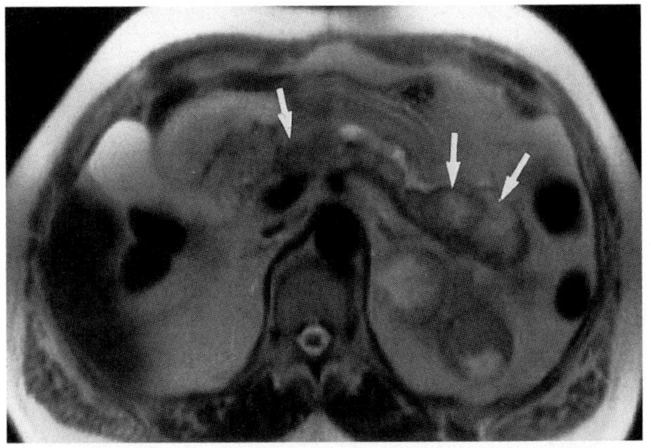

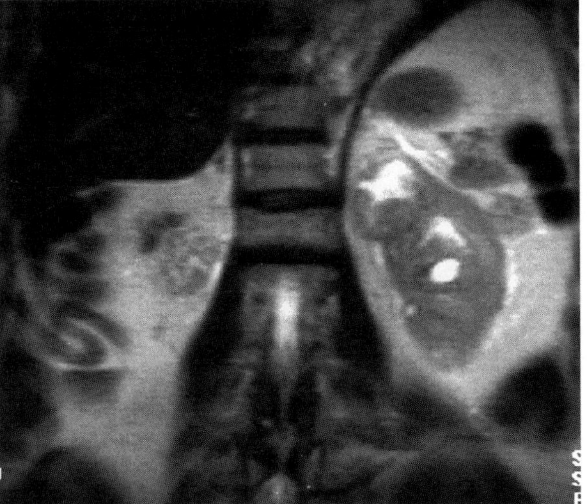

Fig. 4.21 a,b. MRI; metastases from RCC. In this patient a radical right nephrectomy had been performed a few years earlier for an RCC. At least two tumors are visualized in the left kidney (a,b). In addition, multiple lesions with similar signal characteristics can be recognized in the tail of the pancreas (*arrows*, b): multiple pancreatic metastases and metastases in the left kidney

exact preoperative staging, a simple chest radiograph is probably insufficient, because up to 20% of nodules smaller than 1 cm will not show up. Chest CT directed specifically to detection of small pulmonary nodules is much more sensitive than chest radiography.

## 4.5
## Follow-up After Therapy

For follow-up after therapy, which is usually radical nephrectomy or partial nephrectomy, CT scanning remains the best imaging procedure. MRI may be a substitute for CT under appropriate circumstances (Fig. 4.21). Renal bed recurrence of neoplasm occurs in about 5% of patients after radical nephrectomy. It is most likely to occur within 2 years after nephrectomy (LEVINE 1995). Interpretational errors can be avoided by ensuring adequate bowel opacification with oral contrast medium. The detection of a recurrent RCC at the operative site carries a poor prognosis, but CT is often the preferred imaging test and may serve as a guidance mechanism for biopsy if necessary.

## References

Akhtar M, Kardar H, Linjawi T, McClintock J, Ali MA (1995) Chromophobe cell carcinoma of the kidney. A clinicopathologic study of 21 cases. Am J Surg Pathol 19:1245–1256

Amin MB, Crotty TB, Tickoo SK (1997) Renal oncocytoma: a reappraisal of morphologic features with clinicopathologic findings in 80 cases. Am J Surg Pathol 21:1–12

Baert J, Vandamme B, Sciot R, Oyen R, Van Poppel H, Baert L (1995) Benign angiomyolipoma involving the renal vein and vena cava as a tumor thrombus: case report. J Urol 153:1205–1207

Barbaric ZL (1996) Imaging work-up: is it renal carcinoma and is it operable? Semin Urol Oncol 14:196–202

Bell ET (1950) Renal disease, 2nd edn. Lea & Febiger, Philadelphia, p 435

Bennington JL (1987) Renal adenoma. World J Urol 5:66–70

Birnbaum BA, Bosniak MA, Krinsky GA, Cheng D, Waisman J, Ambrosino MM (1994) Renal cell carcinma: correlation of CT findings with nuclear morphologic grading in 100 tumors. Abdom Imaging 19:262–266

Bosniak MA (1986) The current radiological approach to renal cysts. Radiology 158:1–10

Bosniak MA (1991) The small (≤3.0 cm) renal parenchymal tumor: detection, diagnosis, and controversies. Radiology 179:307–317

Bosniak MA (1997) Diagnosis and management of patients with complicated cystic lesions of the kidney. AJR 169:819–821

Bosniak MA, Megibow AJ, Hulnick DH, Horii S, Raghavendra BN (1988) CT diagnosis of renal angiomyolipoma: the importance of detecting small amounts of fat. AJR 151:497–501

Carriero A, Iezzi A, Ciccotosto C, Filippone A, D'Ettore L, Sollecito AM, Bonomo L (1994) The superior and inferior venae cavae: angiography by TOF 2D magnetic resonance versus spin-echo sequences. Radiol Med Torino 87:768–774

Castillo OA, Boyle AT, Kramer SA (1991) Multilocular cysts of kidney: a study of 29 patients and review of literature. Urology 37:156–161

Choyke PL, Walther MM, Wagner JR, Rayford W, Lyne JC, Linehan WM (1997) Renal cancer: preoperative evaluation with dual-phase three-dimensional MR angiography. Radiology 205:767–771

Cittadini G, Pozzi-Mucelli F, Danza FM, Derchi LE, Pozzi-Mucelli RS (1996) "Aggressive" renal angiomyolipoma. Acta Radiol 37:927–932

Cohan RH, Sherman LS, Korobkin M, Bass JC, Francis IR (1995) Renal masses: assessment of corticomedullary-phase and nephrographic-phase CT scans. Radiology 196:445–451

Cohen C, McCue PA, Derose PB (1988) Histogenesis of renal cell carcinoma and oncocytoma. An immunohistochemical study. Cancer 62:1946–1951

Coleman BG, Arger PH, Mintz MC, Pollack HM, Banner MP (1984) Hyperdense renal masses: a computed tomographic dilemma. AJR 143:291–294

Cristol DS, McDonald FR, Immell FL (1946) Renal adenomas in hypernephromatous kidneys: a study of their incidence, nature and relationship. J Urol 55:18–27

Crotty TB, Farrow GM, Lieber MM (1995) Chromophobe cell renal carcinoma: clinicopathological features of 50 cases. J Urol 154:964–967

Curry NS, Schabel SI, Garvin AJ, Fish G (1990) Intratumoral fat in a renal oncocytoma mimicking angiomylipoma. AJR 154:307–308

DalCin P, Gaeta J, Huben R, Li FP, Prout GR, Sandberg AA (1989) Renal cortical tumors. Am J Clin Pathol 134:27–34

Davidson AJ, Hayes WS, Hartman DS, McCarthy WF, Davis JC (1993) Renal oncocytoma and carcinoma: failure of differentiation with CT. Radiology 186:693–696

Davidson AJ, Choyke PL, Hartman DS, Davis CJ (1995) Renal medullary carcinoma associated with sickle cell trait: radiologic findings. Radiology 195:83–85

Davidson AJ, Hartman DS, Choyke PL, Wagner BJ (1997) Radiologic assessment of renal masses: implications for patient care. Radiology 202:297–305

Davis CJ, Sesterhenn IA, Mostofi FK, Ho CK (1992) Renal oncocytoma: clinicopathological study of 166 patients. J Urogen Pathol 1:41–52

Delahunt B, Eble JN (1997) Papillary renal cell carcinoma: a clinicopathologic and immunohistochemical study of 105 tumors. Mod Pathol 10:537–544

Denys A, Hélénon O, Souissi M, Attlan E, Chretien Y, Dufour B, Moreau JF (1991) Color and pulsed Doppler of renal masses. Angiographic and anatomo-pathological correlation. J Radiol 72:599–608

De Wever W, Ghijselings L, Cassiman S, Baert AL (1996) Selective embolization of an aneurysm in a massive angiomyolipoma of the kidney. J Belge Radiol 79:137–138

Dinney CPN, Awad SA, Gajewski JB, Belitsky P, Lannon SG, Mack FG, Millard OH (1992) Analysis of imaging modalities, staging systems, and prognostic indicators for renal cell carcinoma. Urology 39:122–129

Droz D, Zachar D, Charbit L, Gogusev J, Chretien Y, Iris L (1990) Expression of the human nephron differentiation molecules in renal carcinomas. Am J Pathol 137:895–905

Eilenberg SS, Lee JKT, Brown JJ, Mirowitz SA, Tartar VM (1990) Renal masses: evaluation with gradient-echo Gd-DTPA-enhanced dynamic MR imaging. Radiology 176:333–338

Fein AB, Lee JKT, Balfe DM, Heiken JP, Ling D, Glazer HS, McClennan BL (1987) Diagnosis and staging of renal cell carcinoma: a comparison of MR imaging and CT. AJR 148:749–753

Fleming S (1993) The impact of genetics on the classification of renal carcinoma. Histopathology 22:89–92

Fleming S, Lewi HJE (1986) Collecting duct carcinoma of the kidney. Histopathology 10:1131–1141

Forman HP, Middleton WD, Melson GL, McClennan BL (1993) Hyperechoic renal cell carcinoma: increase in detection at US. Radiology 188:431–434

Fukuya T, Honda H, Goto K, et al. (1996) Computed tomography findings of Bellini duct carcinoma of the kidney. J Comput Assist Tomogr 20:399–403

Füzesi L, Cober M, Mittermayer C (1992) Collecting duct carcinoma: cytogenetic characterization. Histopathology 21:155–160

Gohji K, Minayoshi K, Higuchi A, Fujii A, Gotoh A (1994) A case of papillary renal cell carcinoma suggestive of Bellini duct origin. Hinyokika Kiyo 40:329–332

Goncharenko V, Gerlock AJ, Kadir S (1979) Incidence and distribution of venous extension in 70 hypernephromas. AJR 133:263–265

Grieten M, Van-Poppel H, Baert L, Baert AL, Oyen R (1992) Renal pseudotumor due to a retained perirenal sponge: CT features. J Comput Assist Tomogr 16:305–307

Habboub HK, Abu-Youssef MM, Williams RD, See WA, Schweiger GD (1997) Accuracy of color-Doppler sonography in assessing venous thrombus extension in renal cell carcinoma. AJR 168:267–271

Haddad DS, Mufarrij AA (1992) 33-year follow-up after simple excision of a giant renal oncocytoma with calcifications: case report and review of the literature. Hum Pathol 23:324–327

Harmon WJ, King BF, Lieber MM (1996) Renal oncocytoma: magnetic resonance imaging characteristics. J Urol 155:863–867

Harris DD, Ruckle HC, Gaskill DM, Wang Y, Hadley HR (1994) Intraoperative ultrasound: determination of the presence and extent of vena caval tumor thrombus. Urology 44:189–193

Hartman DS, Davidson AJ, Davis CJ, Goldman SM (1988) Infiltrative renal lesions: CT-sonographic-pathologic correlation. AJR 150:1061–1064

Hartman DS, Weatherby E, Laskin WB, Brody JM, Corse W, Baluch JD (1992) Cystic renal cell carcinoma: CT findings simulating a benign hyperdense cyst. AJR 159:1235–1237

Hayakawa M, Hatano T, Tsuji A, Nakajima F, Ogawa Y (1996) Patients with renal cysts associated with renal cell carcinoma and the clinical implications of cyst puncture: a study of 223 cases. Urology 47:643–646

Helenon O, Chretien Y, Paraf F, Melky P, Denys A, Moreau JF (1993a) Renal cell carcinoma containing fat: demonstration with CT. Radiology 188:429–430

Helenon O, Denys A, Chretien Y, et al. (1993b) Role of MRI in the diagnosis of kidney cancer. J Radiol 74:105–115

Helenon O, Merran S, Paraf F, Melki P, Correas JM, Chretien Y, Moreau JF (1997) Unusual fat-containing tumors of the kidney: a diagnostic dilemma. Radiographics 17:129–144

Herr HW (1994) Partial nephrectomy for renal cell carcinoma with a normal opposite kidney. Cancer 73:160–162

Hricak H, Amparo E, Fisher MR, Crooks L, Higgins CB (1985) Abdominal venous system: assessment using MR. Radiology 156:415–422

Hricak H, Thoeni RF, Carroll PR, Demas BE, Marotti M, Tanagho EA (1988) Detection and staging of renal neoplasms: a reassessment of MR imaging. Radiology 166:643–649

Hughson MD, Johonson LD, Silva FG, Kovacs G (1993) Non papillary and papillary renal cell carcinoma: a cytogenetic and phenotypic study. Mod Pathol 6:449–456

Imaide Y, Saitoh M (1995) Clinical implication of selective renal tumor biopsy. Hinyokika Kiyo 41:745–752

Jamis-Dow CA, Choyke PL, Jennings SB, Linehan WM, Thakore KN, Walther MM (1996) Small (≤3 cm) renal masses: detection with CT versus US and pathologic correlation. Radiology 198:785–788

Jinzaki M, Tanimoto A, Narimatsu Y, et al. (1997) Angiomyolipoma: imaging findings in lesions with minimal fat. Radiology 205:497–502

Johnson CD, Dunnick NR, Cohan RH, Illescas FF (1987) Renal adenocarcinoma: CT staging of 100 tumors. AJR 148:59–63

Kabala JE, Penry B, Chadwick D (1990) Magnetic resonance imaging of renal masses. Br J Radiol (congress supplement) 63:15

Kallman DA, King BF, Hattery RR, Charboneau JW, Ehman RL, Guthman DA, Blute ML (1992) Renal vein and inferior vena cava tumor thrombus in renal cell carcinoma: CT, US, MRI and vena cavography. J Comput Assist Tomogr 16:240–247

Klein MJ, Valensi QJ (1976) Proximal tubular adenoma of the kidney with so-called oncocytic features. Cancer 38:906–914

Knudson AG (1987) A two mutational model for human cancer. Adv Virol Oncol 7:1–17

Kovacs G (1989) Papillary renal cell carcinoma: a morphologic and cytogenetic study of 11 cases. Am J Pathol 134:27–34

Kovacs G (1993) Molecular differential pathology of renal cell tumors. Histopathology 22:1–8

Kovacs G, Fuzesi L, Emmanuel A, Kung H (1991) Cytogenetics of papillary renal cell tumors. Genes Chromosomes Cancer 3:249–255

Kovacs A, Storkel S, Thoenes W, Kovacs G (1992) Mitochondrial and chromosomal DNA alterations in human chromophobe renal cell carcinomas. J Pathol 167:273–277

Kreft BP, Müller-Miny H, Sommer T, et al. (1997) Diagnostic value of MR imaging in comparison to CT in the detection and differential diagnosis of renal masses: ROC analysis. Eur Radiol 7:542–547

Kutta A, Schoenfeld B, Martin W, Haupt G (1993) Multifocal renal cell carcinoma of collecting duct origin. Scand J Urol Nephrol 27:531–533

Lager DJ, Huston BJ, Timmerman TG, Bonsib SM (1995) Papillary renal tumors: morphologic, cytochemical and genotypic features. Cancer 76:669–673

Lemaitre L, Provost M, Sault MC (1990) Tumeurs papillaires du parenchyme rénal: particularités de l'imagerie. A propos de 18 observations. Rev Im Med 2:615–623

Lemaitre L, Robert Y, Dubrulle F, Claudon M, Duhamel A, Danjou P, Mazeman E (1995) Renal angiomyolipoma: growth followed up with CT and/or US. Radiology 197:598–602

Levine E (1995) Renal cell carcinoma: clinical aspects, imaging diagnosis, and staging. Semin Roentgenol 30:128–148

Lieber MM, Tomera KM, Farrow GM (1987) Renal oncocytoma. J Urol 125:481–485

London NM, Messios, Kinder RB, Smart JG, Osborn DE, Watkin EM, Flynn JT (1989) A prospective study of the value of conventional CT, dynamic CT, ultrasonography and arteriography for staging renal carcinoma. Br J Urol 64:209–217

Long JP, Choyke PL, Shawker TA, Robertson CA, Pass HI, Walther MM, Linehan WM (1993) Intraoperative ultrasound in the evaluation of tumor involvement on the inferior vena cava. J Urol 150:13–17

MacLennan GT, Farrow GM, Bostwick DG (1997) Low-grade collecting duct carcinoma of the kidney: report of 13 cases of low-grade mucinous tubulocystic renal carcinoma of possible collecting duct origin. Urology 50:679–684

Madayag MA, Ambos MA, Lefleur RS (1979) Involvement of the inferior vena cava in patients with renal cell carcinoma. Radiology 133:321–326

Mancilla-Jimenez R, Stanley RJ, Blath RA (1976) Papillary renal cell carcinomas. Cancer 38:2469–2480

Mauro MA, Wadsworth DE, Stanley RJ, McClenan BL (1982) Renal cell carcinoma: angiography in the CT-era. AJR 139:1135–1138

Mevorach RA, Segal AJ, Tersegno ME, Frank IN (1992) Renal cell carcinoma: incidental diagnosis and natural history: review of 235 cases. Urology 39:519–522

Narumi Y, Hricak H, Presti JC, et al. (1997) MR imaging evaluation of renal cell carcinoma. Abdom Imaging 22:216–225

Nguyen BD, Westra WH, Zerhouni EA (1996) Renal cell carcinoma and tumor thrombus neovascularity: MR demonstration with pathologic correlation. Abdom Imaging 21:269–271

Outwater EK, Bahtia M, Siegelman ES, Burke MA, Mitchell DG (1997) Lipid in renal clear cell carcinoma: detection on opposed-phase gradient-echo MR images. Radiology 205:103–107

Parks CM, Kellett MC (1994) Staging renal cell carcinoma. Clin Radiol 49:223–230

Peppercorn PD, Reznek RH (1997) State-of-the-art CT and MRI of the adrenal gland. Eur Radiol 7:822–836

Polascik TJ, Meng MV, Epstein JI, Marshall FF (1995) Intraoperative sonography for the evaluation and management of renal tumors: experience with 100 patients. J Urol 154:1676–1680

Press GA, McClennan BL, Melson GL, Weyman PJ, Mauro MA, Lee JKT (1984) Papillary renal cell carcinoma: CT and sonographic evaluation. AJR 143:1005–1009

Roberts SC, Winick AB, Santi MR (1997) Papillary renal cell carcinoma: diagnostic dilemma of a cystic renal mass. Radiographics 17:993–998

Rofsky NM, Weinreb JC, Bosniak MA, Libes RB, Birnbaum BA (1991) Renal lesion characterization with gadolinium-enhanced MR-imaging: efficacy and safety in patients with renal insufficiency. Radiology 180:85–89

Rominger MB, Kenney PJ, Morgan DE, Bernreuter WK, Listinsky JJ (1992) Gadolinium-enhanced MR imaging of renal masses. Radiographics 12:1097–1116

Roubidoux MA, Dunnick NR, Sostman HD, Leder RA (1992) Renal carcinoma: detection of venous extension with gradient-echo MR imaging. Radiology 182:269–272

Rueckforth J, Rhode D, Baba H, Adam G (1995) Renal capsular hemangioma: unusual MR findings. J Comput Assist Tomogr 19:817–818

Sanchez-Chapado M, Angulo-Cuesta J, Rodriguez-de-Bethencourt-Codes F, Ontoria J, Prieto-Chaparro L, Dehaini A (1995) Synchronous bilateral renal oncocytoma. Arch Esp Urol 48:909–913

Sasaki S, Hayashi Y, Tsugaya M, Okamura T, Sakakura T, Kohri K (1995) Radiological diagnosis of renal oncocytoma. Hinyokika Kiyo 41:731–735

Semelka RC, Hricak H, Stevens SK, Finegold R, Tomei E, Carroll PR (1991) Combined gadolinium-enhanced and fat-saturation MR imaging of renal masses. Radiology 178:803–809

Semelka RC, Shoenut JP, Kroeker MA, MacMahon RG, Greenberg HM (1992) Renal lesions: controlled comparison between CT and 1.5-T MR imaging with nonenhanced and gadolinium-enhanced fat-suppressed spin-echo and breath-hold flash techniques. Radiology 182:425–430

Semelka RC, Shoenut JP, Magro CM, Kroeker MA, MacMahon R, Greenberg HM (1993) Renal cancer staging: comparison of contrast-enhanced CT and gadolinium-enhanced fat-suppressed spin-echo and gradient-echo MR imaging. J Magn Reson Imaging 3:597–602

Siegel CL, McFarland AG, Brink JA, Fisher AJ, Humphrey P, Heiken JP (1997) CT of cystic renal masses: analysis of diagnostic performance and interobserver variation. AJR 169:813–818

Silverman SG, Lee BY, Seltzer SE (1994) Small (≤3 cm) renal masses: correlation of spiral CT features and pathologic findings. AJR 163:597–605

Smith SJ, Bosniak MA, Megibow AJ, Hulnick DH, Horii SC, Raghavendra BN (1989) Renal cell carcinoma: earlier discovery and increased detection. Radiology 170:699–703

Soyer P, Dufresne A, Klein I, Barbagelatta M, Herve JM, Scherrer A (1997) Renal cell carcinoma of clear type: correlation of CT features with tumor size, architectural pattern, and pathologic staging. Eur Radiol 7:224–229

Steiner M, Quinlan D, Goldman SM, Millmond S, Hallowell MJ, Stutzman RE, Korobkin M (1989) Leiomyoma of the kidney: presentation of 4 new cases and the role of computed tomography. J Urol 143:994–998

Strotzer M, Lehner KB, Becker K (1993) Detection of fat in a renal cell carcinoma mimicking angiomyolipoma. Radiology 188:427–428

Studer UE, Scherz S, Scheidegger J, Kraft R, Sonntag R, Ackermann D, Zingg EJ (1990) Enlargement of regional lymph nodes in renal cell carcinoma is often not due to metastases. J Urol 144:243–245

Sussman S, Cochran ST, Pagani JJ, et al. (1984) Hyperdense renal masses: a CT manifestation of hemorrhagic renal cyst. Radiology 150:207–211

Szolar DH, Kammerhuber F, Altziebler S, Tillich M, Breinl E, Fotter R, Schreyer HH (1997) Multiphasic helical CT of the kidney: increased conspicuity for detection and characterization of small (<3-cm) renal masses. Radiology 202:211–217

Takase K, Takahashi S, Tazawa S, Terasawa Y, Sakamoto K (1994) Renal cell carcinoma associated with chronic renal failure: evaluation with sonographic angiography. Radiology 192:787–792

Thoenes W, Störkel S, Rumplet HJ (1986) Histopathology and classification of renal cell tumors (adenomas, oncocytomas and carcinomas). Pathol Res Pract 181:125–143

Tikkakoski T, Paivansalo M, Alanen A, Nurmi M, Taavitsainen M, Farin P, Apaja-Sarkkinen M (1991) Radiologic findings in renal oncocytoma. Acta Radiol 32:363–367

Vandeputte A, Oyen R, Van Poppel H (1996) Large egg-shell-like calcified cyst in a case of renal cell carcinoma. Eur Radiol 6:462–464

Van Poppel H, Baert L (1992) The case for conservative surgery for renal cell carcinoma (RCC). Prog Clin Biol Res 378:33–143

Van Poppel H, Vandendriessche H, Boel K, et al. (1997) Microscopic vascular invasion is the most relevant prognosticator after radical nephrectomy for clinically nonmetastatic renal cell carcinoma. J Urol 158:45–49

Warshauer DM, McCarthy SM, Street L, et al. (1988) Detection of renal masses: sensitivities ans specificities of excretory urography/linear tomography, US, and CT. Radiology 169:363–365

Webb JAW, Murray A, Bary PR (1987) The accuracy and limitation of ultrasound in the assessment of venous extension in renal carcinoma. Br J Urol 60:14–17

Weiss LM, Gelb AB, Medeiros LJ (1995) Adult renal epithelial neoplasms. Am J Clin Pathol 103:624–635

Weyman PJ, McClennan BL, Lee JK, Stanley RJ (1982) CT of calcified renal masses. AJR 138:1095–1099

Yamashita Y, Takahashi M, Watanabe O, et al. (1992) Small renal cell carcinoma: pathologic and radiologic correlation. Radiology 184:493–498

Yamashita Y, Ueno S, Makita O, Ogata I, Hatanaka Y, Watanabe O, Takahashi M (1993) Hyperechoic renal tumors: anechoic rim and intratumoral cysts in US differentiation of renal cell carcinoma from angiomyolipoma. Radiology 188:179–182

Yamashita Y, Watanabe O, Miyazaki T, Yamanmoto H, Harada M, Takahashi M (1994) Cystic renal cell carcinoma: imaging findings with pathologic correlation. Acta Radiol 35:19–24

Yamashita Y, Miyazaki T, Hatanaka Y, Takahashi M (1995) Dynamic MRI of small renal cell carcinoma. J Comput Assist Tomogr 19:759–765

Yamashita Y, Honda S, Nishirau T, Urata J, Takahashi M (1996) Detection of pseudocapsule of renal cell carcinoma with MR imaging and CT. AJR 166:1151–1155

Zeman RK, Cronan JJ, Rosenfield AT, Lynch JH, Jaffe MH, Clark LR (1988) Renal cell carcinoma: dynamic thin-section CT assessment of vascular invasion and tumor vascularity. Radiology 167:393–396

Zincke H, Engen DE, Henning KM, McDonald MW (1985) Treatment of renal cell carcinoma by in situ partial nephrectomy and extracorporeal operation with auto transplantation. Mayo Clinic Proc 60:651–662

# 5 Radical Nephrectomy

J.P. STEIN and D.G. SKINNER

CONTENTS



## 5.1
## Introduction

In 1996, it was estimated that nearly 30 600 people would be diagnosed with renal cell carcinoma with approximately 12 000 deaths from this disease

J.P. STEIN, MD, Assistant Professor, Department of Urology, University of Southern California, Norris Comprehensive Cancer Center, MS #74, 1441 Eastlake Ave., Suite 7414, Los Angeles, CA 90033, USA

D.G. SKINNER, MD, Professor and Chairman, Department of Urology, University of Southern California, Norris Comprehensive Cancer Center, 1441 Eastlake Ave., Suite 7414, Los Angeles, CA 90033, USA

(PARKER et al. 1996). Although this tumor most frequently occurs in patients in their fifth and sixth decades of life, it is not uncommon for it to occur in young, productive, and otherwise healthy adults or even children (ECKSCHLAGER and KODET 1994). This disease clearly constitutes an important health problem in the United States. Currently, over 30% of patients diagnosed with renal cell carcinoma have metastatic disease at presentation. An additional 30%–50% of patients initially diagnosed with local disease will demonstrate locally advanced or even metastatic disease at the time of radical nephrectomy. These statistics, coupled with the lack of an effective adjuvant form of chemotherapy, radiotherapy, or immunotherapy (despite the initial enthusiasm) for renal cell carcinoma, emphasize that this is a surgical disease that needs to be detected and aggressively treated at an early curable stage.

## 5.2
## Indications for Radical Nephrectomy

Radical nephrectomy, by definition, is the en bloc removal of the kidney, adrenal gland, and Gerota's fascia intact, with an ipsilateral retroperitoneal lymphadenectomy and early ligation of the renal artery and vein. Renal cell carcinoma may be a very vascular tumor and early ligation of the blood supply prior to any manipulation is important to avoid excessive blood loss and to avoid any potential tumor seeding or spill. Proper patient selection and identifying the appropriate surgical candidate is critical to the successful outcome of this disease. Candidates for radical nephrectomy include those with (1) potentially curable lesions (stage I–III) and a reasonable life expectancy; (2) stage IV disease with solitary or limited metastases; (3) stage IV disease with refractory pain, bleeding, or paraneoplastic symptoms; and (4) stage IV disease considered for various adjuvant protocols.

## 5.3
## Presentation of Patients with Renal Cell Carcinoma

Although renal cell carcinoma generally occurs in adults with a median age at diagnosis of 59 years, 30% of patients in one series of over 268 patients were less than 50 years of age at diagnosis (STEIN et al. 1998). Renal cell carcinoma predominately affects males by a ratio of 2:1 (KANTOR 1977; BRETHEAU et al. 1995; STEIN et al. 1998). Renal cell carcinoma may present with a myriad of signs and symptoms suggestive of other illnesses. This masquerade of diseases can often delay or make the diagnosis of renal cell carcinoma very difficult, and is often the reason it has been referred to as the "internist tumor." Patients with this tumor may present with signs and symptoms classic for renal cell carcinoma such as hematuria, pain, or a palpable abdominal mass. This triad, although classic for renal cell carcinoma, is present in only about 10% of patients (SKINNER et al. 1971; STEIN et al. 1998). Alternatively, patients may present with nonspecific, obscure signs and symptoms including: fever of unknown origin, malaise, weight loss, anemia, erythrocytosis, hypercalcemia, hypertension, congestive heart failure, acute onset of a scrotal varicocele, lower extremity edema, and pathologic fractures, just to mention a few (SKINNER et al. 1971; STEIN et al. 1998).

Many symptoms of renal cell carcinoma are caused by the elaboration of specific polypeptide hormones by the tumor itself. These substances are responsible for the "paraneoplastic" effects of the tumor, present in a significant number of patients diagnosed or treated for renal cell carcinoma (McDOUGAL and GARNICK 1995; GOLD et al. 1996). These paraneoplastic syndromes may occur in curable patients with renal cell carcinoma, and do not necessarily imply incurability or represent metastatic disease. Effective therapy of the underlying tumor generally induces regression of the paraneoplastic syndrome. Few paraneoplastic syndromes respond to medical therapy alone; hypercalcemia may be the exception. Importantly, recurrence of a paraneoplastic syndrome should raise suspicion for relapse of disease, either local or metastatic.

To avoid delays in the diagnosis and effectively treat patients, it is important to recognize the paraneoplastic syndromes associated with renal cell carcinoma, which are present sometime during the illness in 10%–40% of patients (McDOUGAL and GARNICK 1995; GOLD et al. 1996). The most commonly observed paraneoplastic syndromes in patients with renal cell carcinoma include: cachexia, hypertension, anemia, hyperglycemia, nonmetastatic hepatic dysfunction (Stauffer's syndrome), erythrocytosis, and amyloidosis.

Presenting signs, symptoms, and clinical and laboratory findings, according to their incidence from two large series of patients with renal cell carcinoma, are shown in Table 5.1 (SKINNER et al. 1971; STEIN et al. 1998). These data represent 309 patients treated over a 30-year period at the Massachusetts

**Table 5.1.** Presenting signs, symptoms, and laboratory findings in patients with renal cell carcinoma: the MGH[a] and USC[b] series; individual and collective experience

| Presentation: signs and symptoms and abnormal laboratory findings | MGH series[a] Number (%) | USC series[b] Number (%) | Total number (%) |
| --- | --- | --- | --- |
| No. of patients | 309 | 264 | 573 |
| Hematuria (micro or gross) | 183 (57%) | 128 (48%) | 311 (54%) |
| Classic triad | 29 (9%) | 13 (5%) | 42 (7%) |
| Pain | 127 (41%) | 101 (38%) | 228 (40%) |
| Abdominal mass | 139 (45%) | 68 (25%) | 207 (36%) |
| Fever | 21 (7%) | 20 (8%) | 41 (7%) |
| Weight loss | 85 (28%) | 51 (19%) | 136 (24%) |
| Anemia | 64 (21%) | 119 (45%) | 183 (32%) |
| Erythrocytosis | 10 (3%) | 3 (1%) | 13 (2%) |
| Hypercalcemia | 11 (3%) | 16 (6%) | 27 (5%) |
| Varicocele | 7 (2%) | 13 (5%) | 20 (3%) |
| Incidental finding | 20 (7%) | 20 (8%) | 40 (7%) |
| Known metastases (clinical or radiographic) | 31 (10%) | 38 (14%) | 69 (12%) |

[a] From SKINNER et al. (1971): Massachusetts General Hospital (MGH).
[b] From STEIN et al. (1998): University of Southern California (USC).

General Hospital (MGH) (SKINNER et al. 1971) as well as 264 patients treated over a 25-year period at the University of Southern California (USC) (STEIN et al. 1998). The similarities of these two large series is striking. The most common presentation in both series was hematuria (microscopically or gross), collectively seen in 311 of 573 patients (54%). The classic triad of hematuria, pain, and abdominal mass was seen collectively in only 42 of 573 patients (7%).

Anemia (hematocrit less than 33%, or hemoglobin less than 10.0 ng/ml) was the most common laboratory abnormality in both series. Anemia was present in 21% of the MGH patients and 45% of the USC patients; collectively it was seen in 183 patients (32%) from the two series. This anemia is generally not a result of hematuria-related blood loss or hemolysis, but rather a result of a hypoproliferative nature that creates a low total iron-binding capacity and low levels of serum iron. It has also been postulated that the anemia seen in patients with renal cell carcinoma may be due to the toxic effects of an unknown circulating substance (possibly a cytokine) that results in bone marrow suppression (GIBBONS et al. 1976; ROBSON 1982; LASKI and VUGRIN 1987).

Renal cell carcinoma is the most common cause of ectopic erythropoietin production; elevated levels are found in nearly two-thirds of patients with erythrocytosis and renal cell carcinoma (SUFRIN et al. 1977). Secondary erythrocytosis (hematocrit greater than 50% or hemoglobin greater than 15.5 ng/dl) upon admission was found in ten patients (3%) in the MGH series, and three patients (1%) in the USC series, i.e., it was collectively seen in 13 of 573 patients (2%). This incidence of erythrocytosis is similar to rates in other series of 1%–5% (GIBBONS et al. 1976; ROBSON 1982; SAMAAN 1979). More recently, GROSS et al. (1994) reported elevated levels of erythropoietin in 1 of 49 patients (2%) diagnosed with renal cell carcinoma. Erythrocytosis differs from polycythemia, in which there is no elevation of the platelet or leukocyte count, and no splenomegaly. The erythrocytosis observed in patients with renal cell carcinoma is thought to be related to a circulating substance similar to eythropoietin, secreted by the tumor. In patients without evidence of metastatic disease, resolution of the erythrocytosis should occur following removal of the tumor. The late reappearance of erythrocytosis (following nephrectomy) may imply recurrence or metastatic disease, and indicates a poor prognosis (ROBSON 1982; ROSENBLUM 1987).

In 1941, Allbright first reported a case of renal cell carcinoma associated with hypercalcemia (ALLBRIGHT 1941). Hypercalcemia (serum calcium level greater than 10.5 mg/dl) is one of the most common paraneoplastic syndromes, affecting as many as 20% of patients with renal cell carcinoma (MUGGIA 1990). Hypercalcemia was found on admission in 11 patients (3%) in the MGH series, and 16 patients (6%) in the USC series; collectively it was seen in 27 of 573 patients (5%). Hypercalcemia may be attributed to skeletal metastases, but more commonly is related to ectopic hormone production of either a parathyroid hormone (PTH)-like substance or prostaglandin secretion by the tumor (CUMMINGS and ROBERTSON 1977; SAMAAN 1979; LYTTON et al. 1965; O'GRADY et al. 1965). More recently, a molecularly cloned PTH-like peptide, purified from a variety of cancer cell lines with near homology with PTH, has been identified (SUVA et al. 1987; STREWLER et al. 1987). Although no correlation to serum calcium was observed, GOTOH and associates identified a PTH-related peptide using a specific monoclonal antibody in 40 of 42 cases of renal cell carcinoma (GOTOH et al. 1993).

In general, hypercalcemia associated with renal cell carcinoma (without evidence of metastatic disease) is best managed by surgical resection or debulking of the primary tumor (GOLDBERG et al. 1980; RITCH 1990).

Hypercalcemia associated with renal cell carcinoma may also imply the presence of bony metastases, reported in 52% of patients in one series (CHASAN et al. 1989). In this situation, the hypercalcemia does not represent a true paraneoplastic syndrome; rather it is related to the direct osteolytic bone activity of the metastatic process. The presentation of these patients may be similar to that of those with humoral hypercalcemia; however, patients with metastatic hypercalcemia may have bony pain and may not respond to nephrectomy. Radiotherapy may help ameliorate the bony pain and hypercalcemia in this situation.

Constitutional symptoms such as fever, weight loss, and cachexia may also suggest the diagnosis of renal cell carcinoma, and are present in over 50% of patients (McDOUGAL and GARNICK 1995). Fevers upon presentation were observed in 21 patients (7%) in the MGH series, and 20 patients (8%) in the USC series; collectively they were seen in 41 of 573 patients (7%). Fever associated with renal cell carcinoma has been reported to occur in up to 25% of patients (CHERUKURI et al. 1977). Although the exact etiology is unknown, it is thought to be related to an unknown circulating pyrogen secreted by the tumor (CRANSTON et al. 1973). More recently interleukin-6 has been implicated as a potential cause of the fever in these patients. Interleukin-6, a cytokine that may stimulate acute phase reactants, has been found to be secreted by several human renal cell carcinoma cell lines, and has also been found to be elevated in 25% of patients with renal cell carcinoma in one study; 78% of those patients with elevated interleukin-6 levels had documented fevers (TSUKAMOTO et al. 1992). Fevers in patients with renal cell carcinoma are frequently intermittent, and may resolve following nephrectomy (TSUKAMOTO et al. 1992). However, return of a fever following treatment may indicate the presence of recurrent or metastatic disease (KEILY 1966).

Weight loss and cachexia are constitutional symptoms commonly seen in patients presenting with renal cell carcinoma. Weight loss was observed in 85 patients (28%) in the MGH series, and 51 patients (19%) in the USC series; collectively it was seen in 136 of 573 patients (24%). Although the mechanism is not well understood, the cancer-related weight loss and cachexia-may be related to a cytokine-mediated factor such as tumor necrosis factor (LASKI and VUGRIN 1987).

Seven men (2%) in the MGH series presented with acute onset of a scrotal varicocele (in six of these cases it occurred on the left side), while 13 patients (5%) in the USC series had a varicocele on presentation. Collectively, 20 of 573 patients (3%) were found to have a varicocele upon presentation. This condition generally occurs secondary to obstruction of the gonadal vein by tumor thrombus (most common) or by tumor compression. On the left side, obstruction occurs at the level of the left renal vein, whereas on the right side obstruction generally involves the vena cava. Obstruction or tumor thrombus involvement of the inferior vena cava may also lead to lower extremity swelling or edema, present in 10 of 264 patients (4%) in the USC series.

Hypertension has been associated with renal cell carcinoma in up to 25% of patients (McDOUGAL and GARNICK 1995). Although the exact etiology of the hypertension is unclear, it is thought to be related to one of the following mechanisms: renin production by the tumor itself, relative ischemia to adjacent normal renal parenchyma, altered renal blood flow, a decreased rate of renin degradation, or the increased production of renin by nonrenal sources (SUFRIN et al. 1977). Several reports have actually demonstrated renin secretion by the tumor itself (NIELSEN 1973; HOLLIFIELD et al. 1975; SUFRIN et al. 1977; LINDOP

and FLEMING 1984). Nephrectomy should relieve this tumor-induced hypertension.

Another unique paraneoplastic syndrome of reversible hepatosplenomegaly with hepatic dysfunction (without clinical evidence of liver metastases) was described in 1935 by CREEVY and in 1961 by STAUFFER. This syndrome (characterized by abnormal hepatic dysfunction in the absence of hepatic tumor involvement), is referred to as Stauffer's syndrome (HANASH et al. 1971; HANASH 1982; RAMOS and TAYLOR 1972; UTZ et al. 1970; WALSH and KISSANE 1968; BOXER et al. 1978).

Diagnosis of this syndrome was initially based on abnormal liver function tests with elevated levels of serum alkaline phosphatase in the absence of hepatic metastases (STAUFFER 1961). Other biochemical abnormalities may include elevated transaminases, hypoprothrombinemia, prolonged partial thromboplastin time, and elevated $\alpha$-globulin levels (LASKI and VUGRIN 1987; ROSENBLUM 1987). This syndrome of reversible hepatic dysfunction has also been described in patients with xanthogranulomatous pyelonephritis (MALEK and ELDER 1978; SAMAAN 1979). However, despite the presence of a renal mass, patients with xanthogranulomatous pyelonephritis are clinically distinct; symptoms of urinary tract infection are commonly present, patients are commonly anemic with hypoalbuminemia, and an obstructed collecting system (kidney stone) is almost always present (FIGUEROA et al. 1995; CHUANG et al. 1992).

Although the exact etiology of the hepatic dysfunction in Stauffer's syndrome is unknown, theories of metabolic hepatic damage by a circulating tumor toxin, and lymphocyte-mediated immunologic hepatic damage mechanism have been suggested (HANASH 1982). Stauffer's syndrome should disappear following nephrectomy in patients with renal cell carcinoma, unless metastatic disease is present. Furthermore, recurrence of this syndrome following therapy, or persistence of the hepatic dysfunction despite treatment, suggests the presence of recurrent or metastatic disease, and indicates a poor prognosis (HANASH 1982; ROBSON 1982).

Elevated levels of other hormones, glycoproteins, and hormone-related syndromes have been associated with renal cell carcinoma. These substances and syndromes include: serum human chorionic gonadotropin (GOLDE et al. 1974), prolactin (TURKINGTON 1971), human placental lactogen, calcitonin (SAMAAN 1979), carcinoembryonic antigen (GUINAN et al. 1975), feminization, masculinization, and Cushing's syndrome (RIGGS and SPRAGUE 1961;

CRONIN et al. 1976). Hyperglycemia has also been associated with renal cell carcinoma and may represent yet another paraneoplastic manifestation of the disease (PALGON et al. 1986; JOBE et al. 1993).

## 5.4
## The Incidentally Discovered Renal Cell Carcinoma

The initial presentation of patients with renal cell carcinoma has shown some change over the past 20 years. The number of incidentally diagnosed renal cell carcinomas has increased considerably due to recent advances, and increased use of ultrasonography and computed tomography (BRETHEAU et al. 1995; ASO and HOMMA 1992; THOMPSON and PEEK 1988; VALLANCIEN et al. 1990; KESSLER et al. 1994). In a large multicenter survey in Japan, ASO and HOMMA (1992) clearly demonstrated an increased detection rate of incidental renal tumors since 1980: 20 cases in 1980, and 338 in 1988. In 1993, a national epidemiological survey on 516 patients from the Association Francaise d'Urologie revealed a 45% rate of incidentally discovered renal cell carcinomas (COULANGE 1993). BRETHEAU and associates (1995) reported a significantly increased detection rate of incidentally discovered renal tumors over a 10 year period: 17% in 1980 to approximately 50% in 1991. Similar detection rates have been reported by others (ASO and HOMMA 1992; VALLANCIEN et al. 1990; KONNACK and GROSSMAN 1985; TSUKAMOTO et al. 1991; KESSLER et al. 1994). In fact, the incidentally discovered renal cell carcinoma may now be the most common form of presentation in up to 50% of patients.

Several series report that incidentally discovered renal tumors are more commonly diagnosed in the right kidney, i.e., in about two-thirds of the patients (BRETHEAU et al. 1995; VALLANCIEN et al. 1990; NAKANO et al. 1992). This may be a consequence of the increased frequency of right upper quadrant (hepatobiliary) evaluation with ultrasound, and the fact that the right renal fossa is more easily examined by ultrasonography than the left side.

Several series also report lower staged tumors with an improved prognosis in patients with incidentally discovered renal cell carcinomas (BRETHEAU et al. 1995; THOMPSON and PEEK, 1988; KONNACK and GROSSMAN 1985; TSUKAMOTO et al. 1991; NAKANO et al. 1992). BRETHEAU and associates (1995) reported on 236 patients with renal cell carcinoma; 74 of these patients were found to have inci-

dentally discovered renal tumors. In this group of patients, the reported 10-year survival rate was 85% for patients, versus 44% for those with symptomatic tumors. Similarly, in an evaluation of 188 patients surgically treated for renal cell carcinoma, the disease-free 5-year survival for 121 patients incidentally diagnosed by ultrasound and/or computed tomography was 80%, compared with only 40% survival at 5 years for 67 symptomatic patients diagnosed by intravenous pyelography ($P < 0.001$) (KESSLER et al. 1994). In this series, the incidence of small renal tumors (<5 cm in diameter) was also significantly higher in patients incidentally diagnosed with ultrasound and/or computed tomography than in those diagnosed by intravenous pyelography (47.9% vs 25.4%, respectively, $P < 0.01$). Smaller tumor size and lower pathologic stage in patients with incidentally discovered tumors have been reported by others, and may relate to an improved prognosis (BRETHEAU et al. 1995; THOMPSON and PEEK 1988; TSUKAMOTO et al. 1991; NAKANO et al. 1992).

This recent change in presentation of patients with renal cell carcinoma differs from our experience. Incidentally discovered tumors were found in only 20 of 309 patients (7%) in the MGH series; most of these renal tumors were discovered intraoperatively. In the more contemporary USC series, still only 20 of 264 patients (8%) had incidentally discovered renal cell carcinomas. These findings are similar to other recent reports (DINNEY et al. 1992). This may be explained by the fact that ultrasonography and computed tomography were either not available or less commonly performed during the particular era under study. Furthermore, the incidence of incidentally discovered renal tumors may differ in series from large tertiary referral centers where more advanced and complicated renal tumors are referred and managed.

## 5.5
## Prognosis of Patients with Renal Cell Carcinoma

Despite extensive research, effective adjuvant forms of therapy for renal cell carcinoma are still lacking. Surgical extirpation remains the only truly effective means of curing this disease. Dedicated efforts have been made to identify various morphologic, molecular, and pathologic features that may provide prognostic information regarding survival in patients with renal cell carcinoma. In addition, better prognostic markers may also help identify patients with increased risk for recurrence and/or disease progression, who may benefit from adjuvant treatment strategies.

Pathologic tumor staging following surgical resection remains the most important prognostic variable in patients with renal cell carcinoma (THRASHER and PAULSON 1993). It has been shown that patients with pathologically organ-confined tumors demonstrate better clinical outcomes (recurrence and survival) than those with nodal or distant metastases (DINNEY et al. 1992; GIULIANI et al. 1990; GOLIMBU et al. 1986; McNICHOLOS et al. 1981; MEDEIROS et al. 1987, 1988; NURMI 1984; ROBSON et al. 1968, 1969; SELLI et al. 1983; SIMINOVITCH et al. 1983; SKINNER et al. 1971; STEIN et al. 1998). The staging system most commonly used is ROBSON's modification (ROBSON 1963) of the system described by FLOCKS and KADESKY (1958). Although still commonly used today, this staging system is limited by collectively designating venous tumor thrombus involvement (renal vein or vena cava) and lymph node involvement to stage III. These two entities have different prognostic implications. Those tumors with thrombus extension into the renal vein or even vena cava completely resected, without perinephric fat or regional lymph nodes, have a similar prognosis to tumors confined to the kidney (stage I) (BOXER et al. 1979; LIBERTINO et al. 1987; MRSTIK et al. 1992; SELLI et al. 1983; SKINNER et al. 1972a). In contrast, lymph node involvement has been shown to be a much worse prognostic variable (SIMINOVITCH et al. 1983; BOXER et al. 1979; SKINNER et al. 1972b; GIULIANI et al. 1990; GOLIMBU et al. 1986). To further complicate matters, although venous tumor thrombus involvement may not affect patient survival, local microscopic tumor infiltration of the wall (endothelium) of the vein appears to adversely impact upon survival (MRSTIK et al. 1992; HATCHER et al. 1991).

These limitations of Robson's staging system were addressed by the TNM staging system proposed by the International Union Against Cancer (BEAHRS and MYERS 1983) and modified by HERMANEK and SCHROTT (1990), taking into consideration tumor size, extent of local invasion, degree of extension into the vein, and extent of lymph node metastases.

Although the accumulated data suggest that the pathologic stage of renal cell carcinoma at the time of surgical resection is the most important single variable in determination of survival, other factors may also be involved. Additional features of a particular renal cell carcinoma may also provide prognostic information including: nuclear grade, histologic pattern, tumor size, cell type, DNA content, and nuclear morphometry (THRASHER and PAULSON 1993).

## 5.6
## The USC Surgical Experience with Renal Cell Carcinoma

We have recently evaluated our experience with the surgical management of renal cell carcinoma over the past 25 years (STEIN et al. 1998). From 1972 through 1997, a total of 264 patients underwent surgical management for renal cell carcinoma. Of these patients, 174 (65%) were male and 90 (35%) were female. The median age at diagnosis was 59 years (range 19–90 years); 25% of patients were less than 50 years of age and 17% greater than 70 years of age at the time of presentation. The median follow-up in these 264 patients was 6.8 years (range 1–21 years).

The median survival for the entire group of patients was 7 years. The most important prognostic variable regarding outcome was pathologic stage (Table 5.2) Overall, the recurrence-free survival for Robson's pathologic stage I ($n = 68$), II ($n = 54$), III ($n = 76$), and IV ($n = 70$) tumors was 95%, 85%, 54%, and 19% at 5 years respectively, and 78%, 80%, 40%, and 19% at 10 years respectively.

Of the 76 patients with stage III tumors: 14 had lymph node only involvement (stage IIIb), 51 had tumor thrombus involvement only (stage IIIa), and 11 had both lymph node and tumor thrombus involvement (stage IIIc). Interestingly, no patient in this series was found to have only tumor extension through Gerota's fascia (stage III) without evidence of lymph node or tumor thrombus involvement or metastatic disease. The 5-year recurrence-free survival in patients with stage IIIb was 54%, compared to a 59% 5-year recurrence-free survival for stage IIIa, and a 33% 5-year recurrence-free survival for stage IIIc. Furthermore, of the 25 patients with lymph node involvement (stage IIIb and stage IIIc), the 5- and 10-year recurrence-free survival was 46% and 25% respectively.

Nuclear tumor grade and the histologic cell type were also found to significantly influence recurrence-free survival in our series of patients (Table 5.2). The 5-year recurrence-free survival for renal tumors with nuclear grade I and II tumors ($n = 87$) was 78%, compared to a 62% and 37% 5-year recurrence-free survival for nuclear grade III ($n = 136$) and IV ($n = 45$) tumors respectively ($P < 0.0001$). Furthermore, renal tumors with clear cell features ($n = 149$) demonstrated an improved 5-year

**Table 5.2.** Recurrence-free survival at 5 and 10 years: relationship with pathologic stage, nuclear grade, and cell type

| Prognostic variable | Number of patients | Recurrence-free survival (%) | | P value |
| --- | --- | --- | --- | --- |
| | | 5-year | 10-year | |
| Pathologic stage[a] | 264 | | | <0.0001 |
| I | 68 | 95% | 78% | |
| II | 54 | 84% | 80% | |
| III | 76 | 54% | 40% | |
| IV | 70 | 19% | 19% | |
| Nuclear grade | 264 | | | <0.0001 |
| I + II | 87 | 78% | 75% | |
| III | 136 | 62% | 51% | |
| IV | 45 | 37% | 20% | |
| Cell type | 264 | | | $P = 0.01$ |
| Clear cell | 149 | 71% | 63% | |
| Clear + granular | 90 | 50% | 30% | |
| Spindle | 19 | 58% | 58% | |

[a]Robson's staging system.

**Table 5.3.** Significance of demographic features related to recurrence-free survival

| Prognostic variable | P value |
| --- | --- |
| Gender of patient | 0.59 |
| Age of patient | 0.66 |
| Number of symptoms | 0.001 |
| Anemia (serum Hct < 35%) | 0.01 |
| Serum LDH | 0.01 |
| Serum alkaline phosphatase | 0.001 |
| Presence of gross hematuria | 0.3 |
| Presence of microhematuria | 0.3 |
| Weight loss | 0.001 |
| Presence of pain | 0.64 |
| Presence of an abdominal mass | 0.3 |
| Hypercalcemia | 0.03 |
| Serum transaminase levels | 0.4 |

recurrence-free survival of 72%, compared to rates of 50% with clear cell and granular features, and 58% with spindle cell features ($P = 0.01$).

When evaluating the demographic features of these 264 patients, certain prognostic indicators were also found to impact upon recurrence-free survival (Table 5.3). Adverse demographic factors significantly affecting survival included: the number of symptoms at the time of presentation, anemia (hematocrit less than 35%), elevated serum lactase dehydrogenase (LDH) level, elevated serum alkaline phosphatase level, hypoalbuminemia, hypercalcemia, and weight loss. Demographic features that did not significantly affect survival included: age at the time of presentation, gender of patient, the presence of gross or microscopic hematuria, the presence of pain, the presence of an abdominal mass, and serum transaminase levels.

## 5.7
## The Current Role of a Retroperitoneal Lymphadenectomy

The current role of a retroperitoneal lymphadenectomy in the management of renal cell carcinoma remains controversial. As previously mentioned, lymph node involvement is an adverse prognostic factor in patients with renal cell carcinoma. Most investigators would agree that a retroperitoneal lymphadenectomy assists in the accurate pathologic staging of the disease and also provides valuable prognostic information based on the presence or absence of nodal involvement. In addition, those patient identified with lymph node involvement may benefit from some form of adjuvant therapy. This, however, is contingent on the efficacy of an effective adjuvant form of therapy; unfortunately, most have been disappointing. Although the authors firmly believe there may be a therapeutic benefit from a properly performed lymph node dissection, this remains conjectural and will continue to be a source of debate until a well-designed, randomized, prospective trial is performed. Currently, it is our policy to perform a lymphadenectomy on all patients for whom radical nephrectomy is potentially curative (stages I, II, and III). This is based on the assumption that, if lymph node dissection were to have any therapeutic benefit, it would be for those with minimal lymph node involvement. This is in addition to the fact that there is no truly effective form of adjuvant therapy currently available for renal cell carcinoma.

Although poorly understood, the lymphatic drainage of the kidney is thought to parallel its vascular architecture. A review by MARSHALL and

Powell (1982) demonstrated that the regional lymph node drainage of the right kidney includes the lateral caval lymph nodes, the pre- and postcaval lymph nodes, and the interaortocaval lymph nodes. The lymph node drainage of the left kidney consists of the upper left lateral lumbar nodes, the pre- and postaortic lymph nodes, the nodes lying on the left crus of the diaphragm (posterior and medial to the adrenal vein), and the lymph nodes along the left renal vein. It has been suggested that the lymphatic drainage from the kidney is predictable at the level of the hilum, but that beyond the immediate region of the kidney, lymphatic drainage is unpredictable (Tsukamoto et al. 1990; Wood 1991).

Of patients undergoing radical nephrectomy, nearly 25% will have metastatic lymph node involvement at the time of surgery, a figure that increases as the limits of the dissection (lymphadenectomy) are extended (Robson et al. 1969; Herrlinger et al. 1991) In addition, this incidence of lymphadenopathy may also depend upon the diligence of the pathologist in accurately identifing and evaluating all nodal tissue removed. In one prospective series, 511 patients with renal cell carcinoma were surgically treated; 320 underwent an extended retroperitoneal lymphadenectomy, while 191 had a limited or no lymph node dissection (Herrlinger et al. 1991). The incidence of positive lymph nodes was found to be 17.5% in the group undergoing a lymph node dissection compared to 10% in those who did not undergo this procedure. In our series of 264 patients at USC, a total of 57 patients (21%) were found to have lymph node involvement: 25 patients (44%) without evidence of distant metastases (stages IIIb and IIIc), and 32 patients (56%) with associated metastatic disease (stage IV). The 5- and 10-year recurrence-free survival in the 25 patients with stage III disease was 46% and 24%, respectively.

In most instances, patients with lymph node involvement have microscopic disease (Peters and Brown 1980). Computed tomography can detect retroperitoneal lymphadenopathy with approximately 95% sensitivity. However, it cannot determine the internal contents of the lymph nodes. In one report, it was found that greater than 50% of patients with renal cell carcinoma and retroperitoneal lymphadenopathy as evaluated by computed tomography, histologically had reactive changes that did not represent metastatic tumor involvement of the lymph node (Studer et al. 1990). This was particularly true when tumor necrosis was present in the primary lesion. Given that microscopic tumor in-

volvement of the lymph nodes occurs in a significant number of patients, coupled with the significant false-positives (even with the best of imaging studies), an unequivocal diagnosis of lymph node involvement with tumor can only be made on resected tissue.

Benefits of an extended lymphadenectomy may include: (1) more accurate pathologic staging which should help to dictate adjuvant treatment protocols; (2) potential curability if disease is limited to the primary tumor and regional lymph nodes; and (3) reduction in the incidence of renal fossa recurrences. Data from retrospective studies and nonrandomized prospective studies suggested that patients who underwent an extended retroperitoneal lymphadenectomy had an improved long-term survival when compared to patients who either did not have a retroperitoneal lymph node dissection, or in whom the dissection was limited (Giuliani et al. 1983, 1990; Herrlinger et al. 1991; Pizzocaro and Piva 1990). Herrlinger and associates (1991) reported a significantly improved survival in 320 patients undergoing an extended lymphadenectomy for renal cell carcinoma. The overall 5- and 10-year survival was 66% and 56%, respectively in patients undergoing a lymphadenectomy compared to 58% 5-year and 40% 10-year survival without lymphadenectomy ($P < 0.01$). This survival benefit was found to be highest among patients with Robson's stage I and II disease.

Skeptics to performing an ipsilateral retroperitoneal lymphadenectomy mention the following: (1) renal cell carcinoma metastasizes via both lymphatic and hematogenous routes; (2) the lymphatic drainage from the kidney is variable; (3) there is no effective adjuvant therapy for patients with lymph node-positive disease; and (4) an extended lymphadenectomy may increase the morbidity of the operation. Although renal cell carcinoma can metastasize by hematogenous and lymphatic channels, there are a substantial number of patients with isolated lymph node involvement only (25%) without clinical evidence of metastatic disease. Secondly, although the lymphatic drainage of the kidney is variable, an extended lymphadenectomy should include the majority of regional lymph nodes draining the ipsilateral kidney. Thirdly, regarding the lack of effective adjuvant therapy for patients with nodal disease, this is precisely the reason an extended lymphadenectomy should be performed as it may cure a significant number patients without the need for additional therapy. Lastly, we and others (Herrlinger et al. 1991; Swanson and Borges

1983; Sago et al. 1979) believe that there is little additional morbidity when a properly performed regional lymphadenectomy is executed. In fact, to safely perform a radical nephrectomy a regional lymphadenectomy may help set up the operative field. Therefore, since a retroperitoneal lymphadenectomy allows for improved surgical staging of the tumor, with some therapeutic benefit, and may lower the local tumor recurrence rate without increasing the operative morbidity and mortality, we firmly believe that it should be an integral component of a radical nephrectomy.

## 5.8
## Surgical Technique of Radical Nephrectomy

Radical nephrectomy is defined as early control of the vascular pedicle with en bloc removal of the kidney and ipsilateral adrenal gland within an intact Gerota's fascia. A regional retroperitoneal lymphadenectomy is routinely performed. Suitable candidates for this procedure should include those with potentially curable tumors (stages I–III) and those in good medical condition whose life expectancy would be reasonable without cancer of the kidney. Radical exenterative surgery is probably not advisable for poor-risk patients; rather, simple palliative nephrectomy may be indicated to control pain, bleeding, and refractory paraneoplastic syndromes (i.e., hypercalcemia), and in those patients considered for adjuvant experimental protocols. Age alone is not a contraindication to the procedure, provided the patient is a reasonable operative candidate. In selected patients with limited, resectable metastases (one or two metastatic deposits), aggressive surgical treatment combining radical nephrectomy and simultaneous excision of all metastatic lesions may be appropriate. Approximately 35% of these carefully selected patients may live 5 or more years (Middleton 1980; O'Dea et al. 1978; Skinner et al. 1971). This may be particularly true for patients with metastatic renal cell carcinoma to the lungs. Several reports have demonstrated an aggressive surgical approach can be performed safely with excellent survival outcomes in this group of patients (deKernion 1983; Tanguay et al. 1996).

The thoracoabdominal incision was initially employed for gastroeosphageal resections in the 1940s (Sweet 1947). Subsequently, this surgical approach was adopted for resection of large renal cell carcinomas (Chute et al. 1949). Cooper and associates first described the use of this approach in retroperitoneal dissections for testis tumors (Cooper et al. 1950).

The thoracoabdominal approach is the authors' preference for nearly all retroperitoneal tumors and employing this incision in the management of renal cell carcinomas is routine. We strongly believe that this incision provides the best possible exposure and visualization. The thoracoabdominal incision provides a versatile approach to either the retroperitoneum solely, or can be combined with an intra-abdominal approach for extensive tumors or in complicated cases. In addition, the thoracoabdominal approach allows evaluation of the intra-abdominal contents. This approach provides the ideal means to gain early vascular control of a renal tumor and allows for a safe, en bloc dissection. This is critical, particularly in large tumors with extensive collateral vessels, or those tumors with venous tumor thrombus involvement. We believe there are no absolute contraindications to the thoracoabdominal approach and routinely perform this incision for many indications including: radical nephrectomy, nephroureterectomy, all retroperitoneal tumors, retroperitoneal node dissections for testes tumors, and ileoureteral substitutions.

## 5.8.1
## Preoperative Preparation

Preoperative preparation is relatively routine. In older patients (>60 years), prophylactic preoperative digitalization is usual unless there is a specific contraindication to its use. We routinely give 0.5 mg of digoxin in the morning the day before surgery, followed by 0.25 mg that afternoon and 0.125 mg the evening before surgery. Patients with large renal tumors, in whom we anticipate a combined intra-abdominal approach with possible resection of a portion of the colonic mesentery, should undergo a short but effective bowel preparation the day before surgery. Several hours following breakfast on the day before surgery, 120 ml of emulsified castor oil is administered and the patient is placed on a clear liquid diet, and made NPO after midnight. Overnight hydration with intravenous fluids is important, particularly in patients undergoing a bowel preparation to ensure adequate hydration upon arrival at the operating room.

## 5.8.2
## Patient Positioning

Patient positioning is critical, and attention to detail facilitates all phases of the operation (Fig. 5.1). The patient should be positioned on the ipsilateral side of the operating table with the break of the table located immediately above the iliac crest. The contralateral leg (lower) is flexed 90° at the knee, and the hip is flexed about 30°. The ipsilateral shoulder is then torqued approximately 30° off the horizontal, and brought across the chest to be placed in an adjustable arm rest. The authors prefer to use a padded airplane arm rest, which provides an ideal positioning of the ipsilateral arm without pressure or stretch to the axillary structures. The contralateral arm is extended on to an arm board ensuring avoidance of hyperextension of the limb. The pelvis remains nearly supine or slightly rotated 10° off the horizontal plane. A rolled sheet is placed longitudinally under the ipsilateral back, ensuring avoidance of any pressure to

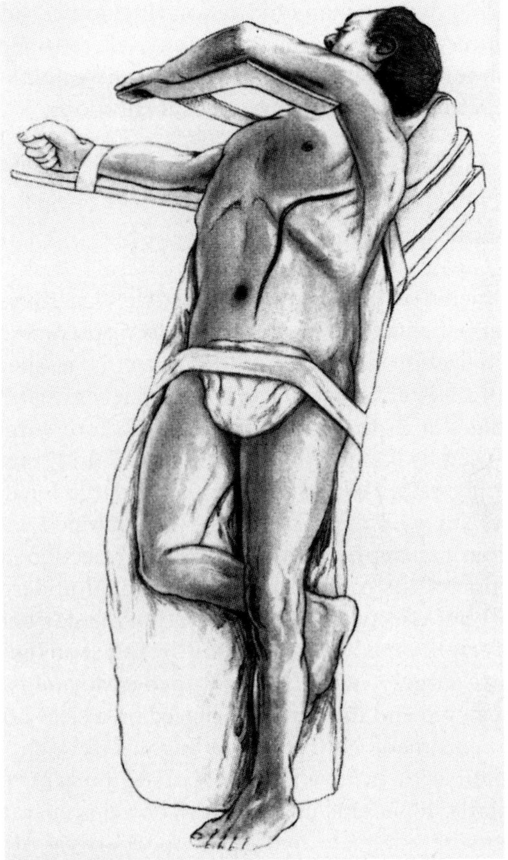

**Fig. 5.1.** Proper patient positioning for a right thoracoabdominal radical nephrectomy. Note that the patient's right side is adjacent to the ipsilateral edge of the operating table. A right paramedian incision is made

the buttocks. A similar roll is positioned under the contralateral abdomen to help secure the position. The table is then fully hyperextended and the patient secured with wide (3-inch) adhesive tape at the shoulder, hip, and leg. The table is tilted in the Trendelenburg position until the abdomen is in the horizontal plane. The ipsilateral leg remains extended (straight) along the lateral edge of the table, supported by a pillow behind the knee. All pressure points are padded.

## 5.8.3
## Surgical Dissection

Generally, an incision is made along the ninth rib. The size and location of the tumor, possible contiguous organ involvement, along with the body habitus of the patient, may otherwise dictate a higher or lower rib incision. The incision begins at the middle axillary line, and extends across the costochondral junction to the epigastrium in a transverse nature. The incision is then directed inferiorly as either a midline or paramedian incision. For very large tumors or bilateral tumors, a T-shaped incision may be employed, extending the horizontal portion of the epigastric incision across to the contralateral costochondral junction and then dropping an ipsilateral paramedian or midline extension inferiorly. This approach may also be employed when a vena caval tumor thrombus is associated with the tumor, requiring vascular control of the vena cava above the diaphragm at the level of the right atrium. For tumors associated with a vena caval tumor thrombus, and when control of the vena cava above the diaphragm or at the level of the right atrium is desired, a higher incision along the eighth or seventh rib is preferred.

We prefer a rib resection to an intercostal incision. Careful comparison of these two techniques reveals no difference in degree of pain or postoperative requirements for analgesics; rib resection is quicker, easier to close, and provides a wider exposure without fracturing adjacent ribs. The subcutaneous tissues and muscles overlying the rib and periosteum are incised using diathermy, and a subperiosteal rib resection is performed in the standard fashion.

The anterior rectus fascia is incised, the rectus muscle retracted laterally, and the rectus muscle transected in the epigastrium with control of the epigastric vessels. Lateral retraction of the muscle prevents denervation of the rectus muscle with resultant diastasis and weakness of the abdominal wall.

The costochondral junction is then divided with heavy scissors after careful and bluntly passing a Mayo scissors under the cartilage. Care must be taken to ensure that the abdominal peritoneum has been swept off the transversalis fascia posteriorly. This is an important step in order to identify the plane between the muscle and fascia of the abdominal wall (anteriorly) and the peritoneum (posteriorly), and in fact is the hallmark to performing an exclusively retroperitoneal dissection without entering the peritoneal cavity.

An exclusively retroperitoneal dissection is appropriate for small, less complicated renal tumors, or tumors of the renal pelvis or ureter. Development of the plane between the anterior surface of Gerota's fascia and the colonic mesentery and parietal peritoneum with large or vascular tumors may lead to considerable venous bleeding if the renal artery has not been previously ligated, and should be avoided. Therefore, when performing a radical nephrectomy for large, vascular renal cell carcinomas, it is preferable to enter the peritoneum after dividing the costochondral junction to gain early vascular control. When the peritoneum is opened widely, the pleura is incised and the diaphragm divided in the direction of its fibers. It is helpful to first dissect the peritoneum off the diaphragm posteriorly before dividing. This maneuver facilitates later mobilization of the liver for right-sided, and the spleen for left-sided tumors. A self-retaining Finochietto retractor is positioned, with the costochondral junction placed through the holes in the blades of the retractor and secured with towel clamps.

At this time, the peritoneum may or may not be entered, depending upon the surgeon's preference. Intra-abdominal access allows one to explore the intra-abdominal contents, including the liver, and also allows palpation of the regional lymph nodes to determine in advance the extent of the primary tumor. Moreover, opening the peritoneum may prove useful to the surgeon to determine accurately the plane between the lateral peritoneal reflection and the anterior surface of Gerota's fascia (Fig. 5.2). Definition of this plane is one of the most important aspects of the operation; its proper identification is achieved by developing a loose fibroareolar tissue plane that separates the anterior surface of Gerota's fascia from the posterior peritoneum. Once the plane is identified, it is further developed medially beyond the great vessels by both sharp and blunt dissection. Medial and superior retraction on the peritoneal envelope around the liver on the right side, and the spleen on the left side, facilitates and

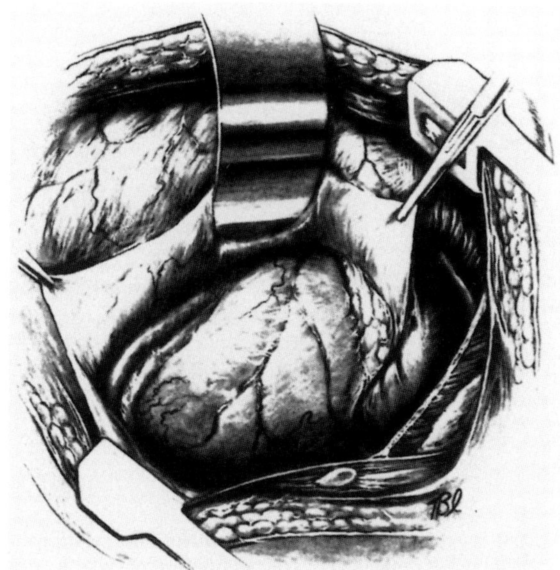

Fig. 5.2. For small, left-sided renal tumors, the transversalis fascia can be divided in the groove between the descending colon and the anterior surface of Gerota's fascia. This will allow the peritoneal envelope to be swept medially off the anterior surface of Gerota's fascia. The inferior mesenteric vein, splenic vein, and origin of the superior mesenteric artery should be identified. Immediately below the superior mesenteric artery is the left renal vein crossing the aorta anteriorly

enhances exposure to the ipsilateral kidney and retroperitoneum.

For left-sided tumors, the only limiting factor that prevents one from completely crossing the midline in this avascular plane is the inferior mesenteric artery. This artery may be ligated and divided to facilitate exposure. Once this plane has been completely developed on either side, certain important landmarks must be identified. The inferior mesenteric vein can be traced to its junction with the splenic vein. Just lateral to this structure is the superior mesenteric artery, an important anatomic landmark. In all cases, this artery should be located as it originates form the anterior surface of the aorta. Immediately caudal or posterior to the superior mesenteric artery is the left renal vein. The left renal vein and the superior mesenteric are the two most important anatomic structures to identify for both right- and left-sided dissections. For left-sided tumors, ligation and division of the three principal branches of the left renal vein should be performed; the left gonadal, the left adrenal, and the normally present ascending (posterior) lumbar vein that enters posteriorly. Control of these veins will facilitate retraction of the left renal vein and expose the left renal artery at its origin from the aorta (Fig. 5.3).

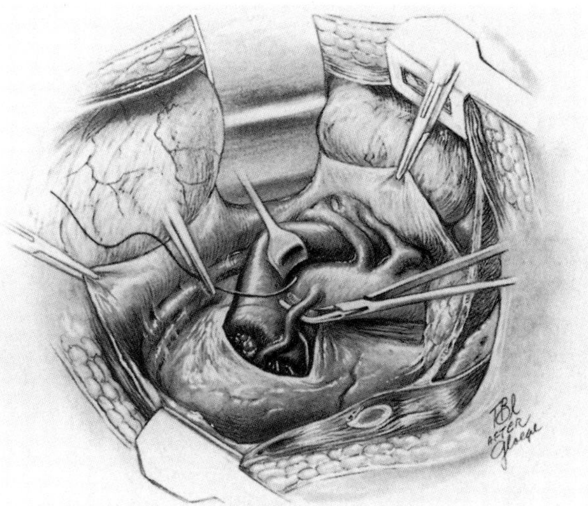

Fig. 5.3. Ligation of the left renal vein. Note the relationship between the left renal vein (retracted inferiorly) and the origin of the superior mesenteric artery and celiac artery

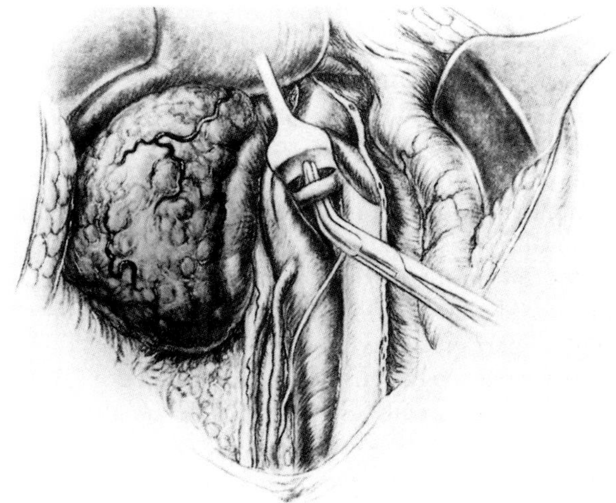

Fig. 5.4. Ligation of the right renal artery. The fibroareolar and lymphatic tissue is divided directly over the aorta. The left renal vein is mobilized and retracted to identify the renal artery. Note that ipsilateral lumbar arteries may also be divided to further mobilize the aorta and facilitate ligation and division of the right renal artery

For right-sided tumors, sufficient mobility of the left renal vein can usually be achieved to expose the aorta and right renal artery without ligating or dividing the left gonadal, adrenal, or ascending lumbar veins. If additional mobility of the left renal vein is required, ligation of the left adrenal branch (most medial) should provide the necessary mobility.

For large right-sided renal tumors, a combined intra-abdominal approach is routinely performed. Attention is directed toward ligation of the renal artery. First, the small bowel contents are retracted to the right and the ligament of Treitz is identified. The duodenum is kocherized to the right and the ligament of Treitz divided. This dissection should begin medial to the junction of the splenic and the inferior mesenteric vein. This maneuver also permits identification of the origin of the superior mesenteric artery. The aorta can be readily palpated below the region of the left renal vein, cephalad to the inferior mesenteric artery. Identification of the aorta is made possible with careful dissection of the fibroareolar lymphatic tissue surrounding it. Using right-angle clips, all fibroareolar and lymphatic tissue immediately over the aorta is divided. Dissection begins at the level of the inferior mesenteric artery and continues cephalad, taking care to ensure that one stays directly on top of the aorta. For right-sided tumors the inferior mesenteric artery need not be ligated. This is particularly important in elderly patients with some component of atherosclerosis; it is best to preserve this vessel. A gonadal artery is frequently encountered and can be clipped and divided. Imme-

diately cephalad to the gonadal artery, the left renal vein should be identified as it crosses over the vena cava. A Gil-Vernet or vein retractor can elevate the left renal vein and allow for dissection to continue up the aorta to the origin of the superior mesenteric artery. The right renal artery can then be identified medial to the aorta and posterior to the left renal vein (Fig. 5.4).

Prior to ligating the renal artery it is sometimes helpful to sweep all fibroareolar lymphatic tissue off the top and side wall of the aorta to the intervertebral ligaments and to ligate the ipsilateral lumbar arteries, usually two or three lumbar arteries exist below the ipsilateral renal artery. This maneuver provides additional mobility to the aorta and may facilitate safe ligation of the renal artery. Furthermore, ipsilateral lumbar arteries may also provide additional blood supply to large renal tumors. Following ligation of the renal artery and ipsilateral lumbar arteries, dissection continues medially down the right common iliac artery, which is below the lowest level of Gerota's fascia. The ureter and gonadal vessels are ligated and divided at this level.

The avascular plane of Toldt is then further incised and the ascending colon, small bowel attachments, and duodenum completely mobilized off Gerota's fascia and reflected medially (Fig. 5.5). Dissection of the small bowel mesenteric attachments is directed toward the previously kocherized duodenum; care must be taken not to extend this dissection

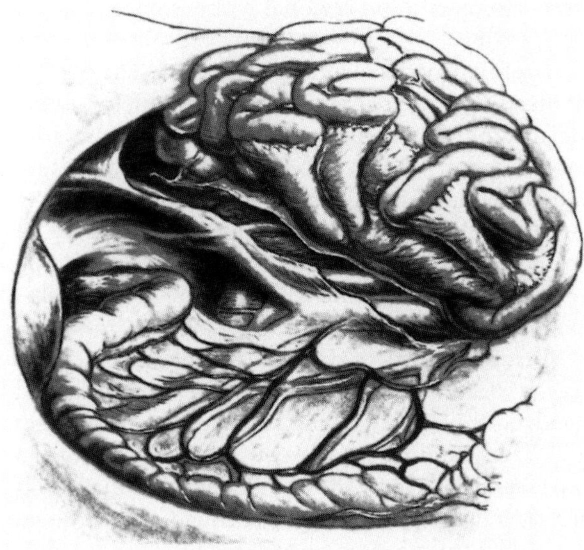

**Fig. 5.5.** Access to the right renal artery. The cecum and ascending colon are mobilized along the avascular line of Toldt, while the retroperitoneal attachments to the small bowel are mobilized and divided in a cephalad direction from the ileocecal junction to the ligament of Treitz (medial to the descending colonic mesentery). This maneuver kocherizes the duodenum and pancreas off the great vessels. Note that the inferior mesenteric vein (lateral to the aorta) is used to help identify the origin of the superior mesenteric artery from the aorta

cephalad into the hepatoduodenal ligament or portal structures. Once completed, this mobilization provides excellent exposure to the vena cava and entire retroperitoneum. The ascending colon and small bowel contents can be placed in a Lahey bowel bag and positioned on the patient's chest.

Next, the vena cava is skeletonized, beginning anteriorly and dividing all fibroareolar and lymphatic tissue over the vena cava extending in a cephalad direction. The gonadal vein is ligated and divided at the insertion into the vena cava. If the renal vein is free of tumor extending into the vena cava, it should be ligated. If a tumor thrombus is present, the nephrectomy should follow the technique described later; the renal vein should be dealt with only after the kidney is totally freed up from the surrounding tissues. Otherwise, the renal vein is ligated at this time. For right-sided tumors, all lumbar veins running to the vena cava (bilateral) below the level of the renal vein should be individually ligated so that the vena cava is entirely skeletonized. Dissection of the vena cava is then extended upward to the level of the insertion of the most inferior hepatic vein, representing the cephalad limit of dissection. Once the vena cava has been skeletonized, it

can be elevated with a vein retractor and all tissue (lymph node packet) from between the aorta and vena cava swept to the ipsilateral side, thus exposing the intervertebral ligaments posterior to the great vessels. Hemoclips should be placed on the ascending lumbar plexus, which passes posteriorly immediately adjacent to the sympathetic chain ganglion.

Attention is then directed toward the cephalad extent of Gerota's fascia, and the prominent right adrenal vein. When the peritoneum is mobilized off the diaphragm, the liver can be elevated and retracted medially. This maneuver allows one to visualize the adrenal and to dissect Gerota's fascia off the diaphragm, the quadratus lumborum, the psoas muscles from a lateral to medial direction. The right adrenal vein can then be easily ligated, thus exposing the right crus of the diaphragm. Once this is accomplished, the entire specimen can be removed en bloc with the regional nodes and with Gerota's fascia intact.

The sympathetic grooves should be carefully inspected as numerous veins course between these nerves, including the lumbar veins and the ascending lumbar venous trunk. These may require suture ligature if bleeding cannot be controlled by hemoclips. Generally, it is possible to preserve the ipsilateral sympathetic chain but this is usually of little consequence in most patients afflicted by renal cell carcinoma. The cisterna chyli should be identified and carefully clipped where it passes medial to the right crus of the diaphragm, posterior to the origin of the right renal artery. This will prevent lymph leak during the postoperative period. Inspection of the origin of the superior mesenteric artery may also reveal some lymph leak from dilated lacteals that run parallel to the artery in this area. These should also be individually clipped.

If the primary right renal tumor is small, a radical nephrectomy and regional lymph node dissection can be performed entirely via the retroperitoneal approach. The advantage of a pure retroperitoneal dissection is the lack of subsequent adhesions and prevention of possible small bowel obstruction. In addition, there is less of an ileus with earlier postoperative return of bowel function.

For small left-sided tumors, it is usually possible to incise the transversalis fascia at the junction of the peritoneum and Gerota's fascia laterally, so that the descending colon and its mesentery can be swept off the anterior surface of Gerota's fascia medially. The inferior mesenteric vein should be identified and traced to its junction with the splenic vein in order to identify the superior mesenteric artery. The left renal vein passes immediately below the origin of this artery. Once identified, the left renal vein is mobilized by ligation of the adrenal, gonadal, and posterior ascending lumbar veins, allowing access to the left renal artery.

For large or vascular left-sided tumors, it is best to approach the dissection again via an intraperitoneal route. The duodenum can be mobilized near the ligament of Treitz, with intraperitoneal identification of the inferior mesenteric vein. One should then divide all tissue directly over the aorta with attention focused on the crossing left renal vein. Once the renal left vein has been identified, it should be mobilized by ligating the adrenal, gonadal, and posterior ascending lumbar veins. In addition, ligation of the ipsilateral lumbar arteries will also provide some added mobility to the aorta and allow for early and safe ligation of the left renal artery. The renal vein can then be elevated and the left renal artery ligated and divided. If no tumor thrombus is present, the left renal vein can then be ligated at its insertion into the vena cava. All fibroareolar and lymphatic tissue is then swept off the top of the vena cava medially, thus cleaning the ipsilateral side wall of the vena cava. The ipsilateral left lumbar veins are ligated at this point. They should be ligated at the junction of the vena cava down to the level of where the right common iliac artery crosses. The left gonadal vessels and ureter are divided where they cross the common iliac vessels.

Gerota's fascia can be mobilized off the quadratus lumborum and psoas muscle posteriorly. The vascular communications between the adrenal and phrenic vessels are clipped and divided superiorly; the celiac ganglion is also clipped and divided, thus exposing the left crus of the diaphragm.

The aorta should then be skeletonized by dividing all fibroareolar and lymphatic tissue immediately over the aorta down to its bifurcation. For most left-sided tumors, the inferior mesenteric artery must be ligated and divided unless there is marked evidence of atherosclerotic disease of the aorta, in which case a wide regional node dissection is probably not indicated and preservation of the inferior mesenteric artery should performed. The uppermost lumbar arteries are ligated off the aorta. Usually, it is not necessary to ligate the lumbar vessels distal to the inferior mesenteric artery, an exception being the relatively young patient in whom an aggressive dissection is performed. The aorta can then be elevated and all fibroareolar and lymphatic tissue swept from underneath the great vessels over the intravertebral ligaments to the ipsilateral side. This provides removal of the kidney within Gerota's fascia along with the regional lymph nodes in an en bloc fashion.

Careful inspection should be made to ensure that all bleeding is well controlled. We routinely inspect the origins of the lumbar arteries and veins and ensure that they are well secured with a silk ligature and a medium-sized hemoclip. We also inspect the renal pedicle and the inferior mesenteric artery (if ligated), and ensure that they too are secured with a hemoclip along with the silk ligature. The wound is then irrigated with sterile water.

Retroperitoneal drains are not necessary; however, a size 22 chest tube is routinely inserted and removed the day following surgery. The diaphragm is closed with a running size 0 absorbable suture in two layers. Closure of the remainder of the incision is performed by figure-of-eight, through-and-through, nonabsorbable sutures, securing all muscular layers of the chest and abdomen in one layer. Care should be taken to ensure that the knots are inverted, particularly in thin individuals. Medially, the diaphragm must be incorporated in several of the closing sutures to ensure separation of the pleural and abdominal or retroperitoneal cavities.

## 5.8.4
## Technical Considerations

Several comments regarding the operative technique deserve specific mention. Proper patient selection and good surgical judgment are essential prerequisites. Patients with extensive atherosclerosis of their aorta are best managed without extensive mobilization of the aorta and an aggressive regional lymph node dissection is probably not indicated.

Ligation and division of the ipsilateral lumbar arteries below the level of the renal pedicle facilitates aortic mobilization and allows easier and safer vascular control of the renal artery. In addition, only ipsilateral lumbar arteries need to be ligated and divided on right-sided tumors. Bleeding from an avulsed lumbar vessel can occur and result in a troublesome problem. Placement of hemoclips on the distal portion of each vessels facilitates this portion of the operation. We feel it is best to ligate the lumbar vessels (arteries and veins) at their origin from the great vessels and place a medium hemoclip to doubly secure the vessel. Occasionally, bleed from a torn lumbar artery or vein may occur despite all precautions, in which case the use of an Allis forceps clamp is helpful. An arterial suture should be available at all times to help control bleeding from a torn or avulsed lumbar vessel.

The cisterna chyli should be identified behind the right renal artery, located in the region medial to the right crus of the diaphragm, between the aorta and vena cava. This should be ligated or secured with a hemoclip to prevent significant loss of protein during the postoperative period and possible chylous ascites. Major hemorrhage from the renal hilum is potentially the most serious complication during a radical nephrectomy. Should this occur, it can almost always be controlled by direct posterior compression of the renal pedicle against the vertebral bodies. Complete dissection of this area and mobilization of the aorta will allow identification of the bleeding vessel and facilitate vascular control.

## 5.8.5
### Postoperative Considerations

The routine use of chest tubes will help to avoid the 30%–35% incidence of hemopneumothorax, with consequent prolonged hospitalization, that occurs when chest tubes are not used. In general, the tube is maintained on suction until significant drainage ceases (usually within 24h), at which time it is removed. Other postoperative complications following a radical nephrectomy are similar to those following any major surgical procedure. Several critical points, however, should be emphasized. When an ipsilateral lymphadenectomy is performed, the sympathetic ganglia may occasionally be removed unilaterally, resulting in a warm ipsilateral lower extremity, a consequence of peripheral vasodilation of the leg, compared with the normal but relatively cool contralateral extremity. This event may occasionally cause a panic-stricken call from the intensive care unit; the anxiety can be relieved if the contralateral distal pulses are predictably intact. Occasionally, diarrhea may result from ischemia of the large bowel following ligation of the inferior mesenteric artery. This is a rare event in younger patients, and is usually managed conservatively without consequences or long-term sequelae.

Concern over possible devascularization of the spinal cord is not warranted, provided that no lumbar arteries are ligated above the renal pedicle. The spinal cord ends at the level of the first lumbar vertebral body. The nutrient arteries to the spinal cord, the anterior and posterior longitudinal spinal arteries, arise from the vertebral arteries and receive additional blood supply from the intercostal and high lumbar arteries through radicular branches. The main lower anterior radicular artery provides collateral blood supply to the anterior spinal area and is called the arteria radicularis magna or artery of Adamkiewicz (Ferguson et al. 1975). This artery originates from the thoracic aorta in 50% of patients, and from the lumbar region in the other 50% (Adams and van Geetruyden 1956; Coupland and Reeve 1968). However, it has been shown that in those patients in whom the arteria radicularis magna originates in the lumbar region, there is an important radicular artery from the lower thoracic aorta that is consistently present and provides adequate collateral circulation to the anterior spinal artery (Adams and van Geetruyden 1956; Coupland and Reeve 1968). We believe that extensive aortic mobilization with ligation of the lumbar arteries is safe and an integral component of a properly performed radical nephrectomy. Again, patients with extensive atherosclerotic vessels are not the ideal candidates for this excessive dissection and good surgical judgment is important to determine the appropriate candidate. In qualified hands, the technique of a thoracoabdominal radical nephrectomy is safe and extremely well tolerated by the patient.

## 5.9
### Management of Tumors Involving the Vena Cava

Renal cell carcinomas may invade surrounding parenchyma directly and extend through the capsule to invade the perinephric fat and/or contiguous visceral structures. They may also expand into the areas of least resistance such as the renal vein and vena cava. It has become apparent that tumors with venous tumor thrombus extension, even into the vena cava, do not necessarily carry an ominous prognosis if they are completely excised and are not associated with perinephric fat, contiguous visceral invasion, or regional nodal or distant metastases (Skinner et al. 1971, 1989; Glazer and Novick 1996; Libertino et al. 1987; Swierzewski et al. 1994). An exception to this is when the tumor thrombus actually infiltrates into the endothelial wall of the vessel, an adverse prognostic factor (Hatcher et al. 1991; Mrstik et al. 1992).

With our extensive experience with renal cell carcinoma and venous tumor thrombus involvement, we have developed a right thoracoabdominal approach to remove extensive venous tumor thrombi en bloc with the primary tumor that we believe provides optimal exposure to the upper vena cava and allows vascular control of all venous inflow to the cava (Skinner et al. 1989). Experience with the midline transabdominal approach with median sternotomy extension has not been as good owing to poor exposure of the vena cava and difficulty in getting around the liver. Only a few patients demonstrate significant venous tumor thrombus extension into the atrium which will demand cardiopulmonary bypass. Usually, small tumor extensions into the atrium can be managed without the need for bypass, thereby avoiding the need to administer heparin and the potential for increased blood loss above and beyond what is already a bloody operation under the best circumstances.

The thoracoabdominal approach that we routinely use involves excising the seventh rib, and extending the incision in the epigastrium to the midline and then inferiorly as a midline or paramedian incision to a level below the umbilicus. For left-sided tumors, the transverse portion of the incision in the epigastrium can be extended to the left costochondral junction (T-shaped) as previously mentioned. Early ligation of the renal artery is again essential to this procedure along with complete isolation of the vena cava with ligation of all lumbar veins. This is accomplished by dividing the ascending colon and peritoneal attachments to the small bowel mesentery so that the bowel, duodenum, and pancreas can be elevated on the superior mesenteric artery pedicle. This allows access and early ligation of the renal artery. The vena cava can then be mobilized by ligating and dividing all lumbar veins and applying a Rummel tourniquet loosely around the distal vena cava and the contralateral left renal vein (for right-sided tumors) or the right renal artery (for left-sided tumors). Note that for right-sided tumors, the collateral branches to the left renal vein should be preserved if possible. The kidney and Gerota's fascia are then completely mobilized, with en bloc dissection of the periaortic and renal hilar lymph nodes. The only remaining attachments at this time are the renal vein and the intracaval thrombus.

Patients with tumor thrombus extending to the level of the inferior hepatic veins (level II) or higher (level III, to the level of the right atrium) will require proximal vascular control of the vena cava in the pericardium, at the junction of the vena cava and right atrium. A vertical pericardiotomy is made, ensuring avoidance of the phrenic nerve. A Rummel tourniquet is applied loosely around the vena cava just below its insertion into the right atrium (interpericardial). Patients with a subhepatic tumor thrombus (level I) require only a Rummel tourniquet placed around the vena cava at a level below the liver.

Patients with intrahepatic tumor thrombus (level II) or higher (level III) will require isolation and control with soft Fogarty vascular clamps of the superior mesenteric artery. The inferior mesenteric artery is similarly occluded. Two Crafoord vascular clamps are placed across the hepatoduodenal ligament (porta hepatis), after which the Rummel tourniquets on the distal vena cava, the contralateral renal vein, and the intrathoracic cava are tightened, effectively isolating the vena cava from all venous inflow (Fig. 5.6). For left-sided tumors, a soft Fogarty vascular clamp is place on the right renal artery, thus obviating the need to occlude the right renal vein.

Patients with tumor thrombus extension to the level of the right atrium (level III), with only a small intra-atrial component, can have a purse-string suture placed around the atrial appendage. A finger inserted into the atrium can gently milk or push the tumor thrombus down the vena cava so the Rumel tourniquet can be tightened above the thrombus extension at the junction of the vena cava and right atrium (Fig. 5.7). A large or patulous tumor thrombus extending into or involving a greater portion of the atrium will require cardiopulmonary bypass to prevent intraoperative embolization.

Once complete vascular control has been performed, a longitudinal incision is made into the posterior portion of the renal vein, just proximal to the junction with the vena cava. This incision is carefully extended first posteriorly and then anteriorly along the renal vein, ensuring that this incision is not extended into or along the vena cava. Generally, the tumor thrombus can be gently extracted, intact from the cava (Fig. 5.8). Occasionally, the thrombus is adherent to the wall of the vena cava, requiring instrument dissection for complete removal.

The patient should be placed in the "head-down" position during the extraction of the tumor thrombus to prevent subsequent air embolization. Trial occlusion of the vena cava should be performed prior to the incision into the renal vein to ensure the patient has sufficient intravascular volume to sustain the systemic pressure at appropriate levels during this portion of the procedure. The anesthesiologist is critical in these events and to the success of the procedure. Mannitol should be given prior to occluding the venous inflow into the vena cava. Overall, the surgeon has about 20 min of safe, warm, hepatic ischemia time during which time the tumor and thrombus can be extracted and the venotomy closed (Fig. 5.9). We routine place a fenestrated vascular clip (DeWeess) on the infrarenal vena cava to prevent pulmonary emboli in patients who have had clot

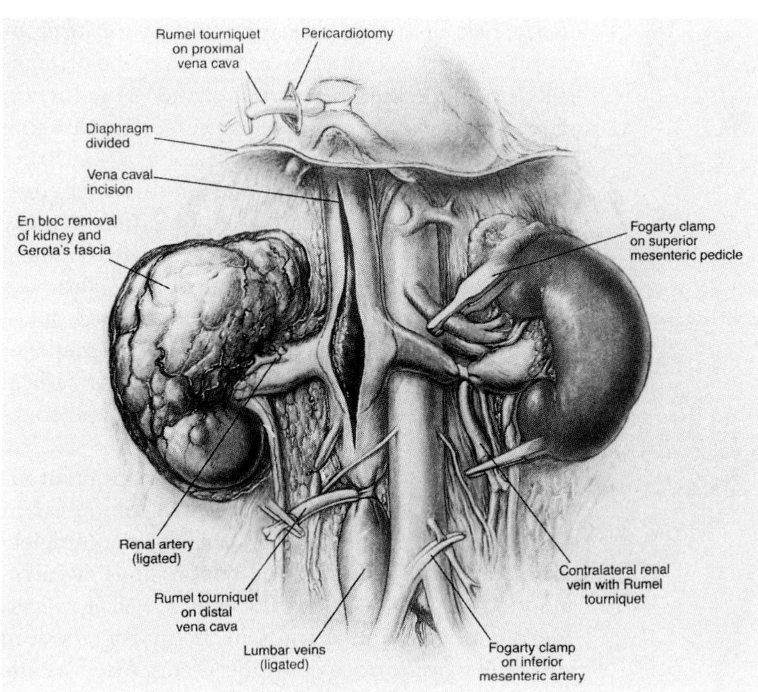



**Fig. 5.6.** Surgical maneuvers necessary for a safe and effective method of removing a level II or III tumor thrombus

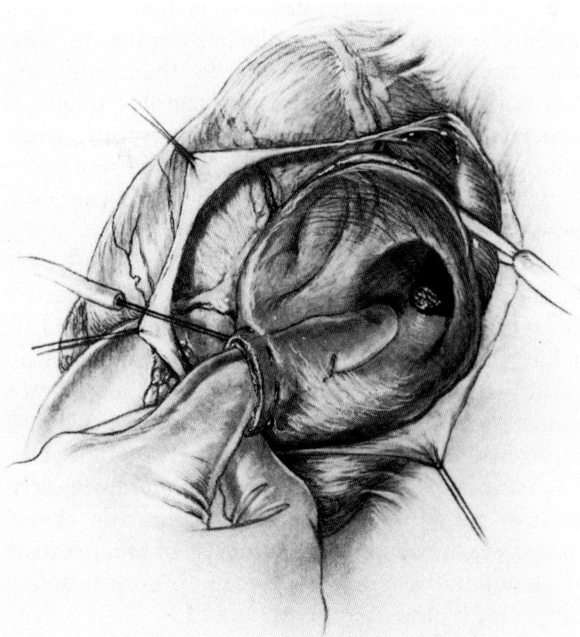

**Fig. 5.7.** The cardiac surgeon can insert a finger through the atrial appendage and into the right atrium in order to milk the tumor thrombus out of the atrium at the time the primary renal tumor and thrombus are simultaneously extracted from the abdominal vena cava. Once the thrombus has descended out of the atrium into the proximal inferior vena cava, a Rumel tourniquet is tightened around the inferior vena cava at its junction with the atrium. This provides proximal venous control, prevents intraoperative embolization, and obviates the need for cardiopulmonary bypass

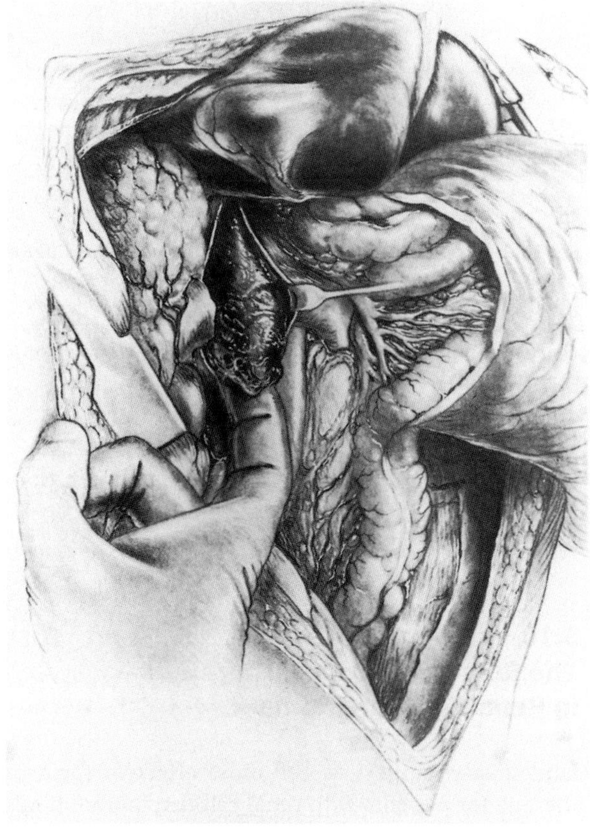

**Fig. 5.8.** Tumor thrombus enucleation. Note that the venotomy should be made in the renal vein (initially posterior) just adjacent to the vena cava. This helps to prevent extension of the venotomy up the vena cava with loss of vascular control

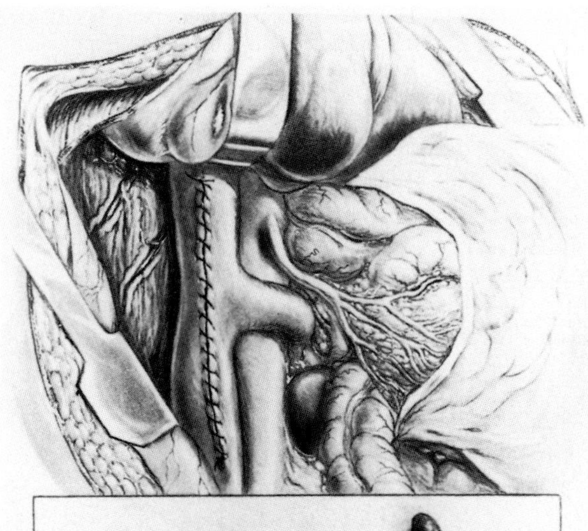

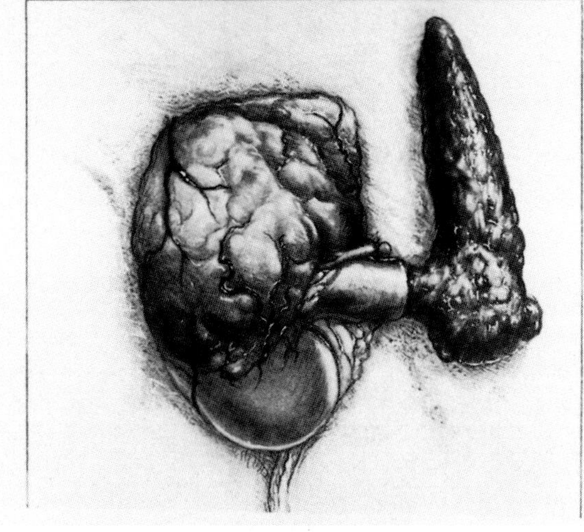

**Fig. 5.9.** Illustration of operative field following tumor removal. We routinely place a fenestrated DeWeese caval clip (infrarenal) in patients whose tumor preoperatively completely occluded the vena cava, in those who had prior evidence of pulmonary embolism, and in those in whom clot is encountered in the distal vena cava

below the level of the tumor thrombus. In addition, postoperative anticoagulation should also be instituted in these patients.

## 5.10
## The Role of Radiation Therapy in Renal Cell Carcinoma

Undeniably, surgery is the most effective form of therapy for patients with renal cell carcinoma. It has been proposed that preoperative radiation therapy may provide several benefits to patients with renal cell carcinoma (Rafla 1970; Rost and Brosig 1977; Flocks and Kadesky 1958; Riches 1966). These benefits were to include the following: (1) reduction

of the risk of tumor dissemination at the time of nephrectomy; (2) reduction of the size of the primary lesion; (3) increased resectability; and (4) reduction of tumor vascularity. Based on some encouraging preliminary retrospective data (Cox et al. 1970), a prospective randomized, national, multicenter clinical trial, comparing preoperative radiation therapy followed by radical nephrectomy with radical nephrectomy alone, was launched and, although the data were never published (unpublished data), this study failed to demonstrate any benefit to preoperative adjuvant radiotherapy versus radical nephrectomy alone (Cox E.C. 1998, personal communication).

Postoperative radiation therapy has the theoretical benefit of providing local control of tumor in patients with positive surgical margins, incompletely resected primary tumors, or lymph node involvement (Riches 1966; Mantyla et al. 1977). However, the role of radiation therapy in the management of renal cell carcinoma has not been supported by the literature (Juusela et al. 1977; van der Werf-Messing 1973; Finney 1973; Peeling et al. 1969). The problem with radiotherapy is that renal cell carcinoma is a relatively radioresistant tumor. This resistance is probably related to the significant degree of necrosis, cystic, and anaerobic qualities associated with the tumor. Furthermore, the large volume of normal (surrounding) tissue likely included in the radiation field may be significant and increase the potential for morbidity.

Currently, radiation therapy in renal cell carcinoma is generally reserved for palliation, most often for symptomatic bony metastases (see Chap. 10). It has been shown that symptomatic responses or improvements following radiation for bony metastases are excellent; 77% of those with bone pain respond at the treatment site (Halperin and Harisiadis 1983). Overall, radiation therapy clearly has a palliative role for symptomatic bony metastases; however, the routine use of preoperative or postoperative radiation therapy is currently not supported by the literature.

## 5.11
## The Role of Chemotherapy in Renal Cell Carcinoma

Despite the remarkable improvements and response rates of single and combination chemotherapy in some solid tumors, renal cell carcinoma remains a chemoresistant tumor. The most common agents, vinblastine and floxiuridine, have response rates of

7% and 16%, respectively (YAGODA et al. 1995). In an excellent review of 72 agents, evaluated in 3500 patients, between 1983 and 1992, an overall objective response rate of 5.6% was found, mostly of short duration (YAGODA et al. 1995). Furthermore, hormone therapy has also been found to be equally ineffective (DEKERNION 1982). Currently, there is no role for chemotherapy or hormone therapy in the treatment of renal cell carcinoma.

## 5.12
## Role of Surgery in Patients with Metastatic Renal Cell Carcinoma

The role of surgery in patients with metastatic renal cell cancer continues to evolve. There will be a number of patients with renal cell carcinoma who present with solitary or limited metastases. The 5-year survival following complete resection of the primary and metastatic deposit is approximately 25%–35% (MIDDLETON 1980: O'DEA et al. 1978; SKINNER et al. 1971). Patients who respond best to this aggressive form of surgical therapy are those with solitary pulmonary lesions (MALDAZYS and DEKERNION 1986; TANGUAY et al. 1996).

Palliation of symptoms from advanced renal cell carcinoma is a reasonable indication for nephrectomy in the face of multiple metastases granted that the primary tumor can be removed without excessive morbidity or mortality. Patients with paraneoplastic syndromes may also benefit from palliative resection. Although most would agree that palliative nephrectomy in this setting is justified, only 10% of patients can be expected to survive for 1 year with nephrectomy alone and 50% of these patients die within 4 months (BELLDEGRUN and DEKERNION 1988).

Advances in immunotherapy for renal cell carcinoma have raised the issue of surgery in the treatment of patients with metastatic disease. There is evidence to suggest that there are improved response rates to immunotherapy when it is administered following the removal of the primary lesion (WALTHER et al. 1993; MINASIAN et al. 1993; UMEDA and NIIJIMA 1986; BELLDEGRUN et al. 1991). Although there is evidence to suggest that patients receiving immunotherapy respond better when nephrectomy is performed prior to treatment, the timing of nephrectomy is a topic of debate. In a large National Cancer Institute study, 40% of patients who underwent nephrectomy were unable to start IL-2 therapy due to progression of disease or postoperative complications (WALTHER et al. 1993). Adjuvant nephrectomy is also currently performed on patients who are on protocols that require tumor-infiltrating lymphocytes (BELLDEGRUN et al. 1993). Obviously, further trials will be important to determine the exact role of surgery in the treatment of patients with metastatic renal cell carcinoma.

## References

Adams HD, van Geetruyden HH (1956) Neurologic complications of aortic surgery. Ann Surg 144:547–610

Allbright F (1941) Case records of the Massachusetts General Hospital – case 39061. N Engl J Med 225:789–796

Aso Y, Homma Y (1992) A survey on incidental renal cell carcinoma in Japan. J Urol 147:340–343

Beahrs OH, Myers MH (eds) (1983) American Joint Committee on Cancer: manual for staging cancer, 2nd edn. Lippincott, Philadelphia, 178

Belldegrun A, deKernion JB (1988) Renal tumors. In: Walsh P, et al. (eds) Campbell's urology. Saunders, Philadelphia, pp 2283–2326

Belldegrun A, Abi-Aad AS, Figlin RA, deKernion JB (1991) Renal cell carcinoma: basic and current approaches to therapy. Semin Oncol 18:96–101

Belldegrun A, Pierce W, Kaboo R, et al. (1993) Interferon-alpha primed tumor-infiltrating lymphocytes combined with interleukin-2 and interferon-alpha as a therapy for metastatic renal cell carcinoma. J Urol 150:1384–1390

Boxer RJ, Waisman J, Lieber MM, Mampaso FM, Skinner DG (1978) "Non-metastatic" hepatic dysfunction associated with renal cell carcinoma. J Urol 119:468–471

Boxer RJ, Waisman J, Lieber MM, Mampaso FM, Skinner DG (1979) Renal carcinoma: computer analysis of 96 patients treated by nephrectomy. J Urol 122:598–601

Bretheau D, Lechevallier E, Eghazarian C, Grisoni V, Coulange C (1995) Prognostic significance of incidental renal cell carcinoma. Eur Urol 27:319–323

Chasan SA, Pothel RL, Huben RP (1989) Management and prognostic significance of hypercalcemia in renal cell carcinoma. Urology 33:167–170

Cherukuri SV, Johenning PW, Ram MD (1977) Systemic effects of hypernephroma. Urology 10:93–97

Chuang C-K, Lai M-K, Chang P-L, et al. (1992) Xanthogranulomatous pyelonephritis; experience in 36 cases. J Urol 147:333–336

Chute R, Soutter L, Kerr WS (1949) The value of the thoracoabdominal incision in the removal of kidney tumors. N Engl J Med 241:951–960

Cooper JF, Leadbetter WF, Chute R (1950) The thoracoabdominal approach for retroperitoneal gland dissection: its application to testis tumors. Surg Gynecol Obstet 90:486–496

Coulange C (1993) Enquete epidemiologique sur les tumeurs du rein. In: Abbou CC, Lobel B (eds) Synthese et Recommendations en Onco-Urologie. Monogr Prog Urol Paris, pp 200–202

Coupland GA, Reeve TS (1968) Paraplegia: a complication of excision of abdominal aortic aneurysm. Surgery 64: 879–881

Cranston WI, Luff RH, Owen D, Rawlins MD (1973) Studies on the pathogenesis of fever in renal carcinoma. Clin Sci Mol Med 45:459–467

Creevy CD (1935) Confusing clinical manifestations of malignant renal neoplasms. Arch Intern Med 55:895–916

Cronin RE, Kaehny WD, Miller PD, et al. (1976) Renal cell carcinoma: unusual systemic manifestations. Medicine 55:291–311

Cummings KB, Robertson RP (1977) Prostaglandin: increased production by renal cell carcinoma. J Urol 118:720–723

deKernion JB (1982) Treatment of advanced renal cell carcinoma – traditional methods and innovative approaches. J Urol 130:2–7

Dinney CPN, Awad SA, Gajewski JB, et al. (1992) Analysis of imaging modalities, staging systems, and prognostic indicators for renal cell carcinoma. Urology 39:122–129

Eckschlager T, Kodet R (1994) Renal cell carcinoma in children; a single institution's experience. Med Pediatr Oncol 23:36–39

Ferguson LRJ, Bergan JJ, Conn J Jr, Yao JST (1975) Spinal ischemia following abdominal aortic surgery. Ann Surg 181:267–272

Figueroa AJ, Stein JP, Cunningham JA, Ginsberg DA, Skinner DG (1995) Xanthogranulomatous pyelonephritis in a pregnant woman: a case report and review of the literature. Urology 48:294–297

Finney R (1973) The value of radiotherapy in the treatment of hypernephroma – a clinical trial. Br J Urol 45:258–269

Flocks RH, Kadesky MC (1958) Malignant neoplasms of the kidney: an analysis of 353 patients followed five years or more. J Urol 79:196–201

Gibbons RP, Montie JE, Correa RJ Jr, Mason JT (1976) Manifestations of renal cell carcinoma. Urology 8:201–206

Giuliani L, Martorana G, Giberti C, Pescatore D, Magnani G (1983) Results of radical nephrectomy with extensive lymphadenectomy for renal cell carcinoma. J Urol 130:664–668

Giuliani L, Giberti C, Martorana G, Rovida S (1990) Radical extensive surgery for renal cell carcinoma: long-term results and prognostic factors. J Urol 143:468–474

Glazer AA, Novick AC (1996) Long-term followup after surgical treatment for renal cell carcinoma extending into the right atrium. J Urol 155:448–450

Gold PJ, Fefer A, Thompson JA (1996) Paraneoplastic manifestations of renal cell carcinoma. Semin Urol Oncol 14:216–222

Goldberg RS, Pilcher DB, Yates JW (1980) The aggressive surgical management of hypercalcemia due to ectopic parathormone production. Cancer 45:2652–2654

Golde DW, Schambelan M, Weintraub BD, et al. (1974) Gonadotropin-secreting renal carcinoma. Cancer 33:1048–1053

Golimbu M, Joshi P, Sperber A, Tessler A, Al-Askari S, Morales P (1986) Renal cell carcinoma: survival and prognostic factors. Urology 27:291–301

Gotoh A, Kitazawa S, Mizuno Y, et al. (1993) Common expression of parathyroid hormone-related protein and no correlation of calcium levels in renal cell carcinoma. Cancer 71:2803–2806

Gross AJ, Wofff M, Fandrey J, et al. (1994) Prevalence of paraneoplastic erythropoietin production by renal cell carcinomas. Clin Invest 72:123–130

Guinan PD, Ablin RJ, Dubin A, Nourkayhan S, Bush IM (1975) Carcinoembryonic antigen test in renal cell carcinoma. Urology 5:185–187

Halperin EC, Harisiadis L (1983) The role of radiation therapy in the management of metastatic renal cell carcinoma. Cancer 51:614–617

Hanash KA (1982) The nonmetastatic hepatic dysfunction syndrome associated with renal cell carcinoma (hypernephroma); Stauffer's syndrome. Prog Clin Biol Res 100:301–316

Hanash KA, Utz DC, Ludwig J, et al. (1971) Syndrome of reversible hepatic dysfunction associated with hypernephroma: an experimental study. Invest Urol 8:399–404

Hatcher PA, Anderson EE, Paulson DF, Carson CC, Robertson JE (1991) Surgical management and prognosis of renal cell carcinoma invading the vena cava. J Urol 145:20–24

Hermanek P, Schrott KM (1990) Evaluation of the new tumor, nodes, and metastases classification of renal cell carcinoma. J Urol 144:238–242

Herrlinger A, Schrott KM, Schott G, Sigel A (1991) What are the benefits of extended dissection of the regional renal lymph nodes in the therapy of renal cell carcinoma? J Urol 146:1224–1227

Hollifield JW, Page DL, Smith C, et al. (1975) Renin-secreting clear cell carcinoma of the kidney. Arch Intern Med 135:859–864

Jobe BA, Bierman MH, Mezzacappa FJ, et al. (1993) Hyperglycemia as a paraneoplastic endocrinopathy in renal cell carcinoma: a case report and review of the literature. Nebr Med J 78:348–351

Juusela HM, Malmio K, Alfthan O, Oravisto KJ (1977) Preoperative irradiation in the treatment of renal adenocarcinoma. Scand J Urol Nephrol 11:277–281

Kantor AF (1977) Current concepts in the epidemiology and etiology of primary renal cell carcinoma. J Urol 131:1053–1055

Keily JM (1966) Hypernephroma – the internist's tumor. Med Clin North Am 50:1067–1083

Kessler O, Mukamel E, Hadar H, Gillon G, Konechezky M, Servadio C (1994) Effect of improved diagnosis of renal cell carcinoma on the course of the disease. J Surg Oncol 57:201–204

Konnack JW, Grossman HB (1985) Renal cell carcimom as an incidental finding. J Urol 134:1094–1096

Laski ME, Vugrin D (1987) Paraneoplastic syndromes in hypernephroma. Semin Nephrol 7:123–130

Libertino JA, Zinman L, Watkins E Jr (1987) Long-term results of resection of renal cell cancer with extension into inferior vena cava. J Urol 137:21–24

Lindop GBM, Fleming S (1984) Renin in renal cell carcinoma – an immuno-cytochemical study using an antibody to pure human renin. J Clin Pathol 37:27–31

Lytton B, Rosof B, Evans JS (1965) Parathyroid hormone-like activity in a renal carcinoma producing hypercalcemia. J Urol 93:127–131

Maldazys JD, deKernion JB (1986) Prognostic factors in renal carcinoma. J Urol 136:376–379

Malek RS, Elder JS (1978) Hypernephroma in the solitary kidney: experience with 20 cases and review of the literature. J Urol 116:553–556

Mantyla M, Nordman E, Minkkinen J (1977) Postopertive radiotherapy of renal adenocarcinoma. Ann Clin Res 9:252–256

Marshall FF, Powell KC (1982) Lymphadenectomy for renal cell carcinoma: anatomical and therapeutic considerations. J Urol 128:677–681

McDougal WS, Garnick MB (1995) Clinical signs and symptoms of renal cell carcinoma. In: Vogelzang NJ, Shipley WU, Scardino PT, et al. (eds) Comprehensive textbook of genitourinary oncology. Williams & Wilkins, Baltimore, pp 154–159

McNicholos DW, Segura JW, DeWeerd JH (1981) Renal cell carcinoma: long-term survival and late recurrence. J Urol 126:17–23

Medeiros LJ, Gelb AB, Weiss LM (1987) Low-grade renal cell carcinoma: a clinicopathologic study of 53 cases. Am J Surg Pathol 11:633–642

Medeiros LJ, Gelb AB, Weiss LM (1988) Renal cell carcinoma: prognostic significance of morphologic parameters in 121 cases. Cancer 61:1639–1651

Middleton AW Jr (1980) Indications for and results of nephrectomy for metastatic renal cell carcinoma. Urol Clin North Am 7:711–717

Minasian LM, Motzer RJ, Gluck L, Mazumdar M, Valamis V, Krown SE (1993) Interferon alpha-2a in advanced renal cell carcinoma. Treatment results and survival in 159 patients with long-term follow-up. J Clin Oncol 11:1368–1375

Mrstik S, Salamon J, Weber R, Stogermayer F (1992) Microscopic venous infiltration as predictor of relapse in renal cell carcinonoma. J Urol 148:271–274

Muggia FM (1990) Overview of cancer-related hypercalcemia: epidemiology and etiology. Semin Oncol 17:3–9

Nakano E, Iwasaki A, Seguchi T, et al. (1992) Incidentally diagnosed renal cell carcinoma. Eur Urol 21:294–298

Nielsen HO (1973) Arterial hypertension due to a renin-producing renal carcinoma. Scand J Urol Nephrol 9:293–296

Nurmi MJ (1984) Prognostic factors in renal carcinoma: an evaluation of operative findings. Br J Urol 56:270–275

O'Dea MJ, Zincke H, Utz DC, Bernatz PE (1978) The treatment of renal cell carcinoma with solitary metastasis. J Urol 120:540–542

O'Grady AS, Morse LJ, Lee JB (1965) Parathyroid hormone-secreting renal carcinoma associated with hypercalcemia and metabolic alkalosis. Ann Intern Med 63:858–868

Palgon N, Greestein F, Novetsky AD, Lichter SM, Rosen Y (1986) Hyperglycemia associated with renal cell carcinoma. Urology 28:516–517

Parker SL, Tong T, Bolden S, Wingo PA (1996) Cancer statistics, 1996. CA Cancer J Clin 46:5–27

Peeling WB, Mantell BS, Shepheard BGF (1969) Post-operative irradiation in the treatment of renal cell carcinoma. Br J Urol 41:23–31

Peters PC, Brown GL (1980) The role of lymphadenectomy in the management of renal cell carcinoma. Urol Clin North Am 7:705–709

Pizzocaro G, Piva L (1990) Pros and cons of retroperitoneal lymphadenectomy in operable renal cell carcinoma. Eur Urol 18:22–23

Rafla S (1970) Renal cell carcinoma – natural history and results of treatment. Cancer 25:26–40

Ramos CV, Taylor HB (1972) Hepatic dysfunction associated with renal carcinoma. Cancer 29:1287–1292

Riches E (1966) The place of radiotherapy in the management of parenchymal carcinoma of the kidney. J Urol 95:313–317

Riggs BL, Sprague RG (1961) Association of Cushing's syndrome and neoplastic disease. Arch Intern Med 108:841–849

Ritch PS (1990) Treatment of cancer-related hypercalcemia. Semin Oncol 17:26–33

Robson CJ (1963) Radical nephrectomy for renal cell carcinoma. J Urol 89:37–42

Robson CJ (1982) The natural history of renal cell carcinoma. Prog Clin Biol Res 100:447–452

Robson CJ, Churchill BM, Andersen W (1968) The results of radical nephrectomy for renal cell carcinoma. Trans Am Assoc Genitourin Surg 60:122–129

Robson CJ, Churchill BM, Andersen W (1969) The results of radical nephrectomy for renal cell carcinoma. J Urol 101:297–301

Rosenblum SL (1987) Paraneoplastic syndromes associated with renal cell carcinoma. JSC Med Assoc 83:375–378

Rost A, Brosig W (1977) Preoperative irradiation of renal cell carcinoma. Urology 10:414–417

Sago AL, Ball TP, Novicki DE (1979) Complications of retroperitoneal lymphadenectomy. Urology 13:241–243

Samaan NA (1979) Paraneoplastic syndromes associated with renal cell carcinoma. In: Johnson DE, Samuels ML (eds) Clinical conference on cancer – cancer of the genitourinary tract. Raven Press, New York, pp 73–78

Selli C, Hinshaw WM, Woodard BH, Paulson DF (1983) Stratification of risk factors in renal cell carcinoma. Cancer 52:899–903

Siminovitch JMP, Montie JE, Straffon RA (1983) Prognostic indicators in renal adenocarcinoma. J Urol 130:20–23

Skinner DG, Colvin RB, Vermillion CD, et al. (1971) Diagnosis and management of renal cell carcinoma: a clinical and pathologic study of 309 cases. Cancer 28:1165–1177

Skinner DG, Pfister RF, Colvin R (1972a) Extension of renal cell carcinoma into the vena cava: the rationale for aggressive surgical management. J Urol 107:711–716

Skinner DG, Vermillion CD, Colvin RB (1972b) The surgical management of renal cell carcinoma. J Urol 107:705–710

Skinner DG, Pritchett TR, Lieskowsky G, Boyd SD, Stiles QR (1989) Vena caval involvement by renal cell carcinoma. Ann Surg 210:387–394

Stauffer MH (1961) Nephrogenic hepatosplenomegaly (abstract). Gastroenterology 40:694

Stein JP, Esrig D, Eastham J, et al. (1998) The surgical management for renal cell carcinoma: long-term results in a large group of patients. J Urol (accepted for publication)

Strewler GJ, Stern PH, Jacobs JW, et al. (1987) Parathyroid hormone-like protein from human renal carcinoma cells. J Clin Invest 80:1803–1807

Studer UE, Scherz S, Scheidegger J, et al. (1990) Enlargement of regional lymph nodes in renal cell carcinoma is often not due to metastases. J Urol 144:243–245

Sufrin G, Mirand EA, Moore RH, et al. (1977) Hormones in renal cancer. J Urol 117:433–438

Suva LJ, Winslow REH, Wettenhall RG, et al. (1987) A parathyroid hormone-related protein implicated in malignant hypercalcemia: cloning and expression. Science 237:893–896

Swanson DA, Borges PM (1983) Complications of transabdominal radical nephrectomy for renal cell carcinoma. J Urol 129:704–707

Sweet RH (1947) Carcinoma of the esophagus and the cardiac end of the stomach. JAMA 135:485–490

Swierzewski DJ, Swierzewski MJ, Libertino JA (1994) Radical nephrectomy in patients wth renal cell carcinoma with venous, vena caval and atrial extension. Am J Surg 168:205–209

Tanguay S, Swansom DA, Putnam JB Jr (1996) Renal cell carcinoma metastatic to the lung: potential benefit in the combination of biological therapy and surgery. J Urol 156:1586–1589

Thompson IM, Peek M (1988) Improvement in survival of patients with renal cell carcinoma – the role of the serendipitously detected tumor. J Urol 140:487–490

Thrasher JB, Paulson DF (1993) Prognostic factors in renal cancer. Urol Clin North Am 20:247–262

Tsukamoto T, Kumamoto Y, Miyao N, Yamazaki K, Takahashi A, Satoh M (1990) Regional lymph node metastasis in renal cell carcinoma: incidence, distribution and its relation to other pathological fingings. Eur Urol 18:88–93

Tsukamoto T, Kumamoto Y, Yamazaki K, et al. (1991) Clinical analysis of incidentally found renal cell carcinomas. Eur Urol 19:109–113

Tsukamoto T, Kumamoto Y, Miyao N, Masumori N, Takahashi A, Yanase M (1992) Interleukin-6 in renal cell carcinoma. J Urol 148:1778–1782

Turkington RW (1971) Ectopic production of prolactin. N Engl J Med 285:1455–1461

Umeda T, Niijima T (1986) Phase II study of alpha interferon on renal cell carcinoma: summary of three collaborative trials. Cancer 58:1231–1235

Utz DC, Warren MM, Gregg JA, Ludwig J, Kelalis PP (1970) Reversible hepatic dysfunction associated with hypernephroma. Mayo Clin Proc 45:161–169

Vallancien G, Torres LO, Gurfinkel E, Veillon B, Brisset JM (1990) Incidental detection of renal tumors by abdominal ultrasonography. Eur Urol 18:94–96

van der Werf-Messing B (1973) Carcinoma of the kidney. Cancer 32:1056–1061

Walsh PN, Kissane JM (1968) Nonmetastatic hypernephroma with reversible hepatic dysfunction. Arch Intern Med 122:214–222

Walther MM, Alexander RB, Weiss GH, et al. (1993) Cytoreductive surgey prior to interleukin-2-based therapy in patients with metastatic renal cell carcinoma. Urology 42:250–258

Wood DP Jr (1991) Role of lymphadenectomy in renal cell carcinoma. Urol Oncol 18:421

Yagoda A, Abi-Rached B, Petrylak D (1995) Chemotherapy for advanced renal cell carcinoma: 1983–1993. Semin Oncol 22:42–60

# 6 Nephron-Sparing Surgery

H.P. Van Poppel and L. Baert

CONTENTS



## 6.1
## Introduction

Adenocarcinoma of the kidney remains a challenge in urologic oncology. While prostate cancer and bladder neoplasms are much more frequent than kidney cancer, the mortality from kidney cancer can be estimated to be twice as high as that from bladder and 3 times as high as that from prostate cancer. The clinical picture of renal cell carcinoma has, however, changed completely during the last decade. Most tumors are no longer presenting at a locally advanced or disseminated stage with hematuria or pain. Indeed, early diagnosis of the disease has been much

H.P. Van Poppel, MD, PhD, Professor of Oncologic Urology, Department of Urology, University Hospitals Gasthuisberg, Catholic University of Leuven, Herestraat 49, B-3000 Leuven, Belgium
L. Baert, MD, PhD, Professor and Chairman, Department of Urology, University Hospitals Gasthuisberg, Catholic University of Leuven, Herestraat 49, B-3000 Leuven, Belgium

more common since the development of ultrasound, computerized axial tomography (CT), and magnetic resonance imaging (MRI). Nowadays more frequently asymptomatic and often low-stage tumors are routinely detected with the use of modern imaging techniques (see Chap. 4). This raises questions about the extent of surgery that is performed with curative intent.

Surgical resection of renal cell carcinoma remains the only effective therapy available in the management of this disease. Other treatments such as radiotherapy, cytotoxic drugs, or immunotherapy are not very effective and the gold standard therapy for kidney cancer is radical nephrectomy. Classically this procedure is performed through an abdominal incision, allowing early ligation of the renal artery and vein with subsequent removal of the kidney and adrenal gland within an intact Gerota's fascia. Several aspects of these surgical guidelines remain controversial. There is no definite proof that a simple nephrectomy is less optimal than a radical nephrectomy, that an en bloc lymph node resection improves survival, or that an adrenalectomy has to be performed in every radical nephrectomy. More recently it has become questionable whether the same treatment has to be applied in patients with large locally advanced tumors as in those with small incidentally diagnosed lesions. As in other surgical disciplines, the concept of radical surgery has been challenged, and more conservative surgery that spares a certain amount of the organ but offers the same results with respect to tumor control and survival has been proposed.

## 6.2
## Kidney-Sparing Surgery

### 6.2.1
### Rationale

The number of clinically detected incidental renal cell carcinomas is increasing. This recent evolution has become an important factor in the improvement of survival of patients with renal cell carcinoma (THOMPSON and PEEK 1988; TOSAKA et al. 1990). Several reports of excellent results after kidney-sparing surgery in an imperative situation have been published. The term "imperative nephron-sparing surgery" is used when a radical nephrectomy for the same tumor would result in renal failure necessitating peritoneal or hemodialysis, as in patients with a solitary kidney, patients with bilateral tumors, and those with poor function of the contralateral kidney (NOVICK 1995). More recently some investigators have reported early results of conservative surgery for small kidney cancers in the presence of a normal contralateral kidney. This represents an elective indication for conservative surgery.

There is no doubt that even small adenocarcinomas of the kidney have metastatic potential. A watchful waiting policy as proposed by some (BOSNIAK 1995) is not justified (TALAMO and SHONNARD 1980). It has been clearly shown that a small adenocarcinoma of the kidney is not a benign disease and that a tumor size of ≤3 cm does not mean that there is no risk of metastatic disease (ESCHWEGE et al. 1996).

A certain number of small solid tumors prove to be benign. Renal oncocytoma, angiomyolipoma, angiomyoma, metanephric adenoma, and complicated cysts can be found on definitive pathologic examination without having been recognized prior to surgery (MONTIE 1991). Preoperative needle biopsy of kidney tumors has to be avoided. The procedure can result in bleeding or tumor seeding and is not diagnostically reliable because of the high incidence of false-negative and false-positive results obtained with this technique (GOETHUYS et al. 1996). Therefore fine-needle aspiration biopsy of renal masses is only advocated when there is clinical or radiologic evidence to suggest a diagnosis other than primary renal cell carcinoma, such as metastatic disease, lymphoma, or renal abscess (HERTS and BAKER 1995). If all suspicious solid tumors were to be treated by radical surgery, a significant number of kidneys without malignancy would be resected.

As stated above, the number of patients being diagnosed with incidental renal cell carcinoma is increasing (ASO and HOMMA 1992). The routine use or abuse of ultrasound and CT scan for many medical conditions may be at least partially responsible for this higher detection rate (BOSNIAK 1991) but there may also be a real increase in the prevalence of renal cell carcinoma (RITCHIE et al. 1984). In the face of an increasing number of small, mostly inciden-

tally found renal tumors it seems appropriate to evaluate the feasibility of nephron-sparing surgery, even in patients who could easily have radical nephrectomy.

## 6.2.2
## Imperative Kidney-Sparing Surgery

A partial nephrectomy for renal cell carcinoma was first performed more than a century ago, by Czerny in 1887 (CZERNY 1890). One had to wait more than 60 years until Vermooten reported on the indications for conservative surgery in certain renal tumors (VERMOOTEN 1950). He described the histologic growth pattern of a small clear cell carcinoma that is well encapsulated and therefore amenable to local resection. Most renal cell carcinomas are located in the upper or the lower pole of the kidney and this location is also particularly suitable for attempts at local resection.

For more than 20 years kidney-sparing surgery has been considered an acceptable therapeutic option for selected patients with renal cancer (WICKHAM 1975). Major technical advances have been made in the application of this conservative surgery. Nowadays it is even possible to locally resect centrally located tumors that would normally require radical nephrectomy. This is possible because of the experience gained with kidney perfusion and cooling, and with knowledge obtained through extensive laboratory studies.

Many investigators have reported their experience with nephron-sparing surgery for imperative indications (BAZEED et al. 1986; BELUSSI et al. 1997; BRISSET et al. 1989; CARINI et al. 1981; CIANCIO et al. 1994; COLSTON 1960; GRABER 1991; GRAHAM and GLENN 1979; JACOBS et al. 1980; JAEGER et al. 1985; JOHANSSON and WAHLQVIST 1981; LICHT and NOVICK 1993; MALEK et al. 1976; MARBERGER et al. 1981; MARSHALL et al. 1986; MOLL et al. 1993; MONTIE and NOVICK 1988; MORGAN and ZINCKE 1990; NOVICK et al. 1977, 1989; PALMER and SWANSON 1978; PETRITCH et al. 1990; PROVET et al. 1991; ROSENTHAL et al. 1984; SCHÄRFE et al. 1988; SCHIFF et al. 1979; SELLI et al. 1991; SMITH et al. 1984; STAEHLER and ERNST 1985; STEINBACH et al. 1991b, 1992; STEPHENS and GRAHAM 1990; TAARI et al. 1993; TOPLEY et al. 1984; TRASHER et al. 1994; VAN POPPEL et al. 1986, 1991; VIETS et al. 1977; ZECHNER et al. 1988; ZINCKE and SWANSON 1992).

The published reports on kidney-sparing surgery in patients who could not have undergone radical nephrectomy have clearly demonstrated the validity of this surgical approach. The survival data resulting from the use of this procedure have been excellent. The 5-year tumor-specific survival rate has been reported by many authors to be about 88% (CARINI et al. 1981; LICHT et al. 1994; MORGAN and ZINCKE 1990; STEINBACH et al. 1991a; PETRITCH et al. 1990; PROVET et al. 1991). One group reported a much lower 5-year survival rate (67%) but the patients treated had larger tumors, higher stage at diagnosis, and the presence of metastatic tumor in lymph nodes (BRKOVIC et al. 1997). Those patients who have progression after imperative conservative surgery often present metastatic disease that was probably present, but not yet recognizable, at the time of surgery. A number of these conservatively treated patients, however, present with local recurrence that could have been avoided by performing a radical instead of a partial nephrectomy. An analysis of all the reports concerning imperative conservative resections showed that local recurrence occurred in about 7.5% (0%–12%) (VAN POPPEL and BAERT 1994).

In these retrospective studies it is difficult to establish whether the local recurrences were due to incomplete resections, i.e., tumor persistence (true local recurrence), or to multifocality of the tumor (kidney recurrence). One should remember that in these imperative indications often locally advanced tumors are treated, with the intention of preserving sufficient nephrons to avoid hemodialysis. In the published reports, however, where only patients with smaller tumors (<4 cm) underwent partial nephrectomy, no local (or systemic) recurrences were reported (LICHT et al. 1994; VELAGAPUDI et al. 1993). In a comparative study (nonrandomized) of partial and radical nephrectomy in patients with small and low-stage tumors, the cancer-specific 5-year survival rates were 100% following kidney-sparing surgery and 97% after radical nephrectomy (BUTLER et al. 1995).

The prognosis of tumor progression after kidney-sparing surgery is generally poor (MORGAN and ZINCKE 1990). In patients with local or kidney recurrence the incidence of simultaneous metastases has been reported to range from a low of 25% to a high of 67% (BRKOVIC et al. 1994; LICHT et al. 1994). In those with local recurrence only and without metastases, the disease should not be considered incurable and successful salvage surgery has been routinely performed (BRKOVIC et al. 1997; NOVICK et al. 1991; NOVICK and STRAFFON 1987).

As expected, complication rates in patients treated with imperative kidney-sparing surgery are higher than in those treated by radical nephrectomy. Complications such as arteriovenous fistula or pseudoaneurysm formation, urinary fistula, or bleeding from the partial nephrectomy edges are known to occur after partial nephrectomy. Radical nephrectomy, on the other hand, is devoid of these complications although no comparative study on hemorrhagic complications is available for review. Radical nephrectomy and dialysis with possible subsequent transplantation has to be considered as a last resort for lesions that are anatomically unresectable, even using an ex vivo technique (MORGAN and ZINCKE 1991).

With the acceptable results of imperative conservative surgery in bilateral tumors or in patients with solitary kidney, the indications for the use of this approach have continued to increase over the past several years. It is now widely accepted that patients with von Hippel-Lindau disease or hereditary renal cell carcinoma can be effectively managed by kidney-sparing surgery. There is, however, a need for close follow-up, because many of these patients will present with a recurrence (STEINBACH et al. 1995a). It is debatable whether patients with multifocal and often bilateral papillary renal cell carcinoma are suitable candidates for kidney-sparing surgery. In such patients we have noted that lesions are disseminated throughout the kidney and not only located underneath the renal capsule (DAL CIN et al. 1996).

One might also propose conservative surgery in patients with a poorly functioning contralateral kidney, or even a contralateral kidney in which function is expected to deteriorate in the future (MORGAN and ZINCKE 1990). By applying these additional indications, urologists are enlarging the spectrum of imperative and relative indications for nephron-sparing surgery to encompass patients with diabetes, arterial hypertension, and renal artery stenosis (BERG et al. 1981; RIEDASCH et al. 1996). In view of the expansion in the indications for conservative surgery, it is expected that even in the presence of a normal contralateral kidney this surgical technique will become more and more popular.

## 6.2.3
## Elective Kidney-Sparing Surgery

The results of kidney-sparing surgery in imperative situations have demonstrated that this approach can be cancer curing, even in the case of larger and locally advanced or centrally located tumors, where surgery is often very demanding. However, the classical selection criteria for nephron-sparing surgery in an elective setting are relatively narrow and limited to clinically low-stage tumors that are located underneath the renal capsule without an obvious exorenal component. These are exactly the cases where radical nephrectomy will be curative in nearly 100% of patients while radical surgery would be expected to have a lower morbidity than a conservative surgical approach (ZINCKE and SWANSON 1982). It is therefore mandatory to evaluate the results of an elective kidney-sparing approach, to discuss the controversies concerning recurrence rates, and to define the surgical technique to be used in the treatment of these patients.

Some investigators have been advocating the use of nephron-sparing resection of the primary tumor in patients with metastatic renal cell carcinoma (KRISHNAMURTHI et al. 1996). This will be discussed in detail in Chap. 7.

## 6.3
## Results of Elective Kidney-Sparing Surgery

Several medical centers have published treatment results with nephron-sparing surgery in patients with a normal contralateral kidney and without any urologic disease that could lead to renal failure in the future (BAZEED et al. 1986; BUTLER et al. 1995; LICHT and NOVICK 1993; MOLL et al. 1993; SELLI et al. 1991; STEINBACH et al. 1992; PETRITCH et al. 1990; PROVET et al. 1991; VAN POPPEL et al. 1991). There are cur-

rently 13 medical centers that have presented relevant data on treatment outcomes in patients managed with nephron-sparing surgery who had elective indications for this procedure. Some of these results have already been reviewed (LICHT and NOVICK 1993; VAN POPPEL and BAERT 1994; VAN POPPEL et al. 1997). Table 6.1 summarizes the most recent data in this group of patients.

The data of two reports were not included (BAZEED et al. 1986; CARINI et al. 1981) since the same medical centers later reported on a larger group of patients (STEINBACH et al. 1991b; SELLI et al. 1991). Eleven out of the 13 reports emerged from single centers with data that could be compared in respect of tumor size, follow-up duration, disease-free survival, and the incidence of local recurrence. Two other papers reported a multicenter experience (BELUSSI et al. 1997; PETRITCH et al. 1990) where data on tumor size or follow-up or disease-free survival were lacking. Although these reports represent a considerable number of patients, they will not be discussed further. Our own results presented here are not those earlier reported (VAN POPPEL et al. 1991). Our study was recently updated in order to include a total of 50 patients treated with nephron-sparing surgery with the longest mean follow-up reported.

From single-center reports it can be concluded that the disease-free survival is nearly 100% and local recurrences are exceptional events. Among a total of 435 renal cell carcinomas with a mean size ranging from 2.6 to 4.0 cm treated by nephron-sparing procedures and followed for a mean duration ranging

**Table 6.1.** Results of elective nephron-sparing surgery for renal cell carcinoma

|  | Number | Mean size (cm) | Follow-up (mos) | Disease-free survival | Local recurrence |
|---|---|---|---|---|---|
| SELLI et al. (1991) | 20 | 3.4 | 31 | 90% | 0 |
| PROVET et al. (1991) | 19 | 2.6 | 35 | 100% | 0 |
| HERR (1994) | 41 | 3.5 | 36 | 95% | 1 (2.4%) |
| LICHT et al. (1994) | 17 | 3.6 | 38 | 100% | 0 |
| BELUSSI et al. (1997)[a] | 320 | <5.0 | 12–60 | ? | 5 (1.4%) |
| BRISSET et al. (1989) | 15 | 3.5 | 40 | 100% | 0 |
| STEINBACH et al. (1991b) | 72 | 3.2 | 40 | 90% | 2 (2.8%) |
| TAARI et al. (1993) | 10 | 3.7 | 48 | 100% | 0 |
| MOLL et al. (1993) | 105 | 4.0 | 42 | 100% | 0 |
| PETRITSCH et al. (1990)[a] | 52 | ? | 42 | 96% | 2 (4.0%) |
| MORGAN and ZINCKE (1990) | 20 | 3.1 | 46 | 100% | 0 |
| D'ARMIENTO et al. (1997) | 19 | 3.34 | 70 | 96% | 0 |
| VAN POPPEL et al. (1991)[b] | 50 | 3.6 | 76 | 100% | 0 |

[a] Multicenter study.
[b] Recently updated in 1997.

from 31 to 76 months, only three (0.7%) patients had local recurrences. This is a 10 times lower recurrence rate than that obtained following kidney-sparing surgery with imperative indications. However, the mean follow-up in this series is relatively short and a longer follow-up will be necessary to allow more accurate assessment of these results (CAMPBELL and NOVICK 1995). It is apparent that a proper selection of patients is at least partly responsible for these excellent treatment results. In the aforementioned single-center reports it was not clarified whether the local recurrences were due to incomplete resections or to tumor multifocality, the former being an avoidable and the latter an unavoidable event.

### 6.3.1
### Arguments in Favor of Elective Kidney-Sparing Surgery

The first argument in favor of a conservative approach for an easily resectable tumor suspected to be renal adenocarcinoma in the presence of a normal contralateral kidney is the unknown malignant potential of small solid renal tumors (AMENDOLA et al. 1988; BOSNIAK 1991; CURRY et al. 1986; FOSTER et al. 1985). While a large oncocytoma may be suspected on CT scan, and a huge angiomyolipoma will be recognized without problems on ultrasound or CT, it is much more difficult to predict the pathologic diagnosis of very small solid kidney tumors. As has already been stated, fine-needle aspiration cytology (HELM et al. 1983) or biopsy, which has been proposed by some authors (AMIS et al. 1987; JUUL et al. 1985), is not advisable when surgery will in any case be performed (GOETHUYS et al. 1996; KISER et al. 1986; WEHLE and GRABSTALD 1986). Secondly, the presence of a tumor pseudocapsule, as surrounds most smaller renal cell carcinomas, makes a nephron-sparing approach very appealing. It was shown that the pseudocapsule is intact in 80% of all renal cell cancers smaller than 7 cm (ROCCA ROSSETTI 1980). Other investigators have shown that in more than 90% of kidney cancers there is no peritumoral infiltration (COSTANTINI et al. 1996).

A third argument for the use of conservative surgery might be the impairment of renal function caused by radical nephrectomy. The risk of contralateral kidney function loss after total nephrectomy, however, is limited and about two-thirds of the renal parenchyma has to be removed before damage is induced in the remaining nephrons (NOVICK et al. 1991; WISHNOW et al. 1990).

The fourth but rather weak argument used in favor of nephron-sparing surgery is the risk of development of a metachronous contralateral renal cell carcinoma. The risk of developing a contralateral cancer is reported to be 1%–4% (MONTIE and NOVICK 1988). Moreover in these rare cases imperative kidney-sparing surgery could still be performed in order to avoid the anephric state.

The possible need for cytotoxic treatment for one or another intercurrent malignancy has been the fifth argument in favor of the kidney-sparing approach (VAN POPPEL and BAERT 1992).

The authors, however, believe that the most important argument in favor of kidney-sparing surgery for easily resectable tumors and in carefully selected patients is, as mentioned earlier, the nearly 100% tumor control rate.

### 6.3.2
### Controversial Issues Concerning Elective Kidney-Sparing Surgery

The major controversy regarding elective nephron-sparing surgery is the risk of local recurrence, which can occur up to 20 years following surgery. Review of the literature does not permit distinction between recurrence due to incomplete resection and recurrence due to the presence of tumors arising elsewhere in the kidney that either were not detected at the time of surgery or developed subsequently. Both these situations are related to the multifocal behavior of renal cell carcinoma. The latter situation cannot be considered a true local recurrence but rather a "kidney" recurrence.

### 6.4
## Multifocality and Kidney Recurrence

The multifocal nature of renal cell carcinoma has been well documented in the literature not only in the case of larger tumors but also in those measuring 3 cm or less in diameter. On the one hand there may be genetically determined tumor multicentricity, as in von Hippel-Lindau disease and hereditary renal cell carcinoma and probably also papillary tumors (DAL CIN et al. 1996, Chap. 3). On the other hand, sporadic renal cell carcinoma can also present with secondary or satellite lesions. The reports on the occurrence of multifocality in renal cell carcinoma are summarized in Table 6.2. The wide variation in the reported occurrence of multifocality is probably due

**Table 6.2.** Occurrence of multifocality in renal cell carcinoma

| Author | No. of kidneys examined | Secondary RCC: No. (%) | Secondary RCC with primary ≤ 3 cm: No. (%) |
|---|---|---|---|
| MUKAMEL et al. (1988) | 66 | 13 (19.7) | 2 (3) |
| CHENG et al. (1991) | 100 | 7 (7) | 0 |
| JACQMIN et al. (1992) | 727 | 53 (7.3) | 10 (1.8) |
| OYA et al. (1995) | 108 | 7 (6.5) | 2 (1.9) |
| KLETSCHER et al. (1995) | 100 | 16 (16) | 5 (5) |
| WHANG et al. (1995) | 44 | 11 (25) | ? |
| NISSENKORN and BERNHEIM (1995) | 27 | 3 (11.1) | 1 (3.7) |
| CHINAGLIA and BELLUSSI (1997) | 387 | 12 (3) | 3 (0.8) |
| Total | 1559 | 122 (7.8) | 23 (1.5) |

to two factors. The first is the completeness of the pathologic examination of the kidneys, which is difficult to evaluate in different medical centers. The second factor is the possible presence of hereditary or papillary renal cell carcinoma, the incidence of these conditions not being accurately reported in different studies. In a recent study the occurrence of multicentricity was shown not to be related to pathologic grade of the tumor, tumor stage, the presence of vascular invasion, or infiltrative tumor pattern (SAIKI et al. 1995).

At the present time it can be anticipated that secondary renal cell carcinomas will be found in about 8% of patients with renal cancers and in 1.5% of those with small (<3 cm in diameter) primary tumors. This multifocality could then be responsible for kidney recurrences after nephron-sparing surgery. As is shown in Table 6.2, however, the incidence of recurrence is even lower. It should therefore be acknowledged that the natural history of a small multifocal renal cell carcinoma remains undetermined.

Tumor multifocality is an unavoidable problem when employing kidney-sparing surgery. With the use of optimal preoperative diagnostic tools such multifocality will often be recognized prior to surgery. This preoperative recognition of multifocality allows the surgeon to plan to perform a radical or a partial nephrectomy, or at the least these important issues can be discussed with the patient prior to surgery. When a satellite lesion is recognized during surgery it can still be decided whether a conservative procedure or a radical nephrectomy is indicated. Finally, when the multifocal behavior is responsible for a late kidney recurrence, salvage is still possible with repeat partial nephrectomy or total excision of the renal remnant (CAMPBELL and NOVICK 1994).

In recent studies, examination of the healthy parenchyma surrounding renal cell carcinoma showed abnormal cells, with abnormal ploidy or altered expression of tumor-associated antigens being revealed in nearly 60% when compared with the normal renal tissue (ANTON et al. 1995; KOVACS and BRUSA 1989; EMANUEL et al. 1992). We have been investigating the origin of chromosomal abnormalities such as trisomy 7 and trisomy 10 that were found in the healthy parenchyma of tumor-bearing kidneys. We have demonstrated that trisomy 7 or 10 is not present in renal parenchymal cells but in a subtype of tumor-infiltrating lymphocytes. We therefore concluded that the chromosomal abnormalities seen were not cancer related (DAL CIN et al. 1992, see Chap. 3). It is apparent that these issues will need further study because it is of utmost importance to recognize multifocal tumors or those which are very likely to become multifocal. This knowledge would prevent consideration of elective nephron-sparing surgery.

## 6.5
## Local Recurrence

Local tumor recurrence after partial nephrectomy is due to tumor persistence during surgery followed by new tumor growth that becomes detectable during the period of follow-up. Local recurrence, as would be expected, is much more common after imperative nephron-sparing surgery. This difference in the incidence of local tumor control between imperative and elective cases is not due to the synchronously unsuspected tumor or the metachronously developing tumor (which can also develop in the contralateral kidney) but to the incomplete resection. This occurs when larger tumors are treated, which are less well circumscribed and less easily resectable. Many of these tumors would, in the presence of a normal contralateral kidney, not be treated by nephron-sparing means (NOVICK 1991). Although small renal cell carcinomas often have a well-defined pseudocapsule (ROCCA ROSSETTI 1980), it has been shown that this pseudocapsule can be absent or may be incomplete or invaded by adenocarcinoma (BLACKLEY et al. 1988; MARSHALL et al. 1986; NOVICK and STRAFFON 1987; ROSENTHAL et al. 1984; VAN POPPEL and BAERT 1994). A recent histologic study of the peritumoral tissue after elective organ-preserving surgery found peritumoral infiltration in nearly 10% of the resected specimens (COSTANTINI et al. 1996). Therefore, when tumor resection is not performed within a safe rim of healthy parenchyma this can lead to incomplete resection, leaving behind microscopic residual tumor. Surgeons who perform simple tumor enucleation will take all precautions to avoid local recurrence at the resection site by performing frozen section biopsies at the tumor margins and applying coagulation of the tumor bed with an infrared sapphire coagulator (BAZEED et al. 1996) or an argon laser beam (HERNANDEZ et al. 1990; MORGAN and ZINCKE 1991; STEINBACH et al. 1995b). The authors are convinced on a theoretical basis that a simple enucleation is less adequate than resection within healthy tissue.

## 6.6
## Technical Aspects of Elective Kidney-Sparing Surgery

The technique of conservative renal cancer surgery has already been well described in detail elsewhere (NOVICK 1987; GRIFFIN and FLANIGAN 1996). Based on our experience we would like to add some comments on the preoperative workup, the surgery itself, and the follow-up after partial nephrectomy.

### 6.6.1
### Preoperative Investigations

A renal mass that is suspected to be renal cell carcinoma and is suitable for conservative surgery in the presence of a normal contralateral kidney is most frequently found incidentally on an imaging study (Chap. 4). Differential diagnosis in such patients includes the following conditions: (1) atypical or complicated renal cyst, (2) cystic adenocarcinoma, (3) oncocytoma, (4) angiomyolipoma, (5) metanephric adenoma, (6) metastatic tumor, and (7) pseudotumor. CT scan is the most frequently performed investigation to assist in the diagnostic process (AMENDOLA et al. 1988; BOSNIAK 1991; FROHMÜLLER et al. 1987; LEVINE et al. 1989). MRI has not been found to be superior to CT scan in predicting the pathologic diagnosis for small renal neoplasms (LONDON et al. 1989; TE STRAKE et al. 1988). Nevertheless, the role of MRI will probably continue to increase (SCATTONI et al. 1995, see Chap. 4). MRI has already been found superior to CT in the evaluation of renal masses in patients with compromised renal function or with a history of allergic reaction to the contrast media as well as in the assessment of vascular involvement (GSCHWEND et al. 1996).

The importance of imaging studies with MRI is not limited to the search for the pathologic diagnosis. A study performed in 54 patients with renal carcinoma demonstrated the presence of a pseudocapsule in 66% of tumors measuring 4 cm or less in diameter (YAMASHITA et al. 1996). Therefore MRI could be very helpful in assisting the urologist to establish which tumors can be safely treated by enucleation. Additionally, spiral CT with image reconstruction and MRI can provide a three-dimensional picture of the tumor in coronal and sagittal planes. These three-dimensional images are found very useful for the selection of patients who can undergo a safe local tumor resection. The use of arteriography or digital intravenous subtraction angiography to investigate the arterial blood supply can be relevant for kidney-sparing surgery in imperative situations, especially for midpole tumors (NOVICK 1987). Once major blood vessels supplying the tumor have been identified, they can be selectively ligated during the surgery, thereby minimizing blood loss and simplifying the procedure (CAMPBELL and NOVICK 1995). The authors believe that in elective cases knowledge of the vascular anatomy is of minor interest because these tumors by definition should always be easily accessible and resectable.

Providing the patient with essential information prior to surgery is of major importance. A patient who undergoes a partial nephrectomy has to be warned that during the surgery it may become necessary to proceed with a radical nephrectomy and should also be aware of the greater need for a strict follow-up schedule to help to identify those few patients who present with late kidney recurrence.

## 6.6.2
### Surgical Approach and Field Preparation

Laparoscopic wedge resection of small renal tumors has been performed but its use remains controversial (McDougall et al. 1993). We continue to believe that proper surgical resection for renal cell carcinoma requires open surgical exposure.

All conventional incisions that offer adequate exposure of the upper retroperitoneum can be used for nephron-sparing surgery. Most investigators recommend the use of an extrapleural flank incision to the 11th or 10th intercostal space (Novick 1987; Van Poppel et al. 1991). Others have found a transperitoneal approach appropriate, but in our opinion this seems less than optimal (Morgan and Zincke 1991). The flank incision is preferred because, once the kidney has been completely mobilized on its pedicle, it can be easily brought out of the wound. Other advantages of this surgical approach include easy avoidance of contamination of the peritoneal cavity and its consequences should a urinary fistula develop. Finally, postoperative recovery is faster after an extraperitoneal approach rather than a peritoneal approach because of a decreased incidence of postoperative paralytic ileus (Campbell and Novick 1995).

After the incision has been made, Gerota's fascia is opened and the arteriovenous pedicle is dissected in order that it can be easily clamped off should this become necessary during surgery. This hilar clamping is most often superfluous in elective situations while in imperative indications it is very often used. It may be performed by the use of simple digital compression (Graham and Glenn 1979) or by placing a soft bulldog clamp (Marberger 1986). The use of special clamping devices has also been proposed (Selikowitz 1995). Routine vascular clamping should, however, be avoided to prevent secondary arterial thrombosis, which has been reported (Carini et al. 1981). Although some surgeons have been able to omit renal artery occlusion in only 10%–20% of cases (Campbell and Novick 1995), we succeeded in performing elective resections without vascular clamping in more than 85% of patients and surface hypothermia was never applied.

With adequate preoperative studies, it is easier to establish the tumor location. Approaching the tumor itself, the entire kidney capsule has to be exposed and inspected for the presence of secondary tumors (Montie 1991). The renal capsule should not be stripped off since nearly all multifocal tumors are located immediately beneath the renal capsule (Mukamel et al. 1988). Moreover, this would increase morbidity without permitting the detection of intraparenchymal secondary carcinomas (Holland 1988). Recently some centers have been advocating the use of intraoperative ultrasonography (Assimos et al. 1991; Gilbert et al. 1988; Marshall et al. 1992) and color Doppler studies (Walther et al. 1994). Although ultrasound can be useful for intraparenchymal tumors, these are not an ideal indication for elective kidney-sparing surgery. Neither have we found intraoperative ultrasound to be of any use in the evaluation of the depth of tumor extension into the kidney. This information can be obtained by preoperative three-dimensional imaging with spiral CT or MRI (Chernoff et al. 1994). The perinephric fat adjacent to the primary tumor has to be left behind on the tumor in order to avoid tumor spill (Novick 1987, 1993; Paulson 1988).

## 6.6.3
### Resection and Kidney Closure

In most patients who have elective indications for conservative surgery, an in situ procedure on a well-mobilized kidney is easily performed after adequate dissection of the renal artery and vein. Use may be made of an ultrasound aspiration dissector, an argon laser beam, a microwave tissue coagulator, or a contact neodymium-YAG laser. According to some investigators such techniques offer advantages over the conventional surgical technique (Addonizio et al. 1984; Hernandez et al. 1990; Korhonen et al. 1993; Muraki et al. 1996). However, we feel that the application of these newer techniques makes the surgery more time-consuming without offering any real benefit. There might be an indication for use of these tools in patients with polar tumors or in those who are treated with heminephrectomy. For wedge resection or enucleation resection we believe that conventional surgery is much faster with less risk of losing the stereotactic feeling about the localization of the tumor and its depth of penetration into the renal parenchyma.

Tumor resection should always be attempted within healthy parenchyma. The tumor has to be removed with a rim of normal tissue of at least a few millimeters because of the possibility of pseudocapsule invasion or its perforation, as has been mentioned above. Although the available data do not show a major oncologic benefit for partial nephrectomy as opposed to simple enucleation (relying on the intactness of the pseudocapsule), the latter approach is viewed as unsafe.

Simple tumor enucleation has nevertheless been performed in many centers, in either imperative or elective situations (CARINI et al. 1988; CIANCIO et al. 1994; GRAHAM and GLENN 1979; KUROZUMI et al. 1993; MORGAN and ZINCKE 1991; NOVICK et al. 1986; SELLI et al. 1991; STEPHENS and GRAHAM 1990; TRASHER et al. 1994). Most authors have defended the use of enucleation by stating that both procedures provide viable treatment options with equal outcomes in respect of local tumor control and disease-free survival (CARINI et al. 1981; GRAHAM and GLENN 1979; JAEGER et al. 1985; MORGAN and ZINCKE 1990; STEPHENS and GRAHAM 1990). A well-controlled study, however, has clearly demonstrated that the limited margins achieved by tumor enucleation should not be recommended even in patients with pT1 tumors: even in these small tumors the use of partial nephrectomy should always be recommended in the presence of a normal contralateral kidney (KUROZUMI et al. 1993). These data suggest that tumor excision with a surrounding margin of normal parenchyma may be the safest approach to assure absence of malignancy in the preserved portion of the kidney (LICHT and NOVICK 1993). We believe that although enucleation can still be safely applied in some imperative cases, it should be avoided in elective settings.

The resection of a tumor with a few millimeters of healthy parenchyma around the pseudocapsule has been called enucleoresection (SELLI et al. 1991) or excavation (VAN POPPEL et al. 1991). While it might be expected that pure enucleation will be easier to perform than enucleoresection or excavation, any advantage in this respect is minimal. It is very easy to incise the renal capsule with a cold knife at 5 mm around the exorenal part of the tumor. The excavation can then be continued with both sharp and blunt dissection. Bleeding vessels can be stitched and when a calix is opened it should be meticulously closed to prevent urinary fistula. In order to be able to recognize an open calix it is important to immediately mark the incised urothelium with a stitch while proceeding with the excavation. When this is not performed, the calix will retract and the opening in the calix cannot be easily recognized once the tumor has been completely removed. Double-J catheters or nephrostomy tubes are almost never necessary in elective nephron-sparing surgery. The injection of methylene blue into the collecting system may assist in recognition of an opened calix (POLASCIK et al. 1995). We are convinced that excavation is the pro-

cedure of choice in many patients with small renal tumors (VAN POPPEL et al. 1996). We have no experience with enucleation followed by the application of a sapphire coagulator or an argon laser beam to the tumor bed (STEINBACH et al. 1995b). The value of these measures has not yet been clearly demonstrated.

For larger tumors of the upper or lower pole a partial nephrectomy will be a safe procedure, while for larger midrenal tumors a wedge resection is more advisable. For intrarenal upper and lower pole tumors a polar nephrectomy has also been advocated.

Some authors have suggested use of frozen sections of the resection margins during the conservative procedure. This may be indicated in imperative situations where it is not always possible to obtain macroscopically safe margins. In elective circumstances, however, the tumor should by definition be easily resectable within normal parenchyma so that one can easily rely on sufficiency of macroscopic margins. We use frozen sections relatively infrequently, in cases where there is doubt about resection margins. Other authors, however, continue to advocate the use of frozen sections to confirm the presence of negative surgical margins during nephron-sparing procedures (CAMPBELL and NOVICK 1995; CAMPBELL et al. 1996; LERNER et al. 1995).

In all types of resections control of bleeding can be easily obtained by oversewing the bleeding arteries and veins. If the blood loss is substantial or it cannot be controlled readily, the renal artery can be clamped off (we avoid clamping off the renal vein). Usually the application of this important measure takes no longer than a few minutes. We have no experience in the application of argon laser beam coagulation, which has been found to be helpful by others (CAMPBELL and NOVICK 1995).

Sometimes the defect resulting from tumor removal after pure enucleation or excavation cannot be closed. It can then be filled up with perirenal fat or reabsorbable hemostatic dressing. After major excavations, wedge resection, or polar nephrectomy, we always try to close the renal capsule. It is therefore important to cautiously plan a fish mouth-like incision that enables the surgeon the bring the cut edges together. Rather than using mattress sutures, which do not allow easy approximation of the edges, we apply interrupted sutures to close the renal parenchyma. These sutures can be tightened with the use of bolsters of fatty tissue, pieces of striated muscle, or exogenous material. We have recently gained favorable experience with the use of Goretex strips

(ZINCKE and RUCKLE 1995). Closure of the capsule should never be performed until the parenchymal bleeding has been adequately controlled. Indeed, when arteries or veins are left open there is a high risk of postoperative development of arteriovenous pseudoaneurysm and fistula. When, in addition, the pyelocaliceal system is not closed appropriately, this can result in severe hematuria necessitating urgent selective embolization of the affected blood vessel.

One or two suction drains are left behind in order to prevent the formation of a hematoma or urinoma. These drains are in most cases removed 3–4 days after surgery.

Following placement of the drains the perirenal fat and Gerota's fascia are sutured, keeping in mind the possibility of a later reintervention which may consist in a radical nephrectomy or a second partial resection. The wound is then closed in routine fashion.

## 6.7
## Follow-up After Kidney-Sparing Surgery

### 6.7.1
### Early Postoperative Management

In the immediate postoperative period, hemorrhage is the most common complication. First hemorrhage in the wound is possible and will usually be recognized when the suction drains have been adequately placed. Surgical exploration may then be indicated. When hematuria occurs, it is very likely that a vessel in the tumor bed is bleeding into a not appropriately closed calix. Surgical exploration is not mandatory in the absence of hypotension or shock. Patients can best be managed by transarterial superselective embolization of the feeding vessel of the pseudoaneurysm. In our initial experience we have needed interventional radiology 4 times; each time this modality was successfully applied (see Chap. 4).

The development of a urinary fistula is very uncommon. We have encountered it once in a patient who had developed an arteriocaliceal fistula with blood clots obstructing the ureter and subsequently giving rise to a urinary fistula. The embolization resolved the bleeding and a double-J catheter inserted for 2 weeks resolved the fistula problem. No cases of fistula have occurred among the other patients we have treated with elective kidney-sparing surgery. As reported by others, the treatment of fistulas is mostly conservative. Most fistulas resolve spontaneously,

but some may need endoscopic manipulation, usually consisting in a temporary ureteral stent placement (CAMPBELL et al. 1994). When there is no ureteral obstruction most fistulas will not need any specific treatment.

Renal arterial thrombosis can occur due to lesion of the intima of the renal artery after clamping of the vessel during the surgery. Because this complication, when recognized early, needs immediate reoperation for correction of the problem, we believe that application of a clamp should be avoided whenever possible in elective nephron-sparing surgery. No randomized studies have been performed to compare the complication rates after nephron-sparing surgery and after radical nephrectomy. In general the complications mentioned will occur only after nephron-sparing surgery, although a retrospective analysis reported no significant difference in complications after radical and after partial nephrectomy (BUTLER et al. 1995).

Our own experience supports the suggestion of others that complications occurring in nephron-sparing surgery can be managed conservatively and are associated with minimal serious morbidity. The majority of these complications can be managed nonoperatively or endourologically.

### 6.7.2
### Oncologic Follow-up

The only patients who are offered nephron-sparing surgery are those who, in addition to meeting the strict medical criteria for inclusion, have a clear understanding of the need for a strict follow-up schedule. As in patients with a solitary kidney or bilateral tumors, those who undergo partial nephrectomy there is a need for close monitoring of the residual renal parenchyma in order to detect promptly any local recurrence. In the case of local recurrence, either because of tumor persistence (positive margins) or because of a relapse elsewhere in the kidney, secondary surgical treatment, usually a salvage nephrectomy, can still be performed with a high probability of success (VAN POPPEL and BAERT 1994).

There is no consensus on which laboratory and imaging studies should be performed to assess patients after partial nephrectomy for renal cell carcinoma. In general, there has not been an established follow-up schedule for patients with renal cell carcinoma. At a time when cost-benefit considerations are interfering in the medical debate, this is becoming an important issue.

Recent retrospective studies have shown that a symptom history, serum liver function studies, and chest radiographs obtained every 6 months for the first 3 years and then yearly thereafter are sufficient measures in monitoring of these patients. It has been suggested that in T1 disease only a symptom history is necessary (HAFEZ et al. 1997; SANDOCK et al. 1995). Further investigations by bone scan or CT of the brain or abdomen are considered to be warranted only in cases in which a carefully obtained relevant history and physical examination reveal any suspicious findings (SANDOCK et al. 1995).

Although this very minimal follow-up schedule might be reasonable, we believe that patients should be subjected to a more comprehensive workup given that we are applying a still not generally accepted treatment for renal cell carcinoma (BUIZZA et al. 1997). We recommend ultrasound of both kidneys at 3-monthly intervals in the first year following surgery and at 4-monthly intervals during the second and third years, together with a yearly contrast-enhanced CT scan. The oncologic follow-up is continued lifelong with yearly follow-up examinations which are to include ultrasound and/or CT scan.

## 6.8
## Conclusions and Further Perspectives

Although many urologists still feel reluctant to offer nephron-sparing surgery to patients with small kidney tumors, recent reports on the use of this approach indicate that it is really becoming an accepted treatment modality in properly selected cases, even in the presence of a normal contralateral kidney. Summarizing the reports on elective nephron-sparing surgery, it can be concluded that this type of surgery can be performed safely and with minimal associated moribidity. It is, of course, assumed that the surgeon needs experience and it has been reported that there is indeed an important learning curve for nephron-sparing surgery (CAMPBELL et al. 1994). Nephron-sparing surgery has now been proven to be feasible and is curative in a high proportion of carefully selected patients with renal cell carcinoma. It is the selection of suitable candidates for this type of surgery that is the most important key to a successful outcome. Except in cases of von Hippel-Lindau disease, the tumor should be solitary and well delineated on CT or MRI without invasion of the perinephric fat or pyelocaliceal system (T1 and T2). Although some investigators have been restricting the size limit for nephron sparing surgery to 4 cm

(LERNER et al. 1996), size is not the most important selection criterion. Rather the most important requirement for successful application of nephron-sparing surgery is that the tumor is easily resectable. This means that it should be at least partly exorenal. It is not good policy to take any risk concerning the surgical margins by embarking on particularly difficult procedures. There is a great need for optimal preoperative diagnostic workup which should include imaging studies with CT scan and/or MRI. During the surgical procedure the entire kidney should be explored in order to detect possible multifocality. The tumor must be resected within a rim of healthy parenchyma; simple enucleation is not indicated. Excavation or enucleoresection, wedge resection, or partial nephrectomy are the surgical techniques of choice. Finally the patient must be well informed about the possibility of kidney recurrence or local relapse and must adhere to a strict postoperative follow-up schedule.

Under these circumstances a considerable group of patients will benefit from conservative surgery for a small renal cell carcinoma in the presence of a normal contralateral kidney. In order to definitely establish the role of this approach, a randomized trial is necessary. Such a trial is being conducted by the Genitourinary Group of the European Organization for Research and Treatment of Cancer (EORTC), in protocol 30904, which is being coordinated by the authors.

*Acknowledgements.* Agnes Goethuys is acknowledged for word processing and preparation of the manuscript.

## References

Addonizio JC, Choudhury MS, Sayegh N, Chopp RT (1984) Cavitron ultrasonic surgical aspirator. Urology 13:417–420

Amendola MA, Bree RL, Pollack HM, et al. (1988) Small renal cell carcinoma: resolving a diagnostic dilemma. Radiology 166:637–641

Amis ES Jr, Cronan JJ, Pfister RC (1987) Needle puncture of cystic renal masses: a survey of the Society of Uroradiology. AJR 148:297–299

Anton P, Tanke HJ, Allehoff EP, Kuczyk MA, Stief SC, Jonas U (1995) Localized renal cell carcinoma: detection of abnormal cells in peritumoral tissue. World J Urol 13:149–152

Aso Y, Homma Y (1992) A survey on incidental renal cell carcinoma in Japan. J Urol 147:340–343

Assimos DG, Boyce WH, Woodruff RD, Harrison LH, McCullough DL, Krovand RL (1991) Intraoperative renal ultrasonography: a useful adjunct to partial nephrectomy. J Urol 146:1218–1220

Bazeed MA, Schärfe T, Becht E, Jurincic C, Alken P, Thüroff JW (1986) Conservative surgery of renal cell carcinoma. Eur Urol 12:238–243

Belussi D, Chinaglia D, Micheli E, Lembo A (1997) Conservative surgery of parenchymal renal carcinoma: urologic data from Lombardy. Arch Ital Urol Androl 69:87–91

Berg S, Jacobs SC, Cohen AJ, Li F, Marchetto D, Brown RS (1981) The surgical management of hereditary multifocal renal carcinoma. J Urol 126:313–317

Blackley SK, Ladaga L, Woolfitt RA, Schellhammer PF (1988) Ex situ study of the effectiveness of enucleation in patients with renal cell carcinoma. J Urol 140:6–10

Bosniak MA (1991) The small renal parenchymal tumors: detection, diagnosis and controversies. Radiology 179:307–317

Bosniak MA (1995) Observation of small incidentally detected renal masses. Semin Urol Oncol 13:267–272

Brisset JM, Lugagne PM, Veillon B, Vallencien G, Charton M, André-Bougaran J (1989) Parenchymal-sparing surgery for small renal cell cancer: are there any reasonable arguments? Prog Clin Biol Res 303:153–159

Brkovic D, Riedasch G, Waldherr R, Röhl L, Staehler G (1994) Lokale Recidive nach organerhaltender Nierentumorchirurgie. Urologe A 33:104–109

Brkovic D, Riedasch G, Staehler G (1997) The role of nephron-sparing surgery in renal cell carcinoma. Urologe A 36:103–108

Buizza C, Antonelli D, Chisena S, Bernasconi S, Zaroli A, Belloni M, Mandressi A (1997) Conservative therapy in renal carcinoma. Arch Ital Urol Androl 69:93–100

Butler BP, Novick AC, Miller DP, Campbell SA, Licht MR (1995) Management of small unilateral renal cell carcinomas: radical versus nephron-sparing surgery. Urology 45:34–41

Campbell SC, Novick AC (1994) Management of local recurrence following radical nephrectomy or partial nephrectomy. Urol Clin North Am 21:593–599

Campbell SC, Novick AC (1995) Surgical technique and morbidity of elective partial nephrectomy. Semin Urol Oncol 13:281–287

Campbell SC, Novick AC, Streem SB, Klein E, Licht M (1994) Complications of nephron sparing surgery for renal tumors. J Urol 151:1177–1180

Campbell SC, Fichtner J, Novick AC, et al. (1996) Intraoperative evaluation of renal cell carcinoma: a prospective study of the role of ultrasonography and histological frozen sections. J Urol 155:1191–1195

Carini M, Selli C, Muraro GB, Trippitelli A, Masini G, Turini D (1981) Conservative surgery for renal cell carcinoma. Eur Urol 7:199–201

Carini M, Selli C, Barbanti G, Lapini A, Turini D, Costantini A (1988) Conservative surgical treatment of renal cell carcinoma: clinical experience and reappraisal of indication. J Urol 140:725–731

Cheng WS, Farrow GM, Zincke H (1991) The incidence of multicentricity in renal cell carcinoma. J Urol 146:1221–1223

Chernoff DM, Silverman SG, Kikinis R, Adams DF, Seltzer SE, Richie JP (1994) Three-dimensional imaging and display of renal tumors using spiral CT: a potential aid to partial nephrectomy. Urology 43:125–129

Chinaglia D, Belussi D (1997) Multifocal renal carcinoma: anatomic-clinical aspects. Arch Ital Urol Androl 69:105–107

Ciancio G, Politano VA, Ferrell S, Block NL (1994) Renal parenchyma-sparing surgery as conservative treatment of renal cell carcinoma. Br J Urol 74:422–430

Colston JAC (1960) Operation for tumor in a solitary kidney: a review of the literature and report of cases. West J Surg 68:141–145

Costantini E, Mearini E, Ficola F, Petroni PA, Biscotto S, Monico S, Porena M (1996) Renal cell carcinoma: histological findings in peritumoral tissue after organ preserving surgery. Eur Urol 29:279–283

Curry NS, Schabel SI, Betrill WL (1986) Small renal neoplasms: diagnostic imaging, pathologic features and clinical course. Radiology 158:113–117

Czerny HE (1890) Cited by Herczele: Ueber Nierenexstirpation. Beitr Z Klin Chir 6:484–486

Dal Cin P, Aly MS, Delabie J, et al. (1992) Trisomy 7 and trisomy 10 characterize subpopulations of tumor infiltrating lymphocytes in kidney tumors and in the surrounding kidney tissue. Proc Natl Acad Sci 89:9744–9748

Dal Cin P, Van Poppel H, Van Damme B, Baert L, Van den Berghe H (1996) Cytogenetic investigations of synchronous bilateral renal tumors. Cancer Genet Cytogenet 89:57–60

D'Armiento M, Damiano R, Feleppa B, Perdona S, Oriani G, De Sio M (1997) Elective conservative surgery for renal carcinoma versus radical nephrectomy: a prospective study. Br J Urol 79:15–19

Emanuel A, Szucs S, Weier HU, Kovacs G (1992) Clonal aberrations of chromosomes X, Y, 7 and 10 in normal kidney tissue of patients with renal cell tumors. Genes Chromosom Cancer 4:75–77

Eschwege P, Saussine C, Steicher G, Delepaul B, Drelon L, Jacqmin D (1996) Radical nephrectomy for renal cell carcinoma 30 millimeters or less: long-term follow-up results. J Urol 155:1196–1199

Foster WL, Halvorsen RA, Dunnick NR (1985) The clandestine renal cell carcinoma: atypical appearances and presentations. Radiographics 5:175–192

Frohmüller HGW, Grups JW, Heller V (1987) Comparative value of ultrasonography, computerized tomography, angiography and excretory urography in the staging of renal cell carcinoma. J Urol 138:482–484

Gilbert BR, Russo P, Zirinsky K, Kazam E, Fair WR, Vaughan ED Jr (1988) Intraoperative sonography: application in renal cell carcinoma. J Urol 139:582–584

Goethuys H, Van Poppel H, Oyen R, Baert L (1996) The case against fine needle aspiration cytology for small solid kidney tumors. Eur Urol 29:284–287

Graber P (1991) Partial nephrectomy for renal carcinoma. Urol Int 47:213–215

Graham SD Jr, Glenn JF (1979) Enucleative surgery for renal malignancy. J Urol 122:546–549

Griffin JH, Flanigan RC (1996) Nephron sparing surgery for renal cell carcinoma. Tech Urol 2:43–47

Gschwend JE, Vogel U, Bader C, Mattfeldt T, Hautmann RE (1996) Predictive value of M.R.I. and computerized tomography for conservative renal surgery in an ex vivo tumor enucleation study followed by step-sectioning. J Urol 155:451–454

Hafez KS, Novick AC, Campbell SC (1997) Pattern of tumor recurrence and guidelines for follow-up after nephron sparing surgery for sporadic renal cell carcinoma. J Urol 157:2067–2070

Helm CW, Burwood RJ, Harrison NW (1983) Aspiration cytology of solid renal tumors. Br J Urol 55:249–252

Hernandez AD, Smith JA, Jeppson KG, Terreros DA (1990) Controlled study of the argon beam coagulator for partial nephrectomy. J Urol 143:1062–1065

Herr HW (1994) Partial nephrectomy for incidental renal cell carcinoma. Br J Urol 74:431–433

Herts BR, Baker ME (1995) The current role of percutaneous biopsy in the enucleation of renal masses. Sem Urol Oncol 13:254–261

Holland JM (1988) Editorial comment: incidental small renal tumors accompanying clinically overt renal cell carcinoma. J Urol 140:24

Jacobs SC, Berg SI, Lawson RK (1980) Synchronous bilateral renal cell carcinoma: total surgical excision. Cancer 46: 2341–2345

Jacqmin D, Saussine C, Roca D, Roy C, Bollack C (1992) Multiple tumors in the same kidney: incidence and therapeutic implications. Eur Urol 21:32–34

Jaeger N, Weissbach L, Wahlensieck W (1985) Value of enucleation of tumor in solitary kidneys. Eur Urol 11:369–373

Johansson S, Wahlqvist L (1981) Conservative surgery in renal carcinoma: total surgical excision. Scand J Urol Nephrol Suppl 60:25–27

Juul N, Torp-Pedersen S, Grønvall S, Holm HH, Koch F, Larsen S (1985) Ultrasonically guided fine needle aspiration biopsy of renal masses. J Urol 133:579–581

Kiser GC, Totonely M, Barry JM (1986) Needle tract seeding after percutaneous renal adenocarcinoma aspiration. J Urol 136:1292–1293

Kletscher BA, Qian J, Bostwick DG, Andrews PE, Zincke H (1995) Prospective analysis of multifocality in renal cell carcinoma: influence of histologic pattern, grade, number, size, volume and deoxyribonucleic acid ploidy. J Urol 153:904–906

Korhonen AK, Talja M, Karlsson H, Tuhkanon K (1993) Contact Nd:Yag laser and regional renal hypothermia in partial nephrectomy. Ann Chir Gynaecol Suppl 206:59–62

Kovacs G, Brusa P (1989) Clonal chromosome aberrations in normal kidney tissue from patients with renal cell carcinoma. Cancer Genet Cytogenet 37:289–290

Krishnamurthi V, Novick AC, Bukowski R (1996) Nephron-sparing surgery in patients with metastatic renal carcinoma. J Urol 156:36–39

Kurozumi T, Yagi H, Omoto T, Iwata Y (1993) Extracapsular tumor invasion in renal cell carcinoma: with special reference to limitation of surgical enucleation. Nippon Hinyokika Gakkai Zasshi 84:1943–1947

Lerner SE, Tsai H, Flanigan RC, Trump DL, Fleischmann JF (1995) Renal cell carcinoma: considerations for nephron sparing surgery. Urology 45:574–577

Lerner SE, Hawkins CA, Blute ML, Grabner A, Wollan PC, Eickholt JT, Zincke H (1996) Disease outcome in patients with low stage renal cell carcinoma treated with nephron sparing or radical surgery. J Urol 155: 1868–1873

Levine E, Hunfrakoon M, Wetzel LH (1989) Small renal neoplasms: clinical, pathologic and imaging features. AJR 153:69–73

Licht MR, Novick AC (1993) Nephron sparing surgery for renal cell carcinoma. J Urol 149:1–7

Licht MR, Novick AC, Goormastic M (1994) Nephron-sparing surgery in incidental versus suspected renal cell carcinoma. J Urol 152:39–42

London NJM, Messios N, Kinder RB, Smart JG, Osborn DE, Watkin EM, Flynn JT (1989) A prospective study of the value of conventional CT, dynamic CT, ultrasonography and arteriography for staging renal carcinoma. Br J Urol 64:209–217

Malek RS, Utz DC, Culp OS (1976) Hypernephroma in the solitary kidney: experience with 20 cases and review of the literature. J Urol 116:553–557

Marberger M (1986) Conservative surgery for renal adenocarcinoma. In: deKernion JB, Pavone Macaluso M (eds) Tumors of the kidney. Williams and Wilkins, Baltimore, pp 157–172

Marberger M, Pugh RCB, Auvert J, et al. (1981) Conservative surgery of renal carcinoma: the EIRSS experience. Br J Urol 53:528–532

Marshall FF, Taxy JB, Fishman EK, Chang R (1986) The feasibility of surgical enucleation for renal cell carcinoma. J Urol 135:231–234

Marshall FF, Holdford SS, Hamper UM (1992) Intraoperative sonography of renal tumors. J Urol 148:1392–1395

McDougall EM, Clayman RV, Anderson K (1993) Laparoscopic wedge resection of a renal tumor: initial experience. J Laparoendosc Surg 3:577–581

Moll V, Becht E, Ziegler M (1993) Kidney preserving surgery in renal cell tumors: indications, techniques and results in 152 patients. J Urol 150:319–323

Montie JE (1991) The incidental renal mass. Management alternatives. Urol Clin North Am 18:427–436

Montie JE, Novick AC (1988) Partial nephrectomy for renal cell carcinoma. J Urol 140:129–130

Morgan WR, Zincke H (1990) Progression and survival after renal-conserving surgery for renal cell carcinoma: experience in 104 patients and extended follow-up. J Urol 144: 852–858

Morgan WR, Zincke H (1991) Renal-conserving surgery for renal cell carcinoma. In: Rous Stn (series ed) Urology Annual vol 5. Appleton and Lange, Norwalk, Conn., pp 67–83

Mukamel E, Konichezky M, Engelstein D, Servadio C (1988) Incidental small renal tumors accompanying clinically overt renal cell carcinoma. J Urol 140:22–24

Muraki J, Cord J, Addonizio JC, Eshghi M, Schwalb DM, Armenakas N, Nagamatsu GR (1996) Application of microwave tissue coagulation in partial nephrectomy. Urology 37:282–287

Nissenkorn I, Bernheim J (1995) Multicentricity in renal cell carcinoma. J Urol 153:620–622

Novick AC (1987) Partial nephrectomy for renal cell carcinoma. Urol Clin North Am 14:419–433

Novick AC (1991) Possibilities and limitations of partial nephrectomy for renal cell carcinoma. Curr Opin Urol 1:30–33

Novick AC (1993) Renal-sparing surgery for renal cell carcinoma. Urol Clin North Am 20:277–282

Novick AC (1995) Partial nephrectomy for renal cell carcinoma. Urology 46:149–152

Novick AC, Straffon RA (1987) Management of locally recurrent renal cell carcinoma after partial nephrectomy. J Urol 138:607–610

Novick AC, Stewart BH, Straffon RA, Banowsky LH (1977) Partial nephrectomy in the treatment of renal adenocarcinoma. J Urol 118:932–936

Novick AC, Zincke H, Reves RJ, Topley HM (1986) Surgical enucleation for renal cell carcinoma. J Urol 135:235–238

Novick AC, Streem S, Montie JE, Pontes JE, Siegel S, Montague DK, Goormastic M (1989) Conservative surgery for renal cell carcinoma: a single-center experience with 100 patients. J Urol 141:835–839

Novick AC, Gephardt G, Guz B, Steinmuller D, Tubbs RR (1991) Long-term follow-up after partial removal of a solitary kidney. N Engl J Med 325:1058–1062

Oya M, Nakamura K, Baba S, Hata JI, Tazaki H (1995) Intrarenal satellites of renal cell carcinoma: histopathologic manifestations and clinical implications. Urology 46:161–164

Palmer JM, Swanson DA (1978) Conservative surgery in solitary and bilateral renal carcinoma: indications and technical considerations. J Urol 120:113–118

Paulson DF (1988) Prognostic factors in renal adenocarcinoma. Prog Clin Biol Res 269:359–380

Petritch PH, Rauchenwald M, Zechner O, et al. (1990) Results of organ-preserving surgery for renal cell carcinoma: an Austrian multicenter study. Eur Urol 18:84–87

Polascik TJ, Pound CR, Meng MV, Partin AW, Marshall FF (1995) Partial nephrectomy: technique, complications and pathological findings. J Urol 154:1312–1318

Provet J, Tessler A, Brown J, Golimbu M, Bosniak M, Morales P (1991) Partial nephrectomy for renal cell carcinoma: indications, results and implications. J Urol 145:472–476

Riedasch G, Brkovic D, Möhring K, Staehler G (1996) Conservative surgery for renal cell carcinoma: a 20 years single center experience. J Urol 155 (Suppl):389A

Ritchie AWS, Kemp IW, Chisholm GD (1984) Is the incidence of renal cell carcinoma increasing? Br J Urol 56:571–573

Rocca Rossetti S (1980) Premesse anatomo-pathologico alla nefrectomia radicale conservative. Estratti dal 3° Congresso Nazionale della Societa Italiana di Chirurgia Oncologica Roma, 1980

Rosenthal CL, Kraft R, Zingg EJ (1984) Organ-preserving surgery in renal cell carcinoma: tumor enucleation versus partial kidney resection. Eur Urol 10:222–225

Saiki S, Kinouchi T, Megudo N, Maeda O, Kuroda M, Usami M, Kotake T (1995) Multicentricity and concomitant tumors in renal cell carcinoma: analysis by serial section of resected kidneys. Hinyokika Kiyo 41:725–729

Sandock DS, Seftel AD, Resnick MI (1995) A new protocol for the follow-up of renal cell carcinoma based on pathological stage. J Urol 154:28–31

Scattoni V, Colombo R, Nava L, et al. (1995) Imaging of renal cell carcinoma with gadolinium-enhanced magnetic resonance: radiological and pathological study. Urol Int 54:121–127

Schärfe T, Thüroff JW, Alken P, Riedmiller H, Jacobi GH, Hohenfellner R (1988) Konservative Chirurgie des Nierenzellkarzinoms – Technik und Verlauf von 84 Patienten. Akt Urol 19:67–71

Schiff M Jr, Bagley DH, Lytton B (1979) Treatment of solitary and bilateral renal carcinomas. J Urol 121:581–582

Selikowitz SM (1995) A simple partial nephrectomy clamp. J Urol 154:489–490

Selli C, Lapini A, Carini M (1991) Conservative surgery for kidney tumors. Prog Clin Biol Res 370:9–17

Smith RB, deKernion JB, Ehrlich RM, Skinner DG, Kaufman JJ (1984) Bilateral renal cell carcinoma and renal cell carcinoma in the solitary kidney. J Urol 132:450–454

Staehler G, Ernst G (1985) Organerhaltende operative Therapie bei Nierentumoren. Urologe A 24:330–334

Steinbach F, Stöckle M, Riedmiller H, Weingärtner K, Hohenfellner R (1991a) Tumor enucleation of renal cell carcinoma: operative technique, DNA cytometry, results, complications. Prog Clin Biol Res 370:1–7

Steinbach F, Stöckle M, Thüroff JW, et al. (1991b) Parenchyma-sparing surgery for renal tumors. Experiences in over 120 patients. World J Urol 9:178–183

Steinbach F, Stöckle M, Müller SC, Thüroff JW, Melchior SW, Stein R, Hohenfellner R (1992) Conservative surgery of renal cell tumors in 140 patients: 21 years of experience. J Urol 148:24–30

Steinbach F, Novick AC, Zincke H, et al. (1995a) Treatment of renal cell carcinoma in von-Hippel Lindau disease: a multicenter study. J Urol 153:1812–1816

Steinbach F, Stöckle M, Hohenfellner R (1995b) Current controversies in nephron-sparing surgery for renal cell carcinoma. World J Urol 13:163–165S

Stephens R, Graham SD Jr (1990) Enucleation of tumor versus partial nephrectomy as conservative treatment of renal cell carcinoma. Cancer 65:2663–2667

Taari K, Salo JO, Rannikko S, Karkkainen P, Nordling S, Leatonen T (1993) Parenchyma conserving surgery for renal cell carcinoma. Ann Chir Gynaecol Suppl 206:54–58

Talamo TS, Shonnard JW (1980) Small renal adenocarcinoma with metastases. J Urol 124:132–134

te Strake L, Bloem JL, Falke THM, et al. (1988) Magnetic resonance imaging in the diagnosis and staging of renal masses: a critical appraisal and comparison with computer tomography. World J Urol 6:35–43

Thompson IM, Peek M (1988) Improvement in survival of patients with renal cell carcinoma: the role of the serendipitously detected tumor. J Urol 140:487–490

Topley M, Novick AC, Montie JE (1984) Long-term results following partial nephrectomy for localized renal adenocarcinoma. J Urol 131:1050–1052

Tosaka A, Ohya K, Yamada K, et al. (1990) Incidence and properties of renal masses and asymptomatic renal cell carcinoma detected by abdominal ultrasonography. J Urol 144:1097–1099

Trasher JB, Robertson JE, Paulson DF (1994) Expanding indications for conservative renal surgery in renal cell carcinoma. Urology 43:160–168

Van Poppel H, Baert L (1992) The case for conservative surgery for renal cell carcinoma. Prog Clin Biol Res 378:133–143

Van Poppel H, Baert L (1994) Elective conservative surgery for renal cell carcinoma. AUA Update Series, Lesson 31, vol XIII, pp 246–251

Van Poppel H, Claes H, Baert L (1986) Preoperative evaluation of small renal masses. Proc 3rd Congress European Society of Surgical Oncology, Lisbon, p 71

Van Poppel H, Claes H, Willemen P, Oyen R, Baert L (1991) Is there a place for conservative surgery in the treatment of renal cell carcinoma? Br J Urol 67:129–133

Van Poppel HP, Bamelis BF, Baert LV (1996) Non metastatic renal cell carcinoma. Curr Opin Urol 6:241–244

Van Poppel H, Bamelis B, Baert L (1997) Elective nephron-sparing surgery for renal cell carcinoma. Eur Urol Update Series 6:8–12

Velagapudi S, Ruckle HC, Zincke H (1993) Conservative surgery in patients with unilateral renal cell cancer and a normal contralateral unit: experience with 60 patients. J Urol (Suppl) 149:446A

Vermooten V (1950) Indications for conservative surgery in certain renal tumors: a study based on the growth pattern of the clear-cell carcinoma. J Urol 64:200–221

Viets DH, Vaughan ED Jr, Howards SS (1977) Experience gained from the management of 9 cases of bilateral renal cell carcinoma. J Urol 118:937–939

Walther MM, Choyke PL, Hayes W, Shawker TH, Alexander RB, Linehan WM (1994) Evaluation of color Doppler intraoperative ultrasound in parenchymal sparing renal surgery. J Urol 152:1984–1987

Wehle MJ, Grabstald H (1986) Contra-indications to needle aspiration of a solid renal mass: tumor dissemination by renal needle aspiration. J Urol 136:446–448

Whang M, O'Toole K, Dixon R, et al. (1995) The incidence of multifocal renal cell carcinoma in patients who are candidates for partial nephrectomy. J Urol 154:968–971

Wickham JEA (1975) Conservative renal surgery for adenocarcinoma: the place of bench surgery. Br J Urol 47:25–35

Wishnow KI, Johnson DE, Preston D, Tenney D (1990) Long-term serum creatinine values after radical nephrectomy. Urology 35:114–116

Yamashita Y, Honda S, Nishiharu T, Urata J, Takahashi M (1996) Detection of pseudocapsule of renal cell carcinoma with magnetic resonance imaging and CT. Am J Roentgenol 166:1151–1155

Zechner O, Hofbauer J, Karnel MF (1988) Die Problematik der organerhaltenden Chirurgie solider Nierentumoren. Akt Urol 19:72–77

Zincke H, Ruckle HC (1995) Use of exogenous material to bolster closure of the parenchymal defect following partial nephrectomy. Urology 46:96–98

Zincke H, Swanson SK (1982) Bilateral renal cell carcinoma: influence of synchronous and asynchronous occurrence on patient survival. J Urol 128:913–916

# 7 Palliative Surgical Therapy

H.P. VAN POPPEL and L. BAERT

CONTENTS



## 7.1
## Introduction

Management of metastatic renal cell carcinoma presents a very difficult problem. Thirty percent of patients diagnosed with renal cell carcinoma have metastatic disease at presentation. Following nephrectomy for apparently localized disease, 50% of patients will develop progression with the occurrence of distant metastases or locoregional recurrence. Most of these patients die within 1 year and the reported 5-year survival rates vary between 0% and 5% irrespective of therapy (SKINNER et al. 1971; MARCUS et al. 1993; MCNICHOLS et al. 1981).

The last century has witnessed the transformation of the medical profession from one whose primary


H.P. VAN POPPEL, MD, PhD, Professor of Oncologic Urology, Department of Urology, University Hospitals Gasthuisberg, Catholic University of Leuven, Herestraat 59, B-3000 Leuven, Belgium
L. BAERT, MD, PhD, Chairman, Department of Urology, University Hospitals Gasthuisberg, Catholic University of Leuven, Herestraat 49, B-3000 Leuven, Belgium


role involved sustaining the patient's morale and interpreting the natural history of an illness as it progressed, to one involved in active intervention as a sine qua non (OLIVER 1989).

The role of surgery for synchronous or metachronous metastatic disease of renal cell carcinoma has always been debated although resection of a solitary metastasis can be beneficial to a few patients only. This issue is even more controversial nowadays, when immunomodulating treatments are proving to have an impact on some patients' time to progression and survival. Surgery remains, however, the only effective treatment for renal cell carcinoma. Palliative surgical means are nephrectomy in the presence of metastatic disease, resection of locoregional recurrences, and surgery for metastases. The role of this surgical treatment in improvement the duration or the quality of survival remains highly controversial. Before dealing with any rationale for a surgical approach in metastatic renal cell carcinoma, some considerations on the occurrence of metastatic disease and the natural history of metastatic renal cell carcinoma should be discussed.

## 7.2
## Occurrence and Distribution
## of Metastatic Disease

Different pathways of metastatic spread of renal cell carcinoma are well known (VETTER 1990). First there is a lymphatic pathway responsible for lymph node metastases that occur in 17.5%–26% of patients (DE FORGES et al. 1988; HERRLINGER et al. 1984). The second pathway is the venous-lymphatic pathway, where neoplastic cells reach the veins through intranodal, lymphovascular channels or through the thoracic duct that empties into the inferior vena cava (SAITCH 1981). The third pathway is hematogenous tumor dissemination. Renal cell carcinoma is characterized by an affinity to penetrate the small renal veins. Most classically the neoplastic cells are shed off into the renal vein to reach the inferior vena cava, the right atrium, and the lung. Other cells, however, can circulate in the spermatic or ovarian vein and be responsible for metastatic spread along the ureters, the bladder, and the ovary. Finally, cancer cells can reach the vertebral veins in Batson's plexus and metastasize into the vertebral column, the thyroid gland, or the central nervous system (SLAVES 1988). The distribution of metastases is related to these different mechanisms of metastatic spread.

Metastases are often multiple and involve more than a single organ. In 43%–50% of patients, however, these metastases are confined to one organ and in 2%–4% they are solitary (O'DEA et al. 1978). The organs most commonly involved include: the lungs, lymph nodes, liver, and bone. Tumor spread to the heterolateral kidney, the homolateral or heterolateral adrenal, the spleen, the brain, and the heart is much less common. It is to be noted that nearly all organs have been involved as metastatic sites in renal cell carcinoma. Many unusual sites of metastatic disease have been reported (STENZL and DEKERNION 1989). Besides the common cerebral metastases there have been cases reported of metastases to the choroid plexus of the lateral ventricles (MIZUNO et al. 1992), to a cerebellar hemangioblastoma in a patient with von Hippel-Lindau disease (JAMJOOM et al. 1992), and to the pituitary gland (KOSHIYAMA et al. 1992; NISHIO et al. 1992). Renal cell carcinoma was also described to metastasize to the nose (JOHNSON and CAMPBELL 1993), into the masseter muscle (NAKAGAWA et al. 1996), in the retrobulbar region of the orbit (BERSANI et al. 1994), the iris (STENZL and DEKERNION 1989), the external auditory canal (GOLDMAN et al. 1992), the parotid gland (GUNBAY et al. 1989; OWENS et al. 1989; COPPA and OSZCZAKIEWICZ 1990) the tonsils (GREEN et al. 1997), and the thyroid (ZAHRADKA et al. 1988; HUDSON et al. 1991; MURAKAMI et al. 1993). In the chest endobronchial metastatic lesions have been reported (THEMELIN et al. 1990; YIM et al. 1996). Metastases to the skin were reviewed by WILLIAMS and HEANY (1994). Metastases to the abdominal wall (YANAGIE et al. 1987), to the gallbladder (GOLBEY et al. 1991), to the pancreas (CARINI et al. 1988; OKA et al. 1991; STANKARD and KARL 1992; TAKEUCHI et al. 1993; PAZ et al. 1996; HIROTA et al. 1996), and to the ampulla of Vater (LESLIE et al. 1996) have also been reported. Very often metastases have been found to be solitary and to have occurred many years after a nephrectomy. The genitourinary tract was reported to be the site of metastasis with the urinary bladder (NAIR and LITTLE 1991), the ureteral stump (SHIMURA et al. 1993; IIMORI et al. 1994), the ureter

and renal pelvis (MITTY et al. 1987) as well as the ovary, the epididymis, and the corpus cavernosum. Involvement of the soft tissues of the hand (WITTHAUT et al. 1994) and the index finger (KIERNEY et al. 1994) and rare skeletal sites such as a metacarpal of the hand (KOBUS et al. 1992) have also been reported.

Many of these metastatic sites cause symptoms that are not readily recognized to be related to a metastatic renal cell carcinoma. The previous history of renal cell carcinoma should therefore always be kept in mind when patients are presenting with unusual clinical manifestations. Renal cell carcinoma metastasis are known occasionally to cause symptoms of acute cholecystitis (GOLBEY et al. 1991), intestinal ischemia by arterial embolism (LOW et al. 1989), duodenal hemorrhage by pancreatic metastases (CALMES and MEYER 1993), bronchial obstruction (YIM et al. 1996), hypopituitarism (KOSHIYAMA et al. 1992), hoarseness (GREENBERG et al. 1992), and even epistaxis (JOHNSON and CAMPBELL 1993). Since these metastases can occur more than 20 years after resection of the primary tumor (PAZ et al. 1996), the patient or even the physician may not be aware of the previous history of renal cell carcinoma.

Finally, there can be some histopathological confusion between metastatic renal cell carcinoma and primary clear cell tumors, e.g., of the thyroid (SHIMIZU et al. 1995) or a clear cell odentogenic tumor (EVERSOLE et al. 1995). Specific immunohistochemical stainings need to be applied in order to make an appropriate diagnosis.

## 7.3
## Natural History and Prognostic Factors

The heterogeneous behavior of renal cell carcinoma in general is well recognized. After nephrectomy with curative intent, some patients will present early progression with metastases and death. Others will be alive for many years without progression of an untreated primary tumor (HOROWITZ et al. 1993) and without progression or even with regression of metastases (GRANT et al. 1997). The unpredictable natural history of renal cell carcinoma makes attempts to determine prognostic factors very difficult.

For renal cell carcinoma in general the tumor stage, nuclear grade, tumor size, and presence of venous involvement have been shown to be important prognostic factors. Survival of patients is probably most related to the local extent of the primary tumor, determined at the time of surgery (Bassil et al. 1985). General symptoms such as anemia, weight loss, and fever are considered unfavorable symptoms and signs. Takahashi found that the acute phase reactants (erythrocyte sedimentation rate, increased $\alpha_2$-globulin, and C-reactive protein increase) are reliable predictors of tumor progression (Takahashi et al. 1992). More recently, we have shown that microscopic vascular invasion is the single most significant adverse prognostic factor in patients who undergo surgery for presumably localized nonmetastatic renal cell carcinoma without lymph node or macroscopic venous involvement (Van Poppel et al. 1997).

In metastatic renal cell carcinoma, prognostic factors were also studied (de Forges et al. 1988). The most relevant prognostic factors were: performance status, weight loss, the occurrence of single or multiple metastases, localization of metastatic disease in the lung, bone, brain or liver, the size of the pulmonary metastases, the number of metastases, and the time of their appearance (deKernion 1983). Hypercalcemia was reported to be an unfavorable prognostic factor (Fahn et al. 1991). It is very likely that also the primary tumor characteristics are important for the prognosis of metastatic renal cell carcinoma. It has been shown that tumors smaller than 5 cm in diameter without invasion of the pelvicaliceal system or perirenal fat and with predominance of clear or granular cells are related to a better prognosis (Golimbu et al. 1986). Others, however, have suggested that the grade of the primary tumor has no prognostic value since the metastases are mostly of poorer differentiation or even of a different cell type (Arai et al. 1988).

With so many different prognostic factors it is impossible to predict an individual patient's outcome (Ritchie and Chisholm 1983). No patient can be considered cured, even following an apparently successful nephrectomy and having good prognostic factors. On the other hand, no patient with metastatic disease should be considered in imminent danger of dying although unfavorable prognostic factors in this patient category will mostly be correlated with a poor outcome.

In a malignancy such as renal cell carcinoma, with such a variable natural history, it is extremely important to take all possible measures to prevent the occurrence of disease progression or metastatic tumor spread. We feel that it is insufficiently pointed out that the primary oncologic surgery remains a relevant prognostic factor. A discussion on the need

for lymphadenectomy and resection of the adrenal gland has been ongoing for many years. It is not these patients with clinically detected lymph nodes or adrenal metastases who will likely benefit from resection. Rather, those who will most likely benefit from such a resection are patients with microscopic invasion of lymph nodes where a dissection will not only be a staging procedure but a curative operation (Skinner et al. 1972; Giuliani et al. 1983). We also feel that adrenalectomy should be advocated in patients undergoing radical nephrectomy, certainly in those having tumors of 5 cm or more in diameter. The incidence of having micrometastatic invasion of the adrenal in these patients is being estimated at 7% (Li et al. 1996). Finally, and this remains debated by many, the urologic surgeon should attempt primary control of the artery and vein before manipulating the tumor, which is actually only possible through a transperitoneal approach. All these surgical considerations need more emphasis and remain important mainstays in the appropriate surgery of a renal cell carcinoma.

## 7.4
## Nephrectomy in the Presence of Distant Metastases

Many urologists perform nephrectomy for metastatic renal cell carcinoma although it is obvious that a nephrectomy alone in a patient with metastatic spread cannot yield a cure. This was well illustrated by the results of a questionnaire sent to 55 European urological centers belonging to the European Organization for Research and Treatment of Cancer (EORTC) Genito-Urinary Group. All but two centers perform nephrectomy for selected patients with metastatic renal cell carcinoma (Van Poppel, oral communication, 1993).

Since the operation does not aim to cure, nephron-sparing surgery has been advocated by some authors (Krishnamurti et al. 1996). In most cases, however, metastatic renal cell carcinoma will present with a locally advanced tumor where a conservative surgical approach is not possible (Brkovic et al. 1997).

Many urologists attempt to find arguments in order to convince themselves that a patient with metastatic disease could have a nephrectomy. Either they pretend to treat symptoms caused by the primary tumor or want to be sure that the patient has a renal cell carcinoma and not, for example, a transitional cell carcinoma. Moreover, psychological factors make it difficult for a surgeon to leave an informed patient with an untreated primary tumor (OLIVER 1989). In fact, the only rationale in favor of a nephrectomy in the presence of metastasis should be increased survival or improvement in the quality of life (FOWLER 1987).

## 7.4.1
### Impact on Survival

Life could be prolonged with a nephrectomy because the tumor burden is reduced, and thus a possible source of new metastasis is removed. In studies comparing nephrectomy versus no nephrectomy a survival advantage was demonstrated in the nephrectomy group. It is obvious, however, that only those patients in good general condition and with more favorable prognostic factors underwent a nephrectomy (FLAMM and WOBER 1987). A randomized study is the only way to sort out whether nephrectomy provides any survival advantage.

It has been suggested that nephrectomy can induce spontaneous regression of metastases. Spontaneous regression was first described 70 years ago (BUMPUS 1928) and the reports on this phenomenon were recently summarized (DE RIESE et al. 1991; GEBOERS and DEBRUYNE 1992). The overall incidence of spontaneous tumor regression is estimated to be about 1% (MONTIE et al. 1977; VOGELZANG et al. 1992; KALLMEYER and DITTRICH 1992; MARCUS et al. 1993). Spontaneous regression was not only described for lung and soft tissue metastases but also in rare cases of metastases to the liver (RITCHIE et al. 1988) and even to the bone (MIMS et al. 1966). Spontaneous regression of intestinal, subcutaneous, or skin meta-stases was also reported (FREED 1977). Nevertheless, the indication to perform a nephrectomy in metastatic patients in order to obtain spontaneous regression remains dubious, and the 1% chance of spontaneous regression is much lower than the mortality of a nephrectomy, which in this group of patients is estimated at 3%–5%. Moreover, the spontaneous regression of metastatic lesions has also been reported to occur without surgery (EDWARDS et al. 1996).

Nephrectomy could potentially enhance a response to systemic therapy. Both hormone therapy (progestagens) and chemotherapy (Vinblastin) were reported to induce a response in about 15% of patients (BLOOM 1973; deKERNION 1983). One form of immunotherapy (interferon, interleukin, tumor necrosis factor, lymphokine-activated killer cells, or combinations thereof) induces tumor response in more than 20% of patients (TYKKÄ 1981; BELLDEGRUN et al. 1991; WALTHER et al. 1993; ATZPODIEN et al. 1993). Although the best results obtained need confirmation, it remains unproved that nephrectomy indeed enhances the response to systemic therapy. Current ongoing trials in collaboration between the South Western Oncology Group (SWOG) and the EORTC GU group (protocol 30947), where patients receive either interferon-α alone or nephrectomy followed by interferon-α, will give an answer to this important question. Meanwhile, however, nephrectomy continues to play a role in the management of patients who are scheduled to receive systemic therapy (WOLF et al. 1994; FRANKLIN et al. 1996).

A few years ago immunotherapy with autologous tumor cells was being advocated. In this setting the tumor nephrectomy was necessary in order to obtain the inactivated tumor cells. A similar mechanism was postulated to occur after angioinfarction followed by a nephrectomy, where tumor necrosis induces tumor antigens that are released and solicit an immunologic response. In a joint EORTC-SWOG study one partial and one complete remission were seen in a group of 64 patients treated (KURTH et al. 1984; GOTTESMAN et al. 1985). A review on this matter, however, failed to show a benefit of infarction and/or nephrectomy in metastatic renal cell carcinoma with respect to survival or metastatic regression (FLANIGAN 1987).

A final argument to remove the kidney could be an attempt to resect all tumor, i.e., when a resection of the primary tumor can be completed with a synchronous resection of a metastatic lesion(s). Many reports on resection of a solitary metastasis have shown that this can result in an improved survival and even long-term tumor control (NEVES et al. 1988). The most important problem with this indication for nephrectomy is the uncertainty about the true solitary nature of a metastasis. Since there is no other adequate therapy yielding better results than surgery, nephrectomy in the presence of a solitary metastasis that can be resected at the same time or a short time after the removal of the primary remains defendable.

## 7.4.2
### Impact on Quality of Life

A nephrectomy could be proposed as an attempt to relieve symptoms such as hematuria, pain, or systemic manifestations. Hematuria from a locally advanced primary tumor can be very impressive and be responsible for flank pain and lower urinary tract obstruction. Often blood transfusions are needed to correct severe anemia and the hematuria itself can be responsible for the patient's death. Nevertheless, nephrectomy is not the only available treatment for this problem since embolization is also an effective therapy (FLANIGAN 1996). The ischemic pain that a patient can experience after embolization can be managed successfully with epidural analgesia.

Flank or abdominal pain caused by the primary tumor can result from tumor necrosis and hemorrhage but also from tumor extension into the skeleton or be due to invasion of nerves. In these cases, a symptomatic improvement could be expected from a nephrectomy. The surgery however, will likely be extensive, difficult to perform, and not always succeed in controlling the pain. Pain caused by neural or skeletal invasion will indeed often persist after nephrectomy.

The systemic manifestations of metastatic renal cell carcinoma are general deterioration, anemia, anorexia, weight loss, fever, hypertension, and hypercalcemia. These symptoms, that are partly paraneoplastic, are very likely to improve after nephrectomy under the condition that no metastases are present that by themselves are responsible for the paraneoplastic symptomatology. In a metastatic patient, these systemic manifestations will often not be influenced by the nephrectomy unless metastasis can be treated at the same time.

One could advocate performance of a nephrectomy in a metastatic patient in order to prevent symptoms that could occur later, caused by a non-treated and growing primary tumor. However, most of the symptoms can be treated adequately when they arise, without surgery, and this is therefore not a valid argument for nephrectomy in metastatic patients. Nevertheless, metastatic patients who undergo nephrectomy will often experience an obvious improvement in general condition after resection of the primary tumor. There is at least a temporary improvement of the progressive deterioration that has already started and will continue until death when no treatment is given. In these patients, the morbidity (and mortality) of the surgery will have to be weighed against the general improvement that may be expected to be highly appreciated by patients and their families.

Finally, when leaving the primary tumor behind, psychological factors can decrease the quality of life. The decision for surgery or surveillance often depends on the urologist's ability to talk with a patient with advanced cancer, the willingness to inform the patient on the stage of the disease, and the arguments to treat or not to treat the primary tumor. One should keep in mind that a nephrectomy in advanced stages can be an operation with relevant morbidity, which also decreases the quality of life for a certain period. Some patients will be unable to undergo immunotherapy because of the impact of the surgery on the general condition (WALTHER et al. 1993; FRANKLIN et al. 1996; RACKLEY et al. 1994). Only well-designed randomized trials with quality of life assessment will answer the question as to the value of nephrectomy in patients with metastatic disease.

### 7.4.3 Conclusion

No patient with a renal cell carcinoma and metastases is cured by nephrectomy alone. Some patients unexpectedly survive with metastatic disease for a long period of time. There is still doubt about the priority of a nephrectomy in metastatic patients. Therefore, nephrectomy in patients with metastases will remain a valuable option in just a small and highly selected group of patients (ABI-AAD and DEKERNION 1997).

Since obtaining complete tumor regression at the primary site with systemic therapy is difficult, it may be preferable to consider a nephrectomy after immunotherapy in highly selected patients who have had a major systemic and local response (MOTZER et al. 1996).

In patients with resectable low-volume metastases a combination of nephrectomy with removal of all visible metastases can improve the 5-year survival rate. In patients with nonresectable metastases, nephrectomy can still be recommended for those in whom adjuvant experimental therapy will be used in addition to nephrectomy, in the framework of prospective clinical trials (FLANIGAN 1986).

Concerning the quality of life, most symptoms can be managed with means other than surgery. Besides the morbidity of nephrectomy, many patients will temporarily fare better. This ultimate subjective improvement can be extremely important in patients who, without surgery, are realizing that they will experience continuous deterioration of their condition.

## 7.5
## Locoregional Recurrence

Renal cell carcinoma can involve adjacent organs and contiguous structures. Direct invasion of the duodenum, pancreas, spleen, colon, mesentery, diaphragm, or liver may occur. Incomplete resection, which should be avoided by a correct surgical technique, can result in a local recurrence. When a macroscopically normal appearing adrenal gland or lymph node is not removed during the radical nephrectomy, this can be responsible for regional recurrence.

Patients with locoregional recurrence have less than 5% probability of survival after 5 years and therefore most of them will die before a local recurrence can become clinically relevant (DEKERNION et al. 1978). Recently, however, the use of computed tomography in the follow-up of patients after radical nephrectomy has resulted in a sharp increase in the incidence of early detection of local or regional recurrences. This early detection permits for frequent successful surgical intervention.

### 7.5.1
### Incidence

Although local recurrence rates following nephrectomy of 35% and more have been reported in the radiologic literature (ALTER et al. 1979), it is accepted that after surgery for renal cell carcinoma pathologic stage T2 or T3, the incidence of local recurrence should be about 2.5% (GIULIANI et al.1990).

Patients with invasion of the lymph nodes have a high risk of locoregional relapse (PHILLIPS and MESSING 1993). After a properly performed radical nephrectomy, including resection of the adrenal and lymph nodes, the incidence of local relapse is expected to be very low. For T4 lesions and sarcomatoid tumors, however, there appears to be an increased risk of leaving residual disease in the renal fossa, responsible for local recurrence.

We are convinced that routine lymphadenectomy can reduce the incidence of local recurrence. This is indeed our own experience. In our medical center nearly all patients undergo routinely lymphadenectomy. Since we have participated in EORTC protocol 30881 where patients are randomized to have a radical nephrectomy with or without lymphadenectomy, we were able to follow a number of patients in whom the lymph nodes were left behind. Two out of 36 patients who had no primary lymph

node dissection presented nodal recurrence and died within 2 years of diagnosis despite secondary resection. Late recurrences in the persistent adrenal gland are also well documented (OZGU et al. 1993; MAEDA et al. 1996). Nevertheless, it was recently suggested that adrenalectomy is mandatory only in the case of large upper pole lesions or abnormal-appearing glands on computed tomography scan and magnetic resonance imaging (MOTZER et al. 1996). It was clearly shown, however, that micrometastatic adrenal invasion, which will be responsible for local recurrence when the adrenal is left behind, is present in 7.5% of the tumors of >5 cm in diameter (LI et al. 1996). Moreover, a local recurrence emerging from the remaining gland, was shown to have the worst prognosis (TANGUAY et al. 1996). While adrenalectomy during radical nephrectomy is an easy procedure, a delayed adrenalectomy presents a difficult problem. Therefore we agree that in the absence of long-term data to suggest otherwise, the practice of removing the adrenal gland as part of radical nephrectomy should continue (BELLDEGRUN et al. 1991).

Adjuvant radiotherapy to the renal fossa after radical nephrectomy has been advocated (STEIN et al. 1992; KAO et al. 1994). A randomized trial, however, showed that postoperative radiotherapy in nephrectomized patients with a high risk of local recurrence is without beneficial effect on the relapse rate and survival (KJAER et al. 1987).

### 7.5.2
### Treatment

Patients with local recurrence following radical nephrectomy have a poor prognosis, with less than 15% probability of 1-year survival after diagnosis of recurrence. Surgical resection of a recurrence in the renal fossa is the only effective treatment that can be advocated when the lesion can be totally removed. The results of the use of other treatment modalities such as immunotherapy or chemotherapy are very poor. Radiation therapy can be used as a palliative treatment for symptomatic local recurrences in patients who are not operative candidates. Surgery is, however, the preferred treatment whenever feasible (CAMPBELL and NOVICK 1994).

The literature about resection of locally recurrent renal cell carcinoma is very scarce. Our own experience is limited to four patients. Surgery for local recurrence is a major procedure but can be justified in highly selected patients. The largest series of cases reported also showed that invasion of contiguous organs is common and that very extensive resection and reconstructive surgery are frequently needed. In most cases this kind of surgery, which can include partial hepatectomy or pancreatectomy, splenectomy, resection of part of the diaphragm or the abdominal wall musculature and vena cava, and small or large bowel, has a considerable morbidity and considerable perioperative mortality (ESRIG et al. 1992). Even when the recurrence is considered to be the only tumor site, its resection often will not influence the patient's survival. In some patients, however, a prolonged disease-free survival can be obtained and this alone can justify the use of this aggressive approach in properly selected cases. The use of neoadjuvant immunotherapy needs to be investigated.

We believe that prevention of local recurrence is the most important issue. As already mentioned, (neo)adjuvant radiation therapy will not improve the incidence of local control. The objective of primary surgery is a total tumor removal and the surgeon should not take any risks concerning the resection margins. Primary splenectomy, distal pancreatectomy, or colonic resections are easily feasible. A preventive lymphadenectomy and adrenalectomy will lower the incidence of regional recurrences.

Once a local recurrence occurs in the presence of metastatic disease successful treatment becomes anecdotal. Some investigators have advocated the use of immunotherapy with salvage surgery to be successful in an individual patient. Those rare patients who have benefited from this approach have had only pulmonary metastases (FLEISCHMANN and KIM 1991). Patients with metastases and local recurrence have an extremely poor prognosis. It has even been suggested that immunotherapy is not very effective in patients with retroperitoneal recurrence. The role of this approach should be further defined.

## 7.6
## Surgery for Metastases

### 7.6.1
### General Considerations

An aggressive approach for the management of solitary metastases of renal cell carcinoma was advocated since case reports on prolonged survival after this type of approach were reported. Already in 1939, a 23-year survival was reported after nephrectomy and excision of a solitary metastasis (BARNEY and CHURCHILL 1939) but probably only

1%–3% of patients with renal cell carcinoma have solitary metastases. The incidence of solitary metastasis reported by various authors was 1.6% (MIDDLETON 1967), 2.5% (O'DEA et al. 1978), 3.2% (TOLIA and WHITMORE 1975), and 3.6% (SKINNER et al. 1971). These investigators demonstrated that survival rates of 35%–50% can be achieved in conjunction with aggressive surgical therapy. It is of importance to note that these results were obtained before the use of the more effective systemic therapies that are currently available. As expected, there must be an important selection bias since only patients with good performance status were selected for additional surgery for metastatic disease (ABI-AAD and DEKERNION 1997). Interesting 3- and 5-year survival rates obtained after excision of solitary metastases were reported by a number of investigators (GEBOERS and DEBRUYNE 1997). The 5-year survival rates ranged from a low of 13% to a high of 50% (KLUGO et al. 1977; GOLIMBU et al. 1986; DINEEN et al. 1988).

Pulmonary metastases are considered to be optimally suitable for surgical treatment. The same metastatic site has been reported to respond best to the available immunomodulating agents. The application of surgical resection for solitary pulmonary metastasis was reported to result in a 5-year survival rate of 35% (TOLIA and WHITMORE 1975).

The most important question is how to identify patients with tumors whose biologic activity is compatible with an extended life expectancy. A number of adverse prognostic factors have been recognized. Some of these factors are related to the primary tumor, others are host-related factors, and still others are related to the type and location of metastasis. Prognostic factors related to the primary tumor are: nuclear grade, tumor stage, histologic type and tumor ploidy (GILCHRIST et al. 1984; MARRONCLE et al. 1994; SELLI et al. 1983; LJUNGBERG et al. 1986). The host-related adverse prognostic factors include: poor performance status, weight loss and other signs of nutritional deficiency, elevated sedimentation rate and other acute phase reactants, increased serum calcium, high interleukin-6 levels, and elevated serum ferritin (KOZLOWSKI 1994). A synchronous presentation of metastatic disease is less favorable than a metachronous occurrence of metastasis (MALDAZYS and DEKERNION 1986; NEVES et al. 1988; TALLEY et al. 1969). Although this has not been confirmed by other investigators, the authors of one study found that a subsequent development of metastasis did not affect the prognosis provided that all metastatic lesions were aggressively treated

(GOLIMBU et al. 1986). Survival is also related to the interval between nephrectomy and the development of a metachronous metastasis, a more favorable prognosis being associated with a prolonged interval (GOLIMBU et al. 1986; MALDAZYS and DEKERNION 1986). The presence of residual tumor in the renal fossa was also demonstrated to be of adverse prognostic significance (DEKERNION et al. 1978). Finally, pulmonary metastases have a better prognosis than all other metastatic sites (DEKERNION et al. 1978; MALDAZYS and DEKERNION 1986). The observation that patients with pulmonary metastasis have a better outcome than those with metastasis to other organs has not yet been explained. One possible explanation is that lung metastasis can be detected and treated early and cause less general deterioration than metastasis to other sites.

The analysis of published data on resection of solitary metastases has major drawbacks. All the studies are retrospective and concern small numbers of patients but most of these reports contain at least some patients who benefited from the use of an aggressive surgical approach. It is to be noted that those metastases with small tumor volume tend to be confined to the lungs. Cure after a resection of metastatic deposit remains uncommon although surgery can be justified for highly selected patients (VAN POPPEL and BAERT 1996).

## 7.6.2
## Surgery for Different Metastatic Sites

Surgery has been the most effective treatment in patients with pulmonary metastasis. Other organs also can present solitary metastatic deposits and are amenable for surgical resection. For some metastatic sites the use of radiotherapy has been advocated (see Chap. 10). The combination of these two treatment modalities and immunotherapy will need further investigation.

### 7.6.2.1
### Lung Metastasis

The lung is the most common site of tumor spread of renal cell carcinoma. When a small solitary metastasis appears it might be followed conservatively in order to see whether it progresses rapidly, in which case systemic treatment is considered. It has, however, been shown that, when the tumor doubling time is long, resection of the metastatic lesion can

improve the patient's prognosis (FUKUDA et al. 1987; OKUBO et al. 1993). The most important factor influencing survival is the completeness of resection (PONTES et al. 1989; POGREBNIAK et al. 1992; JET et al. 1993). Some investigators demonstrated no difference in survival among patients with single versus multiple pulmonary metastases provided they were completely resected (POGREBNIAK et al. 1991; TOBISU and KAKIGIE 1990; FOURQUIER et al. 1997). Most pulmonary metastases are amenable to a wedge resection. A margin of 1–2 cm of healthy pulmonary parenchyma is considered to be sufficient (KERN et al. 1987) while lobectomy and pneumonectomy are rarely indicated. In patients with bilateral pulmonary metastases, staged thoracotomies or sternotomy can be used. Thoracoscopic wedge resection may play an increasingly important role in the future management of pulmonary metastasis.

Since the patients reported in the literature had a good performance status and good pulmonary functional tests, the mortality and the morbidity of pulmonary resection of metastases were very low. Good surgical indications are therefore most important in maintaining a low incidence of treatment toxicity.

The management of other intrathoracic metastases has been described. An endobronchial metastasis was treated endoscopically (THEMELIN et al. 1990). Metastases to the pleura are not that uncommon but are in fact not amenable for surgical therapy. Involvement of the heart, pericardium, and diaphragm has also been reported but surgery has a limited role in their management (BENNINGTON and KRADJIAN 1967). Aggressive treatment for solitary pulmonary metastasis should be considered in patients with good performance status, in those with a primary tumor treated curatively, and in the absence of other metastatic involvement.

### 7.6.2.2
### Adrenal Gland

The occurrence of metastasis in the adrenal gland is so common that radical nephrectomy has been defined as an en bloc resection of the kidney, the perirenal fat, and the adrenal gland. Although adrenal metastases occur most frequently in patients with upper pole lesions, no tumor location in the kidney, tumor size, or tumor stage is completely free of this metastatic involvement. Micrometastatic invasion of an adrenal gland that was left behind following nephrectomy is probably responsible for late tumor recurrences. When there is a suspicion of metastatic disease in a primarily resected ipsilateral or in a contralateral adrenal gland and in the absence of other metastatic lesions, a resection should be proposed. A secondary adrenalectomy on the same side as the primary tumor can be difficult while a contralateral adrenalectomy is a much easier procedure to perform. Before undertaking the adrenalectomy, the patient should be informed of the need for lifelong replacement therapy. The prognosis of patients with metachronous adrenal metastasis is relatively poor (TANGUAY et al. 1996).

### 7.6.2.3
### Skeletal Metastasis

Renal cell carcinoma metastatic to the skeleton most commonly involves the spine and flat bones. These metastatic sites are not easily amenable for surgery and palliative radiotherapy should be considered (see Chap. 10). In 8%–12% of patients bone metastases are localized in the long bones, where surgical treatment could be offered (KATZNER and SCHVINGT 1990). Frequently severe pain that is caused by the presence of lytic lesions may lead to a diagnosis of metastatic renal cell carcinoma. If the pain problem is not addressed in these patients in a timely manner, pathologic fractures may result. Surgery for the treatment of metastasis to the bone aims to improve the quality of life by relieving pain and permitting recovery of function (LANGER et al. 1997). For this purpose orthopedic surgery using Ender's nailing, hip or shoulder arthroplasty, Küntsher nailing, bone cement, and methylmetacrylate are used. The results of these symptomatic approaches are good as regards pain relief and function recovery. In patients with disease in long bones postoperative radiotherapy should be applied following surgical therapy.

Patients with multiple skeletal metastases generally have a poor prognosis. The median survival for patients with multiple skeletal metastases is approximately 1 year irrespective of the therapy used in their management.

In contrast, about 30% of patients with solitary bone metastasis survive 5 years (SWANSON et al. 1981). Solitary bone metastases, however, are very rare (HENRIKSSON et al. 1992). Curative surgery is extremely rare but was reported by some investigators (HOSHI et al. 1991). A resection of a pelvic bone lesion and a lesion in the femur was described, resulting in no evidence of disease after 6 and 14 years after treatment, respectively (MARUOKA et al. 1990).

Also a resection of a lumbar vertebra was attempted with good local results but the patient died of other metastatic disease (STENER 1989). Embolization of vertebral metastases for spinal compression can obviate the need for surgery and has been applied with success by some investigators (O'RELLY et al. 1989).

Most skeletal metastases can only be treated palliatively and radiotherapy will be the treatment of choice. Radiotherapy will be effective in obtaining pain relief in a majority of patients (NIELSEN et al. 1991). A cure by radiotherapy of a solitary bone metastasis has not been reported. We have seen one female patient with a metastatic lesion in the calcaneus, explored by the orthopedic surgeon and leading to the diagnosis of renal cell carcinoma. The patient had local radiotherapy and underwent subsequent nephrectomy. She is now at 4 years after treatment without evidence of disease. Therefore, the finding of a solitary bone metastasis from renal cell carcinoma should not by itself be considered a sufficient reason for withholding therapy.

### 7.6.2.4
### Brain Metastasis

Brain metastases secondary to renal cell carcinoma are mainly located within the cerebral hemispheres (DELATTRE et al. 1988). Common clinical presentation includes: headache, motor deficit, seizures, and disorientation (DECKER et al. 1984). More recently, however, brain metastases of renal cell carcinoma are more often detected in the preclinical stage during rigorous follow-up with the use of CT scan or MRI. Brain metastases can be solitary and have been described as late as 18 years after radical nephrectomy (RADLEY et al. 1993).

Whole brain radiation therapy in association with corticosteroids is an acceptable palliative treatment for patients with multiple metastases. Surgery for tumor removal is frequently recommended, particularly in patients with a larger single cerebral metastasis (WRIGHT 1987; WRONSKI et al. 1997). It was suggested that the use of postoperative irradiation can improve local tumor control (DECKER et al. 1984; SAWAYA et al. 1994; BADALAMENT et al. 1990).

For selected patients with metastases that are not accessible or unsuitable for open surgery, stereotactic radiation surgery has become an attractive option (see Chap. 10). This new treatment approach may replace open surgery in the future (LUTZ et al. 1988; FULLER et al. 1992). The prognosis of patients with brain metastases from renal cell carcinoma is poor but surgery and radiation therapy in patients with good performance status will contribute to improved survival and better quality of life (DECKER et al. 1984).

### 7.6.2.5
### Liver Metastasis

While the liver can be invaded by direct tumor extension, the hepatic parenchyma can also be the site of solitary or multiple metastases. The prognosis of patients with hepatic tumor spread is worse than that of those with pulmonary, cerebral, or skeletal metastases. Therefore, these patients need to undergo a particularly thorough evaluation before surgery is considered as a therapeutic option (KOZLOWSKI 1994). At the time of surgical exploration the use of intraoperative ultrasonography is imperative. During tumor resection at least a 1-cm normal tissue margin needs to be obtained, or if this is impossible, a lobectomy has to be performed. Selective preoperative embolization or chemoembolization has been successfully applied in selected patients (SOULEN 1994). A hepatic local resection or lobectomy can be facilitated by the use of ultrasonic aspiration dissectors or argon or neodymium-YAG laser beams (KOZLOWSKI 1994).

### 7.6.2.6
### Pancreatic Metastasis

The pancreas has been shown to be the only site of metastatic disease of renal cell carcinoma in less than 1% of patients. Several cases have been reported where a partial pancreatectomy or duodeno-pancreatectomy was successfully performed (CALMES and MEYER 1993; TAKEUCHI et al. 1993; OKA et al. 1991; GOHJI et al. 1990; CARINI et al. 1988). One patient was reported to develop pancreatic metastasis 17 years after radical nephrectomy (STANKARD and KARL 1992). A review of the literature on the use of surgery for pancreatic metastasis demonstrated that prolonged survival can be achieved in properly selected patients. The extent of surgery should be determined following the localization of metastasis. There is an obvious need for an adequate surgical margin and in appropriate cases care should be taken to preserve enough pancreas to maintain its normal endocrine function.

### 7.6.2.7
### Thyroid Gland Metastases

The thyroid gland is not a common site of metastasis in patients with renal cell carcinoma, with only somewhat more than 100 cases having been reported in the literature. This literature was recently reviewed (HUDSON et al. 1991). In one patient, a metastatic lesion was diagnosed 11 years after radical nephrectomy (ZAHRADKA et al. 1988). In patients with thyroid metastasis who present with hoarseness, swallowing difficulties, or a palpable mass, a total or subtotal thyroidectomy can be performed. Histologic examination of a metastatic lesion can present a problem due to the difficulty in distinguishing it from a primary clear cell carcinoma of the thyroid. Postoperative irradiation is recommended in patients with close surgical margins (KOZLOWSKI 1994).

### 7.6.2.8
### Parotid Metastasis

The parotid gland is infrequently a site of metastasis of renal cell carcinoma (COPPA and OSZCZAKIEWICZ 1990; GUNBAY et al. 1989; OWENS et al. 1989). In one reported patient, parotid metastasis appeared 8 years after nephrectomy (OWENS et al. 1989). Those investigators recommended the use of superficial parotidectomy with preservation of the facial nerve in selected patients with solitary lesions.

### 7.6.2.9
### Other Metastatic Sites

Surgical treatment for very unusual metastatic sites has been described with most of the reported cases presenting with multiple lesions which were diagnosed by excisional biopsy. The vast majority of these patients are expected to have a poor prognosis irrespective of treatment used in their management. The use of systemic therapy should be investigated since surgery alone will only rarely provide long-term disease-free survival (KOZLOWSKI 1994).

### 7.7
## University of Leuven Experience
## with Solitary Metastases

Between 1983 and 1993, 373 radical nephrectomies were performed for renal cell carcinoma in our medical center. Of the 373 patients, 18 (4.8%) had a presumed solitary metastasis at the time of nephrectomy. Table 7.1 provides the sites of metastatic disease and the outcome in this group of patients. The seven patients presenting with pulmonary metastases were not treated surgically. Radiotherapy alone was used in the management of five patients with a skeletal metastasis. Adrenal metastases were present in four patients who were treated with resection at the time of radical nephrectomy. Two patients presented with thyroid or cutaneous metastasis. It should be pointed out that one of the seven patients with a pulmonary metastasis who received no specific therapy has no evidence of disease at 5 years since diagnosis. One of the five patients presenting with metastatic lesion to the calcaneus was treated with radiotherapy and has no evidence of disease at 4 years posttreatment.

An additional two patients who underwent adrenalectomy for metastasis are without evidence of disease at 3 and 8 years posttreatment, respectively, and a patient who was treated by a subtotal thyroidectomy also is without evidence of disease at 3 years posttreatment.

In the same period of time, 19 patients developed solitary metastatic disease from a few months to 8 years after radical nephrectomy. The time of appearance of metastatic disease, the treatment used, and the outcome are summarized in Table 7.2. The thyroid gland was the only organ thought to be involved in six patients and they survived 1 to 6 years after the resection. In the group with solitary pulmonary metastases, one patient remained without evidence of disease at 4 years after interferon-vinblastine therapy and one patient had no evidence of disease for the same period after lobectomy. One patient developed a metastatic bone lesion 14 years after surgery and was treated with intramedullary nail. He unfortunately died of an unrelated disease. These metastatic cases again demonstrated the unpredictable behavior of metastatic renal cell carcinoma.

## 7.8
## General Conclusions

The controversy on the use of nephrectomy for metastatic renal cell carcinoma will remain until randomized trials can provide answers to a number of critically important questions. Radical surgery for

**Table 7.1.** Solitary metastases in 18 patients at diagnosis

| Organ | Outcome |
| --- | --- |
| Lung ($n = 7$) | 6:CRD < 1 yr |
| | 1:NED 5 yr |
| Bone ($n = 5$) | 3:CRD < 1/2 yr |
| | 1:CRD 3 yr |
| | 1:NED 4 yr |
| Adrenal ($n = 4$) | 2:CRD < 1 yr |
| | 1:NED 3 yr |
| | 1:NED 8 yr |
| Thyroid ($n = 1$) | 1:NED 3 yr |
| Skin ($n = 1$) | 1:CRD < 1/2 yr |

NED, No evidence of disease; CRD, cancer-related death.

**Table 7.2.** Management of solitary metastases diagnosed following nephrectomy

| Site | No. | Time of presentation after nephrectomy | Treatment | Outcome |
| --- | --- | --- | --- | --- |
| Thyroid (6) | 1 | 1 yr | Resection | NED 3 yr |
| | 5 | 3–4 yr | Resection | CRD 1–6 yr |
| Lung (4) | 1 | 1 yr | IFα-VLB | NED 4 yr |
| | 1 | <1 yr | None | CRD < 1 yr |
| | 1 | <1 yr | Radiotherapy | CRD 3 yr |
| | 1 | 5 yr | Lobectomy | NED 4 yr |
| Bone (4) | 1 | 1 yr | Radiotherapy | CRD < 1 yr |
| | 1 | 15 mos | Radiotherapy | CRD < 1 yr |
| | 1 | 4 yr | Radiotherapy | CRD 6 yr |
| | 1 | 14 yr | Osteosynthesis | NCRD |
| Pancreas (2) | 1 | 4 yr | Resection | CRD 2 yr |
| | 1 | 8 yr | Biopsy | CRD 2 yr |
| Adrenal (1) | 1 | 1 yr | Resection | CRD < 1 yr |
| Pleura (1) | 1 | 3 yr | None | CRD < 1 yr |
| Spleen (1) | 1 | <1 yr | None | CRD < 1 yr |

NED, No evidence of disease; CRD, cancer-related death; NCRD, not cancer-related disease; IFα-VLB, interferon-α-vinblastine.

locoregional recurrence will have to be considered in patients with good performance status and favorable prognostic factors. Palliative resections in selected cases can provide prolonged disease-free survival and better quality of life of these patients. There is enough evidence that the excision of solitary metastases may result in long-term survival not only in patients with pulmonary metastasis but also in those with other metastatic sites. The outcome in all these patients will be determined more by the tumor and host-related prognostic factors than by the treatment modality used in their management. Since successful treatments of selected cases of metastatic renal cell carcinoma have been well documented in the literature, routine follow-up of patients treated with radical nephrectomy is required. Further clinical research on the value of combined therapeutic strategies is the main challenge for urologists or radiation and medical oncologists who are taking care of renal cell carcinoma patients.

*Acknowledgements.* Miss Sofie Hendriks is greatly acknowledged for word-processing of the text and for typing the manuscript.

# References

Abi-Aad AS, deKernion JB (1997) Surgery in advanced renal cell carcinoma In: Abi-Aad AS (ed) Adjuvant treatment in urological cancer. The Parthenon Publishing Group, New York, pp 41–52

Alter AJ, Uehling DT, Zwiebel WJ (1979) Computed tomography of the retroperitoneum following nephrectomy. Radiology 133:663–668

Arai Y, Kokuho M, Hayashida H, Konami T, Tomoyoshi T (1988) Surgical treatment for metastatic lesions from renal cell carcinoma. Hinyokika Kiyo: 34:623–636

Atzpodien J, Kirchner H, Hanninen EL, Deckert M, Fenner M, Poliwoda H (1993) Interleukin-2 in combination with interferon-alpha and 5-fluoro-uracil for metastatic renal cell cancer. Eur J Cancer 29A(Suppl):6–8

Badalament RA, Gluck RW, Wong GY, et al. (1990) Surgical treatment of brain metastases from renal cell carcinoma. Urology 36:112–117

Barney JD, Churchill EJ (1939) Adenocarcinoma of the kidney with metastasis to the lung. J Urol 42:269–276

Bassil B, Dosoretz DE, Prout GR Jr (1985) Validation of the tumor, nodes and metastasis classification of renal cell carcinoma. J Urol 134:450–454

Belldegrun A, Abi-Aad AS, Figlin RA, deKernion JB (1991) Renal cell carcinoma: basic biology and current approaches to therapy. Semin Oncol 18:96–101

Bennington JC, Kradjian RM (1967) Distribution of metastases from renal carcinoma. In: Renal cancer. W.B. Saunders, Philadelphia, pp 156–170

Bersani TA, Costello JJ Jr, Mango CA, Streeten BW (1994) Benign approach to a malignant orbital tumor: metastatic renal cell carcinoma. Ophthal Plast Reconstr Surg 10:42–44

Bloom HJG (1973) Hormone induced and spontaneous regression of metastatic renal cancer. Cancer 32:1066–1075

Brkovic D, Riedasch G, Staehler G (1997) The role of nephron-sparing surgery in renal cell carcinoma. Urologe A 36:103–106

Bumpus HC Jr (1928) The apparent disappearance of pulmonary metastases in a case of hypernephroma following nephrectomy. J Urol 20:185–188

Calmes JM, Meyer A (1993) Pancreatic hypernephroma manifested by a duodenal hemorrhage. Rev Med Suisse Romande 113:629–631

Campbell SC, Novick AC (1994) Management of local recurrence following radical nephrectomy or partial nephrectomy. Urol Clin North Am 21:593–599

Carini M, Selli C, Barbanti G, Bianchi S, Murado G (1988) Pancreatic late recurrence of bilateral renal cell carcinoma after conservative surgery. Eur Urol 14:258–260

Coppa GF, Oszczakiewicz M (1990) Parotid gland metastases from renal carcinoma. Int Surg 75:198–202

Decker DA, Decker VL, Herskovic A, Cummings GD (1984) Brain metastases in patients with renal cell carcinoma: prognosis and treatment. J Clin Oncol 2:169–173

de Forges A, Rey A, Klink M, Ghosn M, Kramar A, Droz JP (1988) Prognostic factors of adult metastatic renal carcinoma: a multivariate analysis. Semin Surg Oncol 4:149–154

deKernion JB (1983) Treatment of advanced renal cell carcinoma. Traditional methods and innovative approaches. J Urol 130:2–7

deKernion JB, Ramming JB, Smith RB (1978) The natural history of metastatic renal cell carcinoma: a computer analysis. J Urol 120:148–152

Delattre JY, Krol G, Thaler HT (1988) Distribution of brain metastases. Arch Neurol 45:741–745

de Riese W, Goldenberg K, Allhoff E, Stief C, Schlick R, Liedke S, Jonas U (1991) Metastatic renal cell carcinoma: spontaneous regression, long-term survival and late recurrence. Int Urol Nephrol 23:13–25

Dineen MK, Pastore RD, Emrich LJ, Huben RP (1988) Results of surgical treatment of renal cell carcinoma with solitary metastases. J Urol 140:277–279

Edwards MJ, Anderson JA, Angel JR, Harty JI (1996) Spontaneous regression of primary and metastatic renal cell carcinoma. J Urol 155:1385

Esrig D, Ahlering TE, Lieskowsky G, Skinner D (1992) Experience with fossa recurrence of renal cell carcinoma. J Urol 147:1491–1494

Eversole LR, Duffey DC, Powell NB (1995) Clear cell odontogenic carcinoma. A clinicopathologic analysis. Arch Otolaryngol Head Neck Surg 121:685–689

Fahn HJ, Lee YH, Chen MT, Huang JK, Chen KK, Chang LS (1991) The incidence and prognostic significance of humoral hypercalcemia in renal cell carcinoma. J Urol 145:248–250

Flamm J, Wober L (1987) Status of surgery in the treatment of metastatic renal cell carcinoma. Wien Klin Wochenschr 99:838–842

Flanigan RC (1987) The failure of infarction and/or a nephrectomy in stage IV renal cell cancer to influence survival or metastatic regression. Urol Clin North Am 14:757–762

Flanigan RC (1996) Role of surgery in patients with metastatic renal cell carcinoma. Semin Urol Oncol 14:227–229

Fleischmann JD, Kim B (1991) Interleukin-2 immunotherapy followed by resection of residual renal cell carcinoma. J Urol 145:938–941

Fourquier P, Regnard JF, Rea S, Levi JF, Levasseur P (1997) Lung metastases of renal cell carcinoma: results of surgical resection. Eur J Cardiothorac Surg 11:17–21

Fowler JE (1987) Nephrectomy in metastatic renal cell carcinoma. Urol Clin North Am 14:749–756

Franklin JR, Figlin R, Rauch J, Gitlitz B, Belldegrun A (1996) Cytoreductive surgery in the management of metastatic renal cell carcinoma: the UCLA experience. Semin Urol Oncol 14:230–236

Freed SZ (1977) Nephrectomy for renal cell carcinoma with metastases. Urology 9:613–616

Fukuda M, Satomi Y, Senga Y, Suzaki H, Nakahashi M, Ide K, Kondo I (1987) Results of pulmonary resection for metastatic renal cell carcinoma. Hinyokika Kiyo 33: 993–997

Fuller BG, Kaplan ID, Adler J, Cox RS, Bagshaw MA (1992) Stereotaxic radiosurgery for brain metastases: the importance of adjuvant whole brain irradiation. Int J Radiat Oncol Biol Phys 23:413–417

Geboers ADH, Debruyne FMJ (1992) Limitation of surgical curability in renal cell carcinoma. Prog Clin Biol Res 378:175–186

Gilchrist KW, Hogan TF, Harberg J, Sonneland PR (1984) Prognostic significance of nuclear sizing in renal cell carcinoma. Urology 24:122–124

Giuliani L, Martorana G, Giberti C, Pescatore D, Magnani G (1983) Results of radical nephrectomy with extensive lymphadenectomy for renal cell carcinoma. J Urol 130:664–668

Giuliani L, Giberti C, Martorana G, Rovida S (1990) Radical extensive surgery for renal cell carcinoma: long-term results and prognostic factors. J Urol 143: 468–474

Gohji K, Kamidono S, Yamanaka N (1990) Renal carcinoma in a solitary kidney. Br J Urol 66:248–253

Golbey S, Gerard PS, Frank RG (1991) Metastatic hypernephroma masquerading as acute cholecystitis. Clin Imaging 15:293–295

Goldman NC, Hutchison RE, Goldman MS (1992) Metastatic renal cell carcinoma of the external auditory canal. Otolaryngol Head Neck Surg 106:410–411

Golimbu M, Joshi P, Sperber A, Tessler A, Al-Askari S, Morales P (1986) Renal cell carcinoma: survival and prognostic factors. Urology 27:291–301

Gottesman JE, Crawford ED, Grossman HB, Scardino P, McCracken JD (1985) Infarction – nephrectomy for metastatic renal carcinoma. Urology 25:249–250

Grant R, Trevenen C, Hyndman WC, Rubin SZ, Coppes MJ (1997) Metastatic renal cell carcinoma in a child: 11-years' disease free survival following surgery. Med Pediatr Oncol 28:201–204

Green KM, Pantelides E, de Carpentier JP (1997) Tonsillar metastasis from a renal cell carcinoma presenting as a quinsy. J Laryngol Otol 111:379–380

Greenberg RE, Cooper J, Krigel RL, Richter RM, Kessler H, Petersen RO (1992) Hoarseness: a unique clinical presentation for renal cell carcinoma. Urology 40: 159–161

Gunbay MU, Ceryan K, Kupelioglu AA (1989) Metastatic renal cell carcinoma to the parotid gland. J Laryngol Otol 103:417–418

Henriksson C, Haraldsson G, Aldenborg F, Lindberg S, Pettersson S (1992) Skeletal metastases in 102 patients evaluated before surgery for renal cell carcinoma. Scand J Urol Nephrol 26:363–366

Herrlinger A, Schrott KM, Sigel A, Siedl J (1984) Results of 381 transabdominal radical nephrectomies for renal cell carcinoma with partial and complete en-bloc lymphnode dissection. World J Urol 2:114–119

Hirota T, Tomida T, Iwasa M, Takahashi K, Kaneda M, Tamaki H (1996) Solitary pancreatic metastasis occurring eight years after nephrectomy for renal cell carcinoma. Int J Pancreatol 19:145–153

Horowitz M, Herr HW, Reuter V (1993) Untreated hypernephroma of 33 years. Urology 41:278–279

Hoshi S, Orikasa S, Yoshikawa K, et al. (1991) Evaluation of bone metastases from renal cell carcinoma. Nippon Hinyokika Gakkai Zasshi 82:649–654

Hudson MA, Kavoussi LR, Catalona WJ (1991) Bilateral renal cell carcinoma with metastasis to the thyroid. Urology 37:145–148

Iimori H, Nishimoto K, Ikemoto S, Hayahara N (1994) A case report of ureteral stump metastasis from renal cell carcinoma. Hinyokika Kiyo 40:237–240

Ishikawa J, Umezu K, Yamashita K, Maeda S (1990) Solitary brain metastasis from renal cell carcinoma 14 years after nephrectomy. A case report. Hinyokika Kiyo 36:1439–1441

Jamjoom A, Kane N, Nicoll J (1992) Metastasis of a renal carcinoma to a cerebellar haemangioblastoma in a case of von Hippel-Lindau disease. Neurosurg Rev 15:231–324

Jet JR, Hollinger CG, Zinsmeister AR, Pairolero PC (1993) Pulmonary resection of metastatic renal cell carcinoma. Chest 84:442–445

Johnson IJ, Campbell JB (1993) Renal derived epistaxis. J Laryngol Otol 107:144–145

Kallmeyer JC, Dittrich OC (1992) Spontaneous regression of metastases in a case of bilateral renal cell carcinoma. J Urol 148:138–140

Kao GD, Malkowicz SB, Whittington R, D'Amico AV, Wein AJ (1994) Locally advanced renal cell carcinoma: low complication rate and efficacy of postoperative radiation therapy planned with CT. Radiology 93:725–730

Katzner M, Schvingt E (1990) Operative treatment of bone metastases secondary to renal carcinoma. Prog Clin Biol Res 348:151–168

Kern KA, Pass HI, Roth JA (1987) Surgical treatment of pulmonary metastases. In: Rosenberg SA (ed) Surgical treatment of metastatic cancer. J.B. Lippincott, Philadelphia, pp 69–100

Kierney PC, Van Heerden JA, Segura JW, Weaver AC (1994) Surgeon's role in the management of solitary renal cell carcinoma metastases occurring subsequent to initial curative nephrectomy: an institutional review. Ann Surg Oncol 1:345–352

Kjaer M, Frederiksen PL, Engelholm SA (1987) Postoperative radiotherapy in stage II and stage III renal adenocarcinoma: a randomized trial by the Copenhagen Renal Cancer Study Group. Int J Radiat Oncol Biol Phys 13: 665–672

Klugo RC, Detmers M, Stiles RE, Talley RW, Cerny JC (1977) Aggressive versus conservative treatment of stage IV renal cell carcinoma. J Urol 118:244–246

Kobus RJ, Leinberry C, Kirckpatrick WH (1992) Metastatic renal cell carcinoma in the hand: treatment with preoperative irradiation and ray resection. Orthop Rev 21:983–984

Koshiyama H, Ohgaki K, Hida S, Takasu K, Yumitori K, Shimatsu A, Koh T (1992) Metastatic renal cell carcinoma to the pituitary gland presenting with hypopituitarism. J Endocrinol Invest 15:677–688

Kozlowski JM (1994) Management of distant solitary recurrence in the patient with renal cancer. Urol Clin North Am 21:601–624

Krishnamurti V, Novick AC, Bukowski R (1996) Nephron sparing surgery in patients with metastatic renal cell carcinoma. J Urol 156:36–39

Kurth KH, Cinqualbre J, Oliver RTD, Schulman CC (1984) Embolisation and subsequent nephrectomy in metastatic renal cell carcinoma. World J Urol 1: 122–126

Langer W, Hofmockel G, Theiß M, Frohmüller H (1997) Surgical treatment of metastases in patients with renal cell carcinoma. Urologe A: 36:548–551

Leslie KA, Tsao JI, Rossi RL, Braasch JW (1996) Metastatic renal cell carcinoma to ampulla of Vater: an unusual lesion amenable to surgical resection. Surgery 119:349–351

Li GR, Soulie M, Escourrou G, Plante P, Pontonnier F (1996) Micrometastatic adrenal invasion by renal carcinoma in patients undergoing nephrectomy. Br J Urol 78:826–828

Ljungberg B, Stenling R, Roos G (1986) Prognostic value of deoxyribonucleic acid content in metastatic renal cell carcinoma. J Urol 136:801–804

Low DE, Frenkel VJ, Manley PN, Ford SN, Kerr JW (1989) Embolic mesenteric infarction: a unique initial manifestation of renal cell carcinoma. Surgery 106:925–928

Lutz W, Winston KR, Maleki PV (1988) A system of stereotactic radiosurgery with a linear accelerator. Int J Radiat Oncol Biol Phys 14:373–381

Maeda Y, Nakazawa H, Suzuki M, Ohshima T, Ito F, Onitsuka S, Kihara T (1996) Renal cell carcinoma with solitary asynchronous adrenal metastases. Hinyokika Kiyo 42:39–42

Maldazys JD, deKernion JB (1986) Prognostic factors in renal cell carcinoma. J Urol 136:376–379

Marcus SG, Choyke PL, Reiter R, et al. (1993) Regression of metastatic renal cell carcinoma after cytoreductive nephrectomy. J Urol 150:463–466

Marroncle M, Irani J, Dore B, Levillain P, Gonjon JM, Aubert J (1994) A prognostic value of histologic grade and nuclear grade in renal adenocarcinoma. J Urol 151: 1174–1176

Maruoka M, Miyauchi T, Nagayama T (1990) Surgical treatment of renal cell carcinoma with bone metastasis. Hinyokika Kiyo 36:1131–1135

McNichols DW, Segura JW, De Weerd JH (1981) Renal cell carcinoma: long-term survival and late recurrence. J Urol 126:17–23

Middleton RG (1967) Surgery for metastatic renal cell carcinoma. J Urol 97:973–977

Mims MM, Christenson BC, Schlumberger FC, Goodwin WE (1966) A ten-year evaluation of nephrectomy for extensive renal cell carcinoma. J Urol 95:10–12

Mitty HA, Droller MJ, Dikman SH (1987) Ureteral and renal pelvic metastases from renal cell carcinoma. Urol Radiol 1:16–20

Mizuno M, Asakura K, Nakajima S, et al. (1992) Renal cell carcinoma metastasizing to choroid plexus of lateral ventricle: a case report. No Shinkei Geka 20:469–474

Montie JE, Stewart BH, Straffon HA, Banowsky LHW, Hewitt CB, Montague DK (1977) The role of adjunctive nephrectomy in patients with metastatic renal cell carcinoma. J Urol 117:272–275

Motzer RJ, Bander NH, Nanus DM (1996) Renal cell carcinoma. Review article. N Engl J Med 335:865–875

Murakami S, Yashuda S, Nakamura T, Mishima Y, Iida H, Okano H, Nakano M (1993) A case of renal cell carcinoma with metastases to the thyroid gland and concomitant early gastric cancer. Surg Today 23:153–158

Nair HT, Little G (1991) Metastatic renal carcinoma: rare cause of outflow obstruction. J Postgrad Med 37: 232–233

Nakagawa H, Mizukami Y, Kimura H, Watanabe Y, Kuwayama N (1996) Metastatic masseter muscle tumor: a report of a case. J Laryngol Otol 110:172–174

Neves RJ, Zincke H, Taylor WF (1988) Metastatic renal cell cancer and radical nephrectomy: identification of prognostic factors and patient survival. J Urol 139: 1173–1176

Nielsen OS, Monro AJ Tannock IF (1991) Bone metastases: pathophysiology and management policy. J Clin Oncol 9:509–524

Nishio S, Tsukamoto H, Fukui M, Matsubara T (1992) Hypophyseal metastatic hypernephroma mimicking a pituitary adenoma. Neurosurg Rev 15:319–322

O'Dea MJ, Zincke H, Utz DC, Bernatz PE (1978) The treatment of renal cell carcinoma with solitary metastases. J Urol 120:540–542

Oka H, Hatayama T, Taki Y, Ueyama H, Hida S, Noguchi M (1991) A resected case of renal cell carcinoma with metastasis to pancreas. Hinyokika Kiyo 37:1531–1534

Okubo T, Okayasu T, Hasegawa N, Osaka Y, Tanabe T (1993) Surgical analysis for metastatic lung tumor originating from renal cell carcinoma. Nippon Kyobu Geka Gakkai Zasshi 41:614–618

Oliver RTD (1989) Surveillance as a possible option for management of metastatic renal cell carcinoma. Semin Urol 7:149–152

O'Reilly GV, Kleefield J, Klein LA, Blume HW, Dubuisson D, Cossgrove GR (1989) Embolization of solitary spinal metastases from renal cell carcinoma: alternative therapy for spinal cord and nerve root compression. Surg Neurol 31:268–271

Owens RM, Friedman CD, Becker SP (1989) Renal cell carcinoma with metastasis to the parotid gland: case reports and review of the literature. Head Neck 11:174–175

Ozgu I, Sahin A, Ozen H, Gedikoglu G, Remzi D (1993) Should radical nephrectomy include ipsilateral adrenalectomy? Int Urol Nephrol 25:417–422

Paz A, Koren R, Gal R, Wolloch Y (1996) Late solitary pancreatic metastasis from renal cell carcinoma. Isr J Med Sci 32:1319–1321

Phillips E, Messing EM (1993) Role of lymphadenectomy in the treatment of renal cell carcinoma. Urology 41:9–15

Pogrebniak HW, Haas G, Linehan WM, Rosenberg SA, Pass HI (1992) Renal cell carcinoma: resection of solitary and multiple metastases. Ann Thorac Surg 54:33–38

Pontes JE, Huben R, Novick A, Montie J (1989) Salvage surgery for renal cell carcinoma. Semin Surg Oncol 5: 282–285

Rackley R, Novick A, Klein E, Bukowski R, McLain D, Goldfarb D (1994) The impact of adjuvant nephrectomy on multimodality treatment of metastatic renal cell carcinoma. J Urol 152:1399–1403

Radley MG, McDonald JV, Pilcher WH, Wilbur DC (1993) Late solitary cerebral metastases from renal cell carcinoma: report of 2 cases. Surg Neurol 39:230–234

Ritchie AWS, Chisholm GD (1983) The natural history of renal carcinoma. Semin Oncol 10:390–400

Ritchie AW, Layfield LJ, deKernion JB (1988) Spontaneous regression of liver metastasis from renal carcinoma. J Urol 140:596–597

Saitch H (1981) Distant metastases of renal adenocarcinoma. Cancer 48:1487–1491

Sawaya R, Ligon BL, Bindal RK (1994) Management of metastatic brain tumors. Ann Surg Oncol 1:169–178

Selli C, Hinshaw WM, Woodard BH, Paulson DF (1983) Stratification of risk factors in renal cell carcinoma. Cancer 52:899–903

Shimizu K, Nagahama M, Kitamura Y, et al. (1995) Clinicopathological study of clear-cell tumors of the thyroid: an evaluation of 22 cases. Surg Today 25:1015–1022

Shimura H, Miura T, Kondoh I (1993) Ureteral stump metastasis for renal cell carcinoma: a case report. Hinyokika Kiyo 39:257–260

Skinner DG, Colvin RB, Vermillion CD, Pfister RC, Leadletter WF (1971) Diagnosis and management of renal cell carcinoma: a clinical and pathological study of 309 cases. Cancer 28:1165–1177

Skinner DG, Vermillion CD, Colvin RB (1972) The surgical management of renal cell carcinoma. J Urol 107:705–710

Slaves D (1988) Hematogenous dissemination of cells from renal adenocarcinoma. Br J Cancer 57:32–35

Soulen MC (1994) Chemoembolization of hepatic malignancies. Oncology 8:72–84

Stankard CE, Karl RC (1992) The treatment of isolated pancreatic metastases from renal cell carcinoma: a surgical review. Am J Gastroenterol 87:1658–1660

Stein M, Kuten A, Halpern J, Coachman NM, Coher V, Robinson E (1992) The value of postoperative irradiation in renal cancer. Radiother Oncol 24:41–44

Stener B (1989) Complete removal of vertebrae for extirpation of tumors: a 20-year experience. Clin Orthop 245:72–82

Stenzl A, deKernion JB (1989) Pathology, biology and clinical staging of renal cell carcinoma. Semin Oncol 16:3–11

Swanson DA, Orovan WL, Johnson DE, Giacco G (1981) Osseous metastases secondary to renal cell carcinoma. Urology 18:556–561

Takahashi A, Kumamoto Y, Tsukamoto T, Miyao N, Otani N, Yanase M, Masumori N (1992) Influential factors on recurrence of renal cell carcinoma. Nippon Hinyokika Gakkai Zasshi 83:59–65

Takeuchi H, Konaga E, Harano M, Watanabe K, Takeuchi Y, Hara M, Mano S (1993) Solitary pancreatic metastasis from renal cell carcinoma. Acta Med Okayama 47:63–66

Talley R, Moorhead EL, Tucker WG, San Diego EL, Brennan MJ (1969) Treatment of metastatic hypernephroma. JAMA 207:322–326

Tanguay S, Pisters LL, Lawrence DD, Dinney CPN (1996) Therapy of locally recurrent renal cell carcinoma after nephrectomy. J Urol 155:26–29

Themelin D, Duchatelet P, Boudaka W, Lamy V (1990) Endoscopic resection of an endobronchial hypernephroma metastasis using a polypectomy snare. Eur Respir J 3: 732 –733

Tobisu K, Kakigie T (1990) Surgical treatment of metastatic renal cell carcinoma. Jpn J Clin Oncol 20:263–267

Tolia BM, Whitmore WF Jr (1975) Solitary metastases from renal cell carcinoma. J Urol 114:836–839

Tykkä H (1981) Active specific immunotherapy with supportive measures in the treatment of advanced palliatively nephrectomised renal adenocarcinoma: a controlled clinical study. Scand J Urol Nephrol 63:1–9

Van Poppel H, Baert L (1996) Nephrectomy for metastatic renal cell carcinoma and surgery for distant metastases. Acta Urol Belg 64:11–17

Van Poppel H, Vandendriessche H, Boel K, et al. (1997) Microscopic vascular invasion is the most relevant prognosticator after radical nephrectomy for clinically non-metastatic renal cell carcinoma. J Urol 158:45–49

Vetter JM (1990) Metastasis of renal cell carcinoma: a pathologist's theoretical view. Prog Clin Biol Res 348:13–22

Vogelzang NJ, Priest ER, Borden L (1992) Spontaneous regression of histologically proved pulmonary metastases for renal cell carcinoma: a case with 5-year follow-up. J Urol 148:1247

Walther MM, Alexander RB, Weiss GH, et al. (1993) Cytoreductive surgery prior to interleukin-2-based therapy in patients with metastatic renal cell carcinoma. Urology 42:250–257

Williams JC, Heany JA (1994) Metastatic renal cell carcinoma presenting as a skin nodule: case report and review of the literature. J Urol 152:2094–2095

Witthaut J, Steffens K, Koob E (1994) An unusual case of metastasis to the soft tissues of the palm of the hand with compression of the median and ulner nerve by kidney cancer. Case report. Hand Chir Mikrochir Plast Chir 26:137–140

Wolf JS, Aronson FR, Small EJ, Carroll PR (1994) Nephrectomy of metastatic renal cell carcinoma: a component of systemic treatment regimens. J Surg Oncol 55:7–13

Wright DC (1987) Surgical treatment of brain metastases. In: Rosenberg SA (ed) Surgical treatment of metastatic cancer. J.B. Lippincott, Philadelphia, pp 165–222

Wronski M, Maor MH, Davis BJ, Sawaya R, Levin VA (1997) External radiation of brain metastases from renal carcinoma: a retrospective study of 119 patients from the M.D. Anderson Cancer Center. Int J Radiat Oncol Biol Phys 37:753–759

Yanagie H, Miyamoto H, Yoshizaki I, Takahashi T, Sekiguchi M, Fujii G (1987) A case of metastasis of renal cell carcinoma to the abdominal wall 13 years after nephrectomy. Gan-No-Rinsho 33:1950–1953

Yim AP, Abdullah VJ, Chan H (1996) A case of bronchial obstruction by metastatic renal cell carcinoma. Surg Endosc 10:855–856

Zahradka W, Poley F, Franz G (1988) Solitary late thyroid metastasis of a surgically removed kidney cancer. Z Gesamte Inn Med 43:398–399

# 8 Preoperative and Palliative Embolization

L. STOCKX and H. RAAT

## CONTENTS



## 8.1 Introduction

In our medical center, transcatheter embolization of renal cell carcinoma is a well-accepted vascular interventional procedure that is, however, gradually being applied less frequently. A recent survey in Britain and Ireland (1992) confirms the general abandonment by urologists of transcatheter embolization as a routine component of management of renal malignancy. In this survey only 35% of the responding urologists believed that embolization had a role, namely for palliation of bleeding and pain in cases where surgery would be otherwise inappropriate. An earlier similar survey in 1983 indicated that 60% of urologists still employed the embolization technique at that time (LANIGAN et al. 1992).

This decrease in the frequency of application of this procedure is probably related to the advent of new imaging methods like computerized tomography, magnetic resonance imaging, and ultrasound, which have significantly improved the probability of early detection of renal cell carcinoma. The result is a diminished number of patients presenting with advanced (and therefore sometimes inoperable) renal cell carcinoma. Another contributing factor is the fact that selection criteria nowadays are much stricter than they were a decade ago, when all hypervascular tumors larger than 2 cm were considered suitable candidates for embolization prior to nephrectomy (STOESSLEIN and MUENSTER 1991).

The above-mentioned evolution is also reflected by the abundance of literature on this subject in the late 1970s and 1980s, with scarce reports being published in the 1990s.

## 8.2 Indications

### 8.2.1 Preoperative Embolization

Indications for preoperative embolization are as follows:

1. Large tumors with extension into the renal hilum, which can render difficult the dissection of this area and subsequent clamping off of the renal artery. Complete renal artery embolization reduces perfusion of all larger tumors, regardless of vascularity (BAKAL et al. 1993). Embolization must be complete to be effective and includes the treatment of all identified accessory renal arteries and possible hypertrophic tumor-induced retroperitoneal tributaries. Preoperative embolization might make the resection more difficult by


L. STOCKX, MD, Department of Radiology, University Hospitals Gasthuisberg, Catholic University of Leuven, Herestraat 49, B-3000 Leuven, Belgium
H. RAAT, MD, Department of Radiology, University Hospitals Gasthuisberg, Catholic University of Leuven, Herestraat 49, B-3000 Leuven, Belgium

making the pulsation of the renal vessels more difficult to feel (LANIGAN et al. 1992).

2. Tumors with invasion of the renal vein or inferior vena cava and associated secondary elevated venous pressure. These patients are at higher risk for capsular venous bleeding (KAUFMANN et al. 1992). Another contributing empirically derived reason (personal communications with Prof. R. Oyen) is formation of postembolization tumor clot retraction, which makes it easier to extract tumor thrombus and therefore can prevent a cavotomy.

### 8.2.2
### Palliative Embolization

Indications for palliative embolization are as follows:

1. Hematuria, spontaneous bleeding or intolerable pain, associated with an unresectable tumor. In the majority of patients massive hematuria is the main indication for this procedure.
2. Unresectability of the tumor, as determined by diagnostic imaging, or the presence of distant metastases.
3. Inoperability of the patient because of cardiac, pulmonary, or cerebrovascular disease, i.e., increased risk associated with anesthesia or surgery.
4. Patients with paraneoplastic syndromes which may be life endangering, such as severe hypercalcemia.

The criteria for effectiveness in palliative embolization may be symptomatic improvement, decreased tumor size (assessed with follow-up CT scan), and prolonged survival. Whether palliative embolization has any beneficial effect on prolongation of survival remains controversial. KAUFMANN et al. (1989) initially reported exceptionally successful prolongation of survival (mean survival time 3 years) in six patients with renal carcinoma with metastases after palliative embolization by capillary occlusion with Ethibloc. In a subsequent report, however (KAUFMANN et al. 1992), the authors concluded that no change in the natural history of the disease was found. In spite of this finding, in their experience the outcome of patients without metastases compared very well with the results of radical nephrectomy performed in patients at comparable stages of renal cell carcinoma. PARK et al. (1994) presented their single center experience concluding that renal cell carcinoma patients with stage III disease have rela-

tively longer survival after embolization, and in these patients symptomatic relief may improve the quality of life.

A new but still experimental concept is the combination of intra-arterial chemotherapy and peripheral embolization of the arterial supply to the tumor. This could be indicated for tumor nodules in a solitary kidney and for recurrent retroperitonal tumor (KAUFMANN et al. 1992).

### 8.2.3
### Postoperative Embolization

The indication for postoperative embolization after partial nephrectomy is bleeding, which can manifest itself by ongoing or increasing hematuria, persisting or episodic hypotension, and flank bruits. Ancillary studies (such as computerized tomography and ultrasound) may suggest bleeding at the surgical site.

Selective renal embolization is performed if one or more of the following signs of renal vascular injury are seen:

1. Contrast extravasation
2. Pseudoaneurysm formation
3. Arteriocalyceal and arteriovenous fistula formation

We prefer the use of micro coils which are released via a coaxial catheter system. This allows embolization with optimal conservation of the renal parenchyma (Fig. 8.1).

### 8.3
### Contraindications

Relative contraindications to renal cell carcinoma embolization are as follows:

1. The presence of renal infection such as chronic pyelonephritis
2. A renal artery disease of the contralateral kidney

### 8.4
### Embolization Procedure

#### 8.4.1
#### Timing and Patient Preparation

In order to minimize the probability of postocclusive ischemic symptomatology, preoperative embo-

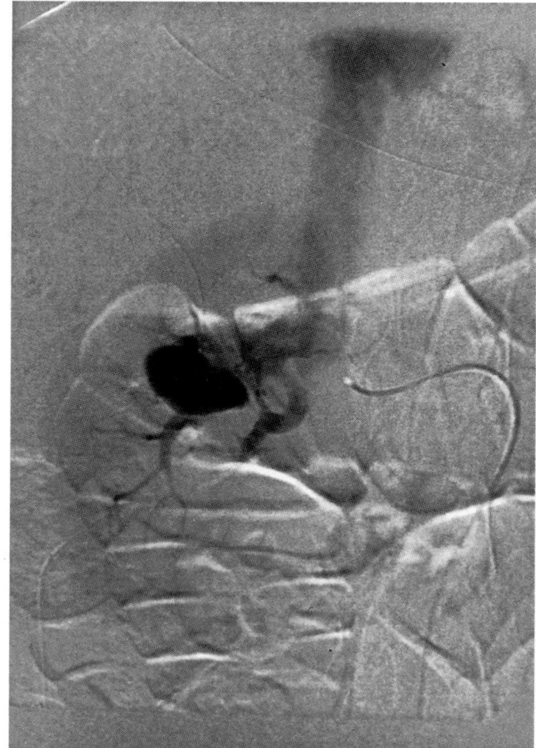

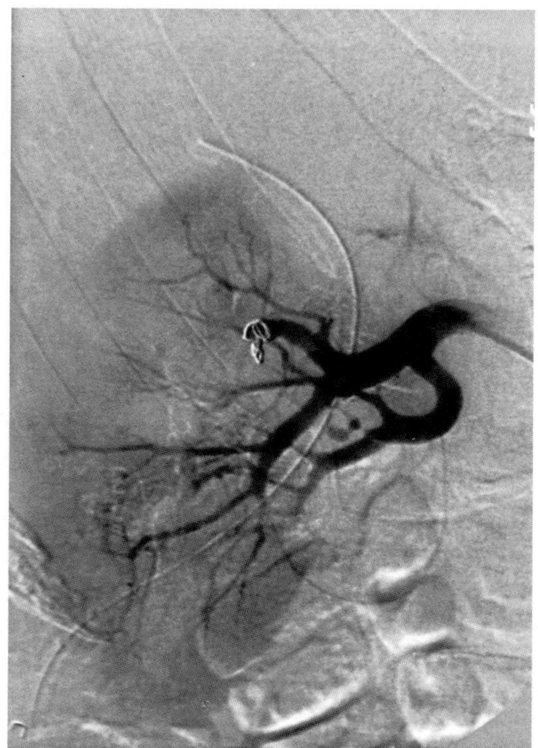

Fig. 8.1. a Large pseudoaneurysm in combination with early venous opacification of the renal vein and inferior vena cava after partial nephrectomy for renal cell carcinoma. b Selective embolization of the feeding artery was performed using two micro coils, thereby preserving the renal parenchyma

lization is usually performed 24 h before the planned nephrectomy. Because of the severity of pain commonly induced by the embolization, the procedure is performed under epidural anesthesia. To eliminate the relatively rare risk of renal abscess formation after embolization, patients receive antibiotics before, during, and after embolization. Elimination of asymptomatic bacteremia or infection of the upper genitourinary tract may prevent a potentially life-threatening renal abscess from developing, which could be a potential risk in the palliative group of patients (TUPPER et al. 1986).

## 8.4.2
## Treatment Technique

An extensive angiographic evaluation, including aortography and selective hepatic and bilateral selective renal arteriography, is performed to delineate the tumoral vascular anatomy and to assess the frequent collateral blood supply to the tumor. The aim of embolization is a peripheral capillary occlusion in combination with a more central occlusion of the renal artery at or close to its division into segmental vessels, but at a safe distance from its aortic origin.

The renal artery is selectively catheterized with a 5-Fr catheter via a transfemoral approach. In most cases a sidewinder (Simmons I or II) or cobra configuration will be optimal for catheterization of the renal artery. In the event of an early bifurcation, it may be necessary to selectively catheterize each branch. If a correct and stable position of the guiding catheter is achieved, a coaxial system with a microcatheter is introduced.

## 8.5
## Embolic Materials

### 8.5.1
### Polyvinyl Alcohol Particles

Polyvinyl alcohol particles (150–250 μm) (Ivalon, Contour Co.) are suspended in pure contrast material, and slowly injected with a 1-ml tuberculin syringe under fluoroscopic control.

Blood flow assists in peripheral embolization, and relative stasis of flow is the endpoint. In the case of rapid arteriovenous shunting (which is illustrated by opacification of the renal vein immediately after contrast injection) larger polyvinyl alcohol particles can be safely used (600 μm), since tumor vessels, even in the event of early shunting, are seldom lager than 100 µm in diameter. There are nonresorbable particles especially useful in the palliative group of patients.

### 8.5.2
### Gelatin Sponge

Gelatin sponge (Gelfoam, Spongostan) is an alternative peripheral embolization agent that can be cut into small cubes (1–3 mm); these are loaded in a 1-ml tuberculin syringe that is subsequently filled with contrast media and injected into the catheter. It is important to realize that this is a resorbable embolization agent, which gives only temporary success. Therefore it is more commonly used in the preoperative group of patients.

### 8.5.3
### Glue (Bucrylate)

The second step is administration of a mixture of tissue adhesive (acrylic glue) which can be mixed

with iodized oil (Lipiodol). This is usually diluted in the ratio 1 : 2 in a 2-ml syringe. The coaxial inner catheter is peripherally positioned, and slowly withdrawn under fluoroscopic control. Prior to the application, the inner catheter is rinsed free of blood, using a 40% glucose solution. The aim of this procedure is to fill with the embolus the intrarenal vascular system at the level of the subsegmental arteries. An attempt is made not to use this material in the proximal part of the main renal artery, since the risk of reflux into the aorta is too great (Figs. 8.2, 8.3).

### 8.5.4
### Steel Coils

The third and final phase may be a central occlusion with deployment of steel coils (diameter range of 3 mm, 5 mm, or 8 mm) in order to occlude the main renal artery. Care must be taken to place the coils distally enough (usually 2–3 cm) to allow the surgeons to tie off the artery at surgery.

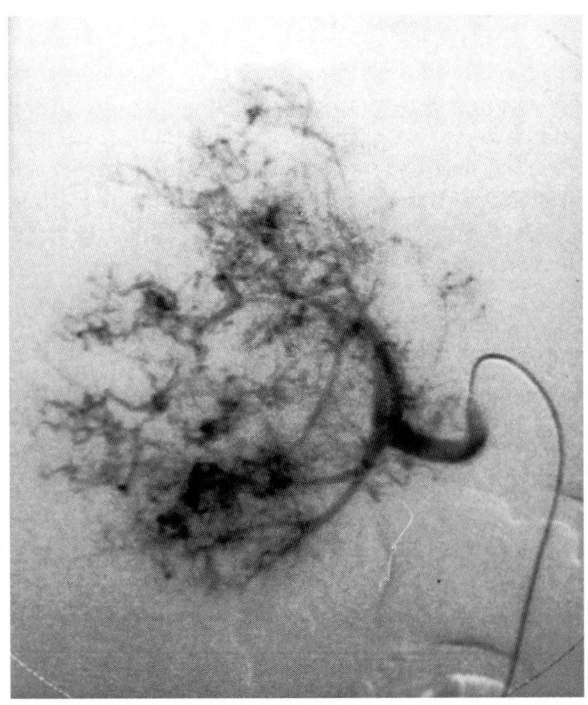

a

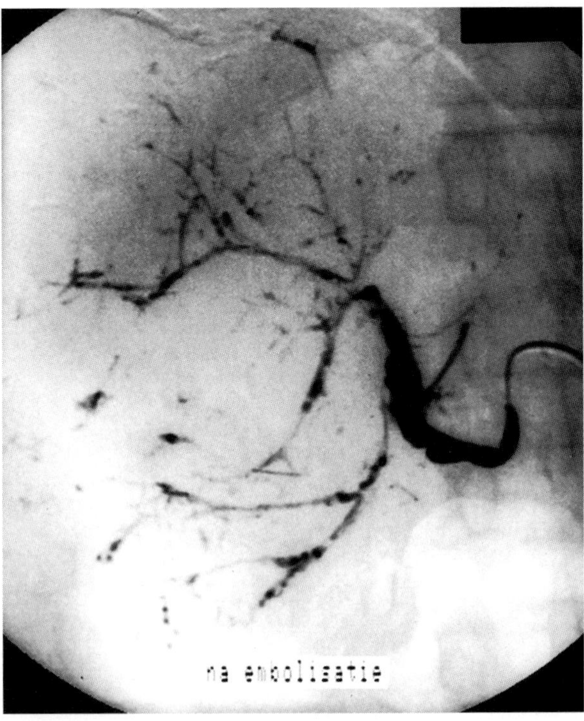


b

**Figure 8.2 a,b.** Renal angiography and preoperative embolization in a 56-year-old male with severe hematuria and nonmetastatic renal carcinoma. **a** Selective renal arteriogram of the right kidney shows a large hypervascular tumor extend- ing beyond the renal capsule. **b** Control after embolization with Ivalon and Histoacryl-Lipiodol at the level of the subsegmental arteries. Note stagnation of contrast and disap- pearance of capillary blush in the tumor

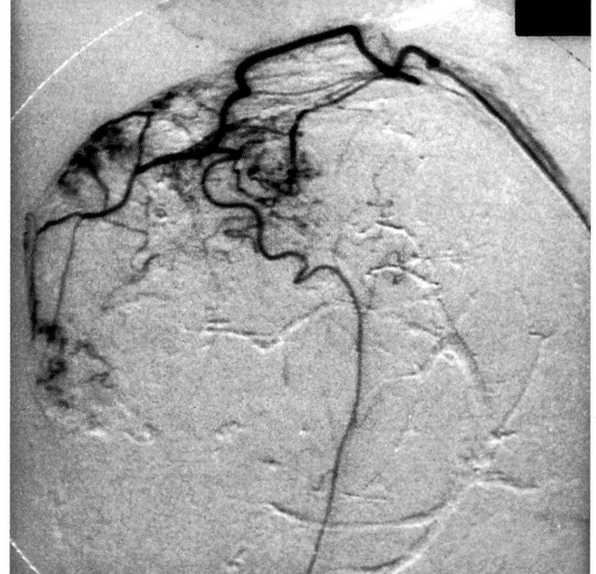

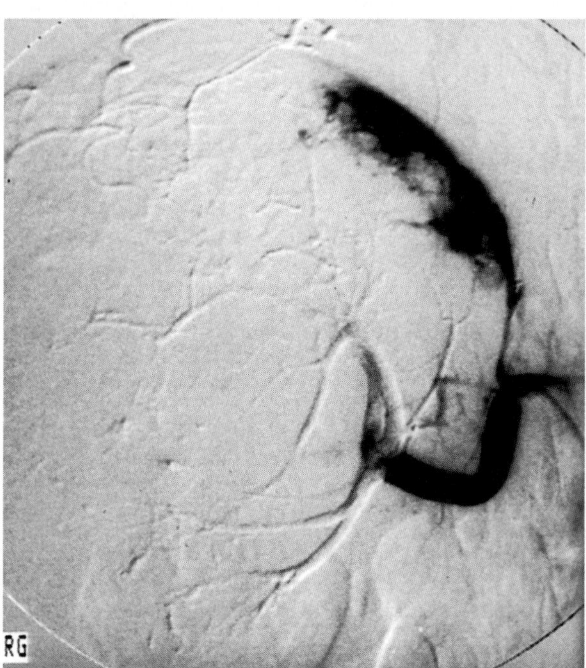

Fig. 8.3. **a** Selective angiography of a hypertrophic capsular artery of the upper pole. **b** Control angiography after embolization with Ivalon and Histoacryl-Lipiodol

## 8.5.5
## Ethanol

Ethanol is a powerful embolic agent, but its use entails a relatively high risk of inadvertent reflux. A total of 0.5 ml/kg of absolute ethanol can be injected into the renal artery. The limitation is the systemic effect of alcohol. It can be rendered radiopaque with iodized oil (Lipiodol). Ethanol produces thrombosis of the renal vascular bed and subsequent infarction of the neoplasm and kidney. It is safer to use a balloon catheter simultaneously. The use of this catheter increases the local concentration of alcohol, decreases the total dose necessary to produce infarction, and minimizes the risk of reflux. Potential hazards of ethanol use such as infarction of the colon (MULLIGAN and ESPINOSA 1983) (reflux in the inferior mesenteric artery) or testes (SINILUOTO et al. 1988) have been described.

## 8.5.6
## Ethibloc

Ethibloc is an "occlusion gel." The characteristic properties of Ethibloc are high viscosity, low speed of intravascular transportation, sufficient radiodensity, and the possibility of occluding arteriovenous shunts.

## 8.5.7
## Detachable Balloons

Detachable balloons are expensive and infrequently used devices primarily because of their relatively high cost. Additionally the use of these balloons results only in central occlusion, further limiting their application in the clinic.

## 8.6
## Treatment Complications

The most common complications of renal artery embolization are pain and the postemobolization syndrome. This syndrome consists of fever, leukocytosis, nausea, and vomiting. It occurs in nearly all patients and can last 1–5 days. To prevent pain the embolization procedure is always performed under epidural anesthesia. To prevent infectious complications the procedure is covered by intravenous administration of antibiotics before, during, and after the procedure. Hypertension occurs in many patients during embolization and may last 2–4 h.

Fever can persist for 2 months due to tumor resorption. Unintentional embolization with the polyvinyl alcohol particles, gelatin sponge, ethanol, and steel coils is always a potential hazard of embolization.

A large retrospective study by LAMMER et al. (1985) showed that in 121 renal tumor embolizations with four different embolic agents (Gelfoam, Ivalon, ethanol, and coils) the mean complication rate was 9.9%, with a mortality of 3.3%.

## 8.7
## Results

During a 5-year period between January 1992 and December 1997, 26 patients with renal cell carcinoma were referred to our department for embolization. This group consisted of six females whose age ranged from 53 to 80 years and 20 males whose age ranged from 34 to 84 years. This procedure turned out to be technically successful in all patients.

In the group of 20 male patients, 16 (80%) were treated preoperatively. Tumor was infiltrating the renal vein and vena cava in 11 of these patients. The remaining four (20%) male patients were treated palliatively for massive hematuria. The four palliatively treated patients showed no recurrence of hematuria during the period of observation ranging from 1 week to 3 months.

Of the six female patients, four (67%) were treated preoperatively. Two of the four treated patients had tumor thrombus extending into the inferior vena cava. The remaining two patients treated preoperatively had hypovascular tumors which on histopathologic examination were diagnosed as an angiomyolipoma and a transitional cell carcinoma, respectively.

An additional two female patients were treated palliatively. No technical complications were recorded in our patients. One of the treated male patients with myocardial disease developed acute pulmonary edema following the embolization.

There were four male patients who presented with bleeding after partial nephrectomy. All four patients were successfully treated with embolization utilizing minicoils.

Two males presented with a combination of pseudoaneurysm and arteriovenous fistula; one patient had an isolated pseudoaneurysm and the second presented with bleeding. Embolization was again successfully applied in the treatment of these four patients.

## 8.8
## Conclusions

Preoperative transcatheter arterial embolization of renal cell carcinoma has been shown to achieve a reliable breakdown of the peritumoral vasculature. This treatment met the surgical requirements for excision of very large tumors associated with abundant retroperitoneal tributaries. Embolization was particularly useful in those patients with tumors infiltrating the renal vein and inferior vena cava. The clinical efficacy of palliative embolization in those patients without metastatic disease may be comparable to palliative nephrectomy. Patients who present with bleeding at the surgical site after a partial nephrectomy will very likely benefit from the use of embolization.

A successful outcome of embolization requires a meticulously applied technique and good communication between urologist and interventional radiologist.

## References

Bakal CW, Cynamon J, Lakritz PH, Sprayregen S (1993) Value of preoperative renal artery embolization reducing blood transfusion requirements during nephrectomy for renal cell carcinoma. JVIR 4:727–731.

Kaufmann GW, Richter GM, Rohrbach R, Wenz W (1989) Prolonged survival following palliative renal tumor embolization by capillary occlusion. Cardiovasc Intervent Radiol 12:22–28

Kaufmann GW, Richter GM, Roeren TK (1992) Nierentumorembolisation. Radiologe 32:127–131

Lammer J, Justich E, Schreyer H, Pettek R (1985) Complications of renal tumor embolization. Cardovasc Interven Radiol 8:31–35

Lanigan D, Jurriaans E, Hammonds JC, Wells IP, Choa RG (1992) The current status of embolization in renal cell carcinoma – a survey of local and national practice. Clin Radiol 46:176–178

Mulligan BD, Espinosa GA (1983) Bowel infarction: complication of ethanol ablation of a renal tumor. Cardiovasc Intervent Radiol 6:55–57

Park JH, Kim SH, Koo Han J, Chung JW, Han MC (1994) Transcatheter arterial embolization of unresectable renal cell carcinoma with a mixture of ethanol an iodized oil. Cardiovasc Intervent Radiol 17:323–327

Siniluoto TM, Hellstrom PA, Paivansalo MJ, Leinonen AS (1988) Testicular infarction following ethanolembolization of a renal neoplasm. Cardiovasc Intervent Radiol 11:162–164

Stoesslein F, Muenster W (1991) Embolization of renal tumors. In: Kadir S (ed) Current practice of interventional radiology. Decker, Philadelphia, pp 625–631

Tupper TB, Cronan JJ, Wald LM, Dorfman GS (1986) Renal abscess: a complication of ethanol embolization. Radiology 161:35–36

# 9 Immunotherapy and Chemotherapy for Metastatic Renal Cell Carcinoma

S.J. Tucker, A. Belldegrun, and R.A. Figlin

CONTENTS



## 9.1 Introduction

Of the 28 800 new cases of renal cell carcinoma (RCC) diagnosed in 1997, approximately 10 000 will present with metastatic disease at the time of diagnosis (Parker et al. 1997). For these patients the prognosis is poor, with an estimated median survival of less than 1 year and an overall 5-year survival of less than 20% (Schwartzentruber et al. 1991). Spontaneous remissions of metastatic lesions have on rare


S.J. Tucker, MD, Fellow, Hematology/Oncology, Division of Hematology/Oncology, Department of Medicine, UCLA School of Medicine, 10945 LeConte Avenue, Suite 2333, Los Angeles, CA 90095, USA
A. Belldegrun, MD, Professor of Urology, Chief, Division of Urologic Oncology, Department of Urology, UCLA School of Medicine, 10945 LeConte Avenue, Suite 2333, Los Angeles, CA 90095, USA
R.A. Figlin, MD, Professor of Medicine, Division of Hematology/Oncology, Department of Medicine, UCLA School of Medicine, 10945 LeConte Avenue, Suite 2333, Los Angeles, CA 90095, USA


occasions been documented to occur after removal of the primary neoplasm (Montie et al. 1977). This documented fact provided one of the first insights into the importance of the immune system in the recognition and destruction of neoplastic cells. There are currently no successful chemotherapy agents for RCC; therefore protocols designed to exploit and modulate the immune system are currently the mainstay of metastatic RCC treatment. Multiple strategies for treatment, both FDA approved and experimental, exist and include infusional biologic response modifiers, adoptive immunotherapy involving transfer of cells with antitumor activity, and active immunotherapy which includes gene therapy, vaccine therapy, and monoclonal antibodies. Chemotherapy still has a role, albeit small, in the treatment of metastatic RCC but it primarily represents an option for palliation.

## 9.2 General Principles of Immunotherapy

The three primary cell types involved in the immune response include B and T lymphocytes, which classically mediate the humoral and cellular responses respectively, and professional antigen-presenting cells of the monocyte-macrophage lineage known as dendritic cells. Antigen-presenting cells activate T lymphocytes through the T-cell receptor in an MHC restricted (CD8+/class I and CD4+/class II) mechanism. Subsequent activity of T lymphocytes is either directed by direct contact with target cells or via secreted cytokines (Braciale et al. 1987; Townsend and Bodmer 1989; Unanue 1992).

Cytotoxic, CD8+, T lymphocytes have been shown to secrete interleukin-3, interferon-γ, and GM-CSF. CD4+ T lymphocytes are described as either Th1 or Th2 and secrete multiple cytokines and growth factors. Manipulation of these T lymphocytes and their products is the main goal of current immunotherapy protocols. In addition to the T lymphocytes, natural killer cells and lymphokine-activated killer cells constitute the effector arm of the immune response. These cells contribute to the constant surveillance and elimination of tumor cells. Successful immunotherapy protocols sensitize these effector cells to tumor antigens and produce a cytolytic response at the site of the cancer. The three major mechanisms by which this goal may be accomplished are: (1) direct infusion of immunostimulants, (2) adoptive immunotherapy with passive transfer of immune cells with antitumor activity to the tumor host, or (3) active immunotherapy by vaccination with tumor cells containing genes or immunostimulants or by transfection of tumor cells with genetic material that results in a cytolytic immune response (gene therapy).

## 9.3
## Biologic Response Modifiers

### 9.3.1
### Recombinant Interleukin-2

High-dose recombinant interleukin-2 (rIL-2) was approved for treatment of metastatic RCC in 1992 and remains the only agent approved for this indication (FYFE et al. 1995; ROSENBERG et al. 1994; ATKINS et al. 1993). rIL-2 does not act directly on tumor cells but activates immune effector cells which then target neoplastic tissues (ROSENBERG 1988). Initial studies with rIL-2 alone performed at the National Cancer Institute demonstrated an overall response rate of 18% and this has been confirmed by multiple other investigators (ROSENBERG 1991; WEST et al. 1987; FISHER 1988; ROSENBERG et al. 1989a, 1994; BUKOWSKI et al. 1990b; GEERTSEN et al. 1992; WEISS et al. 1992; ATKINS et al. 1993). Table 9.1 summarizes the major clinical investigations of rIL-2 in meta-

**Table 9.1.** Representative clinical trials of rIL-2 for the treatment of metastatic RCC

| Authors | Year | Patients | Response |
|---|---|---|---|
| WEST et al. | 1987 | 40 | 32% |
| FISHER | 1988 | 35 | 16% |
| ROSENBERG et al. | 1989a | 54 | 22% |
| BUKOWSKI et al. | 1990 | 41 | 12% |
| ROSENBERG | 1991 | 60 | 18% |
| GEERTSEN et al. | 1992 | 30 | 20% |
| WEISS et al. | 1992 | 94 | 18% |
| ATKINS et al. | 1993 | 71 | 17% |
| ROSENBERG et al. | 1994 | 143 | 20% |
| Total | | 568 | 20% |

static RCC. When these studies were combined, an overall response rate of approximately 15% (complete and partial responses) was demonstrated for high-dose rIL-2 (FYFE et al. 1995). The median survival for patients with metastatic RCC is approximately 40 months for those achieving complete responses and 24 months for those achieving partial responses. Additionally many of the complete responses are highly durable, with 5 or more years' survival. The cumulative experience with rIL-2 has also led to identification of patient characteristics that are associated with favorable responses to therapy with rIL-2: good clinical performance status and either lung, lymph node, or small-volume extrahepatic abdominal disease.

Use of rIL-2 is associated with significant side-effects which are dose-related and reversible. rIL-2 increases capillary membrane permeability and subsequent fluid and colloid losses into soft tissues (ROSENSTEIN et al. 1986; SIEGEL and PURI 1991; BELLDEGRUN et al. 1987, 1993a; WEBB et al. 1988). The most serious side-effect is prerenal azotemia with resultant hypotension, pulmonary edema, renal failure, and fluid retention. Myocardial infarction, gastrointestinal bleeding and perforation, and death may also occur. Less serious but common side-effects include fever, chills, erythroderma, mental status changes, thrombocytopenia, tachyarrythmias, and fluid retention. The majority of these side-effects are spontaneously reversible and resolve within 72 h of discontinuing treatment. Rosenberg has estimated the mortality from therapy at 4% but has also shown that this number declines as greater experience is obtained in using rIL-2 therapy (ROSENBERG et al. 1989a; BUKOWSKI et al. 1990b).

Given the host of serious yet reversible toxicities from rIL-2 therapy, researchers have devised multiple dosing regimens. These regimens include: high-dose intravenous (i.v.) bolus, low-dose i.v. bolus, low-dose subcutaneous, and continuous i.v. YANG et al. (1994) compared multiple dosing schedules in 260 patients in a randomized trial. This trial compared 720 000 international units (IU)/kg/i.v. bolus every 8 h (high-dose i.v. bolus group), 72 000 IU/ kg/i.v. bolus every 8 h (low-dose i.v. bolus group), and a subcutaneous arm 5 days each week similar to LISSONI et al. (1994). The objective response rate was 21% in the high-dose i.v. bolus group compared to 11% in the low-dose i.v. bolus group. Duration of response was significantly greater in the high-dose i.v. bolus group. Toxicity was also greater in the high-dose i.v. bolus group, with more than 50% of patients experiencing significant toxicities requiring treatment of hypotension compared to less than 5% in the low-dose i.v. bolus group. In the subcutaneous arm the response rate and toxicities were similar to those in the low-dose i.v. bolus group. Accrual and follow-up continue on this trial.

High-dose continuous infusion of rIL-2 is frequently used in Europe at doses near 18 million IU/m$^2$ per day. Initial results revealed similar response rates to those achieved using high-dose bolus infusion, but with reduced toxicity profiles (WEST et al. 1987). In a multicenter trial, 57 patients with metastatic RCC were given continuous infusion of 18 million IU/m$^2$ per day for 120 h followed by 6 days of rest prior to a further 108 h of therapy (VAN DER MAASE et al. 1991). An overall response rate of 16% was reported, with two complete responders. Despite three treatment-related deaths the authors reported improved tolerance, with no requirement for monitoring in the intensive care unit. Subsequent studies confirmed the response rates of 15%–20% (GEERTSEN et al. 1992; WEISS et al. 1992) but it is still difficult to demonstrate that continuous infusion high-dose rIL-2 provides a significant benefit to patients over bolus infusion except that toxicities appear to be lessened. Two concerns with delivering rIL-2 by continuous infusion are that serum levels may not approach the maximal tolerated dose and the frequent need to decrease infusion rates secondary to hemodynamic toxicity. A better understanding of the dose-response relationship is required before the implications of these data can be fully evaluated. Overall, high-dose i.v. bolus therapy with rIL-2 appears to be the most effective regimen for metastatic RCC in terms of response rate, duration of response, and overall survival. However, therapy with rIL-2 is associated with significant toxicities that can be avoided by experienced clinicians with adequate monitoring of patients.

## 9.3.2
## Recombinant Interferon-α

Crude preparations of interferon-a have been available since 1980 and by 1983 early clinical trials reported objective responses to intramuscular injection in patients with metastatic RCC. Independently, researchers at the University of California, Los Angeles (UCLA) and at the M.D. Anderson Cancer Center reported regression of metastatic tumor with the partially purified product (DEKERNION et al. 1983; QUESADA et al. 1983). At UCLA, objective responses were seen in 7/43 (16%) evaluable patients with a

median duration of response of approximately 9 months, while at the M.D. Anderson Cancer Center 13/50 (26%) patients had objective responses with a median duration of response of approximately 8 months. Since then multiple studies, using purified recombinant interferon-α (rIFN-α) have demonstrated an objective response rate from the treatment of more than 900 patients in 13 clinical trials of 18.4%, and response durations from 6 to 10 months; however, complete responses are rare (GITLITZ et al. 1996; FIGLIN and GITLITZ 1997). Table 9.2 summarizes the major clinical trials using rIFN-α in the last decade. The optimal dose schedule has not been determined, with responses of good quality (6–10 months' duration) documented when rIFN-α was administered in various dosing regimens. Published data suggest that a dose of 10–20 million IU per day produces optimal response rates with single-agent rIFN-α therapy (WIRTH 1993). Unfortunately, the impact of single-agent rIFN-α on overall survival in patients with RCC has not been demonstrated.

As with rIL-2, certain clinical variables appear to predict the likelihood of response to rIFN-α therapy. Patients with good performance status, prior nephrectomy, and nonbulky pulmonary and/or soft tissue metastases, who are asymptomatic or who exhibit minimal symptoms, have a higher likelihood of response (MINASIAN et al. 1993; MUSS 1988; SARNA et al. 1987). Response rates of up to 30% and response durations of greater than 27 months have been observed in a select subset of patients who have excellent performance status, prior nephrectomy, and no previous therapy. In contrast, patients with unresected primary RCC, extensive prior treatment,

**Table 9.2.** Representative clinical trials of rIFN-α for the treatment of metastatic RCC

| Authors | Year | Patients | Response |
| --- | --- | --- | --- |
| DEKERNION et al. | 1983 | 34 | 16.5% |
| QUESEDA et al. | 1983 | 19 | 26% |
| NEIDART et al. | 1984 | 33 | 15% |
| FIGLIN et al. | 1985 | 23 | 13% |
| QUESEDA et al. | 1985 | 50 | 26% |
| KIRKWOOD et al. | 1985 | 30 | 23% |
| UMEDA and NIIJIMA | 1986 | 226 | 17.7% |
| FOSSA et al. | 1986 | 18 | 33% |
| MUSS et al. | 1987 | 97 | 7% |
| SARNA et al. | 1987 | 65 | 14% |
| CREAGAN et al. | 1988 | 29 | 34% |
| FIGLIN et al. | 1989 | 18 | 26% |
| MINASIAN et al. | 1993 | 159 | 10% |
| Total | | 801 | 20% |

and bulky metastases are less likely to respond (Muss et al. 1987).

Side-effects of rIFN-α therapy include fever, chills, myalgia, anorexia, and headache. These are usually associated with initial dosing and improve spontaneously with continued administration. Occasional reversible hepatic and hematologic changes are encountered, but they, too, usually abate without necessitating change in dosing schedules.

The prognostic findings predicting survival in patients with RCC suggest that those who benefit may have prolonged survival due to the inherent natural history of their tumor. Tumor biology may provide additional factors associated with responsiveness to rIFN-α therapy. Evidence suggests a correlation between rIFN-α responsiveness and expression of a kidney-restricted glycoprotein, gp-160, in tissue culture (Nanus et al. 1990). Further explanations for variable sensitivity may be found in rIFN-α-regulated gene expression. Renal cell carcinoma cell lines sensitive to rIFN-α show a down-regulation of epidermal growth factor receptors upon exposure, while cell lines resistant to rIFN-α show no regulation of their epidermal growth factor receptors (Eisenkraft et al. 1991). Ongoing studies are evaluating both the clinical and the biologic parameters that may predict responsiveness to rIFN-α therapy.

### 9.3.3
### Combination Therapy with Recombinant Interferon-α and Interleukin-2

Combination therapy is a mainstay of most successful chemotherapeutic regimens. This concept can be reasonably applied to therapy with biologic response modifiers as immune surveillance and destruction of tumor is a multistep process involving numerous cytokines and immune cells. While both rIL-2 and rIFN-α produce response rates of 15%–20% as single agents for metastatic RCC, the responses to rIL-2 are considered of "greater quality" based on number of complete responders and duration of responses of several years. This response, however, comes at a greater price in terms of systemic toxicity, which limits the number of patients eligible for therapy. Murine tumor models have shown that the combined administration of rIL-2 and rIFN-α yields synergistic antitumor effects (Cameron et al. 1988; Rosenberg et al. 1988; Chikkala et al. 1990). These biologic agents have different mechanisms of action, with rIL-2 being an immune modulator and rIFN-α having some direct antiproliferative effects (Nanus

et al. 1990; Fidler et al. 1987; Mule et al. 1987). The administration of rIFN-α may augment the immunogenecity of tumor cells by enhancing expression of major histocompatibility antigens and tumor antigens, making them more susceptible to rIL-2-stimulated T lymphocytes (Wan et al. 1987; Heron et al. 1978).

Initial trials of combination therapy at the National Cancer Institute (NCI) demonstrated an overall response rate of 31%; however, the rIL-2 was given in escalating i.v. bolus doses similar to single-agent rIL-2 bolus therapy (Rosenberg et al. 1989b). Since then trials of combination immunotherapy have emphasized low-dose, outpatient-based regimens with lower toxicity profiles. Table 9.3 is a summary of major phase I and II trials of therapy combining rIL-2 and rIFN-α. The data available to date from 1200 patients treated with this combination collectively demonstrate an objective response rate of 20% and a complete response rate of 5%. Responses have occurred at all disease sites including bone, primary tumors, and visceral metastases, and have been observed in patients with bulky tumor burdens. Since 1988, 52 patients at UCLA have been treated with combination therapy and the results compare favorably with high-dose bolus rIL-2 administered alone: the overall response rate was 25%, the median duration of response was 23 months, and the median duration of survival was greater than 34 months (Figlin et al. 1992;

**Table 9.3.** Representative clinical trials of combination of rIL-2 and rIFN-α for the treatment of metastatic RCC

| Authors | Year | Patients | Response |
|---|---|---|---|
| Rosenberg et al. | 1989b | 35 | 31% |
| Budd et al. | 1989 | 12 | 8.3% |
| Lee et al. | 1989 | 5 | 0% |
| Atzpodien et al. | 1990 | 17 | 36% |
| Bergman et al. | 1990 | 10 | 20% |
| Kirchner et al. | 1990 | 17 | 29% |
| Mittleman et al. | 1990 | 18 | 22% |
| Hirsch et al. | 1990 | 15 | 40% |
| Bukowski et al. | 1990a | 20 | 15% |
| Sznol et al. | 1990 | 7 | 43% |
| Figlin et al. | 1992 | 52 | 25% |
| Thomas et al. | 1992 | 34 | 6% |
| Spencer et al. | 1992 | 22 | 5% |
| Budd et al. | 1992 | 21 | 10% |
| Ilson et al. | 1992 | 34 | 12% |
| Vogelzang et al. | 1993 | 42 | 12% |
| Lipton et al. | 1993 | 39 | 33% |
| Atkins et al. | 1993 | 28 | 11% |
| Atzpodien et al. | 1995 | 152 | 25% |
| Total | | 580 | 20% |

HRUSHESKY et al. 1990; FALCONE et al. 1993; SPARANO et al. 1993). In general the frequency of response with this modality is equivalent to or greater than that reported with rIL-2 alone, and durable complete responses are reported with both regimens; however, no large properly performed randomized trial has directly compared the efficacy of rIL-2 alone versus combination of rIL-2 and rIFN-α.

Several studies have also investigated the combination of rIL-2, rIFN-α, and 5-fluorouracil for metastatic RCC. In one study, the combination of these three agents resulted in an overall response rate of 45% with only moderate toxicity (SELLA et al. 1994). A recent study using this regimen (rIL-2 s.c. 20 MIU/m$^2$, rIFN-α 6–9 MIU/m$^2$, 5-FU 750 mg/m$^2$) demonstrated an overall response rate of 39% with 11% complete responses (LOPEZ HANNIEN et al. 1996). Stratification of these patients by risk factors disclosed a significant survival advantage with this combination compared to single-agent rIL-2 in patients at low and intermediate risk. Further confirmation of these data and additional toxicity information are still needed. The addition of other chemotherapeutic drugs such as vinblastine, doxorubicin, floxuridine, and BCNU does not alter the response rate or the duration of response but does result in significant hepatotoxicity and myelosuppression (FIGLIN et al. 1985; FOSSA et al. 1986; MUSS et al. 1985; CREAGAN et al. 1994; HOMMA and ASO 1994).

A combination regimen that has demonstrated synergistic antitumor effects in vitro against several RCC cell lines is the combination of rIFN-α with cis-retinoic Acid (CRA). Results of a phase II trial using this combination in 44 patients with metastatic RCC demonstrate a 30% response rate in 43 evaluable patients with three complete responses and ten partial responses (MOTZER et al. 1995). The median response duration was 22 months. This combination may provide additive therapeutic benefits when compared to rIFN-α alone and currently a multicenter, randomized phase III trial is directly comparing the effect of rIFN-α alone with rIFN-α plus CRA.

### 9.3.4
### Recombinant Interferon-γ and Recombinant Interleukin-12

Interferon-γ, either as a single agent or in combination with rIFN-α therapy, has been disappointing, with little or no improvement over single-agent rIFN-α or rIL-2 (ELLENHORST et al. 1994; RINEHART et al. 1986; QUESADA 1987; SAYERS et al. 1990;

ERNSTOFF et al. 1990). Recombinant interleukin-12 (rIL-12) is currently under investigation in phase I trials in patients with metastatic RCC. Recombinant IL-12 is thought to induce the expression of other cytokines, chemokines, and their receptors (WIGGINTON et al. 1996). In vitro and animal data suggest that pulses of rIL-2 in combination with rIL-12 additively enhance the priming of macrophages for nitric oxide production in culture and delayed growth of tumors in murine systems far more effectively than does either agent alone. There is also evidence to suggest that the combination of these two cytokines may induce a significant antiangiogenic effect. There are two ongoing phase I trials investigating the safety and efficacy of rIL-12 in metastatic RCC. One trial is using a fixed dose of subcutaneous rIL-12 while the second is a dose-escalation trial starting at 0.1 Mg/kg and escalating to the maximum tolerated dose, which has not yet been reached. While regression of tumors has not been observed to date, decreases in the rates of tumor growth have been documented.

## 9.4
## Adoptive Immunotherapy

A variety of adoptive immunotherapeutic strategies have been investigated in RCC, including adoptive transfer of tumor-infiltrating lymphocytes (TILs) and autolymphocyte therapy (ALT). Lymphocytes with potential cytotoxic antitumor activity can be isolated from peripheral blood, tumor-draining lymph nodes, or primary tumor tissue. These cells are subsequently expanded ex vivo and reinfused into the patient, often in combination with biologic response modifiers, in the hope of improving the rate and durability of response.

### 9.4.1
### Tumor-Infiltrating Lymphocytes

Initial approaches to adoptive immunotherapy centered on therapy utilizing lymphokine-activated killer (LAK) cells. These cells, primarily natural killer cells, are generated by cultivating peripheral blood with rIL-2 for 3–4 days. LAK cells mediate tumor lysis in a non-MHC-restricted manner (GRIMM et al. 1993) and have a combined response rate of 24% (WEISS et al. 1992; THOMPSON et al. 1992; FOON et al. 1992; SZNOL et al. 1992; PARKINSON et al. 1990; DILLMAN et al. 1993). However, a randomized trial that compared rIL-2 alone to rIL-2 combined with LAK cells was unable to demonstrate any superiority to the combination therapy (ROSENBERG et al. 1993) and this approach has been abandoned. Whereas LAK cells are nonspecific natural killer cells, TILs are activated cytotoxic T cells, which show a greater specificity in their targets. TILs can be isolated from the patient's tumor, expanded in vitro in rIL-2, and reinfused, typically with rIL-2 or rIFN-α therapy. The ex vivo expanded TILs then mediate tumor cell destruction while leaving nonneoplastic tissues unscathed.

Few clinical studies with TIL immunotherapy have been undertaken. Our experience at UCLA includes 62 patients with a response rate of 35%, an average response duration of 14 months, and an overall median survival of 22 months (FIGLIN et al. 1997). The median survival for responding patients has not yet been reached (range 2–73+ months). As with rIL-2 therapy, survival is greatest in patients with excellent performance status, less metastatic burden, and no prior cytotoxic therapy. The Cleveland Clinic performed two trials with TIL-based immunotherapy (BUKOWSKI et al. 1991). The first study, with TILs harvested from metastatic sites, yielded no clinical responses. The second trial involved retrieving TILs from primary tumor sites (as done at UCLA) and demonstrated a clinical response rate of 25%. At UCLA, response rates were further increased to 43% by enhancing the proportion of cytolytic CD8+ cells in the TIL population (STEGER et al. 1994). Other investigators have reported a decrease in circulating CD8+ cells associated with T-cell-mediated antitumor responses in patients with metastatic RCC (ERNSTOFF et al. 1992).

We have participated in a recently completed trial comparing rIL-2 and rIL-2 plus CD8+ selected TILs following nephrectomy, based upon a pilot study performed at UCLA (FIGLIN et al. 1997). Among the patients treated in this pilot study the overall response rate was 35%, with 9% complete responses and 26% partial responses. Among those who responded to therapy, 43% survived greater than 24 months and median survival among patients achieving complete response was greater than 42 months. In subgroup analysis the cytokine-primed group had an overall response rate of 28% while the CD8+ selection arm had an overall response rate of 43%. However, the overall responses and median durations of response were not statistically different between the two groups. High baseline levels of circulating natural killer cells were the only prognostic factor that correlated with response. These pilot results show that immunotherapy in combination with radical nephrectomy and adoptive transfer of TILs can provide a substantial therapeutic benefit. We await the results of the randomized trial, multiinstitutional, placebo-controlled trial.

## 9.4.2
## Autolymphocyte Therapy

Autolymphocyte therapy (ALT) refers to adoptive immunotherapy with autologous activated memory T lymphocytes that have been expanded and activated ex vivo. The theoretical basis of ALT relies upon activation of memory T lymphocytes in patients with metastatic cancer. These are T cells that have been exposed in vivo to tumor antigens and have the potential for mediating tumor regression following nonspecific activation (GRAY and SPRENT 1990). Memory T cells can then be characterized biologically on the basis of cell surface markers such as CD45RO, specific adhesion molecules, and patterns of circulation and migration. Activation is performed by incubating memory T cells with a monoclonal antibody against the T-cell receptor (anti-CD3) and specificity of the process is due to the inability of anti-CD3 to stimulate antigen naive T cells (SAWCZUK 1993). Triggering of the CD3 component of the T-cell receptor results in clonal T-cell proliferation through an IL-2-dependent autocrine pathway (HERZBERG and SMITH 1987).

Autolymphocyte therapy is a multistep process involving pheresis of peripheral blood mononuclear cells (PBLs) for incubation with anti-CD3 followed by a repeat pheresis for the collection of PBLs for activation. The cells are incubated in both cimetidine and indomethacin, which theoretically blocks subpopulation of suppressor T lymphocytes and inhibits IL-2-mediated T-cell proliferation, respectively (KHAN et al. 1985; WAYMACK et al. 1989). After incubation the cells are briefly irradiated to reduce the activation of suppressor T lymphocytes and infused into patients. Patients continue to receive oral cimetidine during therapy.

Initial reports revealed an approximate 2.5-fold survival advantage in patients receiving ALT compared to patients receiving cimetidine (21 months vs 8.5 months) (OSBAND et al. 1990). The toxicity was mild and patients were treated on an outpatient basis. However, there was no correlation between response and survival. The initial report has been updated (GRAHAM et al. 1993) and there remains a survival advantage in the ALT arm: median survival is greater than 17 months and 22% of patients have survived greater than 44 months. The ability of this therapy to improve survival in patients with metastatic RCC has not been tested; a randomized trial is currently comparing single-agent interferon and ALT, which should conclusively address the benefits of this therapy.

## 9.5
## Active Immunotherapy (Gene Therapy)

The goal of gene therapy is to introduce new genetic material into cells that encodes for specific proteins. The new protein can then either correct an inborn genetic error or provide new function to the native cell. The first gene transfer experiments were begun at the NCI in 1988 and involved transfer of a neomycin resistance gene to TILs in patients with melanoma (ROSENBERG et al. 1990). This study demonstrated that a gene could be successfully inserted and expressed in TILs as well as be safely infused into patients without loss of efficacy. Labeling of TILs allows determination of tumor infiltration and tracking in peripheral blood. Follow-up studies indicated that TILs could be detected in blood and tumor deposits for up to 6 months (CULVER et al. 1991). Gene therapy approaches used in clinical protocols are of three main types: (1) creation of tumor vaccines by in vitro transformation of autologous tumor cells with cytokine genes, (2) generation of potent TILs by transfer of cytokine genes into autologous T cells, and (3) in vivo transfer of genes encoding for MHC class 1 molecules by intralesional injection.

Construction of tumor vaccines involves the transfection of autologous tumor cell lines with genes that render the tumor more immunogenic. One approach involves the introduction of MHC class I or cytokine genes into tumor cells to enhance tumor antigen presentation and activation of tumor-specific cytotoxic T lymphocytes (GOLUMBEK et al. 1991, 1993; DRANOFF et al. 1993). Genetically altered tumor cells can be irradiated and reinfused into the patient, where they will function as a vaccine. Murine models employing this approach have demonstrated prevention of tumor growth, decreased metastatic spread, and prolonged immunologic memory, resulting in rejection of subsequent tumor challenges (ERNSTOFF et al. 1992; WATANABE et al. 1989; GANSBACHER et al. 1990a,b; ASHER et al. 1991; HOCK et al. 1991; GOLUMBEK et al. 1993). Human trials are ongoing at multiple institutions and involve tumor vaccines created by gene transfer of GM-CSF, rIL-2, IFN-γ,

IFN-α, and HLA-A2+ into patient-derived RCC cell lines (GASTL et al. 1992; BELLDEGRUN et al. 1993b; DRANOFF et al. 1993). Phase I trials with genetically engineered tumor cells secreting GM-CSF injected into patients with metastatic RCC have demonstrated an increased delayed-type hypersensitivity response and infiltration of macrophages and dendritic cells at the site of vaccination (JAFFE et al. 1996). While one patient experienced a partial response the methodology is still currently expensive and labor intensive, which limits its overall clinical application.

An alternate approach to gene therapy is the direct transfection of TILs with cytokine genes. The rationale is that since TILs traffic directly to tumor deposits, these cytokine-transfected T cells will concentrate at the tumor sites and locally secrete high levels of cytotoxic cytokines with minimal systemic toxicity. A protocol for the use of tissue necrosis factor (TNF) gene-modified TIL has been approved for patients with advanced cancer (ROSENBERG 1992). Given the severe toxicity of even small doses of TNF, it is hoped that large amounts of TNF will be secreted only at tumor sites with a minimum of systemic toxicity.

Intralesional gene therapy involves the direct transfer of genes encoding cytokines or MHC class I proteins into tumor cells in vivo. One advantage of direct transfer of DNA into tumor cells compared with ex vivo transfer is the simplicity of the procedure, which does not require expensive and laborious manipulation of tumor cells in culture. A distinct disadvantage is the lower efficiency of gene transfer. In vivo transfer of cytokine genes has been shown to reduce tumor growth in murine model systems (SUN et al. 1995). The first phase I clinical trial of in vivo intralesional gene transfer used cationic liposomes to deliver a plasmid harboring the rIL-2 gene. Although no objective responses were recorded, the procedure was demonstrated to be safe. Similar trials are currently underway to examine direct gene transfer of the human lymphocyte antigen-B7 gene (HLA-B7) and the β$_2$-microglobulin gene (NABEL et al. 1995). The HLA-B7 gene was chosen for these studies because of evidence that it is involved in the presentation of tumor-specific antigens in melanoma and RCC. Direct intralesional transfer of HLA-B7 gene into melanoma tumors has produced clinical responses in select patients. However, to date, no clinical responses have been observed in RCC. The injection of the HLA-B7 gene into tumors of 14 RCC patients by Vogelzang and colleagues resulted in HLA-B7 RNA and protein expression in the majority of tumor samples. Although there was evidence of a cellular immune response, no clinical responses were observed (VOGELZANG et al. 1994). Despite these failures, these studies indicate the overall safety and feasibility of intralesional gene transfer for metastatic RCC.

## 9.6
## Novel Therapeutic Approaches

### 9.6.1
### Monoclonal Antibodies

The role of monoclonal antibodies (mAbs) in the treatment of metastatic RCC is evolving. mAbs that bind to tumor-specific antigens can be used for imaging or to deliver cytotoxic agents to the tumor with greater specificity than other anticancer agents. Therapeutic mAbs have demonstrated clinical efficacy in colon cancer and non-Hodgkin's lymphoma (LONGO 1996; PAI et al. 1996). Additionally, mAbs are a powerful tool for identification of tumor antigens that may potentially be exploited as vaccines.

Recently, an RCC-specific antigen, the G250 antigen, was identified and cloned (OOSTERWIJK et al. 1993). The G250 antigen shows homology with a recently cloned cervical carcinoma-associated protein known as MN. Studies are underway to establish whether G250 is immunogenic and has potential for use as an RCC vaccine.

The anti-G250 mAb (mG250) is a murine immunoglobulin-G$_1$ antibody that reacts with 85% of all RCC cell lines, all clear-cell RCCs, and the majority of non-clear-cell RCCs, but does not react with normal kidney cells. In a phase II study investigating the therapeutic use of iodine-131 labeled mG250, 3 of 15 treated patients achieved a partial response (KRANENBORG et al. 1995). A humanized mG250 has been developed and is currently in clinical trials to determine its therapeutic potential. This novel form has demonstrated a high level of tumor uptake with no associated immunogenicity (STEFFENS et al. 1997) and is a promising vehicle for delivery of cytotoxic levels of radiation to renal tumors.

### 9.6.2
### Dendritic Cells

Dendritic cells represent yet another potential tool for generating supercharged tumor-specific cytotoxic T lymphocytes in culture. Dendritic cells, professional antigen-presenting cells, are found in the skin and reticuloendothelial system and can now be propagated in culture from peripheral blood mononuclear cells in the presence of cytokine growth factors (ROMANI et al. 1994). Dendritic cells express high levels of MHC class I and II antigens as well as a variety of cell surface co-stimulatory and adhesion molecules. Consequently, they present antigens effectively to T lymphocytes and produce some cytokines (BHARDWAJ et al. 1996). Research in melanoma and prostate cancer has demonstrated the potential usefulness of dendritic cell cultures for generating antitumor cellular immune responses (MUKHERJI et al. 1995; MURPHY et al. 1996; HSU et al. 1996). Dendritic cells can be pulsed with tumor-specific peptide antigens, whole proteins, or RNA-encoding peptide antigens (MULDERS et al. 1997). Ongoing research is investigating the use of dendritic cells from cancer patients to optimize tumor antigen presentation in culture and to increase production of tumor-specific cytotoxic T cells. Accumulated preclinical data indicate that this approach is applicable to the therapeutic induction of a RCC-specific immune response.

## 9.7
## The Roles of Chemotherapy and Radiation Therapy

Cytotoxic agents are the standard treatment for most solid malignancies but in RCC results have been poor (YAGODA et al. 1995). The resistance to these agents has been ascribed to high levels of expression of the mdr-1 gene product, P-glycoprotein, which actively effluxes drug from tumor cells (NISHIYAMA et al. 1993; KAKEHI et al. 1988). Agents which are frequently cited as having any activity in RCC are vinblastine and floxuridine, which carry response rates of 7% and 16%, respectively. A review of more than 70 agents used in phase II trials in more than 3500 patients between 1983 and 1992 demonstrated an objective response rate of 5%–6%, all with a short duration of response (YAGODA 1989; YAGODA et al. 1995). Hormonal agents including progestational agents, tamoxifen, and flutamide have all been shown ineffective at achieving any objective response rates and are at best anecdotally useful (BLOOM 1973; DEKERNION 1982; FERRAZI et al. 1980). To date, no beneficial effect of radiation therapy has been noted when given as either an adjuvant for surgical debulking or as primary treatment for locally extensive or metastatic disease (RABINOVITCH et al. 1994; VAN DER WERF-MESSING

1973) (see Chap. 10). Palliative radiation therapy has been successful in treating bony pain from osseous metastasis and usually achieves a highly durable response. However, the response rates for use in spinal cord compression have been less good (ONUFREY and MOHIUDDIN 1985; HALPERIN and HARISIADIS 1983) (see Chap. 10).

## 9.8
## Conclusions

Immunotherapy for metastatic RCC has moved from its infancy to young adulthood. Systemic infusion of high-dose bolus rIL-2 remains the reliable standard of care, with predictable and durable complete responses in a select group of patients. Patient characteristics that predict improved responsiveness to therapy have been identified, and treatment protocols that decrease toxicity have been developed. Advances in tumor immunology are rapidly moving from the bench to the bedside as manifest by large numbers of phase I and II trials exploiting both adoptive and active immunotherapies. Still, the development of newer biologic and pharmacologic agents for the treatment of advanced RCC, and their introduction into clinical trials, is necessary. Despite the need for better agents there is no doubt that the natural history of this tumor has been altered by current immunotherapy protocols.

## References

Asher AL, Mule JJ, Kasid A, et al. (1991) Murine tumor cells transduced with the gene for tumor necrosis factor-alpha: evidence for paracrine immune effects of tumor necrosis factor against tumors. J Immunol 146:3227–3234

Atkins MB, Sparano J, Fisher RI, et al. (1993) Randomized phase II trial of high-dose interleukin-2 either alone or in combination with interferon alpha-2b in advanced renal cell carcinoma. J Clin Oncol 11:661–670

Atzpodien J, Hanninen EL, Kirchner H, et al. (1995) Multiinstitutional home-therapy trial of recombinant human interleukin-2 and interferon alpha-2 in progressive metastatic renal cell carcinoma. J Clin Oncol 13:497–501

Atzpodien J, Korfer A, Franks RC, et al. (1990) Home - therapy with recombinant interleukin-2 and interferon alpha-2b in advanced human malignancies. Lancet 35: 1509–1512

Belldegrun A, Webb DA, Austin HA, et al. (1987) Effects of interleukin-2 on renal function in patients receiving immunotherapy for advanced cancer. Ann Intern Med 106:817–822

Belldegrun A, Pierce WC, Kaboo R, et al. (1993a) Interferon alpha-primed tumor infiltrating lymphocytes combined with interleukin-2 and interferon-alpha as a therapy for metastatic renal cell carcinoma. J Urol 150:1384–1390

Belldegrun A, Tso CL, Sakata T, et al. (1993b) Human renal carcinoma line transfected with interleukin 2 and/or interferon alpha gene(s): implications for live cancer vaccines. J Natl Cancer Inst 85:207–212

Bergman L, Wiedmann E, Mitrou PS, et al. (1990) Interleukin-2 in combination with interferon-alpha in disseminated malignant melanoma and advanced renal cell carcinoma: a phase I/II study. Oncologie 13:137–140

Bhardwaj N, Seder RA, Reddy A, et al. (1996) IL-12 in conjunction with dendritic cells enhances antiviral CD8+ CTL responses in vitro. J Clin Invest 98:715–722

Bloom HJ (1973) Hormone-induced and spontaneous regression of metastatic renal cell carcinoma. Cancer 32:1006

Braciale TJ, Morrison LA, Sweetser MT, et al. (1987) Antigen presentation pathways to class I and class II MHC-restricted T lymphocytes. Immunol Rev 98:95–103

Budd GT, Osgood B, Bama B, et al. (1989) Phase I clinical trial of interleukin-2 and interferon: toxicity and immunologic effects. Cancer Res 49:6432–6436

Budd GT, Murthy S, Finke J, et al. (1992) Phase I trial of high-dose bolus interleukin-2 and interferon alpha-2a in patients with metastatic malignancy. J Clin Oncol 10:804–809

Bukowski RM, Murthy S, and Sergi S (1990a) Phase I trial of continuous infusion recombinant interleukin-2 and intermittent recombinant interferon-alpha 2a: clinical effects. J Biol Response Modifiers 9:538–545

Bukowski RM, Goodman P, Crawford ED, et al. (1990b) Phase II trial of high-dose intermittent interleukin-2 in metastatic renal cell carcinoma. J Natl Cancer Inst 82:143–146

Bukowski RM, Sharfman W, Murthy S, et al. (1991) Clinical results and characterization of tumor-infiltrating lymphocytes with or without recombinant interleukin-2 in human metastatic renal cell carcinoma. Cancer Res 51:4199–4205

Cameron RB, McIntosh JK, Rosenberg SA (1988) Synergistic antitumor effects of combination immunotherapy with recombinant interleukin-2 and recombinant hybrid alpha-interferon in the treatment of established murine hepatic metastases. Cancer Res 48:5810–5817

Chikkala NF, Lewis I, Ulchaker J, et al. (1990) Interactive effects of alpha-interferon A/D and interleukin-2 on murine lymphokine-activated killer activity: analysis at the effector and precursor level. Cancer Res 50: 1176–1182

Creagan ET, Kovach JS, Long HJ, et al. (1994) Phase I study of recombinant leucocyte a human interferon combined with BCNU in selected patients with advanced cancer. J Clin Oncol 4:408–413

Creagan ET, Buckner JC, Hahn RG, et al. (1988) An evaluation of recombinant leukocyte-A interferon with aspirin in patients with metastatic renal cell carcinoma. Cancer 61:1787–1791

Culver K, Cornetta K, Morgan R, et al. (1991) Lymphocytes as cellular vehicles for gene therapy in mouse and man. Proc Natl Acad Sci USA 88:3155–3161

DeKernion JB (1982) Treatment of advanced renal cell carcinoma – traditional methods and innovative approaches. J Urol 130:2–7

DeKernion JB, Sarna G, Figlin R, et al. (1983) The treatment of renal cell carcinoma with human leukocyte alpha-interferon. J Urol 130:1063–1066

Dillman RO, Church C, Oldham RK, et al. (1993) Inpatient continuous infusion interleukin-2 in 788 patients with cancer: the National Biotherapy Study Group experience. Cancer 71:2358–2370

                                                                                       

Dranoff G, Jaffee EM, Lazenby A, et al. (1993) Vaccination with irradiated tumor cells engineered to secrete murine GM-CSF stimulates potent, specific, and long lasting antitumor immunity. Proc Natl Acad Sci USA 90: 3539–3544

Eisenkraft BL, Nanus DM, Albino AP, et al. (1991) Alpha-interferon down-regulates epidermal growth factor receptors on renal carcinoma cells: relation of cellular responsiveness to the antiproliferative action of alpha-interferon. Cancer Res 51:5881–5887

Ellenhorst JA, Kilbourne RG, Amato RJ, et al. (1994) Phase II trial of low dose gamma-interferon in metastatic renal cell carcinoma. J Urol 152:841–845

Ernstoff MS, Nair SG, Bahnson RR, et al. (1990) A phase Ia trial of sequential administration of recombinant DNA-produced interferons. J Clin Oncol 8:1637–1649

Ernstoff MS, Gooding W, Nair S, et al. (1992) Immunological effects of treatment with sequential administration of recombinant interferon-gamma and alpha in patients with metastatic renal cell carcinoma during a phase I trial. Cancer Res 52:851–856

Falcone A, Cianci C, Pfanner E, et al. (1993) Floxuridine (FUDR) + alpha-2b interferon (IFN) in metastatic renal cell carcinoma (MRC): a phase II study [abstract]. Proc Am Soc Clin Oncol 12:231

Ferrazi E, Salvagno L, Forasiero A, et al. (1980) Tamoxifen treatment for advanced renal cell cancer. Tumori 66: 601–605

Fidler IJ, Heicappell R, Saiki I, et al. (1987) Direct antiproliferative effects of recombinant human interferon-alpha:B/D hybrids on human tumor cell lines. Cancer Res 47:2020–2027

Figlin RA, Gitlitz BJ (1997) Interferon in urological tumours – renal cell carcinoma. In: Stuart-Harris R, Penny R (eds) The clinical application of interferons. Chapman and Hall, London

Figlin RA, DeKernion JB, Maldazys J, et al. (1985) Treatment of renal cell carcinoma with alpha interferon and vinblastine in combination: a phase I-II trial. Cancer Treat Rep 69:263–267

Figlin RA, Belldegrun A, Moldawer N, et al. (1992) Concomitant administration of recombinant of human interleukin-2 and recombinant interferon alpha-2a: an active outpatient regimen in metastatic renal cell carcinoma. J Clin Oncol 10:414–421

Figlin RA, Dekernion JB, Mukamel E, et al. (1988) Recombinant interferon alpha-2a in metastatic renal cell carcinoma. J Clin Oncol 6:1604–1610

Figlin RA, Pierce WC, Kaboo R, et al. (1997) Treatment of metastatic renal cell carcinoma with nephrectomy, interleukin-2 and cytokine-primed or CD8+ selected tumor infiltrating lymphocytes from primary tumors. J Urol 158:740–745

Fisher RI (1988) Metastatic renal cell cancer treated with interleukin-2 and lymphokine-activated killer cells. Ann Intern Med 108:518

Foon KA, Walther PJ, Bernstein ZP, et al. (1992) Renal cell carcinoma treated with continuous infusion interleukin-2 with ex-vivo activated killer cells. J Immunother 11: 184–190

Fossa SD, deGaris ST, Heier MS, et al. (1986) Recombinant interferon alpha-2a with and without vinblastine in metastatic renal cell carcinoma. Cancer 57:1700–1704

Fyfe G, Fisher RI, Rosenberg SA, Sznol M, Parkinson DR, Louie AC (1995) Results of treatment of 255 patients with metastatic renal cell carcinoma who received high-dose recombinant interleukin-2 therapy. J Clin Oncol 13:688–696

Gansbacher B, Bannerji R, Daniels B, et al. (1990a) Retroviral vector-mediated gamma-interferon gene transfer into tumor cells generates potent and long-lasting antitumor immunity. Cancer Res 50:7820–7825

Gansbacher B, Zier K, Daniels B, et al. (1990b) Interleukin-2 gene transfer into tumor cells abrogates tumorigenecity and induces protective immunity. Exp Med 172:1217–1224

Gastl G, Finstad CL, Guarini A, et al. (1992) Retroviral vector-mediated lymphokine gene transfer into human renal cancer cells. Cancer Res 52:6229–6234

Geertsen PF, Hermann GG van der Maase H, Steven K (1992) Treatment of metastatic renal cell carcinoma by continuous infusion of recombinant interleukin-2: a single center phase II study. J Clin Oncol 10:753

Gitlitz BJ, Belldegrun A, Figlin RA (1996) Immunotherapy and gene therapy. Semin Urol Oncol 14:237–243

Golumbek PT, Lazenby AJ, Levitsky HI, et al. (1991) Treatment of established renal cancer by tumor cells engineered to secrete interleukin 4. Science 254:713–718

Golumbek PT, Levitsky HI, Jaffee L, et al. (1993) The antitumor immune response as a problem of self-nonself discrimination: implications for immunotherapy. Immunol Res 12:183–192

Graham S, Babayan RK, Lamm DL, et al. (1993) The use of ex vivo-activated memory T cells (autolymphocyte therapy) in the treatment of metastatic renal cell carcinoma: final results from a randomized multisite study. Semin Urol 11:27–34

Gray D, Sprent J (1990) Immunological memory. Curr Top Microbiol Immunol 159:1–141

Grimm EA, Mazumder A, Zhang HZ, et al. (1993) Lymphokine-activated killer cell phenomenon. J Exp Med 155: 1823–1841

Halperin EC, Harisiadis L (1983) The role of radiation therapy in the management of metastatic renal cell carcinoma. Cancer 51:614–617

Heron I, Hokland M, Berg K (1978) Enhanced expression of B-2-microglobulin and HLA antigens on human lymphoid cells by interferon. Proc Natl Acad Sci USA 75:6215–6219

Herzberg VL, Smith KA (1987) T cell growth without serum. J Immunol 139:998–1004

Hirsch M, Lipton A, Harvey H, et al. (1990) A phase I study of interleukin-2 and interferon alpha 2a as outpatient therapy for patients with advanced malignancy. J Clin Oncol 8:1657–1683

Hock H, Dorsch M, Diamantstein T, et al. (1991) Interleukin-7 induced CD4+ T-cell dependent tumor rejection. J Exp Med 174:1291–1298

Homma Y, Aso Y (1994) Effect of alpha-interferon alone and combined with other anti-neoplastic agents on renal cell carcinoma determined by the tetrazolium microculture assay. Eur Urol 25:164–170

Hrushesky WJM, Roemeling RV, Lanning RM, et al. (1990) Circadian-shaped infusions of floxuridine for progressive metastatic renal cell carcinoma. J Clin Oncol 8:1504–1513

Hsu FJ, Benike C, Fagnoni F, et al. (1996) Vaccination of patients with B-cell lymphoma using autologous antigen-pulsed dendritic cells. Nat Med 2:52–58

Ilson DH, Motzer RJ, Kradin RL, et al. (1992) A phase II trial of interleukin-2 and interferon-alpha-2a in patients with advanced renal cell carcinoma. J Clin Oncol 10:1124–1130

Jaffe EM, Marshall F, Weber C, et al. (1996) Bioactivity of a human GM-CSF tumor vaccine for the treatment of metastatic renal cell carcinoma [abstract]. Proc Am Soc Clin Oncol 15:237

Kakehi Y, Kanamaru H, Yoshida O, et al. (1988) Measurement of multidrug-resistance messenger RNA in urogenital cancers: elevated expression in renal cell carcinoma is associated with intrinsic drug resistance. J Urol 139:862–865

Khan MM, Sansoni P, Engelman EG, et al. (1985) Pharmacologic effects of autocoids on subsets of T-cells: regulation of expression function of histamine-2 receptors by a subset of suppresser cells. J Clin Invest 75:1578–1583

Kirchner H, Korfer A, Palmer PA, et al. (1990) Subcutaneous interleukin-2 and interferon alpha-2b in patients with metastatic renal cell cancer. The German outpatient experience. Mol Biother 2:145–154

Kirkwood JM, Harris JE, Vera R, et al. (1985) Randomized study of low and high doses of leukocyte alpha-interferon in metastatic renal cell carcinoma. Cancer Res 45:863–871

Kranenborg MH, Boerman OC, Oosterwijk-Wakka JC, et al. (1995) Development and characterization of anti-renal cell carcinoma × antichelate bispecific monoclonal antibodies for two-phase targeting of renal cell carcinoma. Cancer Res 55:5864S–5867S

Lee KH, Talpaz M, Rothenberg JM, et al. (1989) Concomitant administration of recombinant human interleukin-2 and recombinant human interferon alpha-2A in cnacer patients: a phase I study. Cancer Res 49:1726–1732

Lipton A, Harvey H, Givant E, et al. (1993) Interleukin-2 (IL-2) and interferon alpha-2a outpatient therapy for metastatic renal cell carcinoma. J Immunother 13:122–129

Lissoni P, Barni S, Ardizzoia A, et al. (1994) Prognostic factors of the clinical response to subcutaneous immunotherapy with interleukin-2 alone in patients with metastatic RCC. Oncology 51:59–62

Longo DL (1996) Immunotherapy for non-Hodgkin's lymphoma. Curr Opin Oncol 8:353–359

Lopez Hannien E, Kirchner H, Atzpodien J (1996) Interleukin-2 based home therapy of metastatic renal cell carcinoma: risks and benefits in 215 consecutive single institution patients. J Urol 155:19–25

Minasian LM, Motzer RJ, Gluck L, et al. (1993) Interferon alpha-2A in advanced renal cell carcinoma: treatment results and survival in 159 patients with long-term follow-up. J Clin Oncol 11:1368–1375

Mittleman A, Huberman A, Puccio C, et al. (1990) A phase I study of recombinant human interleukin-2 and alpha-interferon-2a in patients with renal cell cancer, colorectal cancer, and malignant melanoma. Cancer 66:664–669

Montie JE, Stewart BH, Stratton RA (1977) The role of adjunctive nephrectomy in patients with metastatic renal cell carcinoma. J Urol 117:272–279

Motzer RJ, Schwartz L, Law TM, et al. (1995) Interferon alpha-2a and 13-cisretinoic acid in renal cell carcinoma: antitumor activity in a phase II trial and interactions in vitro. J Clin Oncol 13:1950–1957

Mukherji B, Chakraborty NG, Yamasaki S, et al. (1995) Induction of antigen-specific cytolytic T cells in situ in human melanoma by immunization with synthetic peptide-pulsed autologous antigen presenting cells. Proc Natl Acad Sci USA 92:8078–8082

Mulders P, Tso C, Kaboo R, et al. (1997) Multi-antigen loaded dendritic cells as potent inducers of a specific anti-tumor response: a novel approach to adoptive immunotherapy for renal cell carcinoma (abstract). J Urol 157:109

Mule JJ, Yang JC, Lafreniere R, et al. (1987) Identification of cellular mechanisms operational in vivo during the regression of established pulmonary metastases by the systemic administration of high-dose recombinant interleukin-2. J Immunol 139:285–294

Murphy G, Tjoa B, Ragde H, et al. (1996) Phase I clinical trial: T-cell therapy for prostate cancer using autologous dendritic cells pulsed with HLA-A0201-specific peptides from prostate-specific membrane antigen. Prostate 29:371–380

Muss HB (1988) The role of biological response modifiers in metastatic renal cell carcinoma. Semin Oncol 15:30–34

Muss HB, Weilander C, Caponera M, et al. (1985) Interferon and doxirubicin in renal cell carcinoma. Cancer Treat Rep 69:721–729

Muss HB, Costanzi JJ, Leavitt R, et al. (1987) Recombinant alpha interferon in renal cell carcinoma: a randomized trial of two routes of administration. J Clin Oncol 5:286–291

Nabel GJ, Yang ZY, Nabel EG, et al. (1995) Direct gene transfer for treatment of human cancer. Ann NY Acad Sci 772:227–231

Nanus DM, Pfeffer LN, Bander NH, et al. (1990) Antiproliferative and antitumor effects of alpha-interferon in renal cell carcinoma: correlation with the expression of a kidney- associated differentiation glycoprotein. Cancer Res 50:4190–4194

Neidhart JA, Gagen MM, Young D, et al. (1984) Interferon-alpha treatment of renal cancer. Cancer Res 44:4140–4143

Nishiyama K, Shirahama T, Yoshimura A (1993) Expression of the multidrug transporter, P-glycoprotein, in renal and transitional cell carcinomas. Cancer 71:3611–3619

Onufrey V, Mohiuddin M (1985) Radiation therapy in the treatment of metastatic renal cell carcinoma. Int J Radiat Oncol Biol Phys 11:2007–2009

Oosterwijk E, Bander NH, Divgi CR, et al. (1993) Antibody localization in human renal cell carcinoma: a phase I study of monoclonal antibody G250. J Clin Oncol 11:738–750

Osband ME, Lavin PT, Babayan RK, et al. (1990) Effect of autolymphocyte therapy on survival and quality of life in patients with metastatic renal-cell carcinoma. Lancet 335:994–998

Pai LH, Wittes R, Setser A, et al. (1996) Treatment of advanced solid tumors with immunotoxin LMB-1: an antibody linked to *Pseudomonas* exotoxin. Nat Med 2:350–353

Parker SL, Tong T, Bolden S, et al. (1997) Cancer statistics, 1997. CA Cancer J Clin 47:5–27

Parkinson DR, Fisher RI, Rayner AA, et al. (1990) Therapy of renal cell carcinoma with interleukin-2 and lymphokine-activated killer cells: phase II experience with a hybrid bolus and continuous infusion interleukin-2 regimen. J Clin Oncol 8:1630–1636

Quesada JR (1987) Phase II studies of recombinant human interferon-gamma in metastatic renal cell carcinoma. J Biol Resp Mod 6:20–27

Quesada JR, Swanson DA, Trinidade A, et al. (1983) Renal cell carcinoma: antitumor effects of leukocyte interferon. Cancer Res 43:940–947

Quesada JR, Swanson DA, Gutterman JU, et al. (1985) Phase II study of interferon alpha in metastatic renal cell carcinoma. J Clin Oncol 3:1086–1092

Rabinovitch RA, Zelefsky MJ, Gaynor JJ, et al. (1994) Patterns of failure following surgical resection of renal cell carcinoma: implications for adjuvant local and systemic therapy. J Clin Oncol 12:206–212

Rinehart J, Young D, Laforge J, et al. (1986) Phase I/II trial of human recombinant beta-interferon serine in patients with renal cell carcinoma. Cancer Res 46:2364–2367

Romani N, Gruner S, Brang D, et al. (1994) Proliferating dendritic cell progenitors in human blood. J Exp Med 180:83–93

Rosenberg SA (1988) Immunotherapy of cancer using IL-2. Immunol Today 9:58–67

Rosenberg SA (1991) The immunology and gene therapy of cancer. Cancer Res 51(18s):5074

Rosenberg SA (1992) Karnofsky Memorial Lecture: the immunotherapy and gene therapy of cancer. J Clin Oncol 10: 180–183

Rosenberg SA, Schwartz S, Spiess PJ (1988) Combination immunotherapy for cancer: synergistic antitumor interactions of interleukin-2, alpha-interferon, and tumor-infiltrating lymphocytes. J Natl Cancer Inst 80:1393–1397

Rosenberg SA, Lotz MT, Yang JC, et al. (1989a) Experience with the use of high-dose interleukin-2 in the treatment of 652 cancer patients. Ann Surg 210:474

Rosenberg SA, Lotze MT, Yang JC, et al. (1989b) Combination therapy with interleukin-2 and alpha-interferon for the treatment of patients with advanced cancer. J Clin Oncol 7:1863–1874

Rosenberg SA, Aebersold P, Cornetta MD, et al. (1990) Gene transfer into humans – immunotherapy of patients with advanced melanoma, using tumor-infiltrating lymphocytes modified by retroviral gene transduction. N Engl J Med 323:570–576

Rosenberg SA, Lotze MT, Yang JC, et al. (1993) Prospective randomized trial of high-dose interleukin-2 alone or in conjunction with lymphokine-activated killer cells for the treatment of patients with advanced cancer. J Natl Cancer Inst 85:622–652

Rosenberg SA, Yang JC, Topalian SL, et al. (1994) Treatment of 283 consecutive patients with metastatic melanoma or renal cell cancer using high dose bolus interleukin-2. JAMA 271:907–913

Rosenstein M, Ettinghausen SE, Rosenberg SA (1986) Extravasation of intravascular fluid mediated by the systemic administration of recombinant interleukin-2. J Immunol 137:1734–1742

Sarna G, Figlin RA, DeKernion J (1987) Interferon in renal cell carcinoma: the UCLA experience. Cancer 59:610–612

Sawczuk IS (1993) Autolymphocyte therapy in the treatment of metastatic renal cell carcinoma. Urol Clin North Am 20:297–301

Sayers TS, Wiltrout TA, McCormick K, et al. (1990) Antitumor effects of alpha-interferon and gamma-interferon in murine renal cell carcinoma in vitro and in vivo. Cancer Res 20:5414–5419

Schwartzentruber DJ, Topalian SL, Mancini M, Rosenberg SA (1991) Specific release of granulocyte-macrophage colony-stimulating factor, tumor necrosis factor-alpha and IFN-gamma by human tumor-infiltrating lymphocytes after autologous tumor stimulation. J Immunol 146: 3674–3681

Sella A, Kilbourn RG, Gray I, et al. (1994) Interleukin-2 combined with interferon-alpha and 5-fluorouracil in patients with metastatic renal cell cancer. Cancer Biotherapy 9:103-111

Siegel JP, Puri RK (1991) Interleukin-2 toxicity. J Clin Oncol 9:694–704

Sparano JA, Wadler S, Diasio R, et al. (1993) A phase I trial of low-dose 5-fluorouracil plus interferon-α: evidence for enhanced 5-fluorouracil toxicity without pharmacokinetic perturbation. J Clin Oncol 11:1609–1617

Spencer WF, Lineham WM, Walter MM, et al. (1992) Immunotherapy with interleukin-2 and alpha-interferon in patients with metastatic renal cell carcinoma with in situ primary cancers: a pilot study. J Urol 147:24–30

Steffens MG, Boerman O, Oosterwijk-Wakka JC, et al. (1997) Targeting of renal cell carcinoma with iodine-131-labeled chimeric monoclonal antibody G250. J Clin Oncol 15: 1529–1537

Steger GG, Pierce WC, Figlin RA (1994) Patterns in cytokine release of unselected and CD8+ selected renal cell carcinoma tumor-infiltrating lymphocytes. Clin Immunol Immunopathol 72:237–247

Sun WH, Burkholder JK, Sun J, et al. (1995) In vivo cytokine gene transfer by gene gun reduces tumor growth in mice. Proc Natl Acad Sci USA 92:2889–2893

Sznol M, Mier JW, Sparano J, et al. (1990) A phase I study of high-dose interleukin-2 in combination with interferon-alpha 2b. J Biol Response Modifiers 9:529–537

Sznol M, Clark JW, Smith JW, et al. (1992) Pilot study of interleukin-2 and lymphokine-activated killer cells combined with immunomodulatory doses of chemotherapy and sequenced with interferon alpha-2a in patients with metastatic renal cell carcinoma. J Natl Cancer Inst 84: 929–937

Thomas H, Batron C, Saini A, et al. (1992) Sequential interleukin-2 and alpha-interferon for renal cell carcinoma and melanoma. Eur J Cancer 28A:1047–1049

Thompson JA, Shulman KL, Benyunes MC, et al. (1992) Prolonged continuous intravenous infusion interleukin-2 and lymphokine-activated killer cell therapy for metastatic renal cell carcinoma. J Clin Oncol 10:960–968

Townsend A, Bodmer H (1989) Antigen recognition by class I-restricted T lymphocytes. Annu Rev Immunol 7:601–631

Umeda T, Niijima T (1986) Phase II study of alpha interferon on renal cell carcinoma: summary of three collaborative trials. Cancer 58:1231–1235

Vogelzang NJ, Lipton A, Figlin RA (1993) Subcutaneous interleukin-2 plus interferon alpha-2A in metastatic renal cancer: an outpatient multicenter trial. J Clin Oncol 11:1809–1816

Unanue ER (1992) Cellular studies on antigen presentation by class II MHC molecules. Curr Opin Immunol 4:63–71

van der Maase H, Geertsen P, Thatcher N, et al. (1991) Recombinant interleukin-2 in metastatic renal cell carcinoma – a European multicentre phase II study. Eur J Cancer 27:1583–1589

Van der Werf-Messing B (1973) Carcinoma of the kidney. Cancer 32:1056–1059

Vogelzang NJ, Lestingi TM, Sudakoff G, et al. (1994) Phase I study of immunotherapy of metastatic renal cell carcinoma by direct gene transfer into metastatic lesions. Hum Gene Ther 5:1357–1370

Wan YJ, Orrison BM, Lieberman R, et al. (1987) Induction of major histocompatibility class I antigens by interferons in undifferentiated F9 cells. J Cell Physiol 130:276–283

Watanabe Y, Kuribayashi K, Miyatake S, et al. (1989) Exogenous expression of mouse interferon-γ cDNA in mouse neuroblastoma C1300 cells results in reduced tumorigenicity by augmented anti-tumor immunity. Proc Natl Acad Sci USA 86:9456–9460

Waymack JP, Guzman RF, Burleson DG, et al. (1989) Effect of prostaglandin E in multiple experimental models. Prostaglandins 38:345–353

Webb DA, Austin HA, Belldegrun A, et al. (1988) Metabolic and renal effects of IL-2 immunotherapy for metastatic renal cell carcinoma. Clin Nephrol 30:141–145

Weiss GR, Margolin KA, Aronson FR, et al. (1992) A randomized phase II trial of continuous infusion interleukin-2 or bolus injection interleukin-2 plus lymphokine-activated killer cells for advanced renal cell carcinoma. J Clin Oncol 10:275–281

West WH, Tauer KW, Vannelli JR (1987) Constant infusion recombinant interleukin-2 in adoptive immunotherapy of advanced cancer. N Engl J Med 316:898–905

Wigginton JM, Kuhns DB, Back TC, et al. (1996) Interleukin 12 primes macrophages for nitric oxide production in vivo and restores depressed nitric oxide production by macrophages from tumor-bearing mice: implications for the antitumor activity of interleukin 12 and/or interleukin 2. Cancer Res 56:1131–1136

Wirth MP (1993) Immunotherapy for metastatic renal cell carcinoma. Urol Clin North Am 20:283–295

Yagoda A (1989) Chemotherapy of renal cell carcinoma: 1983–1989. Semin Urol 7:199–227

Yagoda A, Abi-Rached B, Petrylak D (1995) Chemotherapy for advanced renal cell carcinoma. Semin Oncol 22:42–60

Yang JC, Topalian SL, Parkinson D, et al. (1994) Randomized comparison of high-dose and low-dose intravenous interleukin-2 for the therapy of metastatic renal cell carcinoma: an interim report. J Clin Oncol 12:1572–1576

# 10 The Role of Radiotherapy in the Management of Patients with Renal Cell Carcinoma

Z. Petrovich, G. Jozsef, C. Yu, and C.-S. Zee

CONTENTS



## 10.1
## Introduction

Carcinoma of the kidney is the third most common tumor of the genitourinary tract (Table 10.1). In the United States it represents approximately 11% of all genitourinary tumors in incidence and 18% in mortality rates (Landis et al. 1998). Most (>80%) tumors of the kidneys are renal cell carcinomas (RCCs), which show a predilection to occur in males in their


Z. Petrovich, MD, FACR, Professor of Radiation Oncology and Urology, Chairman, Department of Radiation Oncology, University of Southern California School of Medicine, Kenneth Norris Jr. Cancer Hospital and Research Institute, 1441 Eastlake Ave., Room 34, P.O. 33804, Los Angeles, CA 90033-0804, USA
G. Jozsef, PhD, Department of Radiation Oncology, University of Southern California School of Medicine, Kenneth Norris Jr. Cancer Hospital and Research Institute, 1441, Eastlake Ave., P.O. 33804, Los Angeles, CA 90033-0804, USA
C. Yu, PhD, Assistant Professor of Radiation Oncology, Department of Radiation Oncology, University of Southern California School of Medicine, Kenneth Norris Jr. Cancer Hospital and Research Institute, 1441, Eastlake Ave., P.O. 33804, Los Angeles, CA 90033-0804, USA
C.-S. Zee, MD, Department of Radiology, University of Southern California School of Medicine, Kenneth Norris Jr. Cancer Hospital and Research Institute, 1441, Eastlake Ave., P.O. 33804, Los Angeles, CA 90033-0804, USA


fifth and sixth decades of life, although this tumor is known to occur in much younger patients (Landis et al. 1998; Skinner et al. 1971; Flocks and Kadesky 1958). Multiple environmental factors, including cigarette smoking, have been identified as possible causes for the development of RCC, and a strong association of RCC with von Hippel-Lindau disease is well documented (Christoferson et al. 1961).

Numerous presenting signs and symptoms in patients with RCC have been described. In view of this heterogeneity of symptoms and signs, diagnosis of RCC at times may present a problem (see Chap. 5). "Classic" signs and symptoms including hematuria, pain, or the presence of an abdominal mass were found at diagnosis in only a small fraction (9%) of patients (Skinner et al. 1971; Stein et al. 1998). It is imperative that physicians and surgeons maintain their alertness to the possibility of this diagnosis and include RCC in the differential diagnosis of patients who present with multiple and/or complex signs and symptoms.

### 10.1.1
### Diagnosis

Diagnosis of RCC is usually made based on clinical data with strong supporting evidence provided by modern imaging techniques such as ultrasound, computerized axial tomography, and magnetic resonance imaging (MRI) (see Chap. 4 for relevant details). Once the presumptive diagnosis of RCC is established, patients are evaluated for radical nephrectomy and histological confirmation of RCC is obtained. At the time of initial diagnosis, 20% to nearly 40% of patients have demonstrable metastatic disease (O'Dea et al. 1978; Skinner et al. 1971; Flocks and Kadesky 1958; McNichols et al. 1981; Giuliani et al. 1990). Subsequently, 30%–50% of patients are expected to develop metastasis sometime during the course of their disease. In recent years, with major advances in imaging modalities, patients are increasingly often being diagnosed with

patients treated with radiotherapy for bone metastasis who showed a good response frequently maintained this response for the rest of their life (Halperin and Harisiadis 1983).

Patients with large osteolytic lesions in the weight-bearing axis prior to the consideration of palliative radiotherapy need to undergo evaluation for possible internal stabilization. If such a surgical procedure is felt to be needed, patients should receive a planned course of postoperative radiotherapy to prevent almost certain tumor recurrence. From a review of the literature and our personal experience it is apparent that radiotherapy is a treatment of choice in RCC patients presenting with symptomatic bone metastasis. All patients except those with massive metastatic disease and expected short survival should be treated with well-fractionated radiotherapy with a total dose >45 Gy. Patients treated in this fashion would be expected to maintain a good quality of life for a long period.

## 10.3.2
## Lung Metastasis

Lung is the most common distant site of metastatic disease in patients with RCC. In a large autopsy study of 1451 RCC patients, lung was the site of metastatic involvement in 979 (76%) patients with multiple metastases and in 32% of those with single organ disease (Saitoh 1981). Indications for radiotherapy in patients with pulmonary metastasis include: (1) mediastinal compression syndrome, (2) hemoptysis due to endobronchial involvement, (3) pneumonia refractory to medical therapy due to compression of the bronchus, (4) collapsed lobe due to central bronchial compression, (5) progressive hilar disease refractory to chemo-immunotherapy; and (6) localized severe chest pain due to invasion of the pleura. Relatively high (50 Gy) radiation doses are required to obtain long-lasting tumor remissions. Careful planning of radiotherapy should be performed to minimize the probability of pulmonary toxicity. CT planning with 3-D image reconstruction and 3-D dose delivery using multiple radiation fields should be considered in all patients. This treatment should in fact represent a standard of care rather than to be used only sporadically as it is well tolerated by patients and results in a low incidence of toxicity. High response rates (>70%) are expected in patients treated with palliative radiotherapy for pulmonary metastasis (Fossa et al. 1982; Onufrey and Mohiuddin 1985; Halperin and Harisiadis 1983).

## 10.3.3
## Brain Metastasis

Brain is an uncommon yet very important site of metastatic disease in patients with RCC. At autopsy brain metastases are present in 11% of patients as a part of multiorgan disease and in 7% of those who have solitary organ involvement (Saitoh 1981). In patients with RCC seen in clinical practice the incidence of brain metastasis is probably no higher than 5%. The presence of metastatic brain disease in patients with RCC carries a poor prognosis and this tumor presentation does not respond well to standard external beam radiotherapy or surgery (Maor et al. 1988; Halperin and Harisiadis 1983; Engenhart et al. 1993; Nussbaum et al. 1996). A response to brain radiotherapy measured in symptomatic improvement was reported in 30% of patients with RCC (Halperin and Harisiadis 1983; Maor et al. 1988). Patients were usually treated with a short course of palliative irradiation consisting of 30 Gy given over a period of 2 weeks. Much more optimistic treatment outcomes with the use of external beam radiotherapy were reported by others (Onufrey and Mohiuddin 1985; Yonese et al. 1995). As a result of this low incidence of major palliative benefit in RCC patients with brain metastasis, surgical treatment was investigated (Badalament et al. 1990). At Memorial Sloan-Kettering Cancer Center the authors treated a total of 22 patients with metastatic RCC. The most important parameter influencing treatment response was tumor biology, i.e., the time interval between diagnosis of RCC and the appearance of brain metastasis. The outcome of the study is difficult to evaluate in view of the fact that 20 (91%) of these patients also received radiotherapy. A similar report was published by the group from the National Cancer Center in Tokyo, Japan (Shibui et al. 1990).

Since the prognosis of patients with metastatic RCC to the brain is poor, attempts were made to minimize the need for formal craniotomy. Based on the currently available data craniotomy can be avoided in most of these patients. Stereotactic radiosurgery with a linear accelerator based system, gamma knife, or proton beam has been under active study in patients with metastatic brain disease (Flickinger et al. 1994; Engenhart et al. 1993; Petrovich et al. 1996). The radiobiological rationale for the use of stereotactic radiotherapy in patients with brain tumors has been presented (Leith et al. 1994; Hall and Brenner 1993).

A multi-institutional clinical trial of stereotactic radiosurgery with a gamma knife in 116 patients with brain metastasis, including 14 (12%) patients with RCC, has been reported (FLICKINGER et al. 1994). Of the 116 patients treated, 45 (39%) were failures of prior external beam radiotherapy; 51 (44%) were treated with radiosurgery alone while 65 (56%) received combined treatment which included radiosurgery and external beam radiotherapy with a mean dose of 33.8 Gy. Mean radiosurgery radiation dose was 17.5 Gy. Median survival for all study patients was 11 months and tumor control was obtained in 99 (85%) patients. Tumor control was better for the 28 melanoma and 14 RCC patients than for those with other histological diagnoses ($P = 0.0003$). Treatment was very well tolerated by the study patients with a single patient experiencing focal necrosis. The authors concluded that stereotactic radiosurgery is an effective therapy of low morbidity and should be considered as a useful treatment options in patients with solitary brain metastases including those with RCC.

A group from Heidelberg University reported treatment outcomes in 69 patients treated with linear accelerator radiosurgery for 102 inoperable brain metastases (ENGENHART et al. 1993). Of the 69 patients treated, 14 (20%) had a diagnosis of RCC and 11 (16%) failed prior surgery or external beam radiotherapy. Mean radiosurgery radiation dose was 21.5 Gy. The median survival for all patients was 6 months and neurological improvement was noted in 81%. The incidence of objective tumor regression was as follows: complete regression in 20%, partial regression in 35%, stable disease in 40%, and tumor progression in 5%. There were 15 (22%) patients who died of brain metastasis, including two who had local tumor recurrence and 13 who developed multiple brain lesions. Focal necrosis was seen in one patient. No specific outcomes were provided for the 14 RCC patients. The authors concluded that radiosurgery is an important therapy in the management of brain metastasis.

The management of patients with metastatic RCC to the brain will be discussed based on the USC experience. All patients suspected of having brain metastasis are evaluated by a neurosurgeon, neuroradiologist, and radiation oncologist. Basically, patients with solitary metastatic lesions of 3 cm or less are first considered for stereotactic radiosurgery. External beam irradiation is not given to these patients. Patients presenting with larger (>3.5 cm) solitary tumors are evaluated for craniotomy and tumor resection which can be followed with stereotactic radiosurgery in the event of incomplete tumor removal. RCC patients presenting with multiple metastatic brain lesions receive whole brain irradiation with a total dose of 40 Gy or more given at 200-cGy daily fractions.

A total of 23 gamma knife treatments were given during a 30-month period at USC. Mean patient age was 58 years and 13 (56%) patients were males (Table 10.2). Mean tumor volume was 3.46 cm$^3$ and the mean treated volume was 5.98 cm$^3$. A mean of 2.65 isocenters was used in the treatment of these patients. Radiation doses depended on the tumor volume and tumor location and ranged from 16 to 23 Gy with a mean dose of 20.6 Gy. Symptomatic improvement was noted in 87% while tumor size reduction or a lack of tumor progression was seen in 22 (96%) patients, with only one patient showing tumor progression ultimately leading to his death.

Our treatment policy will be illustrated with specific examples of several treated RCC patients.

Patient 1 was a 52-year-old male who presented in June 1992 with severe headache and dizziness. MRI demonstrated a 26 × 25 × 27 mm enhancing lesion with a collar of edema (Fig. 10.1 a,b). The patient was a well-documented case of RCC who had undergone radical nephrectomy 2 years previously. He was treated with linear accelerator-based stereotactic radiosurgery, receiving a total dose of 22 Gy to the 80% isodose line given with seven arcs (Fig. 10.2). The patient tolerated this treatment well and his symptoms substantially improved during the first 3 weeks posttreatment. Two months later patient was off all medications and was asymptomatic. In July 1993 (13 months later), patient remained symptom-free and a tumor volume reduction was noted on MRI (Fig. 10.3).

Patient 2 (listed as patient 11 in Table 10.2) was a 65-year-old male with RCC who presented in January 1997 with a short history of severe headache. During workup a large right parietal lesion was noted (Fig. 10.4). The patient was treated with gamma knife radiosurgery, receiving a total dose of 18 Gy to the 50% isodose line using nine isocenters. Dose-volume histograms are shown in Fig. 10.5. The patient tolerated radiosurgery very well, and a few weeks after treatment became asymptomatic; he is currently leading a normal life.

Patient 3 (listed as patient 10 in Table 10.2) was a 49-year-old male seen in April 1996 with a history of RCC and progressive headache. MRI demonstrated a 2 cm left frontal lesion (Fig. 10.6). The patient was treated with gamma knife stereotactic radiosurgery, receiving 22 Gy to the 50% isodose line using three

**Table 10.2.** Stereotactic radiotherapy with gamma knife for brain metastasis: USC experience

| No. | Age | Sex | Location | Radiation dose (Gy) | Tumor volume ($cm^3$) | Volume treated ($cm^3$) | Tumor dimension (mm) | No. of isocenters |
|---|---|---|---|---|---|---|---|---|
| 1 | 57 | Female | Occipital | 22 | 2.3 | 3.6 | 14.9 × 14.2 × 16.6 | 1 |
| 2 | 59 | Female | Brain stem | 16 | 0.73 | 0.88 | 10.7 × 15.4 × 10.0 | 4 |
| 3 | 57 | Female | Occipital | 22 | 0.27 | 0.6 | 5.7 × 8.4 × 8.3 | 2 |
| 4 | 45 | Female | Parietal | 22 | 1.8 | 3.0 | 12.8 × 18.7 × 16.5 | 2 |
| 5 | 45 | Female | Parietal | 23 | 0.36 | 1.8 | 11.1 × 8.1 × 16.5 | 1 |
| 6 | 61 | Male | Frontal | 20 | 2.7 | 5.2 | 17.0 × 16.5 × 21.0 | 3 |
| 7 | 66 | Male | Occipital | 20 | 1.5 | 3.4 | 15.3 × 14.2 × 12.6 | 1 |
| 8 | 59 | Female | Frontal | 18 | 19.9 | 32.1 | 33.5 × 32 × 52.7 | 8 |
| 9 | 45 | Female | Occipital | 22 | 1.5 | 3.6 | 13.5 × 13.6 × 18.5 | 1 |
| 10 | 49 | Male | Frontal | 22 | 3.1 | 6.2 | 18.9 × 21.5 × 18.7 | 3 |
| 11 | 65 | Male | Parietal | 18 | 14.4 | 23.0 | 30.0 × 29.0 × 34.0 | 9 |
| 12 | 65 | Male | Frontal | 18 | 20.1 | 28.6 | 40.7 × 33.5 × 47 | 10 |
| 13 | 61 | Male | Occipital | 20 | 0.35 | 1.6 | 9.7 × 9.5 × 8.3 | 1 |
| 14 | 61 | Male | Frontal | 20 | 0.21 | 1.6 | 8.0 × 8.0 × 8.4 | 1 |
| 15 | 65 | Male | Occipital | 22 | 0.21 | 0.43 | 8.5 × 7.8 × 8.2 | 1 |
| 16 | 62 | Male | Occipital | 20 | 5.0 | 10.6 | 20.0 × 24.7 × 24.3 | 4 |
| 17 | 62 | Male | Parietal | 20 | 0.1 | 0.6 | 5.5 × 4.9 × 8.0 | 1 |
| 18 | 62 | Male | Parietal | 20 | 0.01 | 0.32 | 3.7 × 2.4 × 6.0 | 1 |
| 19 | 62 | Male | Frontal | 20 | 0.01 | 0.32 | 2.6 × 2.7 × 6.0 | 1 |
| 20 | 47 | Female | Thalamus | 22 | 0.27 | 1.4 | 6.7 × 7.8 × 8.0 | 1 |
| 21 | 47 | Female | Occipital | 22 | 0.42 | 1.8 | 8.7 × 10.0 × 12.0 | 1 |
| 22 | 55 | Female | Intraventric. | 20 | 4.2 | 6.4 | 19.5 × 18.4 × 27.5 | 3 |
| 23 | 40 | Male | Temporal | 22 | 0.16 | 0.59 | 5.9 × 6.3 × 8.1 | 1 |
| Mean | 58 | | | 20.6 | 3.46 | 5.98 | 14.0 × 14.2 × 17.3 | 2.65 |
| SD 8 | | | | 1.7 | 5.92 | 8.93 | 9.5 × 8.8 × 12.4 | 2.66 |

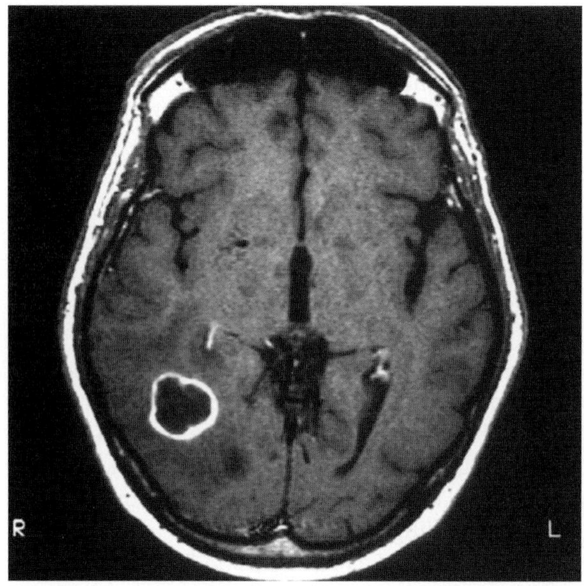

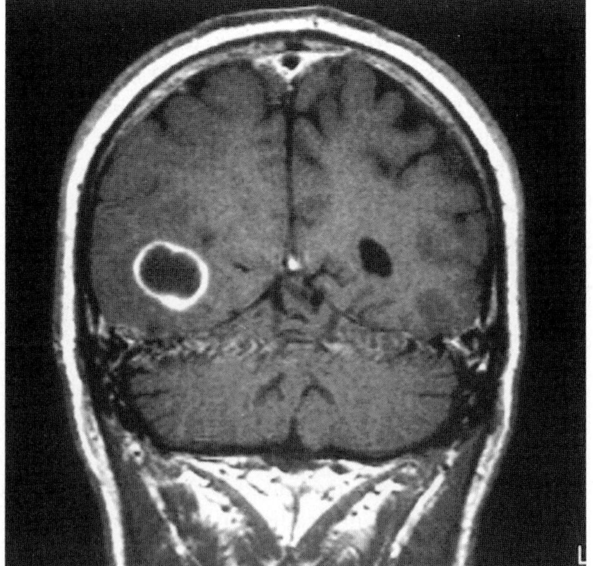

**Fig. 10.1. a** June 1992. 52-year-old male. Axial postcontrast T1-weighted image shows a ring-like enhancing lesion in the right temporo-occipital region with compression of the antrum and occipital horn of the right lateral ventricle clearly demonstrated. **b** June 1992. Coronal postcontrast T1-weighted image demonstrates a ring-like enhancing lesion in the right temporo-occipital region with compression of occipital horn of the right lateral ventricle

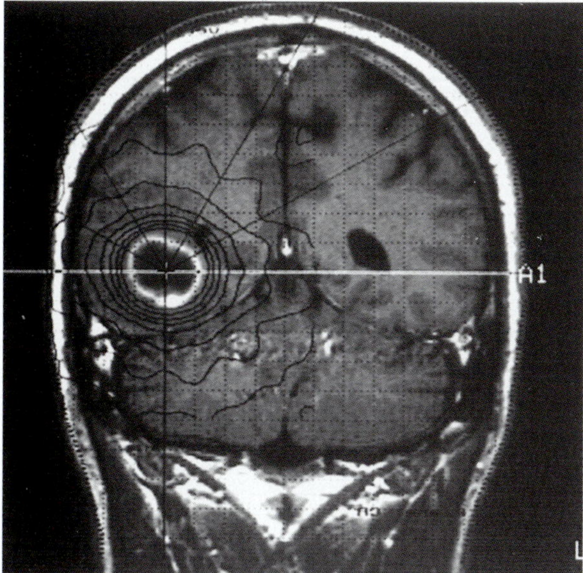

**Fig. 10.2.** Same patient as in Fig. 10.1. June 1992. Coronal postcontrast T1-weighted image shows a ring-like enhancing lesion in the right temporo-occipital region with treatment planning isodose lines seen surrounding the lesion. Dose distribution results from a seven arc treatment plan for this 26 × 25 × 27 mm lesion. The prescribed radiation dose of 22 Gy to the 80% isodose line, relative to the dose maximum, was carried out on a modified Varian 4/100 linear accelerator. Isodose lines shown are the 90%, 80%, 65%, 50%, 35%, 20%, 10%, 5%, and 2%

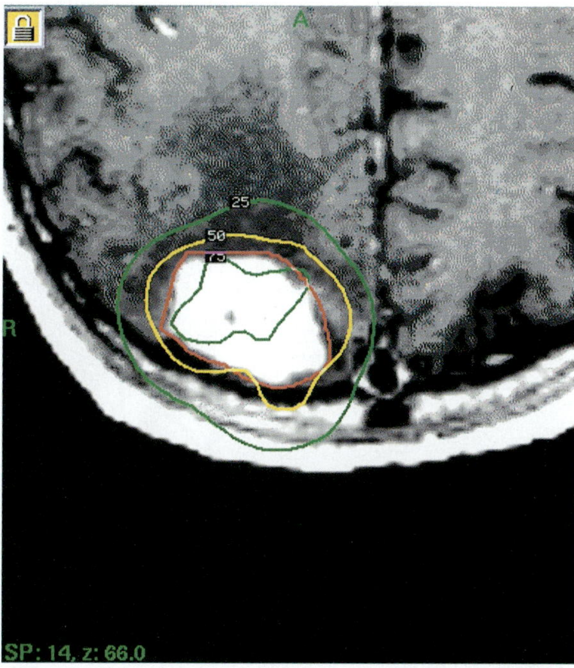

**Fig. 10.4.** January 1997: 65-year-old male. Axial postcontrast T1-weighted image shows an irregular enhancing mass in the right parietal region. Treatment planning isodose lines are seen over and surrounding the mass lesion. Note that the lesion is completely circumscribed by the 50% isodose line. The prescribed radiation dose of 18 Gy to the 50% isodose line, relative to the dose maximum was achieved by using nine isocenter gamma knife treatment plan. The lesion measured 30 × 29 × 34 mm in the three principal axes

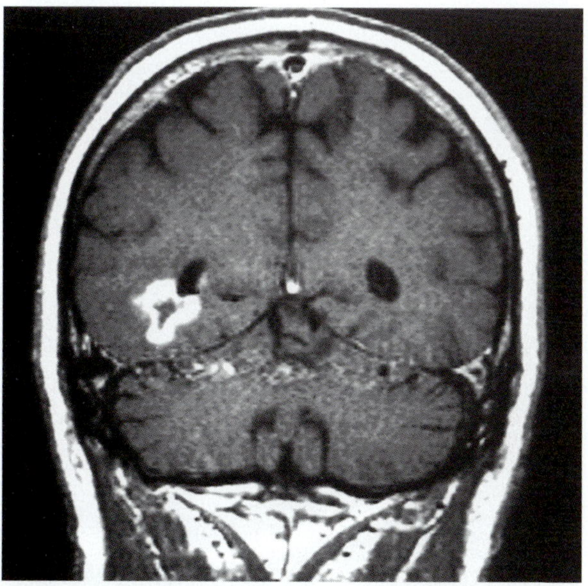

**Fig. 10.3.** Same patient as in Figs. 10.1 and 10.2. July 1993. Coronal postcontrast T1-weighted image reveals an irregular enhancing mass (22 × 22 × 20 mm), which appears to show a decrease in its size since the previous examination of June 1992

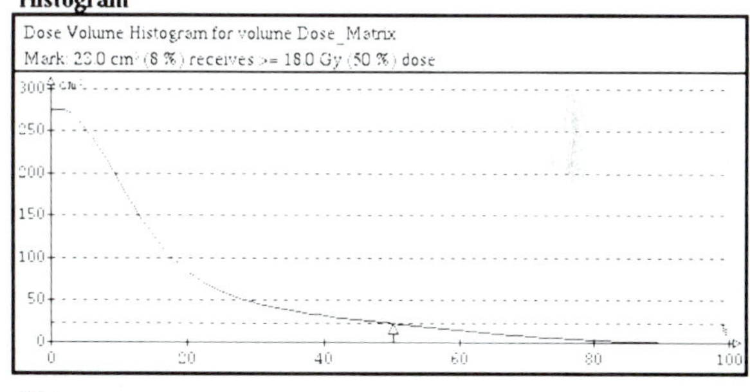

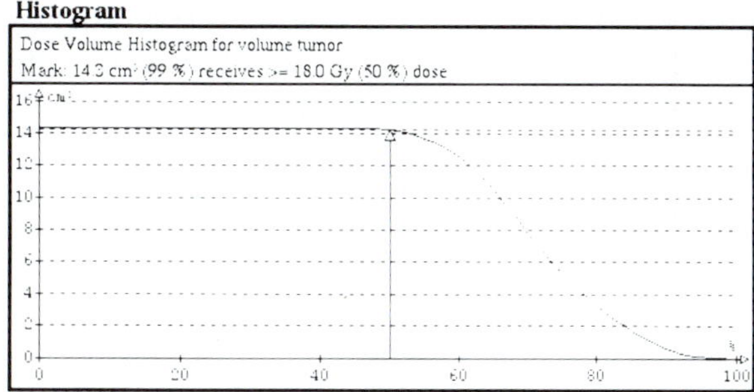

**Fig. 10.5.** Same patient as in Fig. 10.4. Dose-volume histograms calculated for the lesion. *Top*: Dose-volume histogram for the entire brain. A total of 23.0 cm$^3$ of the brain tissue received a radiation dose of 18 Gy or greater. *Bottom*: Dose-volume histogram for the lesion. A total of 14.3 cm$^3$ or 99% of the lesion received the prescribed radiation dose of 18 Gy or greater

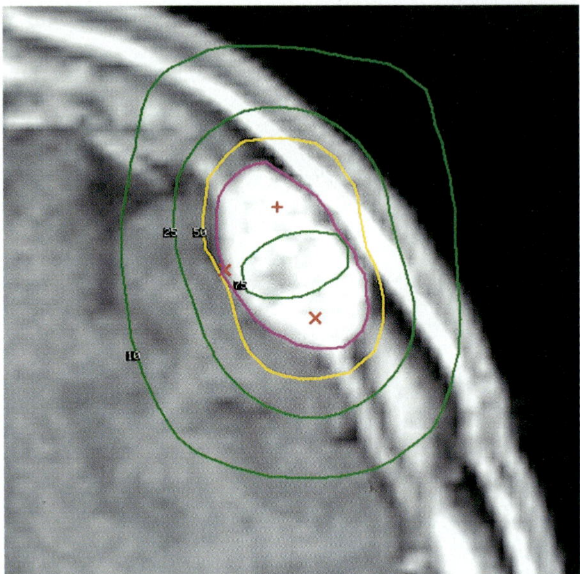

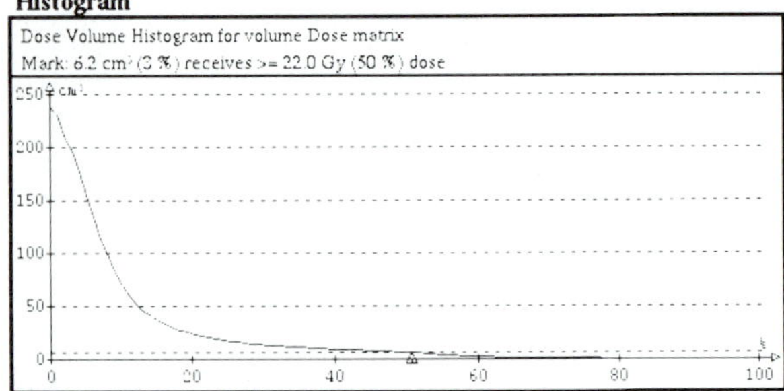



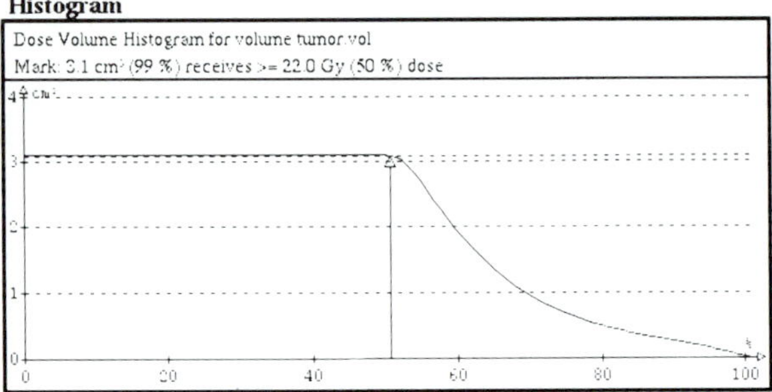



**Fig. 10.6.** April 1996: 49-year-old male. Axial postcontrast T1-weighted image shows an ovoid enhancing mass lesion involving the bony calvarium extradurally. Treatment planning isodose lines are seen over and surrounding the lesion. Note that the lesion is completely circumscribed by the 50% isodose line. The prescribed radiation dose of 22 Gy to the 50% isodose line relative to the dose maximum was achieved by using a three isocenter, gamma knife treatment plan. The tumor measured 18.9 × 21.5 × 18.7 mm in the three principal axes

**Fig. 10.7.** Same patient as in Fig. 10.6. Dose-volume histograms calculated for this 3.1 cm³ tumor. *Top*: Dose-volume histogram for the entire brain. A total of 6.2 cm³ of the brain volume received a radiation dose of at least 22 Gy. *Bottom*: Dose-volume histogram for the tumor volume. A total of 3.1 cm³ or 99% of the tumor received the prescribed dose of 22 Gy or greater

isocenters. Dose-volume histograms are presented in Fig. 10.7. At the present time the patient is doing very well without evidence of recurrence.

Patient 4 (listed as patient 4 in Table 10.2) was a 45-year-old female who was seen in April 1995 with severe headache and dizziness. MRI, dose-volume histogram, and treatment parameters are shown in Figs. 10.8 and 10.9 and Table 10.2. It is of interest to note that this patient developed a contralateral lesion 12 months later which was also successfully treated with gamma knife. This patient died of progressive pulmonary and liver disease in November 1997 without brain tumor recurrence and with nearly complete resolution of the gamma knife treated lesions.

Patient 5 (listed as patient 23 in Table 10.2) was a 40-year-old male who presented in December 1997 with a 2-week history of severe headache and progressively severe dizziness. His MRI demonstrated a large right frontal lesion with a significant "mass effect" (Fig. 10.10 a–d). This patient was treated urgently with craniotomy and tumor resection (Fig. 10.10 e). His condition improved dramatically and a postoperative MRI demonstrated the presence of a small right temporal lesion which was

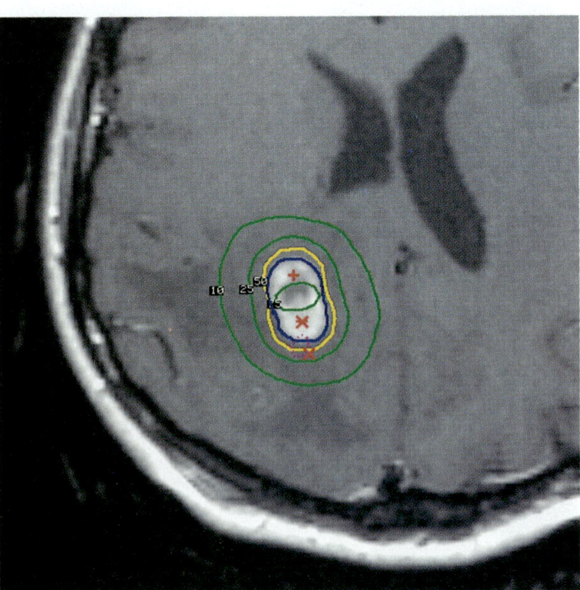

**Fig. 10.8.** April 1995. 45-year-old female. Axial postcontrast T1-weighted image reveals an ovoid, enhancing mass lesion in the right parieto-occipital region. Treatment planning isodose lines are seen over and surrounding the lesion. Note that the lesion is completely circumscribed within the 50% isodose line. The prescribed radiation dose of 22 Gy to the 50% isodose line, relative to the dose maximum, was achieved by using a two isocenter, gamma knife treatment plan. The lesion measured 12.8 × 18.7 × 16.5 mm in the three principal axes

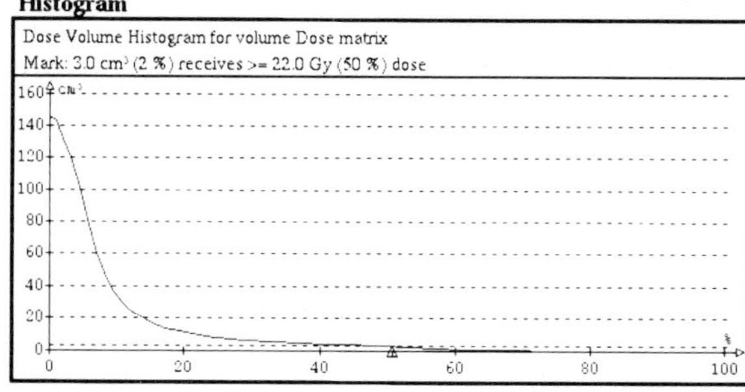

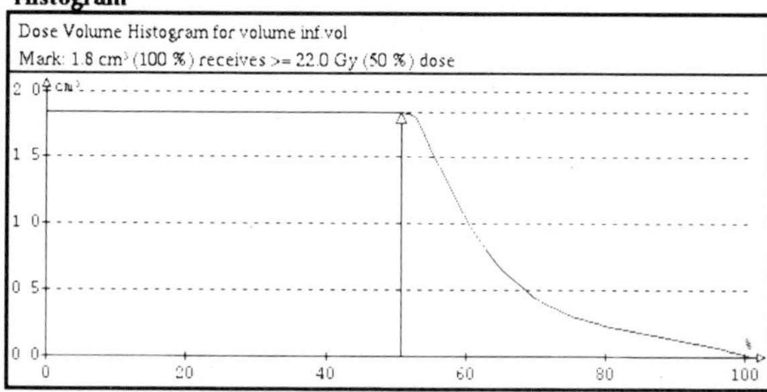

Fig. 10.9. Same patient as in Fig. 10.8. Dose-volume histograms calculated for this 1.8 cm³ lesion. *Top*: Dose-volume histogram for the entire brain. Total volume of 3.0 cm³ received at least 22 Gy of radiation. *Bottom*: Dose-volume histogram for the tumor volume. The entire tumor (100%) received the prescribed radiation dose of 22 Gy or greater)

successfully treated with gamma knife (Fig. 10.10f). It was apparent that stereotactic radiosurgery or external beam irradiation would not be appropriate treatment for the right frontal lesion. This was due to the large size (4.5 cm) of this lesion, the presence of a significant edema, and the acute nature of the problem.

Based on a review of the literature and our medical center experience we believe that stereotactic radiosurgery is the treatment of choice in RCC patients presenting with solitary brain metastasis. This treatment is performed on an outpatient basis under mild systemic sedation with excellent treatment tolerance. Whole brain irradiation should be reserved for patients with multiple metastatic lesions and craniotomy should be used infrequently in carefully selected patients.

## 10.3.4
## Spinal Metastasis

Thoracic and lumbar spine are the two sites of frequent tumor involvement in patients with RCC metastatic to bone (Saitoh 1981). Patients with RCC metastatic to spine and involvement of a single

vertebral body have a better prognosis (and may experience long-term survival) than those with multiple vertebral body involvement (Sioutos et al. 1995). Clinicians need to be alert to make an early diagnosis of spinal metastasis in order to prevent the occurrence of distressing symptoms and signs of spinal cord compression. The presence of even an asymptomatic epidural lesion requires early administration of palliative irradiation. In a study of 125 metastatic RCC patients treated at Thomas Jefferson University, eight (6%) had spinal compression but only one of these patients regained neurological function while five experienced partial neurological improvement (Onufrey aned Mohiuddin 1985). This poor response to radiotherapy of already established spinal cord compression with neurological signs and symptoms was confirmed in a study of 15 patients with metastatic carcinoma to the spine and spinal cord compression (Sioutos et al. 1995). Patients with RCC tend to have more frequently anterior than posterior epidural compression (Sioutos et al. 1995). Those who have rapidly progressing neurological signs and symptoms should be considered for surgical decompression followed by planned postoperative radiotherapy. Patients with already established cord compression of long duration need only a palliative course of irradiation to control pain as an improvement in neurological function is unlikely. Survival of RCC patients with spinal compression in one study ranged from 6 to 84 months with a mean of 21 months and median of 16 months (Sioutos et al. 1995).

Patients with spinal compression should receive a tolerance dose of external beam irradiation consisting of about 50 Gy given in 200 cGy daily fractions. This radiation dose should maintain a response for the rest of the patient's life. At USC patients with involvement of a single vertebral level or those who fail prior irradiation are considered for three-dimensional (3-D) treatment planning and delivery. Typically we use hypofractionated radiotherapy giving 30 Gy in five or six equal fractions using multiple fixed fields. Such a treatment is well tolerated, with the spinal cord receiving 10%–20% of the reference dose. More recently in patients with a single vertebral body involvement we began to use stereotactic radiosurgery. The patient is immobilized and a planning CT in the treatment position is obtained. The obtained images are reconstructed in 3-D and a treatment plan is devised with multiple arcs. This treatment is time consuming and requires substantial time commitment by a radiation oncologist and physicist.

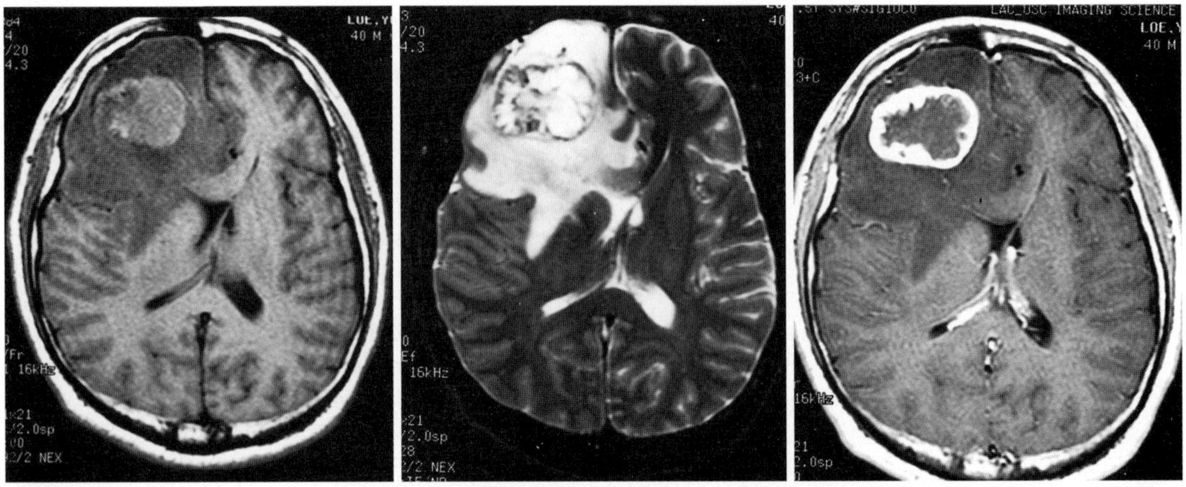

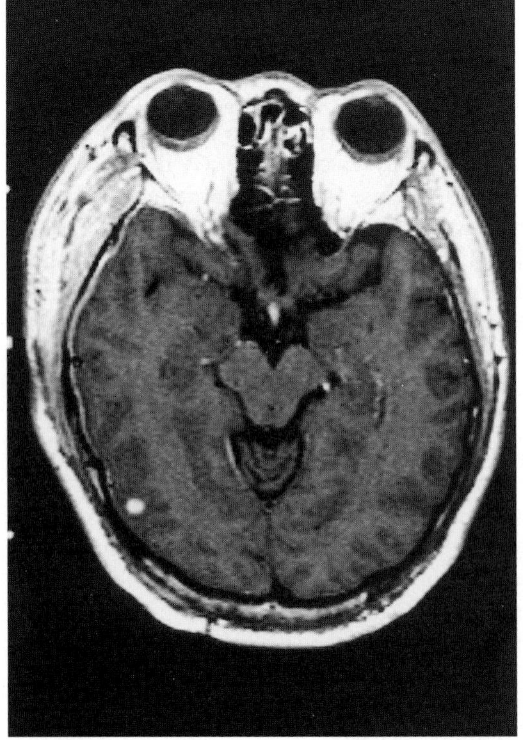

**Fig. 10.10. a** December 1997: 45-year-old male. Axial T1-weighted image shows an ovoid hyperintense mass with surrounding edema and mass effect in the right frontal region. There is marked compression and displacement of the frontal horn of the right lateral ventricle. A marked shift of the midline structure from the right to the left is manifested by the displacement of pericallosal arteries (*arrow*). **b** Axial T2-weighted image reveals the ovoid mass to be predominantly hyperintense. Surrounding edema is better seen on the T2-weighted image. **c** Axial T1-weighted, postcontrast image shows ring-like enhancement of the ovoid lesion with irregular thickness. The central nonenhancing area is probably due to tumor necrosis. **d** Sagittal T1-weighted image again shows the hyperintense, ovoid mass with surrounding edema in the right frontal lobe. **e** Sagittal T1-weighted image obtained following right frontal craniotomy and partial frontal lobectomy with removal of the mass shows postsurgical changes. Extirpation of the mass is achieved surgically. Obviously, this mass was too large for gamma knife treatment (4.5 cm × 3.2 cm 4.0 cm). **f** Axial T1-weighted, postcontrast image at different level in the same patient shows a small (5 mm) nodular enhancing mass in the posterior right temporal lobe. This lesion is ideal for gamma knife treatment

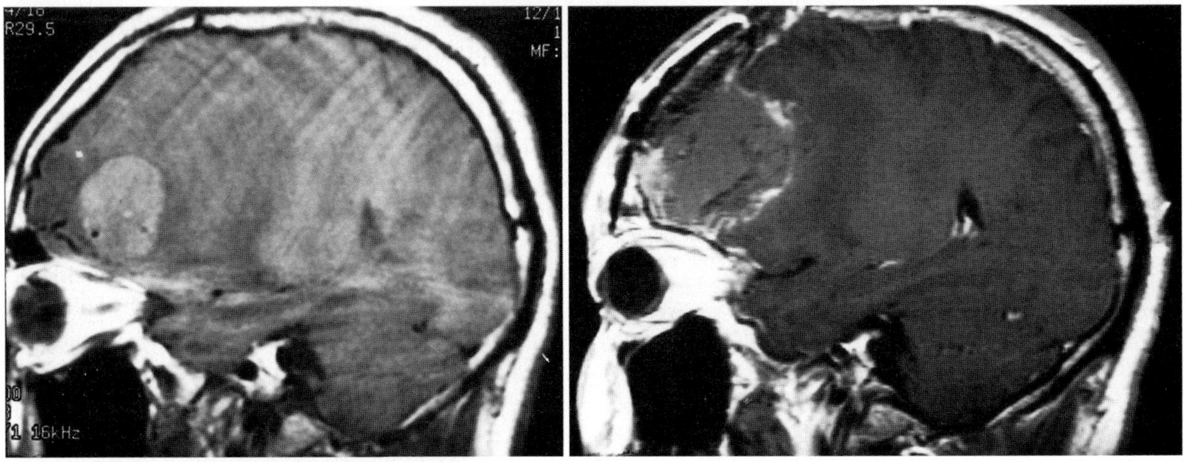

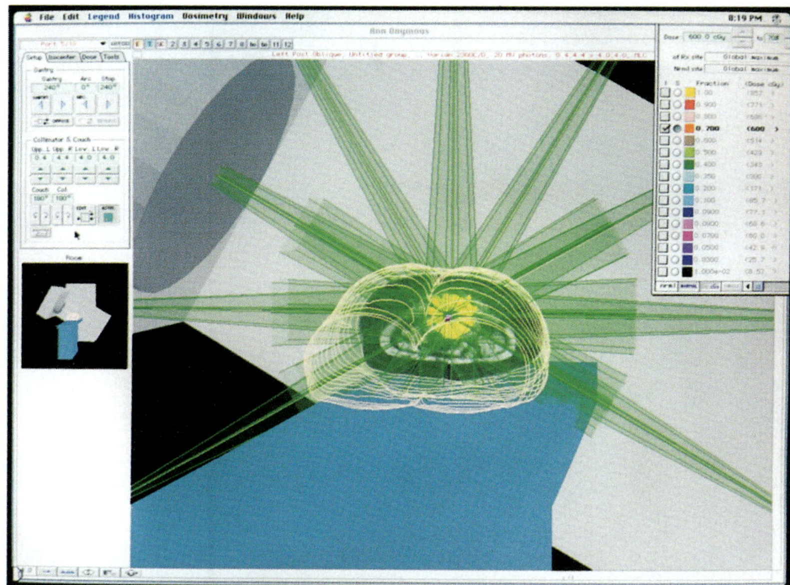

**Fig. 10.11.** The beam directions shown are used with beam angles, expressed in the Varian convention, at 60°, 90°, 120°, 150°, 180°, 210°, 240°, 270°, and 300°. In this convention, for a patient in the prone position the 90°, 180°, and 270° angles represent the right lateral, posterior, and left lateral beams

The USC treatment technique with multiple fixed fields will be illustrated below. The patient in question was a 50-year-old male with a long history of RCC. In April 1996, he presented with severe intractable low back pain and inability to ambulate due to this pain. The patient had had prior spinal irradiation of 40 Gy given at an outside medical center about 9 months previously. The patient was found to have extensive involvement of the L5 vertebral body. Two treatment plans are shown in Figs. 10.11–10.14. A schematic representation of a linear accelerator treatment position is demonstrated in Fig. 10.11. The concept of blocking the spinal cord or cauda equina is shown in Fig. 10.12. Axial and sagittal reconstruction of the treated volume which includes all components of the vertebral body with sparing of the center is shown in Fig. 10.13. A U-shaped radiation dose distribution with relative sparing of the center and the posterior elements of the vertebral body is demonstrated in reconstructed axial and sagittal views (Fig. 10.14), and Table 10.3 shows beam directions and field weights applied.

The treatment resulted in complete pain resolution, allowing the patient to lead a reasonably normal life for the remainder of his life. This patient died 4 months later of rapidly progressing liver and lung metastases.

**Table 10.3.** The field weights applied in the treatment plan shown in Fig. 10.14

| Beam direction | Blocked side | "Ring" distribution | "U" distribution |
| --- | --- | --- | --- |
| 60 | Left | 1.2 | 0 |
| | Right | 1.2 | 1.0 |
| 90 | Left | 1.0 | 0 |
| | Right | 1.0 | 1.0 |
| 120 | Left | 1.0 | 0 |
| | Right | 1.0 | 1.0 |
| 150 | Left | 1.0 | 0 |
| | Right | 1.45 | 1.25 |
| 180 | Left | 1.45 | 1.5 |
| | Right | 1.45 | 1.5 |
| 210 | Left | 1.45 | 1.25 |
| | Right | 1.0 | 0 |
| 240 | Left | 1.0 | 1.0 |
| | Right | 1.0 | 0 |
| 270 | Left | 1.1 | 1.0 |
| | Right | 1.1 | 0 |
| 300 | Left | 1.2 | 1.0 |
| | Right | 1.2 | 1.0 |

### 10.3.5
### Other Metastatic Sites

The application of external beam radiotherapy is of importance in patients with involvement of the left supraclavicular region. This manifestation of metastatic RCC requires attention since tumor invasion of the brachial plexus presents a very difficult management problem and intractable pain. We recommend

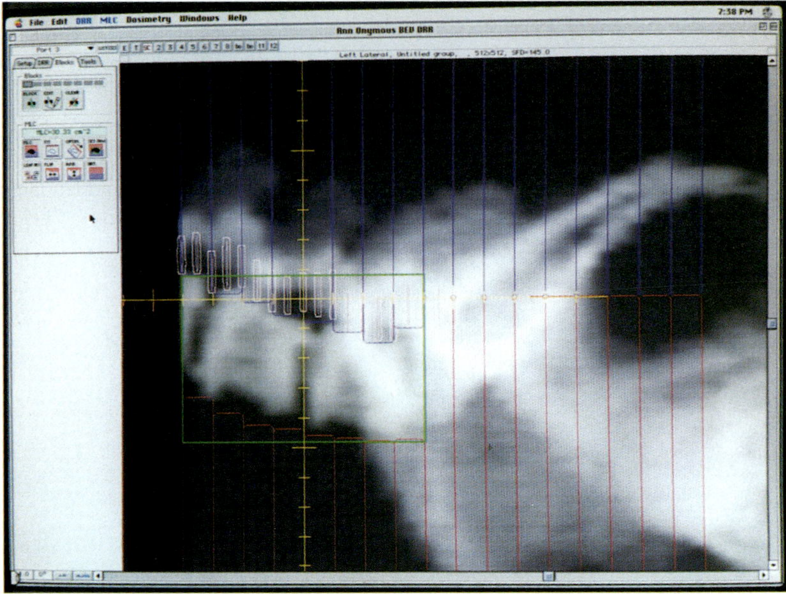

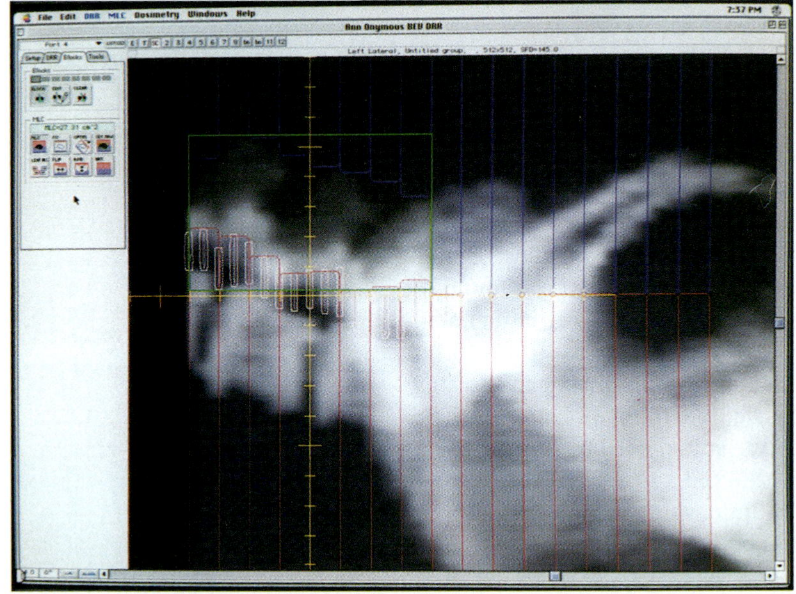

**Fig. 10.12 a,b.** Two fields were designed for each beam direction using different multi-leaf blocking configurations. **a** Looking from the source of the radiation beam, in the first field blocks are covering the left side of the field. This blocking protects the spinal cord or canda equina, leaving the right side of the field open for the treatment. **b** In the second field the right side of the field including the spinal cord is blocked, radiating the left side of the field. The blocking arrangement is illustrated with the computer-generated radiographs of the two lateral fields. Using the 3-D "beam's eye view" capabilities of our virtual simulation program, this alternate shielding can be easily designed. The result is the blocking of the spinal cord from all directions, while radiation dose is delivered to the tumor-involved vertebral body. This in effect represents an irregular central block placed over the spinal cord, conforming to its shape. The length of each radiation field is 6 cm with the width adjusted in each direction to conform to the shape of the treated vertebral body. The 20-MV photon beam generated by the Varian Clinac 2300C linear accelerator was used in this treatment plan

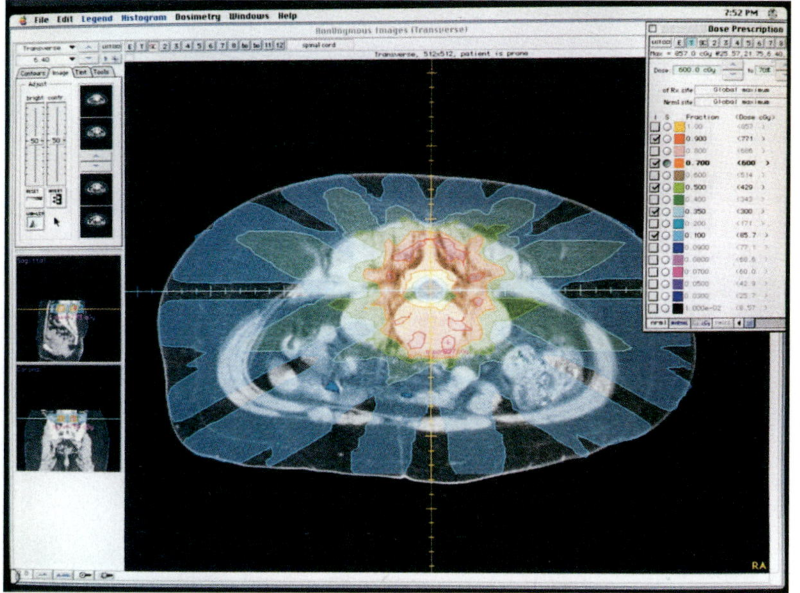

a

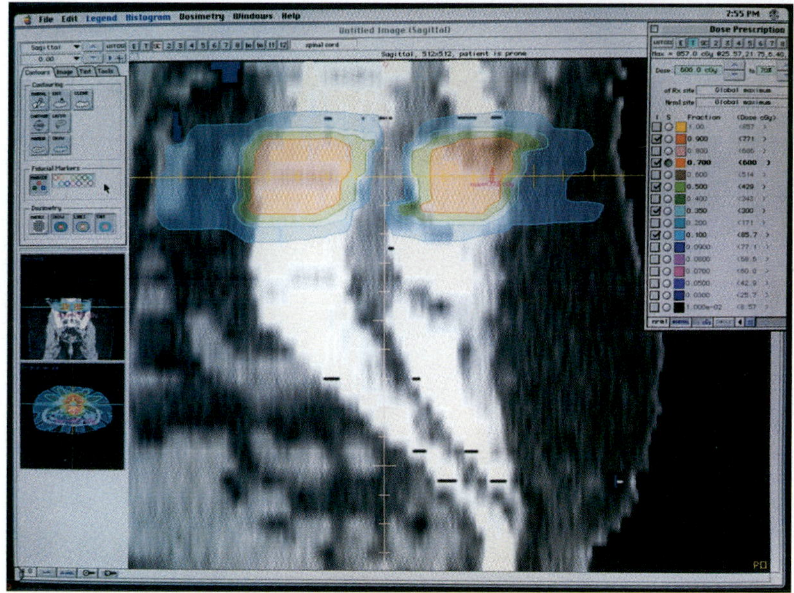

b

**Fig. 10.13 a,b.** The radiation dose distributions as shown here were achieved with the use of the same beam as described in Fig. 10.12. Some adjustments of the beam weights were necessary to close the 70% isodose line into a ring (*red line*). The dose to the spinal cord or cauda equina was less than 20% of the tumor dose, and most of the spinal cord volume received less than 10%, relative to the maximal dose

the use of fractionated >50 Gy external beam irradiation. This radiation dose is likely to result in tumor control of long duration. Other sites of metastatic RCC include the involvement of the upper aero-digestive passages. Unfortunately the dose of radiotherapy required for tumor control will result in short-term treatment toxicity.

## 10.4
## Conclusions

Radiotherapy in an adjuvant setting given prior to or following radical nephrectomy has not been found to be useful and its role has yet to be defined. There is a definite role for radiotherapy as an im-

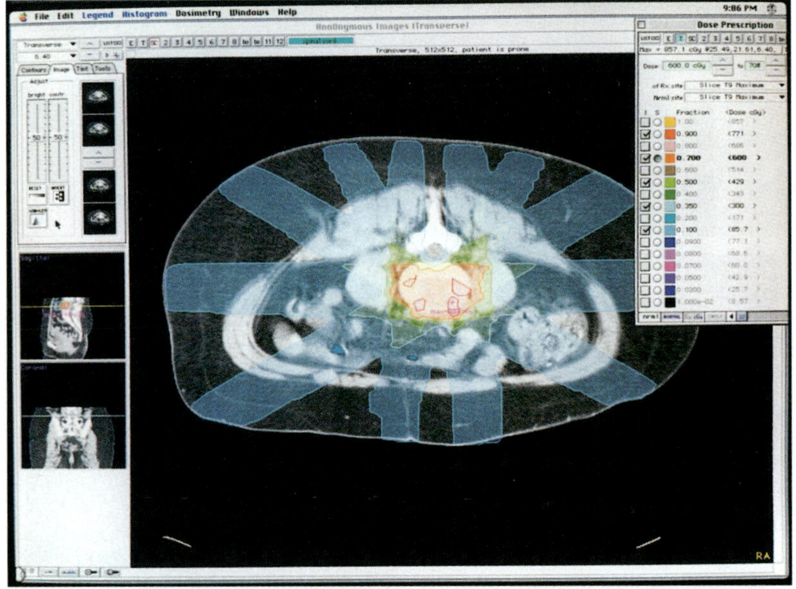

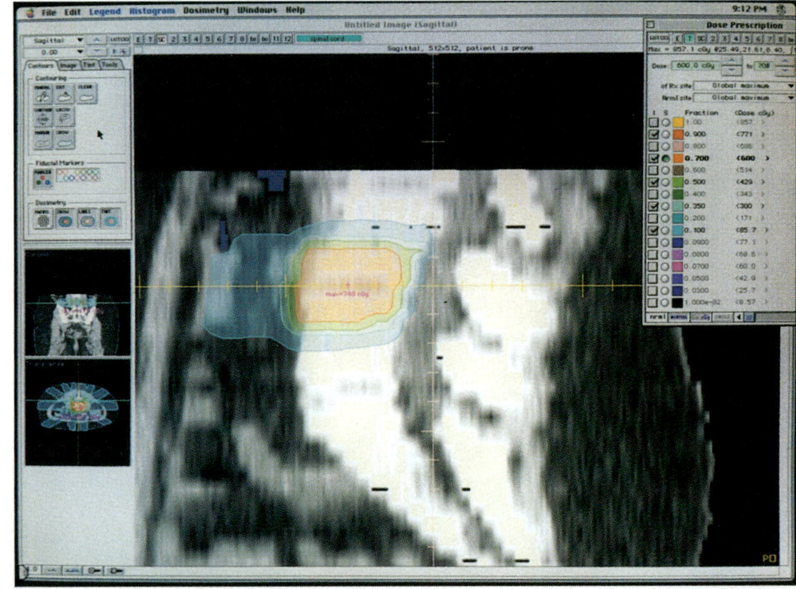

**Fig. 10.14 a,b.** The U-shaped dose distribution was formed by the use of the same beam directions as in Fig. 10.13, but the fields irradiating the posterior part of the vertebral body were omitted. Increased weights from the posterior direction were necessary to achieve a more extended U-shape of the 70% isodose line (*red line*). The dose to the spinal cord is the same as in Fig. 10.13. The field weights as used in this case are shown in Table 10.3

portant palliative treatment in the management of signs and symptoms due to local tumor progression in patients who have contraindications to radical nephrectomy. Radiotherapy with stere otactic radiosurgery is the treatment of choice in patients with solitary brain metastasis and in selected patients with involvement of the spine. Early administration of external beam radiotherapy is required in patients with epidural lesions in order to prevent the development of distressing signs and symptoms of spinal cord compression. For optimal management of patients with RCC there has to be good interaction between a urologist, a medical oncologist, and a radiation oncologist.

# References

Abratt RP, Pontin AR, Ball HS (1993) Activity of a short course of interferon alpha for metastatic renal cell carcinoma – a phase II study. Cancer Immunol Immunother 37:140–141

Badalament RA, Gluck RW, Wong GY, et al. (1990) Surgical treatment of brain metastases from renal cell carcinoma. Urology 36:112–117

Bennett RT, Lerner SE, Taub HC, Dutcher JP, Fleischmann J (1995) Cytoreductive surgery for stage IV renal cell carcinoma. J Urol 154:32–34

Bloom HJG (1973) Adjuvant therapy for adenocarcinoma of the kidney: present position and prospects. Br J Urol 45:237–257

Chiou RK, Vessella RL, Limas C, Shafer RB, Elson MK, Arfman EW, Lange PH (1988) Monoclonal antibody-targeted radiotherapy of renal cell carcinoma using a nude mouse model. Cancer 61:1766–1775

Christoferson LA, Gustafson MB, Petersen AG (1961) Von Hippel-Lindau's disease. JAMA 178:126–129

Coulange C (1993) Enquete epidemiologique sur les tumeurs du rein. In: Abbou CC, Lobel B (eds) Synthese et recommendations en onco-urologie. Monogr Prog Urol, Paris, pp 200–202

deKernion JB, Mukamel E (1987) Selection of initial therapy for renal cell carcinoma. Cancer 60:539–546

Dinney CPN, Awad SA, Gajewski JB, Belitsky P, Lannon SG, Mack FG, Millard OH (1992) Analysis of imaging modalities, staging systems, and prognostic indicators for renal cell carcinoma. Urology 39:122–129

Engenhart R, Kimmig BN, Hover KH, et al. (1993) Long-term follow-up for brain metastases treated by percutaneous stereotactic single high-dose irradiation. Cancer 71:1353–1361

Flanigan RC (1987) The failure of infarction and/or nephrectomy in stage IV renal cell cancer to influence survival or metastatic regression. Urol Clin North Am 14:757–762

Flickinger JC, Kondziolka D, Lunsford LD, et al. (1994) A multi-institutional experience with stereotactic radiosurgery for solitary brain metastasis. Int J Radiat Oncol Biol Phys 28:797–802

Flocks RH, Kadesky MC (1958) Malignant neoplasms of the kidney: an analysis of 353 patients followed five years or more. J Urol 79:196–201

Fossa SD, Kjolseth I, Lund G (1982) Radiotherapy of metastases from renal cancer. Eur Urol 8:340–342

Fossa SD, Droz JP, Pavone-Macaluso MM, Debruyne FJ, Vermeylen K, Sylvester R (1992) Vinblastine in metastatic renal cell carcinoma: EORTC phase II trial 30882. The EORTC Genitourinary Group. Eur J Cancer 28A:878–880

Fossa SD, Kramar A, Droz JP (1994) Prognostic factors and survival in patients with metastatic renal cell carcinoma treated with chemotherapy or interferon-alpha. Eur J Cancer 30A:1310–1314

Fossa S, Jones M, Johnson P, Joffe J, Holdener E, Elson P, Ritchie A Selby P (1995) Interferon-alpha and survival in renal cell cancer. Br J Urol 76:286–290

Frank W, Stuhldreher D, Saffrin R, Shott S, Guinan P (1994) Stage IV renal cell carcinoma. J Urol 152:1998–1999

Frydenberg M, Gunderson L, Hahn G, Fieck J, Zincke H (1994) Preoperative external beam radiotherapy followed by cytoreductive surgery and intraoperative radiotherapy for locally advanced primary or recurrent renal malignancies. J Urol 152:15–21

Gioanni J, Zanghellini E, Mazeau C, et al. (1996) CAL 54, a new cell line derived from a human renal carcinoma: characterization and radiosensitivity. Bull Cancer 83:553–558

Giuliani L, Gilberti C, Martorana G, Rovida S (1990) Radical extensive surgery for renal cell carcinoma: long-term results and prognostic factors. J Urol 143:468–474

Golimbu M, Joshi P, Sperber A, Tessler A, Al-Askari S, Morales P (1986) Renal cell carcinoma: survival and prognostic factors. Urology 27:291–301

Gurney H, Larcos G, McKay M, Kefford R, Langlands A (1989) Bone metastases in hypernephroma. Frequency of scapular involvement. Cancer 64:1429–1431

Hall EJ, Brenner DJ (1993) The radiobiology of radiosurgery: rationale for different treatment regimens for AVMs and malignancies. Int J Radiat Oncol Biol Phys 25:381–385

Halperin EC, Harisiadis L (1983) The role of radiation therapy in the management of metastatic renal cell carcinoma. Cancer 51:614–617

Juusela H, Malmio K, Alfthan O, Oravisto KJ (1977) Preoperative irradiation in the treatment of renal adenocarcinoma. Scand J Urol Nephrol 11:277–281

Kjaer M (1987) The treatment and prognosis of patients with renal adenocarcinoma with solitary metastasis. 10 year survival results. Int J Radiat Oncol Biol Phys 13:619–621

Kjaer M, Frederiksen PT (1987) Postoperative radiotherapy in stage II and III renal adenocarcinoma. A randomized trial by the Copenhagen Renal Cancer Study Group. Int J Radiat Oncol Biol Phys 13:665–672

Kjaer M, Iversen P, Hvidt V, Bruun E, Skaarup P, Bech-Hansen J, Frederiksen PL (1987) A randomized trial of postoperative radiotherapy versus observation in stage II and III renal adenocarcinoma. A study by the Copenhagen Renal Cancer Study Group. Scand J Urol Nephrol 21:285–289

Landis SH, Murray T, Bolden S, Wingo PA (1998) Cancer statistics 1998. CA Cancer J Clin 48:6–29

Leith JT, Cook A, Chougle P, Calabresi P, Wahlberg L, Lindquist C, Epstein M (1994) Intrinsic and extrinsic characteristics of human tumors relevant to radiosurgery: comparative cellular radiosensitivity and hypoxic percentages. Acta Neurochir Suppl 62:18–27

Ljungberg B, Stenling R, Osterdahl B, Farrelly E, Aberg T, Roos G (1995) Vein invasion in renal cell carcinoma: impact of metastatic behavior and survival. J Urol 154:1681–1684

Maldazys JD, deKernion JB (1986) Prognostic factors in metastatic renal carcinoma. J Urol 136:376–379

Maor MH, Frias AE, Oswald MJ (1988) Palliative radiotherapy for brain metastases in renal carcinoma. Cancer 62:1912–1917

McNichols DW, Segura JW, DeWeerd JH (1981) Renal cell carcinoma: long-term results and late recurrence. J Urol 126:17–23

Montie JE, Stewart BH, Straffon RA, Banowsky LHW, Hewitt CB, Montague DK (1977) The role of adjunctive nephrectomy in patients with metastatic renal cell carcinoma. J Urol 117:272–275

Nussbaum ES, Djalilian HR, Cho KH, Hall WA (1996) Brain metastases. Histology, multiplicity, surgery, and survival. Cancer 78:1781–1788

O'Dea MJ, Zincke H, Utz DC, Bernatz PE (1978) The treatment of renal cell carcinoma with solitary metastasis. J Urol 120:540–542

Onufrey V, Mohiuddin M (1985) Radiation therapy in the treatment of metastatic renal cell carcinoma. Int J Radiat Oncol Biol Phys 11:2007–2009

Peeling WB, Mantell BS, Shepheard BGF (1969) Post-operative irradiation in the treatment of renal cell carcinoma. Br J Urol 41:23–31

Petrovich Z, Emami B, Kapp D, et al. (1991) Regional hyperthermia in patients with recurrent genitourinary cancer. Am J Clin Oncol 14:472–477

Petrovich Z, Luxton G, Formenti S, et al. (1996) Stereotactic radiosurgery for primary and metastatic brain tumors. Cancer Invest 14:445–454

Rabinovitch RA, Zelefsky MJ, Gaynor JJ, Fuks Z (1994) Patterns of failure following surgical resection of renal cell carcinoma: implications for adjuvant local and systemic therapy. J Clin Oncol 11:206–212

Rafla S (1970) Renal cell carcinoma. Natural history and results of treatment. Cancer 25:26–40

Robson CJ, Churchill BM, Anderson W (1969) The results of radical nephrectomy for renal cell carcinoma. J Urol 101:297–301

Rubin P, Keller B, Cox C, Eassa EH (1975) Preoperative irradiation in renal cancer. Evaluation of radiation treatment plans. Am J Roentgenol Radium Ther Nucl Med 123:114–121

Saitoh H (1981) Distant metastasis of renal adenocarcinoma. Cancer 48:1487–1491

Salup RR, Back TC, Wiltrout RH (1987) Successful treatment of advanced murine renal cell cancer by bicompartmental adoptive chemoimmunotherapy. J Immunol 138:641–647

Selli C, Hinshaw WM, Woodard BH, Paulson DF (1983) Stratification of risk factors in renal cell carcinoma. Cancer 52:899–903

Shibui S, Nishikawa R, Nomura K (1990) Treatment of metastatic brain tumor from renal cell carcinoma. No Shinkei Geka 18:935–938

Sioutos PJ, Arbit E, Meshulam CF, Galicich JH (1995) Spinal metastases from solid tumors. Analysis of factors affecting survival. Cancer 76:1453–1459

Skinner DG (1989) The value of regional lymph node dissection in genitourinary cancer. Semin Surg Oncol 5:235–239

Skinner DG, Colvin RB, Vermillion CD, Pfister RC, Leadbetter WF (1971) Diagnosis and management of renal cell carcinoma. Cancer 28:1165–1177

Skinner DG, Pritchett TR, Lieskovsky G, Boyd SD, Stiles QR (1989) Vena caval involvement by renal cell carcinoma. Ann Surg 210:387–394

Stein JP, Esrig D, Eastham J, et al. (1998) The surgical management for renal cell carcinoma: long-term results in a large group of patients. J Urol (in press)

Stein M, Kuten A, Halpern J, Coachman NM, Cohen Y, Robinson E (1992) The value of postoperative irradiation in renal cell cancer. Radiother Oncol 24:41–44

Tolia BM, Whitmore WF Jr (1975) Solitary metastasis from renal cell carcinoma. J Urol 114:836–838

Tosaka A, Ohya K, Yamada K, et al. (1990) Incontinence and properties of renal masses and asymptomatic renal cell carcinoma detected by abdominal ultrasonography. J Urol 144:1097–1099

Van Der Werf-Messing (1973) Carcinoma of the kidney. Cancer 32:1056–1061

Waters WB, Richie JP (1979) Aggressive surgical approach to renal cell carcinoma: review of 130 cases. J Urol 122:306–309

Weber W, Rosler HP, Doll G, Dostert M, Kutzner J, Schild H (1992) The percutaneous irradiation of osteolytic bone metastases – a course assessment. Strahlenther Onkol 168:275–280

Yonese J, Kawakami S, Ueda T, et al. (1995) Clinical study of renal cell carcinoma with brain metastasis. Jpn J Urol 86:1287–1293

# 11 Radiation Therapy for Carcinoma of the Renal Pelvis and Ureters

J.E. LAHANIATIS, J.M. MICHALSKI, and L.W. BRADY

CONTENTS



## 11.1 Introduction

Transitional cell carcinoma (TCC) of the upper urinary tract (renal pelvis and ureter) accounts for 7% of all renal neoplasms and 5% of all urothelial malignancies (REITELMAN et al. 1987). The incidence of synchronous and asynchronous bilateral presentation is 2% and 8%, respectively (HUBEN et al. 1988). Patients with tumor in the upper urinary tract have a greater risk of developing TCC elsewhere, especially in the bladder. This multifocal presentation has been reported in up to 30% of patients (CHARBIT et al.

J.E. LAHANIATIS, MD, Department of Radiation Oncology, Allegheny University of the Health Sciences, Allegheny University Hospitals, Hahnemann, 230 North Broad Street, Mail Stop 200, Philadelphia, PA 19102-1192, USA
J.M. MICHALSKI, MD, Department of Radiology, Mallinckrodt Institute of Radiology, Washington University School of Medicine, St. Louis, MO 63110, USA
L.W. BRADY, MD, Hylda Cohn/American Cancer Society Professor of Clinical Oncology, and Professor, Department of Radiation Oncology, Allegheny University of the Health Sciences, Allegheny University Hospitals, Hahnemann, 230 North Broad Street, Mail Stop 200, Philadelphia, PA 19102-1192, USA

1991). This may be due to the fact that the mucosal surfaces of the renal pelvis, ureter, and bladder have the same embryologic origin and many etiologic factors are shared. The most significant risk factor for developing an upper urinary tract malignancy is tobacco use. Other associated etiologic factors include chronic analgesic abuse (especially phenacetin), aminophenol exposure, urban residency, and chronic nephrolithiasis (LAI 1992). A toxic nephropathy endemic to the Balkan peninsula of Eastern Europe is associated with a high frequency of a multifocal, superficial, slow-growing, papillary TCC of the upper urinary tract (PETKOVIC 1975). The list of potential urban toxic agents is extensive and includes: fungal toxins, viruses, silicates, heavy metals, aniline dyes, and waste from textile manufacturing and plastic and rubber industries (CLAYMAN et al. 1983; DROLLER 1986). Tumors of the upper urinary tract are 2–3 times more common in men than in women, with the peak incidence in the fifth to sixth decades of life.

The multifocality of TCC of the upper urinary tract is most frequently seen in patients with large tumors and those with carcinoma in situ. TCC of the upper urinary tract may spread by direct extension, via lymphatics, or through blood-borne metastases. Metastatic disease is present in 40% of these patients (BABAIAN et al. 1980). None of the 43 patients with low-grade tumors had lymph node metastases whereas three (14%) of the 22 patients with high-grade (3–4) tumors in the same study had lymph node metastases (COZAD 1995). Lymph node metastases were reported in nine (35%) of 26 patients selected to receive adjuvant radiation therapy (MAULARD-DURDUX 1996). Squamous cell carcinoma of the renal pelvis is usually associated with chronic inflammation or infection of the renal pelvis and accounts for 8% of renal pelvis tumors. All of the 11 patients with squamous cell carcinoma in a study of 144 patients with tumors of the renal pelvis also suffered from chronically infected staghorn renal calculi of long duration (LI and CHEUNG 1987).

## 11.2
## Diagnosis and Staging

The most common presentation is gross or microscopic hematuria, which has been reported in 70%–95% of patients with TCC of the upper urinary tract. Less common symptoms include pain (8%–40%), flank mass or hydronephrosis (10%–20%), bladder irritation (5%–10%), and other constitutional symptoms (Lai 1992).

### 11.2.1
### Diagnostic Workup

The recommended diagnostic workup for upper urinary tract carcinoma is listed in Table 11.1. A filling defect in the renal pelvis/collecting system is the most common finding with intravenous urography. Accurate cytologic diagnosis on an endoscopically obtained urine sample is made in more than 80% of the cases (Cullen 1972). Retrograde pyelography can be used to define the lower margin of a ureteral lesion, especially if there is a significant proximal lesion obstructing contrast flow from the renal pelvis. Computerized tomography (CT) or magnetic resonance imaging (MRI) of the abdomen and pelvis before and after contrast administration gives useful information regarding the possible extension of tumor outside the collecting system. Bone has been found to be the most frequent site of metastasis outside the pelvis and appropriate studies to demonstrate this tumor spread are indicated in selected patients (Sengelov et al. 1996).

### 11.2.2
### Staging

Grabstald et al. (1971) proposed a staging classification (Table 11.2) for patients with renal pelvis carcinoma based on the extent of primary tumor. The principles of this staging system are similar to the T categories in the American Joint Committee recommended staging system as shown in Table 11.3.

### 11.2.3
### Pathology

More than 90% of upper urinary tract cancers are TCCs. Squamous cell carcinoma accounts for 8% and is often locally advanced and associated with a high

**Table 11.1.** Diagnostic workup for carcinoma of renal pelvis and ureter

General and specific history
Physical examination
Radiographic studies
Standard
    Chest radiographs
    Intravenous excretory urogram
    Retrograde pyelogram
    CT or MRI of abdomen and pelvis
Complementary
    Endoscopic ureteroscopy
    Percutaneous nephroscopy
    CT of chest, brain, or other suspected sites
Special tests
    Urine cytology (endoscopically obtained)
    Retrograde brush cytology or biopsy
Laboratory studies
    Complete blood cell count
    Blood chemistry
    Urinalysis

**Table 11.2.** Staging classification proposed by Grabstald et al. (1971)

| Stage | Description |
| --- | --- |
| Stage I | Superficial, papillary carcinomas without evidence of invasion |
| Stage II | Superficial tumor invasion limited to the l amina propria |
| Stage III | Tumor extension into the muscularis |
| Stage IV | Tumor extension into adventitia, adjacent structures, or metastatic disease |

incidence of local recurrence (Blacher et al. 1985). Adenocarcinoma of the ureter and renal pelvis has been infrequently reported and accounts for 1% of these tumors.

In a study of 98 cases of TCC of the upper urinary tract, including dysplastic lesions, 32 (33%) were positive for human papillomavirus (HPV-16 and HPV-18). Additionally, 26 (26%) of these cases had overexpression of p53 (Furihata et al. 1995). Only three (3%) cases were positive for both HPV DNA and p53 antibody. The study investigators concluded that HPV infection or overexpression (mutation) of p53 may be an early event and be related to tumor cell growth patterns and tumor progression. A similar study by the same group suggested that overexpression of p53 and/or bcl-2 protein may represent early events in tumor genesis and, in particular, p53 alterations are essential for maintenance of a malignant phenotype in tumor development (Furihata et al. 1996).

**Table 11.3.** American Joint Committee staging classification for tumors of the renal pelvis and ureter (from BEAHRS et al. 1992)

*Primary tumor (T)*
TX  Primary tumor cannot be assessed
T0  No evidence of primary tumor
Tis  Carcinoma in situ
Ta  Papillary noninvasive carcinoma
T1  Tumor invades subepithelial connective tissue
T2  Tumor invades muscularis
T3  (For renal pelvis only) Tumor invades beyond the muscularis into peripelvic fat or the renal parenchyma (For ureter only) Tumor invades beyond the muscularis into the periureteric fat
T4  Tumor invades adjacent organs or through the kidney into perinephric fat

*Regional lymph nodes (N)*
NX  Regional lymph nodes cannot be assessed
N0  No regional lymph nodes metastasis
N1  Metastasis in a single lymph node, $\leq 2\,cm$ in greatest dimension
N2  Metastasis in single lymph node, $>2\,cm$ but $<5\,cm$ in greatest dimension, or multiple lymph nodes, $<5\,cm$ in greatest dimension
N3  Metastasis in a lymph node $>5\,cm$ in greatest dimension

*Distant metastasis (M)*
MX  Presence of distant metastasis cannot be assessed
M0  No distant metastasis
M1  Distant metastasis

*Stage grouping*

| Stage 0 | Tis | N0 | M0 | |
|---|---|---|---|---|
| | Ta | N0 | M0 | |
| Stage I | T1 | N0 | M0 | |
| Stage II | T2 | N0 | M0 | |
| Stage III | T3 | N0 | M0 | |
| Stage IV | T4 | N0 | M0 | |
| | Any T | N1,2,3 | M0 | |
| | Any T | Any N | M1 | |

*Histopathologic grade*
GX  Grade cannot be assessed
G1  Well differentiated
G2  Moderately well differentiated
G3–4  Poorly differentiated or undifferentiated

## 11.3
## Prognostic Factors

The most significant prognostic factors for survival of patients with TCC of the upper urinary tract are stage and grade of tumor (GRABSTALD et al. 1971). HENEY et al. (1981) reported 5-year survival rates ranging from 82% to 100% in patients with tumors confined to the mucosa, versus 0%–24% survival rates for patients with more advanced tumors invading through the muscularis. The prognostic importance of histopathologic grade was also evaluated in this study. The investigators reported a 100%, 81%, and 0% 5-year survival for grades 1, 2, and 3–4, respectively. Similar results have been reported by CORRADO et al. (1991) in a series of 127 patients where 5-year survival rates of Ta, T1, T2, T3, and T4 tumors were 80%, 83%, 72%, 51%, and 16%, respectively. In this study, CORRADO et al. reported 5-year survival rates of 83%, 75%, 52%, and 0% for grades 1 through 4, respectively. CHARBIT et al. (1991) noted that lymph node metastases were seen exclusively in patients with high-grade tumors and 90% of tumor-related deaths occurred in patients with high-grade tumors as compared with only 8% of patients without advanced disease.

Flow cytometry and the bromodeoxyuridine labeling index have been used experimentally in estimating long-term prognosis in patients with poor stage and grade criteria. CORRRADO et al. (1991) demonstrated in a multivariate analysis that DNA pattern (diploid versus nondiploid) and the number of lesions (unifocal versus multifocal) identified at initial diagnosis determined prognosis. Patients with diploid tumors had a 79% survival rate while patients with nondiploid tumors had only a 46% survival rate. Similarly, CHIANG et al. (1993), using flow cytometry, identified a group of patients with poor outcome unpredictable by pathologic examination. This study involved a retrospective analysis of 41 formaldehyde/paraffin-treated specimens of TCC of the upper urinary tract. Tumor progression was noted in 82% of the nondiploid lesions but in only 42% of the diploid lesions. Among grade 2 lesions, 85% of the nondiploid DNA tumors showed postoperative tumor progression whereas only 31% of the diploid DNA tumors showed progression. MIYAKAWA et al. (1994) performed a multivariate analysis on a total of 43 upper tract urothelial tumors resected by nephroureterectomy and noted that the single most important factor in predicting prognosis was histologic grade, followed by bromodeoxyuridine labeling index. Actuarial 3-year survival rates according to labeling index in grade 3 tumors were 68.4% and 16.7% in cases of low and high labeling index, respectively. The authors concluded that division of patients with grade 3 upper urinary tract carcinoma into two different prognostic groups based on bromodeoxyuridine DNA analysis is possible.

## 11.4
## General Management

Radical nephroureterectomy is appropriate initial therapy for most patients with TCC of the upper urinary tract. This procedure includes removal of the contents of Gerota's fascia together with the ipsilateral ureter and cuff of the bladder at its distal extent. Less radical surgery has a high local or regional recurrence rate approaching 30%. This is particularly true for patients with higher grade lesions (CLAYMAN et al. 1983). In selected patients treated with conservative resections, postoperative radiation therapy should be considered (BRADY et al. 1968). New treatment strategies for carcinoma in situ involving mitomycin C instillation and immunotherapy with bropirimine and bacillus Calmette-Guérin are currently being investigated (EASTHAM and HUFFMAN 1993; SAROSDY et al. 1996; YOKOGI et al. 1996). Sparse data are available supporting the routine use of adjuvant radiation therapy in patients with TCC of the upper urinary tract. Retrospective data from many institutions suggest that adjuvant radiation therapy in patients with high-stage lesions of the upper urinary tract has been associated with an increase in local tumor control (BABAIAN et al. 1980; BRADY et al. 1968; BROOKLAND and RICHTER 1985; COZAD et al. 1995; MAULARD-DURDUX 1996). Palliation of limited bone metastases with external beam radiation therapy is very effective. Since metastases occur in approximately 40% of all cases, palliative systemic multiagent chemotherapy with MVAC (methotrexate, vinblastine, adriamycin, and cisplatin) and other platinum-based combination chemotherapy regimens has shown overall response rates ranging between 47% and 70% (LI and CHEUNG 1987; SENGELOV et al. 1996; KOBAYASHI and OBATA 1994; LERNER et al. 1996). Combined postoperative chemotherapy and radiation may offer the best chance for long-term tumor control but should be carried out only as a part of clinical study (BRADY et al. 1968).

## 11.5
## Radiation Therapy

### 11.5.1
### Radiotherapy Techniques

Postoperative radiation therapy has been occasionally used in the management of upper urinary tract tumors. The clinical target volume should include the renal fossa and course of the ureter to the ipsilateral trigone. Areas that are at risk of being involved by microscopic disease include paracaval and para-aortic lymph nodes, which should be included in the treated volume. Radiation doses of 45–50 Gy given at 1.8–2.0 Gy per day are used to treat microscopic disease. More extensive disease such as multiple positive lymph nodes or positive surgical margins may require a 5- to 10-Gy boost to a smaller target volume. Higher doses may be necessary for gross residual or unresectable disease. In these cases, multiple fields including laterals and obliques with field reductions are important to minimize surrounding normal tissue toxicity. Preoperative CT-based simulation, three-dimensional treatment planning, and contrast-enhanced radiographic studies are helpful in defining the radiation clinical target volume and improving treatment tolerance. Figure 11.1 shows typical anterior-posterior radiation portals.

### 11.5.2
### Treatment Results

Data supporting the use of adjuvant radiation therapy in tumors of the upper urinary tract are sparse. A report by BROOKLAND and RICHTER (1985) found that poor-risk patients defined as those with high tumor grade, deep tumor invasion, or regional lymph node metastases receiving between 40 Gy and 50 Gy benefited from radiotherapy. A lower incidence of local recurrence (11% vs 46%) and a higher 5-year survival (27% vs 17%) were noted in a group of patients treated adjuvantly with postoperative radiation as compared with those treated by surgery alone. BABAIAN et al. (1980) reported a local recurrence rate of approximately 12% in a group of patients treated with postoperative adjuvant radiation therapy. Similar encouraging results were reported by COZAD et al. (1995). Patients receiving postoperative radiation therapy demonstrated a 90% 5-year actuarial local control rate as compared to 76% for those treated with surgery alone. A report by MAULARD-DURDUX (1996) questioned the benefit of adjuvant radiation therapy because the survival rate in the irradiated patients was comparable to that seen in historical series of patients managed by surgery alone. However, local recurrences were seen in only one patient (4%) and nodal failure in only four patients (15%) in the irradiated group. Two of the five local-regional failures occurred in sites that were not electively irradiated, therefore making the true

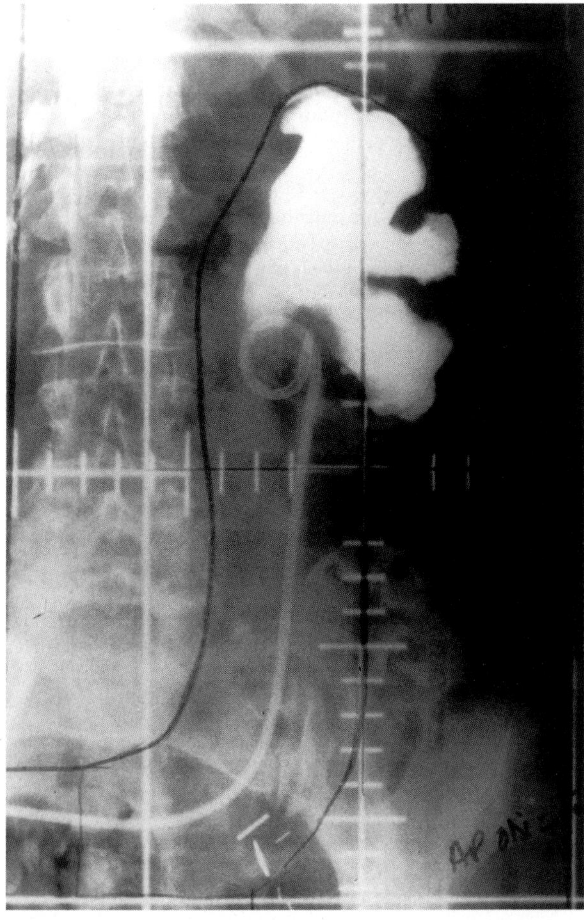

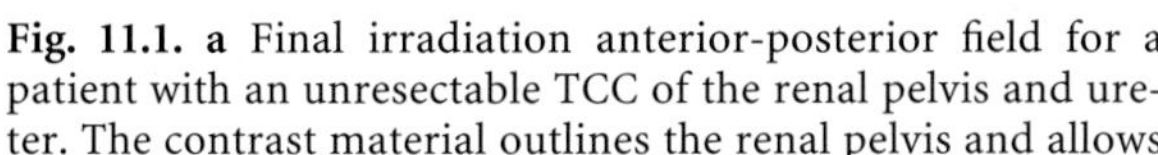

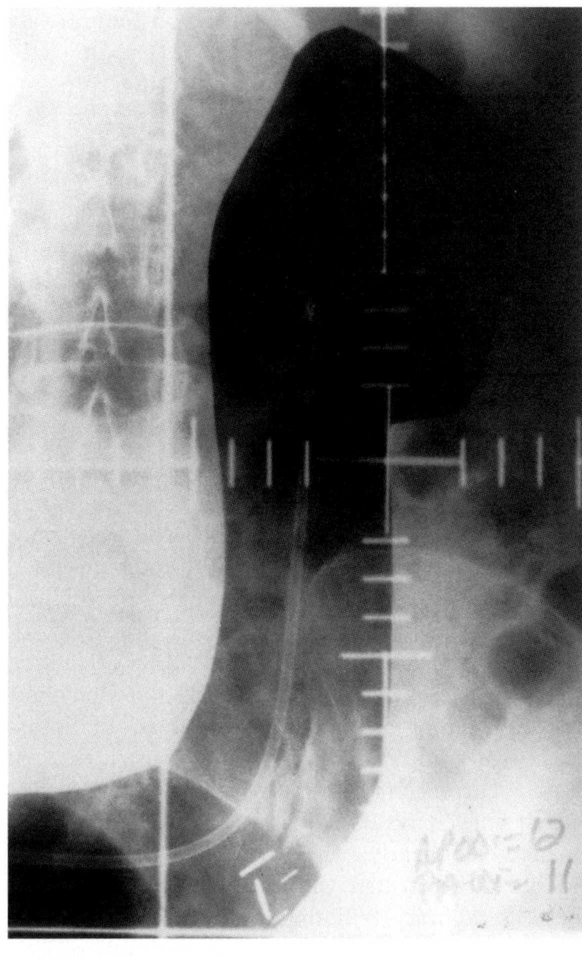

**Fig. 11.1. a** Final irradiation anterior-posterior field for a patient with an unresectable TCC of the renal pelvis and ureter. The contrast material outlines the renal pelvis and allows a block design to spare the renal parenchyma. The ureter is treated up to the insertion in the bladder. **b** The "block check" or port verification film of the field designed in **a**

infield failure rate 11.5% (3 of 26 patients). A multivariate analysis showed that high tumor grade and failure to receive adjuvant radiation therapy were the only significant predictors of local recurrence (COZAD et al. 1995). The overall infield irradiation failure rate among these studies suggests that there is an advantage to carefully planned postoperative local and regional lymph node irradiation.

## 11.5.3
## Sequelae of Radiation Therapy

The possible complications of radiation therapy to the kidney, renal pelvis, and ureters are similar to those seen in patients receiving radiation therapy to other sites of the abdomen and pelvis. They include nausea, vomiting, diarrhea, and abdominal cramping. The complication rate after radiation therapy for tumors of the kidney and upper urinary tract depends on multiple factors including total dose, fraction size, and technique of irradiation. The Copenhagen Renal Cancer Study Group reported a 44% rate of significant complications, including three patients with biochemical liver abnormalities indicating radiation hepatitis and nine patients with duodenal and small bowel stenosis and bleeding. Of the latter nine patients, four required surgery to correct the problem (KJAER et al. 1987). Five of the Danish study patients died of treatment-related complications. The total radiation dose used in this study was 50 Gy at 2.5 Gy per fraction. This particular fractionation schedule alone may account for the high rate of treatment complications. The Copenhagen study was conducted during an era before the routine use of CT-based treatment planning.

Kao et al. (1994) treated 12 patients postoperatively with a median radiation dose of 45 Gy using CT-based treatment planning. No long-term treatment-related morbidity was noted in these 12 patients. We can reasonably conclude that CT-based simulation and three-dimensional treatment planning may decrease the risk of serious complications after elective radiation therapy in patients with upper urinary tract malignancies.

## 11.6 Conclusions

Transitional cell carcinoma of the renal pelvis and ureter is a relatively rare tumor and is frequently associated with carcinoma of the bladder. The poor prognosis of patients with high-stage and high-grade TCC and its association with a high rate of local recurrence warrants adjuvant radiation therapy for carcinoma of the renal pelvis and ureter. Adjuvant radiation therapy has resulted in an improved overall survival in patients with locally advanced disease and high-grade pathology. A lower incidence of local recurrence (11% vs 46%) and a higher 5-year survival (27% vs 17%) was reported in patients treated adjuvantly with postoperative radiation versus those treated with surgery alone. The use of contemporary radiotherapy techniques resulted in a good treatment tolerance without serious treatment-related toxicity. The use of radiotherapy with high dose per fraction should not be undertaken as it is likely to produce severe treatment complications.

## References

Babaian RJ, Johnson DE, Chan RC (1980) Combination nephroureterectomy and postoperative radiotherapy for infiltrative urethral carcinoma. Int J Radiat Oncol Biol Phys 6:1229–1232

Beahrs OH, Henson De, Hutter RVP, Kennedy BJ (eds) (1992) Manual for staging of cancer, 4th edn. Lippincott, Philadelphia, p 205

Blacher EJ, Johnson DE, Abdul-Karim FW, et al. (1985) Squamous cell carcinoma of the renal pelvis. Urology 25:124–126

Brady LW, Gislason GJ, Faust DS, et al. (1968) Radiation therapy: a valuable adjunct in the management of carcinoma of the ureter. JAMA 206:2871–2874

Brookland RK, Richter MP (1985) The postoperative irradiation of transitional cell carcinoma of the renal pelvis and ureter. J Urol 133:952–955

Charbit L, Gendreau MC, Mee S, et al. (1991) Tumors of the upper urinary tract: ten years' experience. J Urol 146:1243–1246

Chiang PH, Huang MS, Tsai CJ, et al. (1993) Transitional cell carcinoma of the renal pelvis and ureter in Taiwan. DNA analysis by flow cytometry. Cancer 71:3988–3992

Clayman RV, Lange PH, Fraley EE (1983) Cancer of the upper urinary tract. In: Javadpour N (ed) Principles and management of urologic cancer. Williams & Wilkins, Baltimore, p 544

Corrado F, Ferri C, Mannini D, et al. (1991) Transitional cell carcinoma of the upper urinary tract: evaluation of prognostic factors by histopathology and flow cytometric analysis. J Urol 145:1159–1163

Cozad SC, Smalley SR, Austenfeld M, et al. (1995) Transitional cell carcinoma of the renal pelvis or ureter: patterns of failure. Urology 46:796–800

Cullen TH, Popham RR, Voss HJ (1972) Urine cytology in primary carcinoma of the renal pelvis and ureter. Aust NZ J Surg 41:230–236

Droller MJ (1986) Transitional cell cancer: upper tracts and bladder. In: Walsh PC, Gittes RF, Perlmutter AD, Stamey TA (eds) Urology. Saunders, Philadelphia, p 1343

Eastham JA, Huffman JL (1993) Technique of mitomycin C instillation in the treatment of upper urinary tract urothelial tumors. J Urol 150:324–326

Furihata M, Yamasaki I, Ohtsuki Y, et al. (1995) p53 and human papillomavirus DNA in renal pelvic and ureteral carcinoma including dysplastic lesions. Int J Cancer 64:298–303

Furihata M, Sonobe H, Ohtsuki Y, et al. (1996) Detection of p53 and bcl-2 protein in carcinoma of the renal pelvis and ureter including dysplasia. J Pathol 178:133–139

Grabstald H, Whitmore WF, Melamed MR (1971) Renal pelvic tumors. JAMA 218:845–854

Heney NM, Nocks BN, Daly JJ, et al. (1981) Prognostic factors in carcinoma of the ureter. J Urol 125:632–636

Highman WJ (1986) Transitional carcinoma of the upper urinary tract: a histologic and cytopathologic study. J Clin Pathol 39:297–305

Huben RP, Mounszer AM, Murphy GP (1988) Tumor grade and stage as prognostic variables in upper tract urothelial tumors. Cancer 62:2016–2020

Kao GD, Malkowicz SB, Whittington R, et al. (1994) Locally advanced renal cell carcinoma: low complication rate and efficacy of postnephrectomy radiation therapy planned with CT. Radiology 193:725–730

Kjaer M, Frederiksen PL, Engelholm SA (1987) Postoperative radiotherapy in stage II and III renal adenocarcinoma: a randomized trial by the Copenhagen Renal Cancer Study Group. Int J Radiat Oncol Biol Phys 13:665–672

Kobayashi H, Obata K (1994) Results of adjacent chemotherapy for invasive urothelial cancer with lymph node metastasis. Cancer Chemother Pharmacol 25 Suppl:514–517

Lai PP (1992) Kidneys, renal pelvis, and ureter. In: Brady LW, Perez CA (eds) Principles and practice of radiation oncology. Lippincott, Philadelphia, p 1025

Lerner SE, Blute ML, Tichardson RL, Zincke H (1996) Platinum-based chemotherapy for advanced transitional cell carcinoma of the upper urinary tract. Mayo Clin Proc 71:945–950

Li MK, Cheung WL (1987) Squamous cell carcinoma of the renal pelvis. J Urol 138:269–271

Loehrer PJ, Einhorn LH, Elson PJ, et al. (1992) A randomized comparison of cisplatin alone or in combination with methotrexate, vinblastine and doxorubicin in patients with metastatic urothelial carcinoma: a cooperative group study. J Clin Oncol 10:1066–1072

Maulard-Durdux C (1996) Postoperative radiation therapy in 26 patients with invasive transitional cell carcinoma of the upper urinary tract: no impact on survival? J Urol 155:122

Miyakawa A, Tachibana M, Nakashima J, et al. (1994) Flow cytometric bromodeoxyuridine/deoxyribonucleic acid bivariate analysis for predicting tumor invasiveness of upper tract urothelial cancer. J Urol 152:76–80

Petkovic SD (1975) Epidemiology and treatment of renal pelvic and urethral tumors. J Urol 114:858–865

Reitelman C, Sawczuk IS, Olsson CA, et al. (1987) Prognostic variables in patients with transitional cell carcinoma of the renal pelvis and proximal ureter. J Urol 138:1144–1145

Sarosdy MF, Pisters LL, Carroll PR, et al. (1996) Bropirimine immunotherapy of upper urinary tract carcinoma in situ. Urology 48:28–32

Sengelov L, Kamby C, von der Massé H (1996) Patterns of metastases in relation to characteristics of primary tumor and treatment in patients with disseminated urothelial carcinoma. J Urol 155:111–114

Sternberg CN, Yagoda A, Scher HI, et al. (1989) Methotrexate, vinblastine, doxorubicin and cisplatin for advanced transitional cell carcinoma of the urothelium. Cancer 64:2448–2458

Yokogi H, Wada Y, Mizutani M, et al. (1996) Bacillus Calmette-Guerin perfusion therapy for carcinoma in situ of the upper urinary tract. Br J Urol 77:676–679

# 12 Diagnosis and Management of Tumors of the Adrenal Gland

A. Van den Bruel, R. Oyen, and R. Bouillon

CONTENTS



## 12.1
## Introduction

The adrenals are small glands with a combined weight of 8–10 g. Numerous conditions result in enlargement of the adrenal gland, and tumors are not an infrequent finding, having an estimated prevalence of 1.4%–8.7% based on autopsy studies (Table 12.1) and 0.7%–3% based on computed tomographic (CT) studies (Table 12.2).

The pathologic conditions resulting in enlargement of the adrenal gland(s) range from cysts through benign (a)functional adenoma and pheochromocytoma to adrenocortical carcinoma. The

A. van den Bruel, MD, Laboratory and Clinic of Experimental Medicine and Endocrinology, University Hospitals Gasthuisberg, Catholic University of Leuven, Herestraat 49, B-3000 Leuven, Belgium
R. Oyen, MD, PhD, Adjunct Clinic Head, Department of Radiology, University Hospitals Gasthuisberg, Catholic University of Leuven, Herestraat 49, B-3000 Leuven, Belgium
R. Bouillon, MD, PhD, Professor and Chairman, Laboratory and Clinic of Experimental Medicine and Endocrinology, University Hospitals Gasthuisberg, Catholic University of Leuven, Herestraat 49, B-3000 Leuven, Belgium

vast majority of adrenocortical tumors are benign and hormonally silent; however, a minority are hormonally active or represent malignancy (adrenocortical carcinoma or metastasis). The approach to the incidentally discovered adrenal mass has to take into account these prevalences and aims to identify these infrequent but serious conditions among the majority of benign silent tumors in a cost-effective way. The situation is analogous to that in respect of incidentally discovered thyroid and pituitary nodules.

## 12.2
## Embryology and Anatomy
## of the Adrenal Gland

From the fifth week of gestational age, the adrenal cortex develops from cells of mesenchymal origin. A first group of cells make up the fetal cortex, which disappears in later life, leaving only the zona reticularis; a second group of cells create the zona glomerulosa and zona fasciculata of the final cortex. The adrenal medulla is derived from the neural crest area (neuroectoderm). Cortical adenomas, carcinomas, and myelolipomas are all of mesenchymal origin. Pheochromocytomas and neuroblastomas originate from neuroectodermal elements (Joffre et al. 1996). Histologically both the cortex and the medulla have a high lipid content and generally cannot be differentiated on CT or magnetic resonance imaging (MRI). The high lipid content of the adrenal cortex is explained by the active low-density lipoprotein cholesterol uptake for the synthesis of the adrenal steroids. Benign lesions of the adrenal cortex contain 10%–30% fat (Leroy-Wilig et al. 1993).

The adrenals usually have a V- or Y-shape and are closely related to the upper pole of the kidneys. In patients with renal agenesis, the ipsilateral adrenal has a flattened and elongated aspect. As mentioned above, the adrenals are tiny organs with a weight of less than 6 g each. The maximum width of the body measured perpendicular to the long axis, at the junc-

**Table 12.1.** Prevalence of adrenal tumors in autopsy studies

| Investigator(s) | No. of patients | No. of adenomas | % | Tumor diameter (cm) |
| --- | --- | --- | --- | --- |
| COMMONS and CALLAWAY (1948) | 7500 | 217 | 2.9 | >3 |
| KOKKO et al. (1967) | 1500 | 22 | 1.4 | >5 |
| ABECASSIS et al. (1985) | 1116 | 73 | 6.5 | – |
| HEDELAND et al. (1968) | 739 | 64 | 8.7 | >2 |
| Total | 10855 | 376 | 3.5 | – |

**Table 12.2.** Prevalence of adrenal tumors in CT studies

| Investigator(s) | No. of patients | No. of adenomas | % |
| --- | --- | --- | --- |
| HERRERA et al. (1991) | 61054 | 259 | 0.4 |
| ABECASSIS et al. (1985) | 14589 | 19 | 0.13 |
| BELLDEGRUN et al. (1986) | 12000 | 88 | 0.7 |
| GLAZER et al. (1982) | 2200 | 16 | 0.7 |
| HENSEN et al. (1994) | – | – | 3.0 |
| Total | 89843 | 382 | 0.4 |

tion of the adrenal body and limb, is 0.79 mm (SD 0.21) on the left and 0.6 mm (SD 0.2) on the right (VINCENT et al. 1994). The thickness of the limbs of the right adrenal is slightly less than that of the left, i.e., 0.14–0.49 mm compared with 0.13–0.52 mm. In practice, the normal adrenal limb should not measure more than 5 mm (VINCENT et al. 1994). The adrenals are enveloped in a fine layer of fibrous tissue. The cortex is divided into three zones: the aldosterone-producing zona glomerulosa, regulated by the renin-angiotensin system; the glucocorticoid-producing zona fasciculata, stimulated by adreno-corticotropic hormone (ACTH); and the zona reticularis, where adrenal sex steroids are synthesized partly under the control of ACTH. The adrenal medulla is the site of catecholamine synthesis (JOFFRE et al. 1996). Co-stored acidic proteins are the chromogranins A and B (AARDAL et al. 1996). Adrenomedullin, a member of the calcitonin gene-related peptide family, is synthesized in the adrenal medulla and in the vascular endothelium. It was first isolated from pheochromocytoma and its physiologic role is unknown (NISHIKIMI et al. 1997).

The left adrenal vein joins the left renal vein; the right adrenal vein typically drains in the inferior vena cava. This may explain the different routes of venous tumor spread in patients with primary adrenocortical carcinoma.

## 12.3
## Tumors of the Adrenal Gland

The vast majority of adrenocortical tumors are benign and hormonally silent. The frequency of benign adrenal tumors increases with age. An inherited predisposition to develop adrenocortical tumors has been reported, and several genetic syndromes have been recognized as associated with adrenocortical neoplasms, including: (1) congenital adrenal hyperplasia, (2) Li-Fraumeni syndrome, (3) Beckwith-Wiedemann syndrome, and (4) the Carney complex (LATRONICO and CHROUSOS 1997). Potential mechanisms of adrenocortical tumorigenesis (activation of proto-oncogenes on the short arm of chromosomes 11 and 17 in adrenocortical carcinomas, inactivation of the tumor suppression gene p53 in adrenal adenomas, and changes in adrenocortical tissue-specific factors) are the subject of current basic research in sporadic adrenocortical tumors (GICQUEL et al. 1995, 1997).

Pheochromocytoma is often diagnosed in the setting of multiple endocrine neoplasia (MEN) type IIA and B, an autosomal dominant disorder arising from mutations on chromosome 10q11.2 in the RET proto-oncogene.

### 12.3.1
### Cortical Adenoma

#### 12.3.1.1
#### Aldosterone-Producing Adenoma

Aldosterone-producing adenoma, first described by Conn in 1955, is diagnosed in 0.45% of outpatient hypertensive patients (TUCK 1995).

Hypertension with suppressed plasma renin activity (PRA) and hypokalemia is present in most patients. Hypokalemia-related symptoms (muscle weakness, polyuria, impaired glucose tolerance) can be present especially in patients on a high sodium intake.

Diagnosis is based on biochemical tests performed to diagnose primary hyperaldosteronism and to differentiate between subsets of primary aldosteronism. Hypokalemia and a suppressed PRA are the most useful clues to diagnosis. Confirmation of the diagnosis is established by demonstrating the autonomous, nonsuppressible plasma aldosterone after expansion of plasma volume.

A second step is the differentiation between subsets of primary aldosteronism [essentially aldosterone-producing adenoma (65%) versus idiopathic hyperaldosteronism (30%)]. In aldosterone-producing adenoma, aldosterone secretion is entirely autonomous whereas in idiopathic hyperaldosteronism there is some dependence on the renin-angiotensin system. A postural aldosterone response test can therefore differentiate between these two conditions: plasma aldosterone 2–4h after adoption of an upright position is lower than the baseline value in aldosterone-producing adenoma and higher than the baseline value in idiopathic hyperaldosteronism (TUCK 1995; BLEVINS and WAND 1992). Elevated levels of serum 18-hydroxycorticosterone and 24-h urinary 18-hydroxycortisol and 18-oxocortisol point to an aldosterone-producing adenoma. Normal levels are present in idiopathic hyperaldosteronism.

The third step is localizing the adenoma. Conn adenomas are usually small (mean size 1.6–1.8 cm), although approximately 15%–20% are micronodules measuring less than 1 cm (YOUNG et al. 1990). On CT they tend to be of low density on precontrast scans [0–10 Hounsfield units (HU)], and display only faint enhancement after intravenous injection of iodinated contrast medium. The sensitivity of CT is 58%–88% (KOROBKIN and FRANCIS 1995). The accuracy of MRI is similar to that of CT. On MRI, adenomas are usually hypointense or isointense compared with liver on T1-weighted images and isointense or slightly hyperintense on T2-weighted images.

Iodine-131-6-β-iodomethyl-19-norcholesterol (NP-59) uptake (after dexamethasone suppression of the normal adrenal gland) can be useful in the localization of (small) tumors and gives additional functional information (SHAPIRO et al. 1990). Adrenal venous sampling for aldosterone should be performed in cases of: (1) biochemically confirmed aldosterone-producing adenoma where CT and NP-59 scan fail to visualize an adenoma, (2) bilateral adrenal nodules, and (3) equivocal cases (DOPPMAN et al. 1992). Unilateral adrenalectomy is the treatment of choice in aldosterone-producing adenoma, whereas medical treatment (spironolactone) is effective in most cases of idiopathic primary hyperaldosteronism (BLEVINS and WAND 1992).

### 12.3.1.2
### Adrenal Adenoma Causing Cushing's Syndrome (Hypercortisolism)

Cushing's syndrome results from excess production of glucocorticoids, which gives rise to the characteristic clinical signs and symptoms. Central obesity, facial plethora, hypertension, hirsutism, and menstrual disorders are common presenting symptoms. Important signs are the presence of purplish-reddish striae and a typical fat accumulation in the supraclavicular and dorsocervical fat pads, which explains the well-known "buffalo hump." Functional adrenal adenomas account for 10%–20% of cases of Cushing's syndrome (ARON 1994).

The demonstration of hypercortisolism is the first step in the diagnosis. Hypercortisolism is suggested by positive screening tests (elevated urinary free cortisol, an elevated evening cortisol value, or a cortisol level not suppressed after an overnight 1 mg dexamethasone test) and is corroborated by the 2-day low-dose dexamethasone test. The diagnosis is further confirmed by the demonstration of low or undetectable levels of ACTH.

Both CT and MRI permit the localization of adrenal adenomas. The size of these tumors generally ranges between 2.0 and 2.5 cm. Adrenal adenomas have a varying appearance on CT scans; they may be of low or soft tissue attenuation and enhance after intravenous contrast medium administration. There is a poor correlation between the CT attenuation value of these tumors and their functional status. On MRI they are typically of low signal on T1-weighted images and produce an intermediate to high signal on T2-weighted images. The contralateral gland is usually normal, but on rare occasions it will be atrophic secondary to decreased ACTH secretion.

Adrenocortical carcinoma accounts for 10%–15% of cases of Cushing's syndrome. On CT the tumors generally exceed 6 cm and are heterogeneous owing to necrosis and calcification. In some cases, however, the tumors are smaller and may have the typical appearance of benign homogeneous tumors with regular contours. The MRI appearance of carcinoma is nonspecific. Tumors are usually hypointense relative to liver on T1-weighted images, and hyperintense on T2-weighted images.

Treatment is essentially surgical with appropriate hormonal substitution.

### 12.3.1.3
### Nonhyperfunctioning Adrenal Adenoma

Nonhyperfunctioning adrenal adenomas are the adrenal masses most frequently encountered as "incidentalomas"; in fact in nonselected series they represent 36%–94% of incidentally discovered adrenal masses (ABECASSIS et al. 1985). On CT benign nodules are characteristically round in shape and less than 3 cm in diameter, with smooth borders and homogeneous internal architecture. Calcification, necrosis, and hemorrhage are uncommon. Typical attenuation values range from −10 to 30 HU. Nonhyperfunctioning adenomas enhance only minimally after intravenous injection of contrast medium.

The signal characteristics of nonhyperfunctioning adenomas are similar to those of the normal adrenal gland. They are typically hypointense on T1-weighted images and isointense or slightly hyperintense on T2-weighted images. However, occasional atypical adenomas can be considerably hyperintense relative to liver on T2-weighted images.

### 12.3.2
### Adrenocortical Carcinoma

Adrenonocortical carcinoma is a rare tumor, with 0.5–2 cases per million people per year. It is present in 8% of patients diagnosed as having Cushing's syndrome. The majority of patients are female (sex ratio 2.5 : 1); the tumor occurs at all ages but with a bimodal age distribution, the first peak occurring before age 5 years and the second in the fourth to fifth decade (FLACK and CHROUSOS 1996).

The most common clinical presentation is an endocrine syndrome, usually Cushing's syndrome with or without virilizing features. Virilization is present in 20%–30% of adults with functional adrenocortical carcinomas; it is the most common hormonal syndrome in pediatric cases (SANDRINI et al. 1997), causing heterosexual pseudoprecocious puberty in girls and pseudoprecocious puberty in boys. Symptoms of the adrenal mass or general malaise can disclose an adrenocortical carcinoma (LUTON et al. 1990). A high proportion of patients (50%–80%)

already have metastatic disease (lungs, liver, lymph nodes, bone) at the time of diagnosis (SCHTEINGART 1992). A minority of cases are detected during evaluation of an unrelated condition, as will be discussed in subsequent sections.

Elevated levels of steroid precursors in serum (DHEAS, 17α-hydroxyprogesterone, 11-deoxycortisol) and elevated 17-hydroxysteroid and/or ketosteroid levels in ·24-h urine specimens represent biochemical clues to the diagnosis and are also important in follow-up.

Adrenocortical carcinomas are of considerable size at the time of diagnosis (3–28 cm, mean 12 cm) (WEISS et al. 1989; CHAPUIS et al. 1995). CT characteristics include heterogeneity (due to areas of necrosis) and heterogeneous enhancement after intravenous contrast administration (FISHMAN et al. 1986; KOROBKIN and FRANCIS 1995; VAN ERKEL et al. 1994). On MRI, adrenocortical carcinomas display heterogeneous signal intensity on both T1- and T2-weighted images (LEE et al. 1994). MRI is superior to CT in the assessment of operability because of the possibility of multiplanar imaging.

Fine-needle aspiration has a poor potency for distinguishing adrenal adenoma and adrenocortical carcinoma. A large number of mitoses is a specific but nonsensitive indicator of malignancy. Cytologic examination gives no information on capsular or venous invasion, which are the more reliable features of endocrine carcinomas (COPELAND 1983).

Primary treatment is surgery and is advised in most patients, offering cure to a few and reducing tumor burden and symptoms of the endocrine syndrome in most. Adjunctive treatment with mitotane (op-DDD) controls the hormonal secretion in 75% of patients and causes tumor regression in 8%–20% of treated patients (LUTON et al. 1990; HOFFMAN and MATTOX 1972; BERTAGNA and ORTH 1981). No clear significant effect on survival has been shown to date. Potential side-effects are anorexia and nausea, a maculopapular exanthem, hepatotoxicity, and neurologic disturbances.

The prognosis is poor (median survival of 50% at 1 year and 20% at 5 years). Favorable prognostic factors are a small tumor (<5 cm diameter) (stage I) and an isolated mass (stage II). Local or lymphatic spread (stage III) and metastases (state IV) worsen the prognosis (CHAPUIS et al. 1995). Children have been found to have a more favorable survival than adults (MENDONCA et al. 1995).

### 12.3.3
### Pheochromocytoma

Pheochromocytomas are the most common tumors of the adrenal medulla in adults. They arise from chromaffin cells and secrete catecholamines. Pheochromocytomas can arise anywhere in the autonomic nervous system. However, 98% originate in the abdomen, predominantly (90%) in the adrenal medulla. The incidence of pheochromocytoma is 2–8 cases per million per year (YOUNG 1997). Most patients present with continuous or episodic hypertension. This is frequently associated with headache (pounding and severe), palpitations (with or without tachycardia), and excessive perspiration (BRAVO and GIFFORD 1984). The "rule of 10's" (10% bilateral, 10% extra-adrenal, 10% malignant, 10% pediatric, 10% nonsporadic) refers to less frequent presentations of pheochromocytomas (MANGER and GIFFORD 1982). Nonsporadic pheochromocytomas include familial pheochromocytoma, MEN IIa and IIb, von Recklinghausen's disease, and von Hippel-Lindau syndrome. Hypertension is relatively refractory to medication. Approximately 10% of pheochromocytomas are malignant; the incidence of malignancy is higher in extra-adrenal masses and in tumors larger than 6 cm in diameter. Malignancy can often be identified only by the presence of metastases, i.e., histology is often insufficient for this purpose.

The diagnosis is based on excessive catecholamine secretion (urinary catecholamines and metabolites: vanillylmandelic acid and metanephrines). Falsely negative measurements can be obtained when the tumor is not continuously hormonally active (10%). In such cases the test should be repeated when the patient becomes symptomatic. Plasma chromogranin A (storage vesicle protein release with catecholamines) is a sensitive marker (NOBELS et al. 1997), though the test specificity is not optimal as this marker is elevated in (mild) renal insufficiency (YOUNG 1997; AARDAL et al. 1996).

Imaging is used primarily to localize the tumor. CT accurately localizes these tumors, which are usually rather large (average 5 cm). Central areas with low attenuation values are present in at least 50% of cases (KOROBKIN and FRANCIS 1995). Rarely pheochromocytomas are completely cystic. Most tumors enhance markedly after intravenous injection of contrast medium, a sign that can be particularly useful in the detection of extra-adrenal pheochromocytomas. Occasionally use of α-adrenergic blockade is appropriate prior to intravenous injection of iodinated ionic contrast medium in order to avoid precipitation of a hypertensive crisis. However, such blockade does not appear necessary when a nonionic contrast medium is employed. CT is very accurate in the detection of adrenal pheochromocytoma, the reported sensitivity ranging from 93% to 100% (QUINT et al. 1987; see Chap. 4).

On MRI most pheochromocytomas are hypointense on T1-weighted images and markedly hyperintense on T2-weighted images. There is some overlap with edematous or necrotic adrenal metastases. The use of gadolinium is rarely necessary; pheochromocytomas enhance markedly following injection. In general, MRI has a higher specificity than CT owing to better tissue characterization. The sensitivity of MRI also seems somewhat higher, especially for extra-adrenal tumors (LUCON et al. 1997; see Chap. 4).

Radiolabeled metaiodobenzylguanidine (MIBG) accumulates in functional chromaffin tissue; this test is less sensitive than CT and MRI, but more specific. The test performance is especially helpful in the demonstration of extra-adrenal, recurrent, or metastatic tumor.

Pheochromocytoma is curable by surgical removal of the tumor. Thorough pre- and peroperative monitoring and treatment are essential prerequisites to minimize the morbidity and mortality, especially since plasma volume is decreased prior to surgery and vascular tone might collapse after surgery.

### 12.3.4
### Myelolipoma

Myelolipoma is a benign nonsecreting tumor of mesenchymal origin which is often asymptomatic and represents 7%–15% of incidentally discovered adrenal masses. A large myelolipoma can cause symptoms through a mass effect or hemorrhage (SANDERS et al. 1995).

These lesions have a typical appearance on CT because of the presence of fat with negative attenuation numbers (KOROBKIN and FRANCIS 1995). Thin sections may be required to demonstrate small amounts of fat. MRI allows for a histologic diagnosis in typical myelolipomas.

Treatment is required in selected cases only. Surgery can be indicated for large masses.

## 12.3.5
## Adrenal Metastases

Extra-adrenal neoplasms known to metastasize frequently to the adrenal(s) are lung, breast, colon, and kidney neoplasms and malignant melanoma. If an adrenal mass is detected during the staging of an extra-adrenal neoplasm, the nature of the adrenal mass is critical in the decision as to the appropriate treatment of the primary tumor when there is no evidence of other metastatic spread (GROSS and SHAPIRO 1993).

Acute adrenal insufficiency is infrequent. The cortisol response at the ACTH challenge test, however, is frequently (33%) subnormal (REDMAN et al. 1987). In many cases, CT allows an equivocal differentiation between adrenal adenoma and adrenal metastases (KOROBKIN and DUNNICK 1995). Metastases tend to be larger than adenomas, to be less well defined, to be of inhomogeneous density, and occasionally to have a thick enhancing rim after intravenous injection of contrast medium.

On MRI metastases are typically hypointense compared to liver on T1-weighted images and relatively hyperintense on T2-weighted images. Some adrenal metastases are atypical and either isointense or hypointense relative to liver on T2-weighted images. MRI using chemical shift imaging enables differentiation between typical fat-containing adrenal adenomas and the absence of fat in metastases (LEE et al. 1994). In equivocal cases, percutaneous biopsy of an adrenal mass is indicated (WELCH et al. 1994; SILVERMAN et al. 1993; KATZ and SHIRKHODA 1985).

## 12.3.6
## Lymphoma

Primary lymphomas arising in the adrenal gland are extremely rare, but secondary involvement of the adrenal gland is reported in 4%–25% of patients with lymphomas (PALING and WILLIAMSON 1983; HARRIS et al. 1989). Adrenal insufficiency is unusual, except in the presence of bilateral adrenal lymphoma.

Neither CT nor MRI provides typical information on adrenal involvement by lymphoma. On T2-weighted images, adrenal lymphoma has a modertely high signal intensity, similar to that of metastatic disease and adrenocortical carcinoma. Percutaneous biopsy or surgery may be required in selected patients.

Tumor response to chemotherapy or radiotherapy confirms the diagnosis.

## 12.4
## Adrenal Hemorrhage

Adrenal hemorrhage deserves some attention because the diagnosis and differential diagnosis may be problematic. Hemorrhage usually originates in the adrenal medulla. Approximately 80% of adrenal hemorrhages are unilateral and most are right-sided. This is thought to be related to the direct drainage of the right adrenal vein into the inferior vena cava, which results in direct exposure to acute rises in central venous pressure. Adrenal hemorrhage may occur during severely debilitating disease, shock, trauma, and anticoagulation therapy. Many cases are clinically silent. Clinical symptoms related to adrenal hemorrhage include flank pain, nausea, and vomiting. The most common findings at physical examination are fever and hypotension.

Acute adrenal hemorrhage can be easily diagnosed by CT. It presents as a round or oval mass of 1.5–3 cm in diameter with a high attenuation number (60–90 Hounsfield units) (KOROBKIN and FRANCIS 1995). There is no enhancement after intravenous administration of contrast medium. The density of the masses and the size decreases with time. Sometimes an adrenal pseudocyst persists from a previous hemorrhage. MRI is indicated in situations where CT is equivocal. In the acute phase, intracellular deoxyhemoglobin typically causes signal loss on both T1- and T2-weighted images. Subacutely, methemoglobin causes bright signal intensity on T1-weighted images. Chronic adrenal hemorrhage often has a low signal intensity on T1- and T2-weighted images owing to calcification and hemosiderin deposition.

After detection, prompt steroid substitution therapy can be life-saving as adrenal hemorrhage frequently causes adrenal insufficiency (LING et al. 1983; WOLVERSON and KANNEGIESSER 1984).

## 12.5
## Granulomatous Disease

Tuberculosis, histoplasmosis, and blastomycosis can occasionally present as an adrenal mass lesion, usually bilaterally but often asymmetrically. Clinical presentation and biochemical tests are usually sufficient to establish the diagnosis. Adrenal insufficiency may occur.

Neither CT nor MRI allows a tissue-specific diagnosis. The glands are usually enlarged and heterogeneous in density, and often show central low attenuation representing caseous necrosis. Calcification is variable and may be seen in the acute phase or during healing. CT-guided percutaneous biopsy may be indicated.

## 12.6
## Adrenal Cyst

Cystic lesions include endothelial-lined (45%) and epithelial-lined cysts, pseudocysts (from previous adrenal hemorrhage), and *Echinococcus* cyst. They occur more often in women than men and are unilateral in more than 80% of cases.

The cystic nature is easily demonstrated by ultrasonography, CT, or MRI. The cysts are of fluid echogenicity or density with a clearly defined margin and a thin wall on CT. On MRI they are usually markedly hypointense on T1-weighted images and markedly hyperintense on T2-weighted images. The presence of proteinaceous fluid, infectious debris, or hemorrhage within a cyst can cause increased signal intensity on T1-weighted images. *Echinococcus* serology is essential in cases of voluminous, septated cysts.

## 12.7
## Diagnostic Approach and Management of the Adrenal Incidentaloma

It is estimated that an incidental adrenal mass of at least 1 cm is discovered in up to 4% of abdominal CT studies (LORIAUX and DAVID 1997). The number and size of these nodules increase with age, and they occur with increased frequency in obese diabetic patients and elderly women. The term "incidentaloma" has to be considered as a definition, not as a diagnosis. It refers to masses sharing the same modality of discovery (ANGELI et al. 1997). A more appropriate definition is a mass lesion of more than 1 cm in diameter, discovered by radiologic examinations in the absence of symptoms or clinical signs of adrenal disease (YOUNG 1997).

As benign adrenal masses are far more common than malignant masses, appropriate management is essential to avoid a "disease of modern technology" with unnecessarily thorough exploration or surgery (COPELAND 1983; CHIDIAC and ARON 1997). Yet there is no simple answer to the question of how clinically silent, incidental masses should be evaluated. Some basic factors, however, to be integrated in an algorithm are described in Sect. 12.7.1. The proposed algorithm in Sect. 12.7.2 is subject to change in a time of fast evolution of imaging techniques, surgical techniques, and molecular biology. One can imagine that more experience with laparoscopic adrenalectomy could influence treatment decisions (GUAZZONI et al. 1994). Advances in molecular biology as described by MARX (i.e., MHC class II expression in the majority of benign adenomas, but not in all carcinomas) could constitute a reason to reintroduce the biopsy technique for differentiating adrenal adenoma from carcinoma (MARX et al. 1996).

## 12.7.1
## Factors To Be Integrated in the Algorithm

### 12.7.1.1
### Function or Biochemical Activity

A careful search for hormonal hypersecretion is a priority as the latter finding indicates the need for surgery independent of the nature of the mass and as some adrenocortical carcinomas are hormonally active (COPELAND 1983). Indeed, hyperfunctioning tumors are a surgical indication whereas incidential masses associated with hypofunction are only exceptionally surgical cases (LORIAUX and DAVID 1997).

Clinical suspicion of Cushing's syndrome, virilization, feminization, or mineralocorticoid and catecholamine excess indicates a need for thorough investigation as described in the previous section.

By definition clinical evidence of hormonally hypersecretion is virtually absent in incidentalomas. Even then screening tests to evaluate "true incidentalomas" are needed; these tests are summarized in Table 12.3.

Pheochromocytoma is extremely rare in the absence of symptoms and of hypertension. However, it

**Table 12.3.** Biochemical screening in incidentaloma

---

Urinary catecholamines (or metanephrines and VMA) and plasma chromogranin A
Serum potassium (PRA and aldosterone in the event of hypokalemia) in hypertensive patients
Urinary 24-h free cortisol excretion or cortisol level after 1 mg dexamethasone overnight
DHEAS, 17-ketosteroids in 24-h urine collection
17α-hydroxyprogesterone (basal and/or ACTH-stimulated value)
Cortisol (basal and/or ACTH-stimulated value)

---

VMA, Vanillylmandelic acid; PRA, plasma renin activity; ACTH, adrenocorticotropic hormone.

is a potentially lethal disorder with an unpredictable course. Assessment of urinary catecholamines, vanillylmandelic acid, or metanephrines, as well as serum chromogranin A, is mandatory (Ross and Aron 1990; Young 1997).

Virtually all patients with hyperaldosteronism have hypertension at the time of diagnosis. In hypertensive patients we propose assessment of serum potassium (in a salt-repleted state); if it is found to be decreased, plasma renin activity and aldosterone measurements are needed (Ross and Aron 1990).

The ongoing debate about the definition, prevalence, morbidity, and natural history of the entity "preclinical" or "subclinical" Cushing's syndrome will influence the screening tests used to detect glycocorticoid hypersecretion (McLeod et al. 1990; Reincke et al. 1992; Chidiac and Aron 1997). Recent evidence suggests that preclinical Cushing's syndrome can contribute to poor glycemic and blood pressure control (Leibowitz et al. 1996) and can have negative effects on bone turnover and density (Ambrosi et al. 1995; Osella et al. 1997). This would indicate a need for a sensitive screening test. The 1 mg overnight dexamethasone test (Reincke et al. 1992) should be performed and/or urinary free cortisol should be determined.

To screen for hormonal precursors in adrenocortical carcinoma, serum DHEAS, 17-hydroxysteroids and 17-ketosteroids in a 24-h urine specimen are determined (Mantero et al. 1997).

Since patients with congenital adrenal hyperplasia have a high incidence of adrenal tumors [82% in homozygous congenital hyperplasia, and 45% in heterozygous congenital adrenal hyperplasia due to 21-hydroxylase deficiency (Jaresch et al. 1992)], a screening test for 17α-hydroxyprogesterone (basal level and/or ACTH-stimulated values) should be performed.

### 12.7.1.2
### Presence or History of Extra-adrenal Malignancy

The presence or history of extra-adrenal malignancy clearly influences diagnostic and treatment options. In the absence of other metastases, the nature of the adrenal mass determines the curability of the primary tumor. We propose two different algorithms, one for patients with a known (history of) extra-adrenal malignancy, and the second for patients without an extra-adrenal malignancy. The workup and management of these patient is shown in Figs. 12.1 and 12.2.

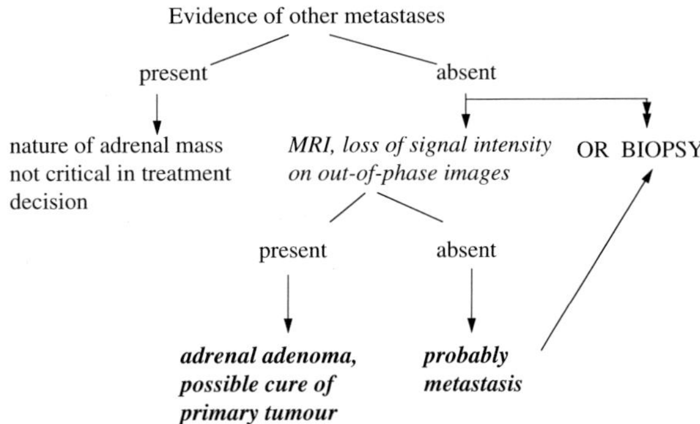


**Fig. 12.1.** Evaluation and management of patients with a history of primary extra-adrenal malignancy

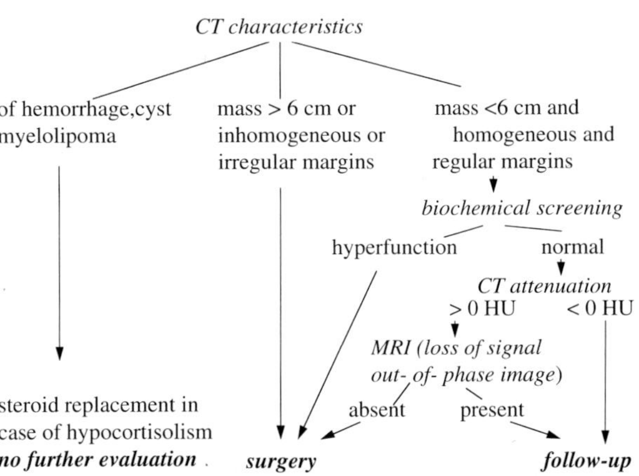


**Fig. 12.2.** Evaluation and management of patients with no history of primary extra-adrenal malignant tumor

### 12.7.1.3
### Size of the Mass

The size of the adrenal mass is important in predicting its behavior. Because of the fast growth rate of adrenocortical carcinoma and metastases, these masses are small for less time. Small lesions are more likely to be benign. Large adrenal masses are more likely to be malignant. One series of masses with a diameter of more than 5 cm showed 15% to be adrenocortical carcinomas (Khafagi et al. 1991). There are two major problems in stipulating a size criterion for evaluation and/or surgery: (1) in individual cases the utility of the size criterion is limited due to the considerable overlap in size between benign and malignant masses (Angeli et al. 1997; Kasperlik-Zaluska et al. 1997; Belldegrun et al. 1986); (2) at some point in their development adrenal adenocarcinomas must have been small and it is early in the course of development that surgical removal of the tumor could improve morbidity and mortality (CHAPUIS et al. 1995; KLOOS et al. 1995).

A mass diameter of more than 6 cm [for some authors 5 cm (ANGELI et al. 1997; KHAFAGI et al. 1991) or 4 cm (ANGELI et al. 1997; KASPERLIK-ZALUSKA et al. 1997; HERRERA et al. 1991)] is an indication for surgical removal of the mass (BOUILLON and OYEN 1997); smaller masses have to be evaluated for their composition.

### 12.7.1.4
### Composition of the Mass

Benign adrenal masses contain fat whereas the fat content of most adrenal metastases and adrenocortical carcinomas is too limited for detection at CT or MRI. Attenuation numbers of less than 10 HU are 96% specific for a benign mass (sensitivity 85%) (LEE et al. 1991). According to KOROBKIN and FRANCIS (1995), masses with attenuation values of less than 18 HU on nonenhanced scans are likely to be benign (specificity 100%, sensitivity 85%). At attenuation values of less than 10 HU the specificity was 100% and the sensitivity 68%. Much greater overlap is seen in attenuation values on enhanced CT. Recent work suggests that CT densitometry, performed on delayed images obtained 14–60 min after enhancement with intravenously injected contrast medium, may be useful in characterizing an adrenal mass as an adenoma (KOROBKIN 1995; KOROBKIN et al. 1996; BOLAND et al. 1997; SZOLAR and KANNERHUBER 1997).

Chemical shift MRI is equally suited to differentiate between adenomas and other masses, and may even be more specific for this purpose. Chemical shift imaging relies on the fact that protons in water molecules recess at a slightly different rate to the protons in lipid molecules in a magnetic field. As a result, water and fat protons cycle in and out of phase with respect to one another. By selecting an appropriate TE, one can acquire an in- and out-of-phase image. The signal intensity of a pixel on an in-phase image is derived from the signal of water plus fat protons. On out-of-phase images, the signal intensity is derived from the difference of the signal of water and fat protons. Therefore, adenomas lose signal intensity on out-of-phase images compared with in-phase images, whereas metastases remain unchanged (BOLAND and LEE 1995; OUTWATER et al. 1995; TSUSHIMA et al. 1993; MITCHELL et al. 1992). The spleen has been shown to be the most reliable internal standard in assessing the degree of loss of signal intensity. Although a specificity of 100% has

been reported, there is some concern about the true specificity of this criterion (REINIG et al. 1994). Metastases from hepatocellular carcinomas, renal cell carcinoma, and liposarcoma can also contain lipid, and even cases of fat-containing adrenocortical carcinoma have been reported. However, in the latter cases, signal loss was heterogeneous. Conversely, it is probable that some functioning and nonfunctioning adenomas contain insufficient lipid to result in loss of signal on out-of-phase imaging. These cases would presumably be identified biochemically. Conventional spin-echo imaging and gadolinium-enhanced MRI are not reliable either: considerable overlap in the characteristics of benign and malignant masses limits the clinical applicability of these techniques in differentiating adenomatous from nonadenomatous masses.

Some authors propose NP-59 scan as a less expensive (KLOOS et al. 1995) examination than MRI. In the presence of normal biochemistry, a concordant NP-59 imaging pattern (uptake of NP-59 at the side of the mass) is diagnostic of a benign adenoma. A discordant NP-59 imaging pattern (low or absent NP-59 uptake at the side of the mass) is suggestive for malignancy (GROSS et al. 1994). Other authors prefer MRI because of the limited specificity of the NP-59 scan (some adrenocortical carcinomas present with NP-59 uptake).

### 12.7.2
### Algorithm for Investigation of Incidentaloma

### 12.7.2.1
### Algorithm for Patients with (a History of) a Primary Extra-adrenal Malignancy

As described in Sect. 12.7.1.4, loss of signal intensity on out-of-phase images is typical of a benign adrenal adenoma. In this case surgical cure of the primary extra-adrenal tumor is possible. No loss of signal intensity on out-of-phase images makes a metastasis highly probable, and confirmation by biopsy will influence the tumor staging from NO to the presence of distant metastasis with the appropriate consequences for treatment decisions.

### 12.7.2.2
### Algorithm for Patients Without (a History of) a Primary Extra-adrenal Malignancy

In patients without a primary extra-adrenal malignancy (or any history thereof), characteristics of the original CT scan indicate the further approach in two situations. First, hemorrhages, cysts, or myelolipoma can be identified with fairly high certainty and need *no further exploration* (except for detection of adrenal insufficiency in cases of adrenal hemorrhage). Second, tumors with a diameter of 6 cm or more and tumors with an irregular appearance on CT scan require *surgical exploration*. Here biochemical screening is limited to cortisol secretion and catecholamine secretion to guide preoperative monitoring and treatment.

In the majority of cases (homogeneous masses smaller than 6 cm in diameter) biochemical screening tests as summarized in Table 12.3 are performed first. Hyperfunction indicates the need for surgery independent of the nature of the mass and some biochemical clues can point to malignancy. The vast majority of incidentalomas are homogeneous masses smaller than 6 cm in diameter, without evidence of hypersecretion. A CT attenuation coefficient of 0 HU or less indicates a benign tumor. Masses with attenuation coefficients of more than 0 HU need further exploration with MRI using the chemical shift technique. Loss of signal on the out-of-phase images indicates the presence of fat in a benign tumor. In these cases in which CT or MRI characteristics are compatible with a benign tumor with a high fat content (≤0 HU, loss of signal intensity on out-of-phase images), follow-up with a CT scan after 6 and 12 months is proposed. In the absence of loss of signal intensity on the out-of phase images, the fat content of the tumor is low, malignancy is probable, and surgery should be considered.

Some authors prefer to use an iodocholesterol scan or an adrenal biopsy instead of MRI in the diagnostic approach. A concordant image on the iodocholesterolscan is typical for a benign adenoma whereas a discordant image is a sign of malignancy. A biopsy provides the only opportunity to obtain histologic proof but the inability to diagnose an adrenocortical carcinoma, the accuracy rate of ca. 90% and the complication rate of ca. 10% are major drawbacks.

## References

Aardal S, Aardal NP, Larsen TH (1996) Human pheochromocytoma: different patterns of catecholamines and chromogranins in the intact tumour, urine and serum in clinically unsuspected cases. Scand J Clin Lab Invest 56:511–523

Abecassis M, McLoughlin MJ, Langer B, Kudlow JE (1985) Serendipitous adrenal masses: prevalence, significance and management. Am J Surg 149:783–788

Ambrosi B, Peverelli S, Passini E, et al. (1995) Abnormalities of endocrine function in patients with clinically "silent" adrenal masses. Eur J Endocrinol 132:422–428

Angeli A, Osella G, Ali A, Terzolo M (1997) Adrenal incidentaloma: an overview of clinical and epidemiological data from the national Italian Study Group. Horm Res 47:279–283

Aron DC (1994) In: Greenspan FS (edn) Basic and clinical endocrinology, IVth edn. Appleton & Lange, Norwalk, Conn., pp 307–346

Belldegrun A, Hussain S, Seltzer SE, Loughlin KR, Gittes RF, Richie JP (1986) Incidentally discovered mass of the adrenal gland. Surg Gynecol Obstet 163:203–208

Bertagna C, Orth DN (1981) Clinical and laboratory findings and results of therapy in 58 patients with adrenocortical tumors admitted to a single medical center (1951 to 1978). Am J Med 71:855–875

Blevins L, Wand GS (1992) Primary aldosteronism: an endocrine perspective. Radiology 184:599–600

Boland GW, Lee MJ (1995) Magnetic resonance imaging of the adrenal gland. Crit Rev Diagn Imaging 36:115–174

Boland GW, Hahn PF, Pena C, Mueller PR (1997) Adrenal masses: characterization with delayed contrast-enhanced CT. Radiology 202:693–696

Bouillon R, Oyen R (1997) Bijnierincidentaloom: Kostefficiënte diagnostiek en therapie. Tijdschr Geneesk 53:123–130

Bravo EL, Gifford RW (1984) Pheochromocytoma: diagnosis, localization and management. N Engl J Med 311:1298–1303

Chapuis Y, Icard P, Louvel A (1995) Le cortico-surrénalome malin. Rev Franç Endocrinol Clin 36:93–104

Chidiac RM, Aron DC (1997) Incidentalomas: a disease of modern technology. Endocrinol Metab Clin North Am 26:233–243

Commons RR, Callaway CP (1948) Adenomas of the adrenal cortex. Arch Intern Med 81:37–41

Copeland PM (1983) The incidentally discovered adrenal mass. Ann Intern Med 98:940–945

Doppman JL, Gill JR Jr, Miller DL, et al. (1992) Distinction between hyperaldosteronism due to bilateral hyperplasia and unilateral aldosteronoma: reliability of CT. Radiology 184:677–682

Fishman EK, Deutch BM, Hartman DS, Goldman SM, Zerhouni EA, Siegelman SS (1986) Primary adrenocortical carcinoma: CT evaluation with clinical correlation. AJR 148:531–535

Flack MR, Chrousos GP (1996) Neoplasms of the adrenal cortex. In: Holland R (edn) Cancer medicine, 4th edn. Lea and Febiger, New York, pp 1563–1570

Gicquel C, Bertagna X, Le Bouc Y (1995) Recent advances in the pathogenesis of adrenocortical tumours. Eur J Endocrinol 133:133–144

Gicquel C, Raffin-Sanson ML, Gaston V, et al. (1997) Structural and functional abnormalities at 11p15 are associated with the malignant phenotype in sporadic adrenocortical tumors: study on a series of 82 tumors. J Clin Endocrinol Metab 82:2559–2565

Glazer HS, Weyman PJ, Sagel SS, et al. (1982) Nonfunctioning adrenal masses: incidental discovery on computed tomography. Am J Roentgenol 139:81–85

Gross MD, Shapiro B (1993) Clinical review 50: clinically silent adrenal masses. J Clin Endocrinol Metab 77:885–888

Gross MD, Shapiro B, Francis IR, et al. (1994) Scintigraphic evaluation of clinically silent adrenal masses. J Nucl Med 35:1145–1152

Guazzoni G, Montorsi F, Bergamaschi F, Rigatti P, Cornaggia G, Lanzi R, Pontiroli AE (1994) Effectiveness and safety of laparoscopic adrenalectomy. J Urol 152:1375–1378

Harris GJ, Tio FO, Von Hoff DD (1989) Primary adrenal lymphoma. Cancer 63:799–803

Hedeland H, Ostberg G, Hokfelt B (1968) On the prevalence of adrenocortical adenomas in autopsy material in relation to hypertension and diabetes. Acta Med Scand 184:211

Hensen J, Stark S, Pavel M, Sachse R, Buchfelder M, Dörr IIG (1994) Non-functioning adrenocortical adenomas (ACA): age and sex dependency [abstract 102]. 76th Annu Meet Endocr Soc p 226

Herrera MF, Grant CS, van Heerden JA, Sheedy PF, Ilstrup DM (1991) Incidentally discovered adrenal tumors: an institutional perspective. Surgery 110:1014–1021

Hoffman DL, Mattox VR (1972) Treatment of adrenocortical carcinoma with o'p'-DDD. Med Clin North Am 999–1012

Jaresch S, Kornely E, Kley HK, Schlaghecke R (1992) Adrenal incidentaloma and patients with homozygous or heterozygous congenital adrenal hyperplasie. J Clin Endocrinol Metab 74:685–689

Joffre F, Colombier D, Otal PH (1996) Imagerie radiologique des surrénales. In: Bléry M (ed) Collection d'imagerie radiologique, Masson, Paris, p 178

Kasperlik-Zaluska AA, Roslonowska E, Slowinska-Srzednicka J, Migdalska B, Jeske W, Makowska A, Snochowska H (1997) Incidentally discovered adrenal mass (incidentaloma): investigation and management of 208 patients. Clin Endocrinol 46:29–37

Katz RL, Shirkhoda A (1985) Diagnostic approach to incidental adrenal nodules in the cancer patient. Cancer 55:1995–2000

Khafagi FA, Gross MD, Shapiro B, Glazzer GM, Francis I, Thompson NW (1991) Clinical significance of the large adrenal mass. Br J Surg 78:823–833

Kloos RT, Gross MD, Francis IR, Korobkin M, Shapiro B (1995) Incidentally discovered adrenal masses. Endocr Rev 16:460–484

Kokko JP, Brown TC, Berman MM (1967) Adrenal adrenoma and hypertension. Lancet I:468

Korobkin M, Dunnick NR (1995) Characterization of adrenal masses. AJR 164:643–644

Korobkin M, Francis IR (1995) Adrenal imaging. Semin Ultrasound CT MR 16:317–330

Korobkin M, Broder FS, Francis IR, et al. (1996) Delayed enhanced CT for differentiation of benign from malignant adrenal masses. Radiology 200:737–742

Latronico AC, Chrousos GP (1997) Adrenocortical tumors. J Clin Endocrinol Metab 82:1317–1324

Lee MJ, Hahn PF, Papanicolaou N, Egglin TK, Saini S, Mueller PR, Simeone JF (1991) Benign and malignant adrenal masses: CT distinction with attenuation coefficients, size and observer analysis. Radiology 179:415–418

Lee MJ, Mayo-Smith WW, Hahn PF, Goldberg MA, Boland GW, Saini S, Papanicolaou N (1994) State-of-the-art MR imaging of the adrenal gland. Radiographics 14:1015–1029

Leibowitz G, Tsur A, Chayen SD, Salameh M, Raz I, Cerasi E, Gross DJ (1996) Pre-clinical Cushing's syndrome: an unexpected frequent cause of poor glycaemic control in obese diabetic patients. Clin Endocrinol 44:717–722

Leroy-Willig A, Bittoun J, Luton JP (1993) A step forward in the characterization of adrenal cortical lesions? Radiology 188:880–881

Ling D, Korobkin M, Silverman PM, Dunnick NR (1983) CT demonstration of bilateral adrenal hemorrhage. Am J Roentgenol 141:307–308

Loriaux DL, David MC (1997) In: Clinical endocrinology update syllabus. The incidental adrenal mass. The Endocrine Society, Bethesda, pp 261–265

Lucon AM, Pereira MAA, Mendonça BB, Halpern A, Wajchenbeg BL, Arap S (1997) Pheochromocytoma: study of 50 cases. J Urol 157:1208–1212

Luton J-P, Cerdas S, Billaud L, et al. (1990) Clinical features of adrenocortical carcinoma, prognostic factors and the effect of mitotane therapy. N Engl J Med 322:1195–1201

Manger MM, Gifford RW Jr (1982) Hypertension secondary to pheochromocytoma. Bull N Y Acad Med 58:148–158

Mantero F, Masini AM, Opocher G, Giovagnetti M, Arnaldi G (1997) Adrenal incidentaloma: an overview of hormonal data from the national Italian Study Group. Horm Res 47:284–289

Marx C, Wolkersdörfer GW, Brown JW, Scherbaum WA, Bornstein SR (1996) MHC class II expression – a new tool to assess dignity in adrenocortical tumours. J Clin Endocrinol Metab 81:4488–4491

McLeod MK, Thompson NW, Gorss MD, Bondeson AG, Bondeson L (1990) Sub-clinical Cushing's syndrome in patients with adrenal gland incidentalomas. Am Surg 7:398–403

Mendoça BB, Lucon AM, Menezes CAV, et al. (1995) Clinical, hormonal and pathological findings in a comparative study of adrenocortical neoplasms in childhood and adulthood. J Urol 154:2004–2009

Mitchell DG, Crovello M, Matteucci T, Petersen RO, Miettinen MM (1992) Benign adrenocortical masses: diagnosis with chemical shift MR imaging. Radiology 185:345–351

Nishikimi T, Kitamura K, Saito Y, et al. (1994) Clinical studies on the sites of production and clearance of circulating adrenomedullin in human subjects. Hypertension 24:600–604

Nobels FRE, Kwekkeboom DJ, Coopmans W, et al. (1997) Chromogranin A as serum marker for neuroendocrine neoplasia: comparison with neuron-specific enolase and the alpha-subunit of glycoprotein hormones. J Clin Endocrinol Metab 82:2622–2628

Osella G, Terzolo M, Borreta G, et al. (1994) Endocrine evaluation of incidentally discovered adrenal masses (incidentalomas). J Clin Endocrinol Metab 79:1532–1539

Osella G, Terzolo M, Reimondo G, et al. (1997) Serum markers of bone and collagen turnover in patients with Cushing's syndrome and in subjects with adrenal incidentalomas. J Clin Endocrinol Metab 82:3303–3307

Outwater EK, Siegelman ES, Radecki PD, Piccoli CW, Mitchell DG (1995) Distinction between benign and malignant adrenal masses: value of T1-weighted chemical-shift MR imaging. Am J Roentgenol 165:579–583

Paling MR, Williamson BJR (1983) Adrenal involvement in non-Hodgkin lymphoma. AJR 141:303–305

Quint LE, Glazer GM, Francis IR, Shapiro B, Chenevert TL (1987) Pheochromocytoma and paraganglioma: comparison of MR imaging with CT and I-131 MIBG scintigraphy. Radiology 165:89–93

Redman BG, Pazdur R, Zingas AP, Loredo R (1987) Prospective evaluation of adrenal insufficiency in patients with adrenal metastasis. Cancer 60:103–107

Reincke M, Nieke J, Krestin GP, Saeger W, Allolio B, Winkelman W (1992) Preclinical Cushing's syndrome in adrenal "incidentalomas": comparison with adrenal Cushing's syndrome. J Clin Endocrinol Metab 75:826–832

Reinig JW, Stutley JE, Leonhardt CM, Spicer KM, Margolis M, Caldwell CB (1994) Differentiation of adrenal masses with MR imaging: comparison of techniques. Radiology 192:41–46

Ross NS, Aron DC (1990) Hormonal evaluation of the patient with an incidentally discovered adrenal mass. N Engl J Med 323:1401–1404

Sanders R, Bissada N, Curry N, Gordon B (1995) Clinical spectrum of adrenal myelolipoma: analysis of 8 tumors in 7 patients. J Urol 153:1791–1793

Sandrini R, Ribeiro RC, DeLacerda L (1997) Extensive personal experience: childhood adrenocortical tumors. J Clin Endocrinol Metab 82:2027–2031

Schteingart DE (1992) Treating adrenal cancer. Endocrinologist 2:149–157

Shapiro B, Fig LM, Gross MD, Khafagi F (1990) Contributions of nuclear endocrinology to the diagnosis of adrenal tumors. Recent Results Cancer Res 118:113–138

Silverman SG, Mueller PR, Pinkney LP, Koenker RM, Seltzer SE (1993) Predictive value of image-guided adrenal biopsy: analysis of results of 101 biopsies. Radiology 187:715–718

Szolar DH, Kannerhuber F (1997) Quantitative CT evaluation of adrenal gland masses: a step forward in the differentiation between adenomas and non-adenomas? Radiology 202:517–521

Tsushima Y, Ishizaka H, Matsumoto M (1993) Adrenal masses: differentiation with chemical shift, fast-low-angle shot MR imaging. Radiology 186:705–709

Tuck ML (1995) Mineralocorticoid hypertension. In: Clinical endocrinology update syllabus. The Endocrine Society, Bethesda, pp 263–272

van Erkel AR, van Gils APG, Lequin M, Kruitwagen C, Bloem JL, Falke THM (1994) CT and MR distinction of adenomas and nonadenomas of the adrenal gland. J Comput Assist Tomogr 18:432–438

Vincent JM, Morison ID, Armstrong P, Reznek RH (1994) The size of normal adrenal glands on computed tomography. Clin Radiol 49:453–455

Weiss LW, Medeiros LJ, Vickery AL (1989) Pathologic features of prognostic significance in adrenocortical carcinoma. Am J Surg Pathol 13:202–206

Welch TJ, Sheedy PF, Stephens DH, Johnson CM, Swensen SJ (1994) Percutaneous adrenal biopsy: review of a 10-year experience. Radiology 193:341–344

Wolverson MK, Kannegiesser H (1984) CT of bilateral adrenal hemorrhage with acute adrenal insufficiency in the adult. AJR 142:311–314

Young WF Jr, Hogan MJ, Klee GG, et al. (1990) Primary aldosteronism: diagnosis and treatment. Mayo Clin Proc 65:96–110

Young WF Jr (1997) Phaeochromocytoma: how to catch a moonbeam in your hand. Eur J Endocrinol 136:28–29

# 13 Surgical Treatment of Adrenal Gland Tumors

J.P. STEIN and D.G. SKINNER

CONTENTS



## 13.1
## Introduction

The adrenal gland is an important structure both anatomically and physiologically. To properly diagnose and treat adrenal disorders, one must have a thorough understanding of the anatomy, the normal physiology, and the pathophysiology of the gland. Adrenal tumors comprise an interesting spectrum of benign and malignant diseases. The most common tumors involving the adrenal gland are metastatic lesions to the adrenal. Management of these metastatic lesions is dependent upon the primary disease entity. The major primary adrenal disorders discussed in this chapter will include: Cushing's syndrome, hyperaldosteronism, pheochromocytoma, an incidentally discovered adrenal mass, and adrenal cortical carcinoma. These tumors can present with a variability of clinical signs and symptoms which often overlap, making the differentiation on the basis of symptoms and physical examination both difficult and unreliable.

With the development of more sensitive biochemical assays, and improved radiologic imaging techniques, the diagnosis, treatment, and surgical approach of adrenal disorders has improved. The appropriate management of a patient with an adrenal tumor requires an understanding of normal adrenal physiology, the functional nature of the endocrinopathy, potential perioperative complications, and a comprehensive understanding of the adrenal anatomy.

## 13.2
## Anatomy of the Adrenal Gland

The adrenal glands are paired organs located in the retroperitoneum adjacent to the upper pole of the kidneys. They are located within the perinephric fat surrounded by Gerota's fascia at the anterosuperior and medial aspects of the kidneys. The adult adrenal gland measures up to 5 cm in length, 3 cm in width, and 1 cm in thickness, and weighs about 5 g. The adrenal weight at birth, in contrast, is much larger because the adrenal cortex plays an important role in fetal embryogenesis and homeostasis (PEPE and ALBRECHT 1990). In addition, the newborn adrenal gland is susceptible to adrenal hemorrhage under stressful situations, particularly during birth. Fetal adrenal regression occurs rapidly during the first 6 weeks of life (SCOTT et al. 1990).

Anatomically, the right adrenal gland is positioned above the kidney, lateral and posterior (cephalad aspect) to the inferior vena cava. The anterior surface of the right adrenal is in immediate contact with the liver and lies slightly higher than the left adrenal gland. The anterior aspect of the right adrenal gland may therefore be approached via a retroperitoneal manner with cephalad traction of the liver within the peritoneal envelope. The left adrenal gland is in more direct contact with the kidney as it overlies its upper pole, the anterior surface and me-


J.P. STEIN, MD, Assistant Professor of Urology, Department of Urology, University of Southern California, Norris Comprehensive Cancer Center, MS #74, 1441 Eastlake Avenue, Suite 7414, Los Angeles, CA 90033, USA
D.G. SKINNER, MD, Department of Urology, University of Southern California, Norris Comprehensive Cancer Center, MS #74, 1441 Eastlake Avenue, Suite 7414, Los Angeles, CA 90033, USA

dial aspect of which are located posterior to the pancreas and splenic vessels. Special consideration must be given to removal of the left adrenal gland because of the intimate relationship with the left renal vasculature. The anterior surface of the left adrenal gland may be exposed via a retroperitoneal approach and by retracting the spleen cephalad within the peritoneal envelope.

The inferior phrenic artery provides the main blood supply to the adrenals superiorly, with additional branches from the aorta laterally and the renal artery inferiorly (ANSON et al. 1947). The arteriole supply to the adrenals is more variable than the venous drainage. The primary venous drainage is usually via a common vein on the right which empties into the side wall of the inferior vena cava. This is a short and fragile vein that can be easily injured or disrupted during surgery, resulting in troublesome bleeding. The major left adrenal vein empties into the superior aspect of the left renal vein. This vein is generally located in between the inferior vena cava (medially) and the left gonadal vein (laterally), draining into the inferior aspect of the left renal vein. Inferior phrenic veins generally provide venous drainage of the adrenals superiorly.

Although rare, congenital anomalies of the adrenal gland, including agenesis, presence of accessory adrenal tissue, and ectopia, can occur. If the kidney is absent or ectopic in location, the adrenal gland is generally found in its normal position. Even in the face of renal agenesis, it is rare to have unilateral absence of the adrenal gland.

The adrenal cortex develops from a mesodermal and the medulla from an ectodermal origin. Histologically, the adult adrenal cortex constitutes 90% of the gland and is divided into three anatomic and functionally distinct zones: zona glomerulosa (outer), zona fasciculata (middle), and zona reticularis (inner). The zona glomerulosa is involved in aldosterone production, the zona fasciculata in glucocorticoid synthesis, and the zona reticularis in sex hormone (androgens and estrogens) production. The centrally located adrenal medulla is involved in catecholamine (norepinephrine and epinephrine) production.

## 13.3
## Cushing's Syndrome

Cushing's syndrome comprises several disease entities that refer to the clinical presentation of excess corticosteroid production. This syndrome can be produced by administration of glucocorticoids, or may result from a pathologic dysfunctional status. Harvey Cushing initially described a basophilic pituitary adenoma as the cause of the syndrome (CUSHING 1912). Adrenocortical hypersecretion can be classified as Cushing's disease (pituitary dependent) or as Cushing's syndrome (pituitary independent) including: adrenal tumors producing cortisol or ectopic tumors (benign or malignant) producing adrenocorticotrophic hormone (ACTH). The term Cushing's syndrome will be used to include both conditions for the remaining portion of the discussion.

The etiology for Cushing's syndrome includes a pituitary tumor (70%), an adrenal adenoma (15%), adrenal carcinoma (5%), adrenal hyperplasia (5%), and ectopic ACTH production (5%) (GOLDFARB 1993). In a series of over 100 patients with Cushing's syndrome, 75% had an elevated ACTH (ORTH and LIDDLE 1971). Of these patients with an elevated ACTH, 80% were pituitary dependent with either a microadenoma (Cushing's disease) or a pituitary macroadenoma (Nelson's syndrome), while 20% demonstrated an ectopic source of ACTH (pituitary independent). In contrast to patients with Cushing's disease (pituitary dependent) with an elevated ACTH, those with an adrenal source (adenoma, carcinoma, hyperplasia) of Cushing's syndrome exhibit excess circulating cortisol and a suppressed circulating serum ACTH.

Virtually all organ systems can be affected by Cushing's syndrome. The clinical presentation of this syndrome may be classic. Prominent clinical signs may include central obesity (with peripheral extremity muscle wasting), moon facies, the buffalo hump, hypertension, purple stria, acne, edema, increased bruising, and muscle weakness. Old photographs are sometimes helpful in documenting these physical changes. In women, amenorrhea and hirsutism may be present. Personality changes or psychiatric symptoms may also be present. Other problems from long-term cortisol excess may include infections and cardiovascular accident.

Although the etiology of Cushing's syndrome (pituitary, adrenal, or ectopic) cannot be determined based on clinical presentation, those with an ectopic ACTH-producing tumor may appear sick, with cachexia, weight loss, or severe hypertension (BAGSHAWE 1960). Patients with pituitary or ectopic ACTH production may demonstrate signs of hyperpigmentation secondary to elevated melanocyte-stimulating hormone (MSH), a breakdown product of ACTH. The majority of children less than 15 years of age presenting with Cushing's syndrome have an adrenal neoplasm. Furthermore, patients with adrenal cortical carcinoma are more likely to demonstrate virilization in the female and feminization in the male.

The clinical suspicion of Cushing's syndrome is confirmed by the laboratory evaluation. The two basic steps in the evaluation of patients with this disease are: (1) establishing whether they have the syndrome, and (2) establishing the etiology.

The diagnosis of Cushing's syndrome can be made by measuring serum and urinary (24-h) cortisol levels. First, a morning and afternoon serum cortisol level should be performed. Patients with Cushing's syndrome lose their normal diurnal variation. This can be confirmed by a 24-h urine free-cortisol determination. In fact, the 24-h urinary excretion of cortisol has recently been shown to be the most direct and reliable test for cortisol hypersecretion (ORTH 1995). This test should provide a reliable diagnosis of Cushing's syndrome.

Once the diagnosis has been established, serum ACTH measurement should be performed. This helps to determine the major subgroups (precise etiology) of Cushing's syndrome: those with a normal or elevated ACTH level suggestive of a pituitary or ectopic source, and those with a low level of ACTH suggestive of an adrenal source. One should suspect an ectopic source in patients with ACTH levels greater than twice normal. Ectopic ACTH-producing tumors include: oat cell carcinoma of the lung (most common), bronchial adenomas, pancreatic tumors, renal cell carcinomas, and carcinoid tumors. If the ACTH is low, an adrenal secreting tumor causing ACTH suppression should be suspected (LIBERTINO 1988).

Additional testing in patients suspected of having Cushing's syndrome may include the dexamethasone suppression test or the administration of corticosteroid synthesis inhibitors such as metyrapone (LIDDLE 1960). The overnight dexamethasone suppression test (low dose) requires administration of 1 mg of dexamethasone at midnight, followed by a cortisol measurement at 8 a.m. Failure to suppress serum cortisol with the low-dose dexamethasone test helps to establish the diagnosis of Cushing's syndrome. Once Cushing's syndrome is confirmed, a high-dose dexamethasone suppression test may be performed to differentiate between a pituitary-dependent and a pituitary-independent cause. Dexamethasone, 2 mg every 6 h for 2–3 days is given, and a serum cortisol level is measured. If the cortisol is suppressed by 50% or more, then

Cushing's disease (pituitary dependent) should be suspected. Lack of cortisol suppression with the high-dose test suggests either an adrenal source (adenoma or carcinoma) or an ectopic ACTH source (CHANDLER et al. 1987). In this situation, a serum ACTH level will identify the source. The high-dose dexamethasone suppression test may also help identify an ectopic ACTH source when there is complete resistance to the test.

Although less commonly performed, the metyrapone test may help distinguish between the various forms of Cushing's syndrome. Metyrapone inhibits the 11β-hydroxylase enzyme in cortisol production, resulting in a decrease in cortisol production and causing an increase in ACTH production through a loss of the normal feedback mechanism. If Cushing's disease is present, an exaggerated response is seen with this test, while no effect is seen with adrenal tumors or with ectopic ACTH secretion (JUBIZ et al. 1970).

The development of computerized axial tomography (CT) and magnetic resonance imaging (MRI) has led to the replacement of older radiographic modalities such as intravenous pyelography, ultrasound, and adrenal arteriography or venography. CT scan has become the primary radiographic test of choice to evaluate for adrenal diseases.

The initial radiologic study should be performed based on the level of ACTH. If the ACTH is elevated and Cushing's disease is suspected, CT or MRI of the brain, with specific interest in the sella turcica, should be performed (MITTY and YEH 1982). Because pituitary microadenomas may be difficult to diagnose radiographically, various forms of CT or MRI have been employed to enhance the detection rate. High-resolution CT may be necessary to demonstrate pituitary tumors greater than 6 mm in diameter (TEASDALE et al. 1986). Recently, both enhanced and gadolinium-enhanced MRI have been employed to detect small pituitary lesions (KLIBLANSKI and ZERVAS 1991; HALL et al. 1994). Despite these modalities, however, approximately 50% of pituitary microadenomas may still be missed. Selective ACTH sampling of the inferior petrosal sinuses, with comparison to peripheral serum ACTH levels, may be useful to confirm the diagnosis in this situation (ZOVICHIAN et al. 1988).

If the ACTH level is low, a pituitary source is unlikely, and a CT scan should be performed with specific attention to the adrenal glands. CT scan is considered the radiographic modality to evaluate for an adrenal tumor (ABRAMS et al. 1983). A functional adenoma greater than 2 cm is generally easily visualized and may result in contralateral adrenal atrophy. Adrenal hyperplasia will usually produce bilateral symmetrical cortical thickening and can be demonstrated on CT scanning. Adrenal carcinomas are sometimes difficult to distinguish from adenoma except for their large size. Adrenal carcinomas are usually larger than 6 cm and may demonstrated non-specific necrosis and/or calcification (BELLDEGRUN and DEKERNION 1989). Metastatic tumors to the adrenal glands may also produce this appearance and must always be considered.

Alternatively, MRI may be employed to evaluated the adrenal gland. On T2-weighted images, adrenal adenomas are isointense whereas adrenal carcinomas appear hyperintense. MRI may also be employed to help evaluate anatomic detail and identify venous tumor thrombus involvement in patients with adrenal tumors (FIGUEROA et al. 1997).

The treatment of Cushing's syndrome is dependent on the etiology. In the case of a pituitary adenoma (Cushing's disease) the treatment is a transsphenoidal resection of the tumor. This is a safe and effective form of therapy with cure rates of 85%–90%, and low recurrence rates (LUDECKE 1991). Following transsphenoidal therapy, some patients may demonstrate a temporary decrease in serum cortisol levels requiring supplementation and careful monitoring for a period of time. Irradiation therapy with approximately 4500 cGy may be employed in patients failing transsphenoidal surgery, salvaging 50%–80% of patients (HALBERG and SHELINE 1987). Alternatively, total hypophysectomy may be considered in patients (adults past the reproductive years) not cured initially via transsphenoidal surgery.

Prior to the advent of transsphenoidal surgery and irradiation therapy, bilateral adrenalectomy was the primary form of therapy for patients with Cushing's disease. Despite the fact that most patients respond to this therapy, adrenal insufficiency is problematic, with approximately 10% of patients developing Nelson's syndrome, a macroadenoma of the pituitary thought to result from the lack of inhibitory feedback mechanism and high ACTH levels (NELSON et al. 1958; MOORE et al. 1976). The tumor associated with Nelson's syndrome may be more aggressive, and less responsive to surgery or radiotherapy, in which case irradiation is generally the treatment of choice (WILSON et al. 1980). Currently, bilateral adrenalectomy is a last resort and should be reserved for those patients with Cushing's disease who fail transsphenoidal surgery, irradiation therapy, and cortisol enzyme inhibitors.

The treatment of an adrenal adenoma is adrenalectomy. The surgical approach (see later discussion) is dictated by several variables including the size of the adrenal tumor. Small adrenal tumors can be treated through a dorsal or flank approach while larger tumors may be best approached through a transverse upper abdominal or thoracoabdominal (author's preference) incision.

Corticosteroid supplementation is critical to the perioperative care of patients with Cushing's syndrome. The variable amount of contralateral adrenal cortex suppression may warrant perioperative monitoring and administration of corticosteroids with gradual tapering over a period of time (may be several months) following surgery.

In the case of ectopic ACTH production, treatment of the primary tumor may be performed. If this is prohibited, medical therapy with cortisol inhibition should be attempted using metyrapone, aminoglutethimide, or ketoconazole. This treatment may result in adrenal insufficiency and require cortisol and mineralocorticoid supplementation.

## 13.4
## Primary Hyperaldosteronism

Primary hyperaldosteronism (Conn's syndrome) was initially described by Conn and included the syndrome characterized by hypertension, hypokalemia, hypernatremia, and metabolic alkalosis resulting from an aldosterone-secreting tumor of the zona glomerulosa (CONN 1955). Primary hyperaldosteronism is a relatively uncommon disorder and accounts for approximately 1% of all cases of hypertension. The clinical manifestations of this syndrome result from the increased total body sodium content, and loss of total body potassium (FERRISS et al. 1978). Hypertension is the most common sign and is related to sodium retention. The metabolic alkalosis is secondary to the hypokalemia. Physical examination generally cannot distinguish hyperaldosteronism and essential hypertension. Most symptoms of primary hyperaldosteronism are related to potassium wasting; they include muscular weakness (most common), urinary frequency, polydipsia, paresthesias, visual disturbances, temporary paralysis, cramps, and tetany.

The etiology of primary hyperaldosteronism is a unilateral adenoma in 80% of patients, and bilateral micronodular hyperplasia in about 20% of patients (DONOHUE 1980). An adenoma is more common in younger patients and in women (NEVILLE and

O'HARE 1982). Adrenal cortical carcinomas rarely produce isolated Conn's syndrome without Cushing's syndrome, virilization, feminization, or a combination of these.

The diagnosis of primary hyperaldosteronism should be suspected in patients who manifest typical signs and symptoms of the disease. Although hypokalemia is the hallmark of the disease, 20% of patients may have normal serum potassium levels (CONN 1967; BRAVO et al. 1983). Hypokalemia may be exaggerated when patients take diuretics or restrict their sodium intake. Importantly, plasma renin activity (PRA) is suppressed secondary to increase blood volume in patients with primary hyperaldosteronism. This is an important test to help distinguish between primary and secondary hyperaldosteronism.

Secondary hyperaldosteronism is found in patients with elevated PRA resulting from a physiologic adjustment to a contracted intravascular volume or a decrease in renal perfusion, leading to increased production of angiotensin II and subsequent increase in serum aldosterone. The most common cause of secondary hyperaldosteronism is renovascular hypertension. Secondary hyperaldosteronism is characterized by an increase in serum aldosterone and PRA.

Serum potassium and PRA should be first performed to screen patients suspected of hyperaldosteronism. If these screening tests suggest hyperaldosteronism, confirmatory tests should be performed. The two most reliable confirmatory tests are: (1) failure to suppress serum aldosterone during sodium loading (saline suppression test), and (2) failure to stimulate PRA even in the face of sodium depletion (negative lasix stimulation test). Therefore, the diagnosis of primary hyperaldosteronism is confirmed when there is failure to suppress plasma aldosterone after saline loading (2 l in 3 h) and failure of PRA to be stimulated by salt and volume depletion (40 mg furosemide q 8 h, 10 mEq sodium diet for 24 h, and 2 h of ambulation) (DONOHUE 1990). The diagnosis of primary hyperaldosteronism is made by identifying hypokalemia, high urinary and plasma aldosterone levels following sodium repletion, and suppressed PRA (despite sodium restriction) in hypertensive patients.

Once the diagnosis of primary hyperaldosteronism is confirmed, radiographic evaluation is performed to determine the etiology, i.e., either unilateral adenoma or bilateral adrenal hyperplasia. CT has evolved as the most accurate method to localize the site of an adrenal adenoma. Refinements in technology have allowed accurate visualization of small (1 cm) adenomas of the adrenal gland. MRI of small adrenal lesions has not been found to be as clinically useful (NEWHOUSE 1990). If CT scanning is unable to identify the adrenal lesion, localization with adrenal vein aldosterone sampling should be performed. Patients with primary hyperaldosteronism will demonstrate an elevated ipsilateral aldosterone concentration (involved gland) with contralateral suppression (normal gland) (GEISINGER et al. 1983). If a solitary, unilateral adrenal mass is unequivocally identified on CT scanning in a patient with biochemically proven primary hyperaldosteronism, then surgery is clearly indicated and further testing with adrenal vein sampling can be avoided.

Primary hyperaldosteronism due to adrenal adenoma is a surgical disease. Prior to surgery it is important that patients undergo several weeks of adequate hypertensive control and correction of any metabolic abnormalities. Spironolactone, administered preoperatively, is helpful to correct the hypokalemia.

Once the patient has been appropriately managed preoperatively, unilateral adrenalectomy should be performed. Generally, these adrenal adenomas are small and can be surgically approached via an ipsilateral extraperitoneal approach, using either a posterior or a flank incision. Results are encouraging with this disease and hypertension is either cured or improved in more than 90% of patients surgically treated for an adrenal adenoma.

Patients with primary hyperaldosteronism secondary to bilateral hyperplasia should be treated with medical therapy employing spironolactone.

## 13.5
## Pheochromocytoma

Pheochromocytoma is an uncommon, but very interesting tumor with signs and symptoms directly related to the biochemical hypersecretion of catecholamines. Although pheochromocytomas are the causative factor of hypertension in less than 1% of the hypertensive population, early and accurate detection is critical for cure and to prevent the potential lethal effects of the tumor, specifically malignant hypertension, cardiac arrhythmias, congestive heart failure, myocardial infarction, cerebral vascular accidents, and hemorrhage.

Pheochromocytomas arise in cells of neural crest origin and can be identified anywhere along the distribution of chromaffin tissue laid down during fetal development. The largest accumulation of chromaffin tissue includes the adrenal medulla, the periaortic sympathetic chain ganglia, and the organ of Zuckerkandl at the origin of the inferior mesentery artery. Ectopic pheochromocytomas have been described in the bladder, vagina, ovaries, testes, spleen, and carotid bodies (LIBERTINO 1988). The majority of pheochromocytomas (90%) are located between the diaphragm and the pelvic floor; 10% are found in the mediastinum or the skull. Most pheochromocytomas (90%) are sporadic (nonfamilial), approximately 90% of which involve a single adrenal gland. Pheochromocytomas are commonly referred to as the "10% tumor" because 10% are familial, 10% are extra-adrenal, 10% are bilateral, and 10% are malignant (HUME 1960). In children, they are often referred to as the 30% tumor; approximately 30% are familial, bilateral, and extra-adrenal (STACKPOLE et al. 1963).

Norepinephrine and epinephrine are catecholamines synthesized from the amino acid tyrosine. The enzyme phenylethylamine $N$-methyltransferase converts norepinephrine to epinephrine, a property almost exclusive of the adrenal medulla. Although 85% of normal adrenal catecholamine secretion is epinephrine, most pheochromocytomas secrete primarily norepinephrine. If a pheochromocytoma is found to be predominantly epinephrine secreting, it is invariably located within the adrenal. A pure epinephrine-secreting pheochromocytoma is rare and may be difficult to diagnose because hypertension is usually minimal in this instance.

The clinical manifestations of pheochromocytomas are a result of the physiologic effects of the type and amount of catecholamine secretion by the tumor, primarily norepinephrine and epinephrine and less commonly dopamine and seritonin. The clinical symptoms of a pheochromocytoma are related to epinephrine secretion, while the clinical signs are related to norepinephrine secretion. Hypertension is the most common sign of the disease (VAN HEERDEN et al. 1982); 10% of patients, however, are normotensive. Half of these patients demonstrate paroxysmal hypertension while 50% have sustained hypertension. Nearly all patients have headaches, palpitations, and excessive sweating. Other symptoms may include chronic fatigue, anxiety, pallor, flushing, nausea, tremor, chest pain, shortness of breath, and abdominal cramps. Other clues to the disease include a sudden elevation of blood pressure during initiation of anesthesia or during pregnancy. Symptoms precipitated with micturition suggest a pheochromocytoma of the blad-

der. A pheochromocytoma should also be suspected when the administration of various drugs such as morphine or methyldopa stimulates a hypertensive crisis.

The diagnosis of a pheochromocytoma is made biochemically. Elevated levels of catecholamines or their metabolic byproducts can be demonstrated in the serum or urine in over 95% of patients (BRAVO 1991). The best screening test for pheochromocytomas is urinary measurements of vanillylmandelic acid (VMA), metanephrines, and free catecholamines. Of these, urinary measurement of the urinary metanephrines is probably the most optimal because it is most stable and less affected by stress (HENGSTMANN 1985). Approximately 95% of patients with a pheochromocytoma will have elevated urinary levels of one of these substances. In addition, serum catecholamine measurements, a sensitive test for pheochromocytoma, should also be performed. Only rarely are the concentrations of plasma and urinary catecholamines not elevated in a patient with a pheochromocytoma; such instances are primarily seen when the patient is normotensive at the time of the evaluation. In this situation, a high index of suspicion and repeat sampling in the face of hypertension are indicated and may resolve the dilemma. Furthermore, the use of imaging studies [MRI or iodine-131 metaiodobenzylguanidine (MIBG)] may be helpful with the diagnosis. Today, provocative tests with histamine, glucagon, or phentolamine are only rarely employed (DOLAN and CAREY 1989).

Some patients with essential hypertension, demonstrating signs and symptoms of pheochromocytoma, have slightly elevated levels of catecholamines. This is probably a result of a neurogenic component to their hypertension. The clonidine suppression test may help differentiate these two groups (BRAVO et al. 1981). Patients with essential hypertension at rest will demonstrate a fall in plasma norepinephrine and epinephrine as clonidine inhibits centrally mediated adrenergic influences (BRAVO 1991). Patients with pheochromocytoma, however, do not demonstrate a fall in the catecholamine levels following a clonidine suppression test.

Pheochromocytomas may be associated with other familial syndromes or neuroectodermal diseases. Pheochromocytomas can occur in the multiple endocrine neoplasia (MEN) II syndrome which includes medullary carcinoma of the thyroid, parathyroid adenomas, and pheochromocytoma (SIPPLE 1961). Neuroectodermal diseases associated with pheochromocytomas include von Recklinghausen's disease (neurofibromatosis), Sturge-Weber disease, and von Hippel-Lindau disease.

Once the diagnosis of pheochromocytoma is made, the location of the tumor must be established. Abdominal CT scanning will detect more than 90% of adrenally located tumors (THOMAS et al. 1980). MRI may also be helpful in diagnosing and localizing pheochromocytomas; a classic high signal intensity is seen on T2-weighted images (GLAZER et al. 1986). In addition, sagittal and coronal views with MRI can provide excellent anatomic information. Some investigators now feel that MRI should be the initial radiographic procedure in patients with the biochemical findings of a pheochromocytoma (VAUGHAN 1997).

Although CT and MRI scanning have greatly improved the localization of a pheochromocytoma, multiple, recurrent, metastatic, and occult tumors may be very difficult to diagnose. MIBG may be helpful in these situations. MIBG it is an analogue of guanethidine and is taken up by adrenergic granules and the adrenal medulla (SHAPIRO et al. 1985). This test has an overall sensitivity of 87%, with a specificity of 99%, and may actually be more sensitive than CT or MRI in identifying small extra-adrenal tumors.

The treatment of a pheochromocytoma is by surgical extirpation. Critical to a successful outcome is appropriate perioperative preparation. Careful preoperative management facilitates treatment for both the surgeon and the anesthesiologist, while maintaining the safety of the patient. Preoperative pharmacological management may also help prevent the potential cardiovascular complications associated with this disease. Most pheochromocytomas secrete norepinephrine, and an α-adrenergic blocker such as phenoxybenzamine (dibenzyline) may help control the hypertension. β-Blockers may help prevent arrhythmias and permit a reduction in the amount of α-blocker used to control the hypertension. To prevent rebound hypertension a β-blocker should only be administered when α-blockade has been firmly established.

Patients with malignant pheochromocytomas, or those with tumors resistant to α-blockade, may be treated with α-methyltyrosine. This drug, which inhibits tyrosine hydroxylation, the rate-limiting step for catecholamine synthesis, helps reduces catecholamine excess and may be valuable in malignant or refractory cases of pheochromocytoma. Administration of this medication, however, does carry some adverse side-effects including extrapyramidal signs, crystalluria, diarrhea, sedation, and anxiety.

Intravascular volume status is another important perioperative consideration. Patients with pheochromocytomas may be severely volume depleted secondary to chronic α-stimulation. Vigorous intravenous hydration may be required in these patients to raise the intravascular volume and accommodate the expanded vascular response produced by α-blockade. Close intraoperative monitoring is critical in these patients and should include a central venous catheter, a Swan-Ganz catheter, and an arterial line. Care must also be taken with induction of anesthesia; blood pressure must be controlled and arrhythmias avoided. Postoperative hypotension should be carefully monitored and treated with vigorous intravenous hydration.

The appropriate surgical approach to a pheochromocytoma must allow for intraoperative abdominal exploration and evaluation of the sympathetic chain. This can be performed through a midline or transabdominal chevron incision, or an ipsilateral thoracoabdominal incision (authors' preference).

## 13.6
## Incidental Adrenal Mass

With the increasing use of modern imaging modalities (abdominal ultrasound, CT, and MRI) incidental adrenal masses ('incidentalomas') are discovered more commonly (BELLDEGRUN et al. 1986). These adrenal masses are found during the evaluation of an unrelated disease, seen in 1% of asymptomatic patients undergoing CT scans (COPELAND 1983; Ross and ARON 1990).

Little controversy exists when an incidental adrenal mass of 5 cm or larger is discovered or when an incidental adrenal mass is found to be functional. Solid adrenal masses greater than 5 cm should be surgically removed. This is based on the finding that adrenal masses greater than 6 cm in size are usually adrenal malignancies (BELLDEGRUN et al. 1986). In a review of six series, Belldegrun and associates found that 105 of 114 adrenocortical carcinomas were more than 6 cm in size. It has also been shown that CT scanning may underestimate the size of an adrenal mass; therefore a solid adrenal tumor of more than 5 cm in size should be considered malignant and be surgically removed (VAUGHAN 1997).

All patients found to have a solid adrenal mass should undergo a biochemical (endocrine) evaluation. The endocrine workup should include urinary cortisol and metanephrines, as well as serum catecholamines, potassium, aldosterone, cortisol, ACTH, estrogen, testosterone, dehydroepiandrosterone sulfate (DHEAS), and pregnenolone (Ross and Aron 1990). If any biochemical abnormality is identified, the adrenal lesion should be surgically removed.

Controversy arises in the management of an incidentally discovered solid adrenal tumor less than 5 cm in size and functionally inactive. Some advocate MRI in this situation (Vaughan 1997). It has been suggested that adrenal adenomas display little change in intensity from T1- to T2-weighted images. They are generally hypointense or isointense relative to the liver or spleen on T1-weighted images and slightly hyperintense or isointense related to hepatic or splenic tissue on T2-weighted images. In contrast, adrenal cortical carcinomas have a higher (>0.8) signal intensity change between T1- and T2-weighted images. They are hypointense to the liver and spleen on T1-weighted images and hyperintense on T2-weighted images (Vaughan 1997). Additionally, fine-needle adrenal biopsy under ultrasound or CT guidance may aid in the diagnosis of a small, nonfunctional adrenal lesion. In one large series, significant histology material was obtained in over 96% of patients, and was 85% accurate in differentiating benign and malignant tumors (Tikkakoski et al. 1991). Care must be taken in this situation as an accurate pathologic diagnosis may be extremely difficult and requires an experienced pathologist.

Another management approach to a solid, nonfunctional adrenal mass less than 5 cm in diameter is to carefully follow the lesion with serial CT scans and biochemical evaluations at 3- or 6-month intervals. During follow-up, any evidence of tumor growth or development of functional activity is observed, then adrenalectomy is clearly indicated. Overall, good clinical judgment and flexibility are key components to the management of the incidentally discovered adrenal mass.

## 13.7
## Adrenocortical Carcinoma

Primary adrenocortical carcinoma is a rare tumor that generally carries a poor prognosis (Luton et al. 1990). The incidence is estimated at one case in over 1.7 million of the population and accounts for approximately 0.02% of all cancers (Brennan 1987). Although adrenocortical carcinoma can occur in patients at any age, the mean age of patients is in the fourth decade. Adrenocortical carcinomas can be classified according to their biochemical (functional) secretion of various hormones. Luton and associates found that nearly 80% of adrenal tumors are biochemically functional; this is a higher incidence than previously reported, thought to be a result of more sensitive assays (Luton et al. 1990).

Patients with adrenocortical carcinoma may present with abdominal or flank pain, fatigue, or other constitutional symptoms. Clinically functional tumors may induce paraneoplastic symptoms including most commonly Cushing's syndrome (50%) and virilization (10%–20%), while aldosterone-producing tumors (2%) are rarely seen without concomitant glucocorticoid or sex hormone production (Barzilay and Pazianos 1989). Clinical signs and symptoms of sex steroid production in males are more subtle than in females because these are usually virilizing tumors. It is more common for women with adrenocortical carcinomas to have a virilizing tumor than it is for men to have a feminizing tumor. In children, adrenocortical carcinoma is the most common cause of Cushing's syndrome.

The diagnostic assessment of an adrenocortical carcinoma includes the proper biochemical and radiographic evaluation. Biochemical assessment should include the evaluation of Cushing's syndrome (serum cortisol and ACTH, and urinary 17-hydroxycorticosteroids), a virilizing syndrome (serum androgens and urinary 17-ketosteroids), a feminizing syndrome (serum estrogens and urinary 17-ketosteroids), and hyperaldosteronism (serum aldosterone, potassium, and PRA).

The radiologic test of choice is an abdominal CT scan. This will assess the tumor size (usually greater than 5 cm), tumor consistency (solid, inhomogeneous), the presence of calcification, and any potential contiguous organ involvement (Dunnick et al. 1982). MRI demonstrates a characteristic high intensity signal on T2-weighted images and may be important to determine the presence of venous tumor thrombus involvement (Figueroa et al. 1997). Arteriography generally provides little additional information and is less commonly performed.

Adrenal carcinomas are generally radio- and chemoresistant tumors. The primary form of therapy is surgical extirpation. Adrenocortical carcinomas tend to be larger, vascular tumors that may involve contiguous organs. The most common sites of metastases include the lung, liver, and lymph nodes (Richie and Gittes 1980). Optimal surgical exposure and visualization are critical when planning the operative approach. An anterior transabdominal chevron or ipsilateral thoracoab-dominal incision (authors' preference) are the optimal surgical approaches. Postoperative steroid replacement may be necessary for hypercortisol-producing tumors.

Despite en bloc resection, even in patients without evidence of metastatic disease, the 5-year survival rate for adrenocortical carcinoma is only 50% with complete resection and 35% overall (POMMIER and BRENNAN 1992). This has generated efforts to pro-vide an effective form of adjuvant therapy. Patients with extra-adrenal local spread, or with metastatic adrenocortical carcinoma may benefit from adjuvant chemotherapy using o,p′-DDD (mitotane) as an adrenolytic agent. This DDT derivative has been shown to induce a tumor response in 35% of patients in a review of 500 reported cases (WOOTEN and KING 1993). Unfortunately, these responses do not appear to improve survival. Furthermore, this is a toxic agent that results in adrenal insufficiency requiring cortisol and mineralocorticoid replacement.

## 13.8
## Surgical Approaches to the Adrenal Gland

There are numerous surgical approaches to the adre-nal gland. Each case must be individualized. The ideal surgical approach depends on several variables including the underlying etiology of the adrenal tumor, the size of the tumor, the potential for con-tiguous organ or venous tumor involvement, the patient's body habitus, and possibly most impor-tantly, the surgeon's experience and personal prefer-ence. Critical to the successful treatment outcome in patients with adrenal disorders is maintenance of a proper surgical technique. Adequate operative expo-sure and visualization along with early and careful

vascular control are important. Malignant tumors should be excised with adequate surgical margins in an en bloc technique. The surgeon should anticipate and be prepared to remove any involved contiguous organs (kidney, pancreas, spleen, or colon) when the need arises. The surgeon must be committed to these principles and to the patient to provide the best sur-gical and clinical outcome.

Prior to surgical extirpation, all patients with adrenal diseases must be carefully evaluated and treated for metabolic and hormonal imbalances. This may include the administration of various medications (cortisone and α-blockers), as well as proper intravenous hydration. Team work and co-operation with an experienced anesthesiologist and critical care team will help optimize the clinical outcome in these difficult patients and minimize perioperative morbidity and mortality.

## 13.8.1
## Posterior (Dorsal) Approach

The posterior or dorsal approach provides an extraperitoneal route to the adrenal glands. This sur-gical approach is generally reserved for small, unilat-eral or bilateral adrenal tumors confined to the adrenal gland. Patient recovery is quick with mini-mal morbidity and postoperative pain. Limitations of the dorsal approach include a smaller operative field with the inability to evaluate an extra-adrenal process.

With the patient in the prone position, rolled tow-els are placed beneath the hips and rib cage. The table may be flexed to widen the intercostal space and provide further exposure (Fig. 13.1). The suit-able rib is chosen (either the 11th or 12th) and a subperiosteal rib resection is performed (Fig. 13.2). The rib is removed as proximal to its articulation

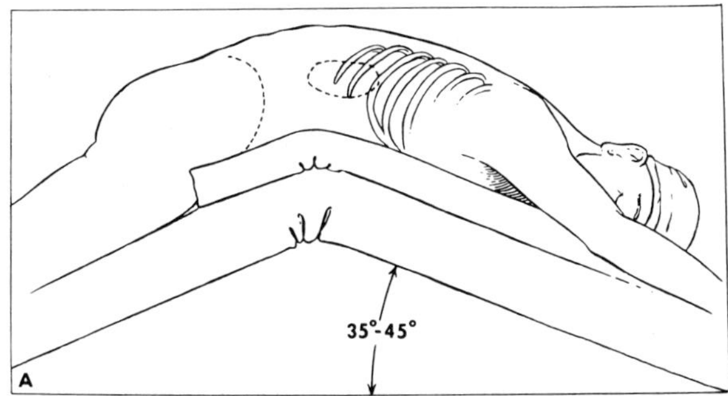


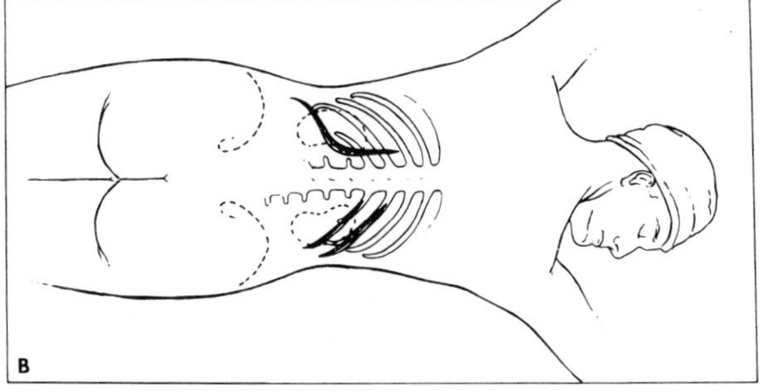


**Fig. 13.1 A,B.** The patient is placed in the prone position and the table flexed. [From Glenn JF (1991) Adrenal surgery. In: Glenn JF (ed) Urologic surgery, 4th edn. Harper & Row, New York, pp 1–22, Fig. 1-17]

(medial) as possible to facilitate exposure. Furthermore, to ensure adequate exposure the costovertebral ligament should be incised by medial palpation on the superior surface of the rib adjacent to the vertebral body. The key is to stay on the superior and dorsal aspect of the rib and to divide the ligamentous attachments with either heavy scissors or diathermy.

The periosteum is then incised and the pleura mobilized superiorly. Superior traction on the diaphragm and pleura, and medial retraction on the

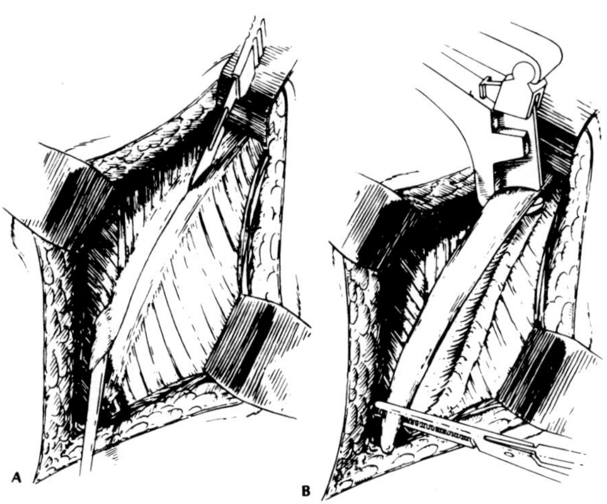

**Fig. 13.2 A,B.** The incision is made over the 11th or 12th rib. Note that the rib is removed in a subperiosteal manner. [From Glenn JF (1991) Adrenal surgery. In: Glenn JF (ed) Urologic surgery, 4th edn. Harper & Row, New York, pp 1–22, Fig. 1-18]

paraspinous muscle group, exposes the adrenal gland and the cephalad portion of the kidney. It is important to mobilize the adrenal and kidney in a caudal direction without entering Gerota's fascia. Caudal and lateral retraction of the kidney will allow separation of the right adrenal from the liver and diaphragm superiorly, and from the cava medially (Fig. 13.3). Similarly, this retraction allows separation of the left adrenal from the diaphragm and pancreas on the left side. Deaver retractors are helpful with medial retraction while a Harrington retractor aids in the superior retraction of the diaphragm, liver, and pancreas. A dedicated effort should be made not to excessively manipulate the adrenal gland. A meticulous dissection employing vascular clips or suture ligatures is critical in maintaining hemostasis (Fig. 13.4).

Control of the prominent left and right adrenal veins as they enter the renal vein on the left and inferior vena cava on the right, respectively, may be the most difficult portion of the dissection and marks the terminal portion of the dissection. Control of prominent adrenal veins should be performed with silk ligatures and then secured with hemoclips. Care should be taken to achieve enough length to double ligate this structure if possible.

To close the incision, the retracted muscles are allowed to return to their original position and the lumbodorsal fascia reapproximated. If the pleural cavity has been entered, it should be closed in two layers with a continuous suture. Air in the pleural space is evacuated with the use of a small catheter;

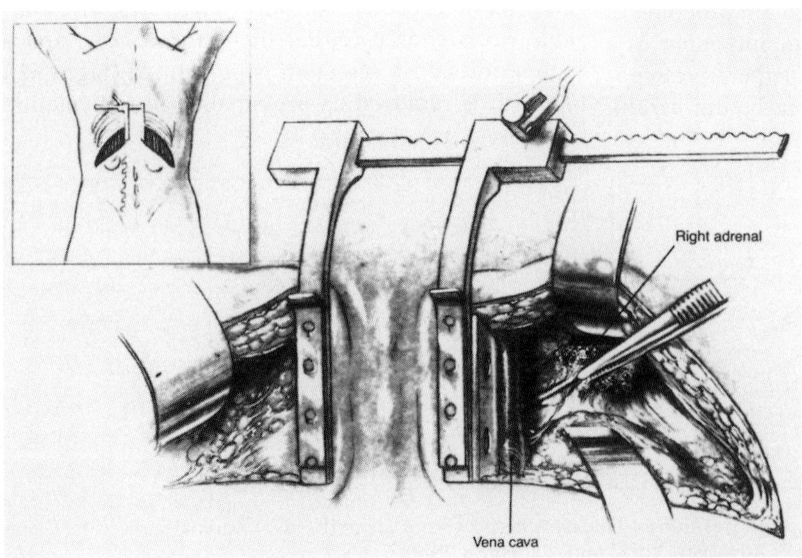


**Fig. 13.3.** With the dorsal approach, the adrenal is exposed carefully by caudal and lateral retraction of the ipsilateral kidney. The adrenal and kidney should not be separated initially. The dissection should be initiated at the superior and medial attachments of the adrenal. [From Donohue JP (1988) Diagnosis and management of adrenal tumor. In: Skinner DG, Lieskovsky G (eds) Diagnosis and management of genitourinary cancer. Saunders, Philadelphia, pp 372–389, Fig. 21-10]

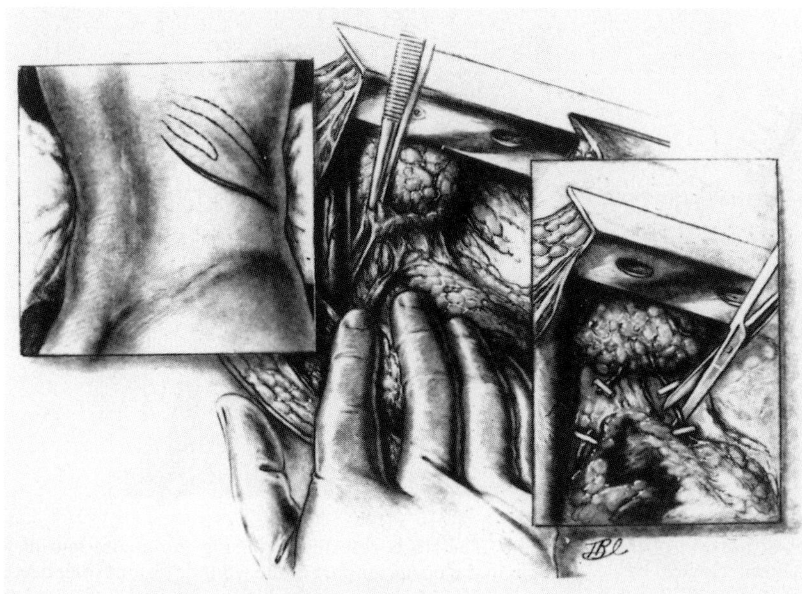

Fig. 13.4. The technique of controlling small vessels with the use of vascular hemoclips. The dorsal approach with inherent limitations of space and wound depth make the use of small vascular clips a practical method of securing hemostasis. It is best to avoid excessive manipulation of the adrenal gland. [From Donohue JP (1988) Diagnosis and management of adrenal tumor. In: Skinner DG, Lieskovsky G (eds) Diagnosis and management of genitourinary cancer. Saunders, Philadelphia, pp 372–389, Fig. 21-11]

with the lung field inflated under positive pressure, the air is evacuated and the catheter is removed. Generally, a chest tube is not required. A chest radiograph should be performed in the recovery room to exclude a pneumothroax.

## 13.8.2
## Flank or Supracostal Approach

The flank approach is an appropriate retroperitoneal route to the ipsilateral adrenal gland for a small, unilateral disorder. Owing to the familiarity of the incision, it is the most common approach to the adrenal gland for small tumors. We caution against a subcostal incision, which may be too low to safely access the ipsilateral adrenal gland. An 11th rib resection is generally suitable for this incision and may result in entry into the pleural cavity. It should be emphasized that entry into the pleural cavity should not prohibit the appropriate surgical approach which maintains best access to the adrenal.

The patient is placed in the lateral position with the back close to the edge of the operating side of the table (Fig. 13.5). The superior iliac crest should be positioned over the break of the table. The bottom leg is flexed 90° with the top leg straight to maintain the distance between the superior iliac crest and the 12th rib. A pillow is placed between the knees and a pad placed under the axilla to prevent compression of the axillary nerves and vessels. The ipsilateral arm is placed in a position that is horizontal to the floor

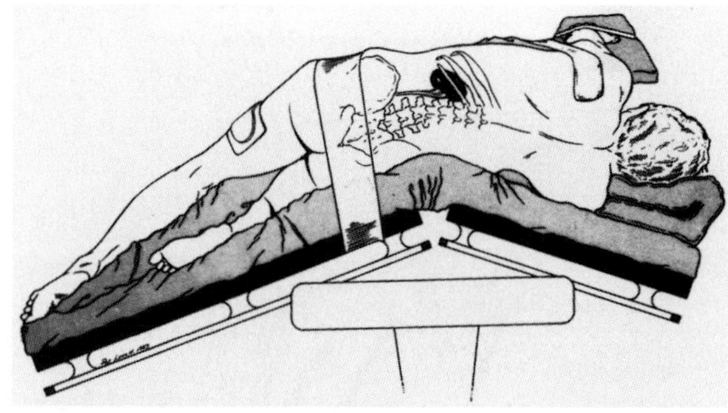

Fig. 13.5. Proper patient positioning for the flank approach. [From Novick AC, Streem SB (1992) Surgery of the kidney. In: Walsh PC, Retick AB, Stamey TA, Vaughan ED (eds) Cambell's urology, 6th edn. Saunders, Philadelphia, pp 2413–2500, Fig. 65-6]

with slight internal rotation at the shoulder. The arm is best supported by a well-padded airplane. After all pressure points are padded the patient is secured with wide cloth tape (3 inch) at the shoulder and superior iliac crest.

The flank incision is made directly over the appropriate rib, extending from the lateral aspect of the sacrospinalis muscle to the lateral aspect of the rectus abdominus muscle. The latissimus dorsi (lateral) and external oblique muscles are divided and the periosteum over the rib is incised (Fig. 13.6). The periosteal elevator is used to elevate the periosteum off the rib anteriorly, and the intercostal muscle fibers superiorly and inferiorly. The intercostal muscle fibers should be dissected off the rib in the

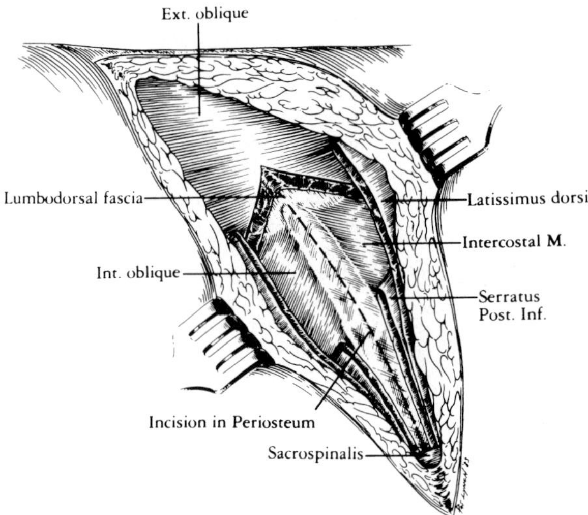



**Fig. 13.6.** The flank muscles in the posterior portion of the incision are divided to expose the rib. [From Novick AC, Streem SB (1992) Surgery of the kidney. In: Walsh PC, Retick AB, Stamey TA, Vaughan ED (eds) Cambell's urology, 6th edn. Saunders, Philadelphia, pp 2413–2500, Fig. 65-8]

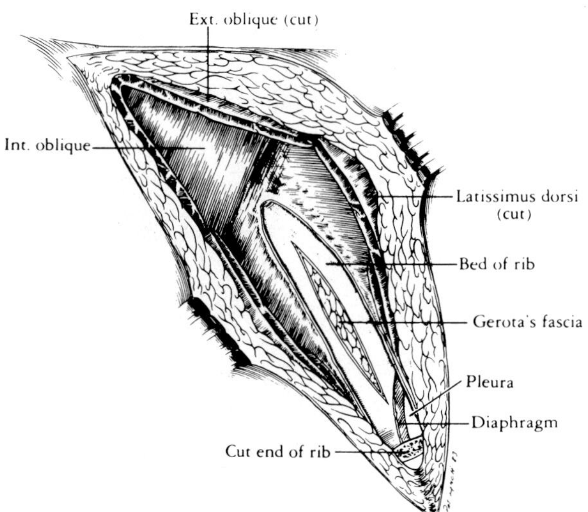



**Fig. 13.8.** The rib is resected, exposing the pleura and diaphragm in the posterior part of the wound. [From Novick AC, Streem SB (1992) Surgery of the kidney. In: Walsh PC, Retick AB, Stamey TA, Vaughan ED (eds), Cambell's urology, 6th edn. Saunders, Philadelphia, pp 2413–2500, Fig. 65-11]

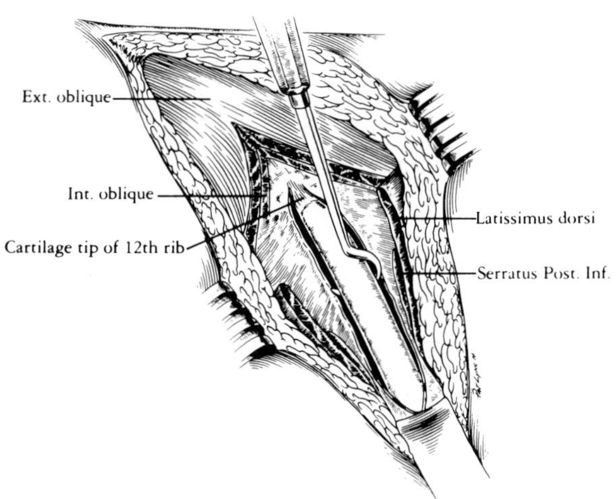



**Fig. 13.7.** The periosteum is dissected off the rib using the Doyen periosteal elevator. [From Novick AC, Streem SB (1992) Surgery of the kidney. In: Walsh PC, Retick AB, Stamey TA, Vaughan ED (eds) Cambell's urology, 6th edn. Saunders, Philadelphia, pp 2413–2500, Fig. 65-10]

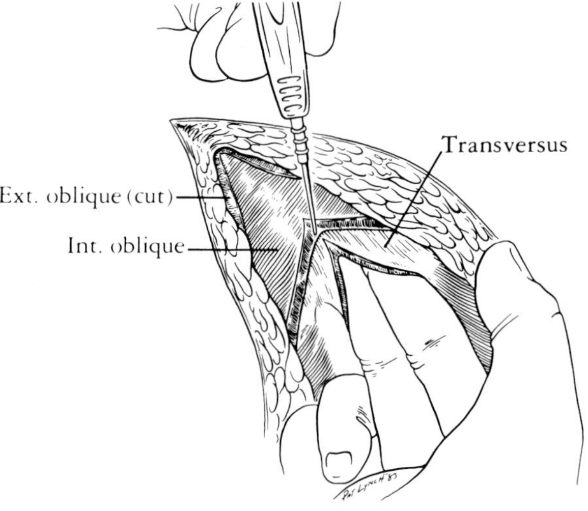



**Fig. 13.9.** The anterior abdominal muscles are incised. Note that the peritoneum is reflected medially. [From Novick AC, Streem SB (1992) Surgery of the kidney. In: Walsh PC, Retick AB, Stamey TA, Vaughan ED (eds) Cambell's urology, 6th edn. Saunders, Philadelphia, pp 2413–2500, Fig. 65-12]

direction of their fibers (inferior-posterior and superior-anterior). Mobilization of the posterior periosteum off the rib is completed with a Doyen periosteal elevator (Fig. 13.7). The rib is transected as far posterior as possible with a guillotine resector (Fig. 13.8).

Care must be taken to avoid entry into the pleura. The pleura should be reflected superiorly by dividing the fascial attachments to the diaphragm. Next, the lateral peritoneum is swept off the posterior aspect of the transversalis fascia. This is easily performed if in the appropriate plane. Next the anterior portion of the incision is completed by dividing the external and internal oblique and the transversus muscles with diathermy (Fig. 13.9). Note that the intercostal neurovascular bundle, which courses between the internal oblique and the transversus muscles, should be identified and preserved if possible.

A Finochietto retractor (authors' preference) is then placed over moistened gauze sponges to maintain exposure. No pressure is applied to the skin edges, which should be rolled outward. Slight caudal and lateral traction of the kidney provides exposure to the superior and medial attachments of the adrenal gland. On the right, the liver (located within the peritoneum) is retracted off the anterior aspect of the adrenal gland. Because the kidney is useful for inferior retraction, the superior dissection should be performed first in a lateral to medial direction. Vascular control is performed with either silk ligatures or hemoclips (authors' preference). Care must be taken to identify the lateral aspect of the inferior vena cava as the dissection is carried more medially on the right. Release of the superior attachments provides better exposure to the medial aspect of the adrenal and the inferior vena cava. The medial aspect of the dissection is performed with vascular control of the main arterial and venous supply to the adrenal gland. Attention to surgical detail allows control of the short right adrenal vein as it drains into the inferior vena cava. The inferior attachments to the kidney are dissected last and the adrenal gland is removed.

On the left, caudal and lateral traction of the kidney will expose the splenorenal ligament, which should be divided. This allows mobilization of the peritoneum (along with the pancreas and spleen), which is then retracted superiorly off the adrenal. Again, dissection is first performed in a lateral to medial direction along the superior aspect of the left adrenal gland. Care must be taken along the superior-medial aspect of the left adrenal; prominent phrenic venous drainage may be encountered and must be carefully controlled. Finally, once the medial attachments are controlled, the inferior dissection is performed. This includes the prominent inferior adrenal vein draining into the left renal vein. Once the inferior attachments have been dissected, the adrenal gland is removed.

The surgical bed is then inspected for hemostasis and irrigated with sterile water. In addition, inspection should be made of the diaphragm and pleura. If entry into the pleura is made, it can be closed with the use of a catheter (previously described) or if larger, may be treated with a chest tube overnight. The flank incision is then closed in two layers with a running internal and interrupted external (external oblique fascia) fashion.

## 13.8.3
## Transabdominal Approach

The transabdominal approach provides simultaneous access to both adrenals and allows for a thorough exploration of the abdomen. Furthermore, it provides exposure and visualization for large, vascular adrenal carcinomas that may involve contiguous organs. The anterior approach may be performed through a midline or a chevron incision. It is the authors' belief that the chevron incision provides better exposure in the epigastrium and access simultaneously to both adrenals than does the midline approach.

The chevron incision extends from the tips of the 12th rib and transverses 1–2 cm below the costal margins (Fig. 13.10). To expose the right adrenal gland, the avascular line of Toldt (lateral to the right colon) and hepatic flexure of the ascending colon are incised. The mesenteric attachments to the cecum and small bowel may then be incised up to the ligament of Treitz. The stomach and duodenum are then drawn medially after development of the

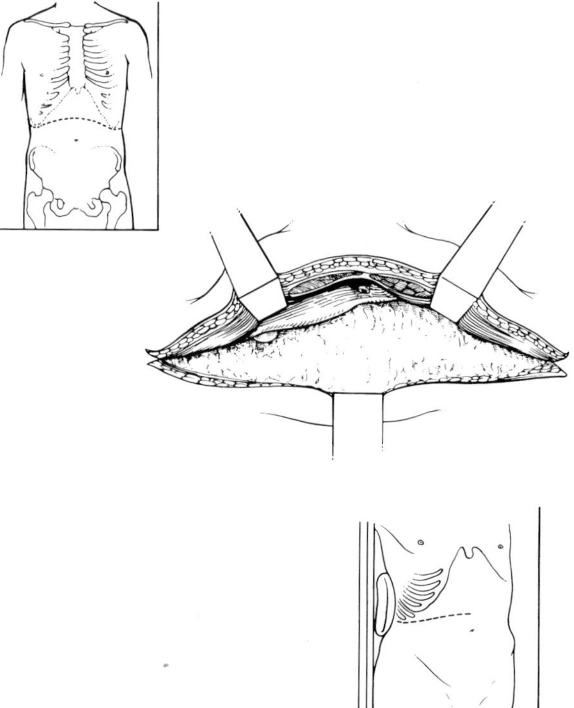

Fig. 13.10. Bilateral anterior subcostal transperitoneal incision (chevron). [From Novick AC, Streem SB (1992) Surgery of the kidney. In: Walsh PC, Retick AB, Stamey TA, Vaughan ED (eds), Cambell's urology, 6th edn. Saunders, Philadelphia, pp 2413–2500, Fig. 65-17]

Kocker maneuver. These maneuvers allow superior traction on the liver, medial retraction of the ascending colon and small bowel, and visualization of the adrenal gland. Once exposed, the adrenal can be removed with minimal manual pressure on the tumor itself.

An incision in the peritoneum is made directly over the inferior vena cava allows mobilization of the inferior vena cava. Gentle, caudal retraction on the kidney and medial retraction of the inferior vena cava provide access to the right adrenal gland and control of the prominent right adrenal vein. The right adrenal artery transverses to the adrenal posterior to the vena cava and can also be controlled. After the medial attachments have been dissected, the superior dissection is performed. The liver is lifted off the adrenal and the small vessels arising from the inferior phrenic blood supply are secured. The terminal step should again be the removal of the adrenal from the kidney (inferior attachments). Silk ligatures and/or hemoclips are used to maintain vascular control and hemostasis throughout the procedure.

Exposure to the left adrenal gland is made by incising the posterior peritoneum (lateral to the left colon) along the avascular line of Toldt up to the splenocolic ligament, which is also incised. This allows medial retraction of the descending colon. The plane between the pancreas and the spleen anteriorly and the adrenal posteriorly is then developed. The pancreas and the duodenum can then be mobilized and reflected medially and in a cephalad direction, providing exposure to the left adrenal. Ideally, the left renal vein should be identified early in the dissection and the prominent adrenal vein ligated as it enters the superior aspect of the renal vein. The superior attachments and the inferior phrenic vessels are then controlled with dissection directed from lateral to medial. Again, with the exception of the previously ligated left adrenal vein, the inferior attachments of the adrenal to the kidney are dissected last.

Following removal of the tumor, careful inspection is made to ensure hemostasis and to exclude injury to surrounding organs. The surgical bed is irrigated with sterile water. Drains are generally not necessary. The wound is closed in two layers; a running suture is used for the transversalis and posterior rectus sheath, while the anterior rectus sheath is closed with interrupted nonabsorbable suture incorporating the external oblique.

## 13.8.4
## Thoracoabdominal Approach

The thoracoabdominal incision is the authors' preferred approach to large adenomas, adrenal carcinomas, and pheochromocytomas. We strongly believe that this incision provides the best exposure and visualization possible. The thoracoabdominal incision provides a versatile approach to the retroperitoneum solely, or it can be combined with an intra-abdominal approach for extensive tumors or in complicated cases. The thoracoabdominal approach allows evaluation of the intra-abdominal contents along with inspection of the contralateral adrenal gland. Furthermore, this approach provides the ideal means to gain early vascular control of a tumor and allows for a safe en bloc dissection. This is critical, particularly in large tumors with extensive collateral vessels or those tumors with venous tumor thrombus involvement. We believe there are no absolute contraindications to this approach and routinely perform this incision for many indications, including radical nephrectomy, nephroureterectomy, all retroperitoneal tumors, retroperitoneal node dissections for testicular tumors, and ileoureteral substitutions.

Patient positioning is critical, and attention to detail facilitates all phases of the operation (Fig. 13.11). The patient should be positioned on the ipsilateral side of the operating table with the break of the table located immediately above the iliac crest. The contralateral leg (lower) is flexed 90° at the knee, and the hip is flexed about 30°. The ipsilateral shoulder is then torqued approximately 30° off the horizontal and brought across the chest to be placed in an adjustable arm rest. The authors prefer to use a padded airplane arm rest which provides an ideal positioning of the ipsilateral arm without pressure or stretch to the axillary structures. The contralateral arm is extended on an arm board ensuring avoidance of hyperextension of the limb. The pelvis remains nearly supine or slightly rotated 10° off the horizontal plane. A rolled sheet is placed longitudinally under the ipsilateral back, ensuring avoidance of any pressure on the buttocks. A similar roll is positioned under the contralateral abdomen to help secure the position. The table is then fully hyperextended and the patient secured with wide (3-inch) adhesive tape at the shoulder, hip, and leg. The table is tilted in the Trendelenburg position until the abdomen is in the horizontal plane. The ipsilateral leg remains extended (straight) along the lateral edge of the table, supported by a pillow behind the knee. All pressure points are padded.

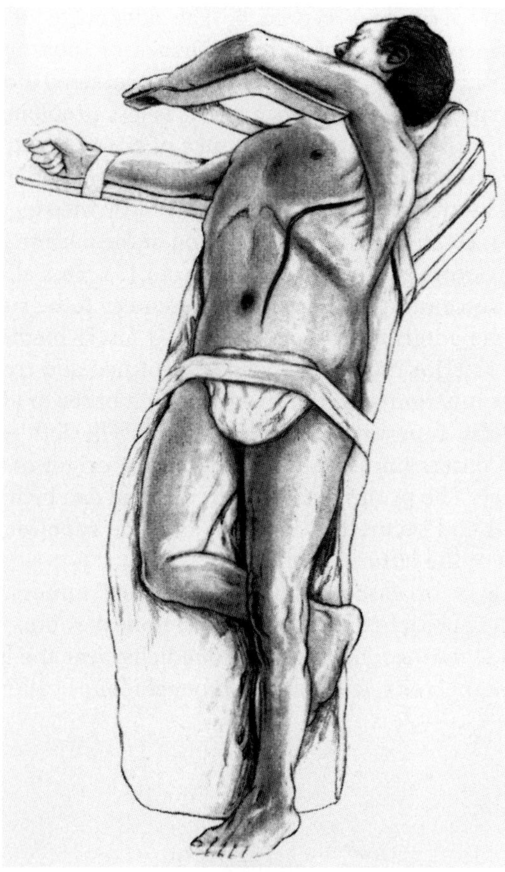

Fig. 13.11. Patient positioning for a right thoracoabdominal incision. Note that the patient's right side is adjacent to the ipsilateral edge of the operating table. [From Skinner DG, Lieskovsky G, Pritchett TR (1988) Technique of radical nephrectomy. In: Skinner DG, Lieskovsky G (eds) Diagnosis and management of genitourinary cancer. Saunders, Philadelphia, pp 684–693, Fig. 48-1]

Generally, an incision is made along the ninth rib. The size and location of the tumor, possible contiguous organ involvement, and the body habitus of the patient may otherwise dictate a higher or lower rib incision. The incision begins at the midaxillary line and extends across the costochondral junction to the epigastrium in a transverse nature. The incision is then directed inferiorly as either a midline or a paramedian incision. For very large tumors or bilateral tumors, a T-shaped incision may be employed, extending the horizontal portion of the epigastric incision across to the contralateral costochondral junction and then dropping an ipsilateral paramedian or midline extension inferiorly. This approach may also be employed when a vena caval tumor thrombus is associated with an adrenal tumor requiring vascular control of the vena cava

above the diaphragm or at the level of the right atrium (FIGUEROA et al. 1997).

The authors prefer a rib resection to an intercostal incision. Careful comparison of these two techniques reveals no difference in degree of pain or postoperative requirements for analgesics; rib resection is quicker, is easier to close, and provides a wider exposure without fracturing adjacent ribs. The subcutaneous tissues and muscles overlying the rib and periosteum are incised using diathermy, and a subperiosteal rib resection is performed in the standard fashion.

The anterior rectus fascia is incised, the rectus muscle retracted laterally, and the rectus muscle transected in the epigastrium with control of the epigastric vessels. Lateral retraction of the muscle prevents denervation of the rectus muscle with resultant diastasis and weakness of the abdominal wall.

The costochondral junction is then divided with heavy scissors after carefully and bluntly passing a Mayo scissors under the cartilage. Care must be taken to ensure that the abdominal peritoneum has been swept off the transversalis fascia posteriorly. This is an important step in order to identify the plane between the muscle and fascia of the abdominal wall (anteriorly) and the peritoneum (posteriorly), and in fact is the hallmark of an exclusively retroperitoneal dissection without entering the peritoneal cavity. An exclusively retroperitoneal dissection is appropriate for smaller, less complicated adrenal tumors. Development of the plane between the anterior surface of Gerota's fascia and the colonic mesentery and parietal peritoneum with large or vascular tumors may lead to considerable venous bleeding if the arterial supply is not first controlled. Therefore, when performing an adrenalectomy for large, vascular tumors, it is preferable to enter the peritoneum after dividing the costochondral junction to gain early vascular control. When the peritoneum is opened widely, the pleura is incised and the diaphragm divided in the direction of its fibers. It is helpful to first dissect the peritoneum off the diaphragm posteriorly before dividing the latter. This maneuver facilitates later mobilization of the liver for right-sided and of the spleen for left-sided tumors. A self-retaining Finochietto retractor is positioned, with the costochondral junction placed through the holes in the blades of the retractor and secured with towel clamps.

In the case of large tumors with extensive collateral blood supply, attention is then directed toward maximizing exposure and providing for early vascular control. For right-sided tumors, the cecum is first mobilized from the right lower quadrant by incising along the avascular line of Toldt and dividing the peritoneal attachments to the small bowel mesentery medially up to the ligament of Treitz (Fig. 13.12). When an ipsilateral nephrectomy is required along with an adrenalectomy, mobilization of the ascending colon overlying the tumor is deferred until the arterial supply is first secured. As the small bowel is elevated, the retroperitoneal aspects of the duodenum come into view and should be elevated off the great vessels along with the pancreas as the dissection continues to the ligament of Treitz (Kocker maneuver). At this point, exposure and visualization of the aorta and inferior vena cava are ideal and provide safe and early vascular control of the adrenal tumor and kidney if necessary. Following the medial dissection and vascular control, dissection of the tumor should continue, employing an en bloc technique with adequate surgical margins.

If the primary right adrenal tumor is small and does not appear to invade the mesentery of the colon, an adrenalectomy can be performed entirely via a retroperitoneal approach. The advantage of the retroperitoneal dissection is the lack of subsequent adhesions and prevention of possible small bowel obstruction. In addition, an ileus is less problematic with earlier postoperative return of bowel function.

For small left-sided adrenal tumors, a retroperitoneal approach can also be employed by incising the transversalis fascia at the junction of the peritoneum and Gerota's fascia laterally (Fig. 13.13). This allows the descending colon and its mesentery to be swept off the anterior surface of Gerota's fascia medially. The inferior mesenteric vein is identified and traced to its junction with the splenic vein in order to identify the superior mesenteric artery. The left renal vein passes immediately caudal to the origin of this artery. The prominent left adrenal vein can be identified and secured as it drains into the superior aspect of the left renal vein.

Large or vascular left-sided adrenal tumors are best approached via an intraperitoneal route. The duodenum can be mobilized medially near the ligament of Treitz, with intraperitoneal identification of

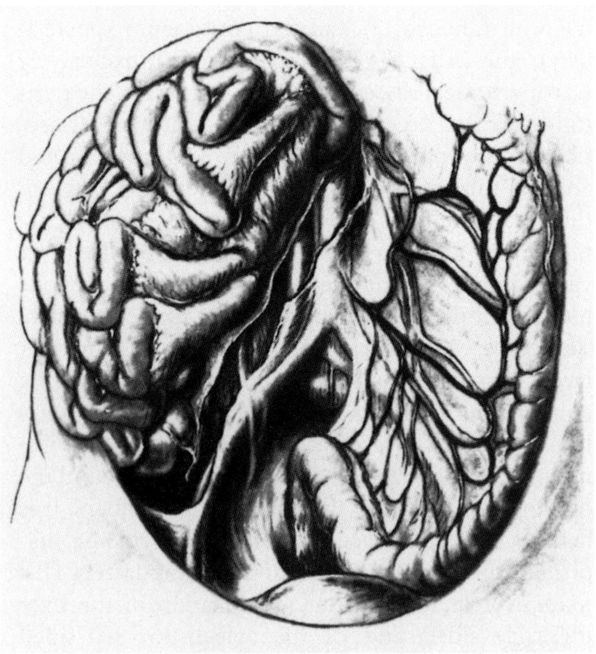

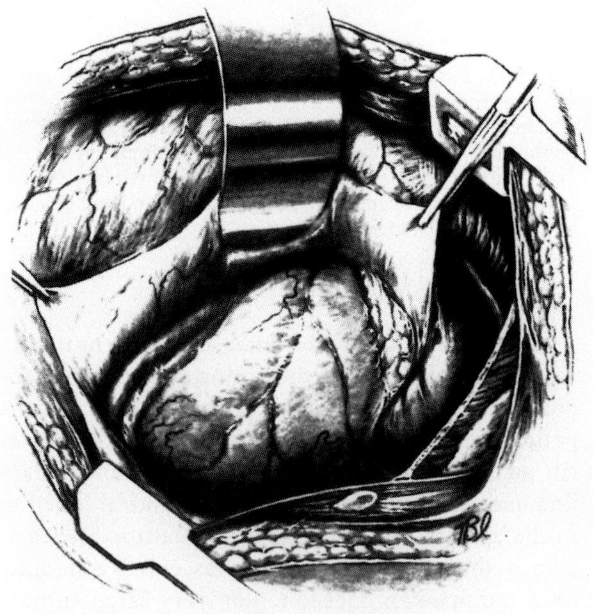

**Fig. 13.12.** Access to the right adrenal. The cecum and ascending colon are mobilized along the avascular line of Toldt. The peritoneal attachments to the small bowel are mobilized. This allows the duodenum and pancreas to be elevated off the retroperitoneal area and exposure to the great vessels. [From Skinner DG, Lieskovsky G, Pritchett TR (1988) Technique of radical nephrectomy. In: Skinner DG, Lieskovsky G (eds) Diagnosis and management of genitourinary cancer. Saunders, Philadelphia, pp 684–693, Fig. 48-2]

**Fig. 13.13.** For small, left-sided tumors the transversalis fascia can be divided in the groove between the descending colon and the anterior surface of Gerota's fascia, allowing the descending colon and its envelope of peritoneum to be swept medially off the anterior surface of Gerota's fascia. [From Skinner DG, Lieskovsky G, Pritchett TR (1988) Technique of radical nephrectomy. In: Skinner DG, Lieskovsky G (eds) Diagnosis and management of genitourinary cancer. Saunders, Philadelphia, pp 684–693, Fig. 48-4]

the inferior mesenteric vein (laterally). In some cases, ligating and dividing the inferior mesenteric vein provides valuable additional exposure. This approach again allows early and safe control of the blood supply to the adrenal tumor. Following the medial dissection and vascular control, dissection of the tumor should continue as previously described.

Once the tumor has been removed, careful inspection should be made to ensure all bleeding is controlled. Retroperitoneal drains are not necessary. A No. 22 chest tube is routinely inserted. The diaphragm is closed with a running size 0 absorbable suture in two layers. Closure of the remainder of the incision is performed by figure-of-eight, through-and-through, nonabsorbable sutures, securing all muscular layers of the chest and abdomen in one layer. Care should be taken to ensure that the knots are inverted, particularly in thin individuals. Medially, the diaphragm must be incorporated in several of the closing sutures to ensure separation of the pleural and abdominal or retroperitoneal cavities.

# References


Abrams HL, Siegelman S, Adam DF, Sanders R, Finberg HJ, Hessel SJ, McNeil BJ (1982) Computed tomography versus ultrasound of the adrenal gland: a prospective study. Radiology 143:121–128

Anson BJ, Caldwell EW, Pick JW, Beaton LE (1947) The blood supply of the kidney, suprarenal gland and associated structures. Surg Gynecol Obstet 84:313–320

Bagshawe KD (1960) Hypokalemia, carcinoma and Cushing's syndrome. Lancet II:284–287

Barzilay JL, Pazianos AG (1989) Adrenocortical carcinoma. Urol Clin North Am 16:457–468

Belldegrun A, Hussain S, Seltzer SE, Loughlin KR, Gittes RF, Richie JP (1986) The incidentally discovered adrenal mass: a therapeutic dilemma – BWH experience 1976–1983. Surg Gynecol Obstet 163:203–208

Belldegrun A, deKernion JB (1989) What to do about the incidentally found adrenal mass. World J Urol 7:117–120

Bravo EL (1991) Pheochromocytoma: new concepts and future trends. Kidney Int 40:544–556

Bravo EL, Tarazi RC, Fouad FM, Bidt DG, Gifford RW Jr. (1981) Clonidine-suppression test: a useful aid in the diagnosis of pheochromocytoma. N Engl J Med 305:623–626

Bravo EL, Tarazi RC, Dustan HP, et al. (1983) The changing clinical spectrum of primary aldosteronism. Am J Med 74:641

Brennan MF (1987) Adrenocorticoid carcinoma. Cancer 37:348

Chandler WF, Schteingart DE, Lloyd RV, McKeever PE, Perez-Ibarra G (1987) Surgical treatment of Cushing's disease. J Neurosurg 66:204–212

Conn JW (1955) Primary hyperaldosteronism: a new clinical syndrome. J Lab Clin Med 45:3–17

Conn JW (1967) The evolution of primary aldosteronism: 1954–1967. Harvey Lect 62:257

Copeland PM (1983) The incidentally discovered adrenal mass. Ann Intern Med 98:940–945

Cushing H (1912) The pituitary body and its disorders. J.B. Lippincott, Philadelphia

Dolan LM, Carey RM (1989) Adrenal cortical and medullary function: diagnostic tests. In: Vaughan ED Jr, Carey RM (eds) Adrenal disorders. Thieme Medical, New York, p 81

Donohue JP (1990) Surgically treatable adrenal disorders. Part I. AUA Update Series 19:146–151

Dunnick NR, Heaston D, Halvorsen R, et al. (1982) CT appearance of adrenal cortical carcinoma. J Comput Assist Tomogr 6:978–982

Ferriss JB, Beevers DG, Brown JJ, et al. (1978) Clinical, biochemical and pathological features of low-renin ("primary") hyperaldosteronism. Am Heart J 95:375–388

Figueroa AJ, Stein JP, Lieskovsky G, Skinner DG (1997) Adrenal cortical carcinoma associated with venous tumor thrombus extension. Br J Urol 80:397–400

Geisinger MA, Zelch MG, Bravo EL, et al. (1983) Primary hyperaldosteronism: comparison of CT, adrenal venography and venous sampling. AJR 141:299

Glazer GM, Woolsey EJ, Borrello J, et al. (1986) Adrenal tissue characterization using MR imaging. Radiology 158:73–79

Goldfarb DA (1993) Surgical adrenal disease in the National Center for Advanced Medical Education. Urology Review, pp 1–13, Cook County Hospital, Chicago

Halberg FE, Sheline GE (1987) Radiotherapy of pituitary tumors. Endocrinol Metab Clin North Am 16:667–684

Hall WA, Luciano MG, Doppman JL, Patronas NJ, Oldfield EH (1990) Pituitary magnetic resonance imaging in normal human volunteers: occult adenomas in the general population. Ann Intern Med 120:817–820

Hengstmann JH (1985) Evaluation of screening tests for pheochromocytoma. Cardiology 72:153–156

Hume DM (1960) Pheochromocytoma and hypertension: an analysis of 207 cases. Int Abstr Surg 99:458–465

Jubiz W, Meikle AW, West CD, et al. (1970) Single dose metyrapone test. Arch Intern Med 125:472–474

Klibanski A, Zervas NT (1991) Diagnosis and management of hormone-secreting pituitary adenomas. N Engl J Med 324:822–831

Libertino JA (1988) Surgery of adrenal disorders. Surg Clin North Am 68:1027–1056

Liddle GW (1960) Tests of pituitary-adrenal suppressibility in the diagnosis of Cushing's syndrome. J Clin Endocrinol Metab 20:1539–1560

Ludecke DE (1991) Transnasal microsurgery of Cushing's disease 1990. Overview including personal experiences with 256 patients. Pathol Res Pract 187:608–612

Luton J-P, Cerdas S, Billaud L, et al. (1990) Clinical features of adrenocortical carcinoma, prognostic factors, and the effect of mitotane therapy. N Engl J Med 322:1195–1201

Mitty HA, Yeh HC (1982) Radiology of the adrenals for sonography and CT. W.B. Saunders, Philadelphia

Moore TJ, Dluhy RG, Williams GH, et al. (1976) Nelson's syndrome: frequency, prognosis and effect of prior pituitary irradiation. Ann Intern Med 85:731–734

Nelson DH, Meakin JW, Dealy JB Jr., Matson DD, Emerson K Jr., Thorn GW (1958) ACTH-producing tumor of the pituitary gland. N Engl J Med 259:161–164

Neville AM, O'Hare MJ (1982) The human adrenal cortex: pathology and biology – an integrated approach. Springer-Verlag, New York Berlin Heidelberg

Newhouse JH (1990) MRI of the adrenal gland. Urol Radiol 12:1

Orth DN (1995) Cushing's syndrome. N Engl J Med 32:791–803

Orth DN, Liddle GW (1971) Results of treatment in 108 patients with Cushing's syndrome. N Engl J Med 285:243–247

Pepe GJ, Albrecht ED (1990) Regulation of the primate fetal adrenal cortex. Endocr Rev 11:151–176

Pommier RF, Brennan MF (1992) An eleven-year experience with adrenocortical carcinoma. Surgery 112:963–971

Richie JP, Gittes RF (1980) Carcinoma of the adrenal cortex. Cancer 45:1957–1964

Ross NS, Aron DC (1990) Hormonal evaluation of the patient with an incidentally discovered adrenal mass. N Engl J Med 323:1401–1405

Scott EM, Thomas A, McGarrigle HHG, Lachelin GC (1990) Serial adrenal ultrasonography in normal neonates. J Ultrasound Med 9:279–283

Shapiro B, Sisson JC, Eyre P, Copp JE, Dmucowski C, Beierwaltes WH (1985) [131]I-MIBG – new agent in diagnosis and treatment of pheochromocytoma. Cardiology 72:137–142

Sipple JH (1961) The association of pheochromocytoma with carcinoma of the thyroid gland. Am J Med 31:163–166

Stackpole RH, Melicow MM, Uson AC (1963) Pheochromocytoma in children. J Pediatr 66:315

Teasdale E, Teasdale G, Mohsen F, Macpherson P (1986) High-resolution computed tomography in pituitary microadenoma: is seeing believing? Clin Radiol 37:227–232

Thomas JL, Bernardino ME, Samaan NA, Hickey RC (1980) CT of pheochromocytoma. AJR 135:477

Tikkakoski T, Taavitsainen M, Paivansalo M, et al. (1991) Accuracy of adrenal biopsy guided by ultrasound and CT. Acta Radiol 32:371–374

van Heerden JA, Sheps SG, Hamberger B, et al. (1982) Pheochromocytoma: current status and changing trends. Surgery 91:367–373

Vaughan DE Jr (1997) Diagnosis of surgical adrenal disorders. AUA Update Series 16:306–311

Wilson CB, Tyrell JB, Fitzgerald PA, Pitts LH (1980) Cushing's disease and Nelson's syndrome. Clin Neurosurg 27:19–30

Wooten MD, King DK (1993) Adrenal cortical carcinoma. Epidemiology and treatment with mitotane and a review of the literature. Cancer 145:3145–3155

Zovickian J, Oldfield EH, Doppman JL, Cutler GB, Loriaux DL (1988) Usefulness of inferior petrosal sinus venous endocrine markers in Cushing's disease. J Neurosurg 68:205–210

# 14 Diagnosis and Management of Retroperitoneal Tumors in Pediatric Patients

G.A. BOGAERT and B.A. KOGAN

CONTENTS



## 14.1
## Introduction

Retroperitoneal masses are considered as a single diagnostic and therapeutic complex because of the similarity of their clinical manifestations. These masses include different well-defined pathologic entities that can be benign or neoplastic. In this chapter, we will focus primarily on the retroperitoneal neoplastic lesions and will briefly discuss the possible benign lesions that should to be considered in the differential diagnosis.

The commonest presenting feature in a child with a retroperitoneal tumor is an abdominal mass. Of


G.A. BOGAERT, MD, Professor of Pediatric Urology, Department of Urology, University Hospitals Gasthuisberg, Catholic University of Leuven, Herestraat 49, B-3000 Leuven, Belgium
B.A. KOGAN, MD, Professor and Chief, Division of Urology, K209/A-108, The Albany Medical College, 47 New Scotland Avenue, Albany, NY 12208-3479, USA


all the children presenting with an abdominal mass, one-third have a retroperitoneal mass. Of the retroperitoneal masses, 40% are cystic or hydronephrotic renal lesions (BELL 1938; SCANLAN 1959). Because of the different nature of a retroperitoneal mass, the child requires specific, precise, and if possible minimally invasive investigations. If an abdominal or retroperitoneal mass is suspected, it is important to localize the tumor precisely. The newer imaging modalities, including ultrasound, nuclear isotoped scan, computed tomography (CT), magnetic resonance imaging (MRI), and positron emission tomography (PET), allow fast and precise localization of the tumor in most cases. Except when fever or acute symptoms are present, a complete and accurate diagnostic workup is important prior to treatment.

## 14.1.1
## Incidence

The incidence of malignancy in children is low, approximately 12/100 000 children. Nonetheless, it is the second most frequent cause of child mortality behind accidents.

Of all malignancies in children, 15%–20% are urologic. These tumors are: nephroblastoma (Wilms) (6%), neuroblastoma of the retroperitoneum or the adrenal gland (5.5%), rhabdomyosarcoma of the bladder, prostate, the paratesticular soft tissue, and the retroperitoneum (5%), testicular tumors (1%), and tumors that secondarily invade genitourinary organs (leukemia and malignant lymphoma) (<1%). Even less common are pheochromocytoma and carcinoma of the medulla of the adrenal gland.

## 14.1.2
## Diagnosis

In examining a child with an abdominal mass, the clinician should try to differentiate an intraperitoneal from a retroperitoneal mass. Intraperitoneal masses, such as hepatomegaly and splenomegaly, usually can be easily distinguished by palpation, and may also be detected during a routine prenatal or postnatal ultrasound examination. Indeed, most tumors are not symptomatic and are detected during a routine physical examination. Ultrasound then serves to confirm the clinical suspicion and facilitate the exact localization of the tumor.

Knowledge of the differential diagnosis is of major importance; not only the clinical findings and the radiographic appearance but also the age of the child and whether tumors are unilateral or bilateral will assist in reaching the correct diagnosis. Blood studies and urinalysis will also be helpful and are of importance for tumor staging.

More precise localization and staging of the tumor can be achieved by means of CT, MRI, or PET (see Chap. 4). These imaging techniques are available at most major medical centers and have largely rendered intravenous pyelography (IVP) obsolete.

## 14.2
## Renal Masses

### 14.2.1
### Multicystic Dysplastic Kidney (Type II Potter)

*Synonym*: Potter II (nongenetic)

#### 14.2.1.1
#### Classification

In Potter IIa the kidney appears as a "bunch of grapes" with little stroma between the cysts (Fig. 14.1a). In Potter IIb the kidney has very small cysts and the stroma predominates ("solid cystic dysplasia").

#### 14.2.1.2
#### Clinical Features

The multicystic kidney is the most common renal mass in the newborn period. It is believed that the original process begins by the 8th week in utero. The disease is more common on the left side and is slightly more common in males. Unless there has been a prenatal diagnosis, these children have no symptoms. Ultrasound will usually demonstrate

multiple cystic areas without apparent connections and of different sizes, with no evidence of renal parenchyma (Fig. 14.1b).

#### 14.2.1.3
#### Diagnostic Workup and Staging

With the routine use of prenatal ultrasound, the overall frequency of diagnosis has increased. The mean age at the time of diagnosis is around the 28th week of gestation. If ultrasound cannot clearly differentiate between cysts (multicystic kidney) and hydronephrosis (ureteropelvic junction (UPJ) obstruction, a postnatal nuclear renal scan (dimercaptosuccinic acid) will help to make the diagnosis. A multicystic kidney has minimal or no function and complete nonfunction in a hydronephrosis is very rare.

It is also important to investigate the contralateral kidney as there is a higher incidence of contralateral abnormalities, especially UPJ obstruction, reflux, and obstructive megaureter.

#### 14.2.1.4
#### Treatment and Prognosis

Treatment is still controversial and includes nephrectomy or observation. As previously stated, a renal scan will have demonstrated minimal or no function, and the general rule states that these kidneys can be ignored unless the volume of the kidney is increased significantly (PATHAK and WILLIAMS 1964). If an underlying malignancy, such as congenital mesoblastic nephroma or a Wilms' tumor, is not completely ruled out, more detailed imaging studies (CT scan or MRI) are the diagnostic tools of choice.

There have been several case reports in the literature of patients who developed cancers in previously unrecognized multicystic kidneys (BARRETT and WINELAND 1980; BURGLER and HAURI 1983; BIRKEN et al. 1985; NAKADA et al. 1985). However, these were case reports and one can argue over whether the correct diagnosis of multicystic kidney was made in the first place. Recently, a larger series of 120 patients was described by NOE et al. If it is accepted that there is a 1% chance of Wilms' tumor and a 5% incidence of nodular renal blastema, one would have to perform 2000 nephrectomies for multicystic kidney disease to prevent one Wilms' tumor (NOE et al. 1989).

Although many clinicians recommend periodic ultrasound studies until the kidney involutes, this

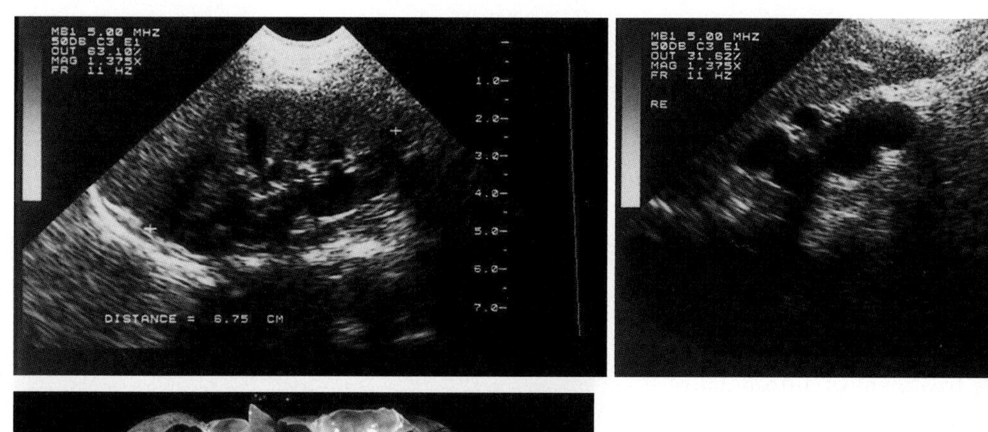

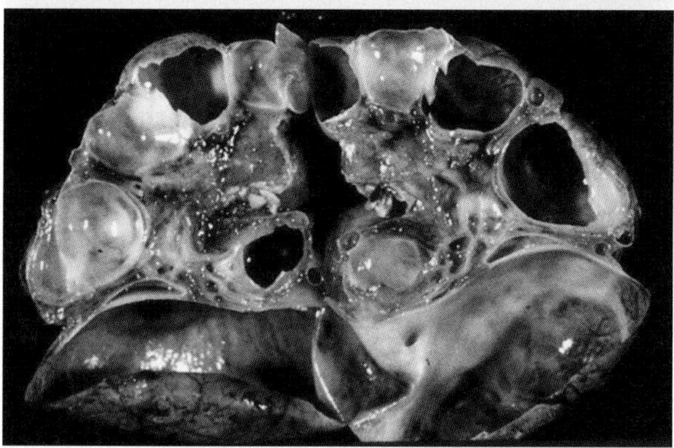

**Fig. 14.1. a** Ultrasound image of both kidneys in a 1-year-old boy with a history of abnormal right kidney on fetal ultrasound. The images show a normal-appearing left kidney and a right multicystic dysplstic kidney. **b** Macroscopic appearance after surgical removal of a multicystic kidney in another patient

leaves dysplastic renal tissue which may still be at risk of malignancy. Ultrasound is not a good diagnostic tool to follow these patients because most kidneys shrink and lose cyst fluid, leaving the dysplastic kidney in the center, which is frequently not well visualized (COLODNY 1995; MINEVICH et al. 1997).

Another concern is the development of hypertension in children with multicystic kidney disease. GORDON et al. (1988) have described in a review article that there is no proof that the incidence of hypertension is higher in children with a retained multicystic dysplastic kidney. Surgical exploration is indicated if the diagnosis becomes equivocal at any point or should concerns exist regarding compliance with follow-up (Minevich et al. 1997).

## 14.2.2
## Autosomal Recessive Polycystic Kidney Disease (Type I Potter)

*Synonyms*: Potter I (genetic form) or (previously) polycystic kidney

This form of polycystic kidney disease is better known as the "infantile" form of renal cystic disease. The incidence is extremely low, 1:40000 live births

(ZERRES et al. 1996). The disease is autosomal recessive and has perinatal, neonatal, infantile, and juvenile forms. The expression and severity of the disease vary markedly. In severe cases, there may be biliary ectasia and periportal fibrosis. In infants in whom the disease is evident at birth, there will be respiratory failure due to pulmonary hypoplasia and prenatal oliguria. The prognosis depends on the age at presentation, but the overall survival rate is very low.

### 14.2.2.1
### Staging

In the absence of prenatal detection by ultrasound, the first sign of disease is the bilateral enormous flank masses. Oliguria and increased serum creatinine are typical findings in severe cases, but they are not specific. Ultrasound examination will demonstrate increased medullary echogenicity and it might even be possible to detect small cysts. If the diagnosis remains in doubt, however, a CT scan or MRI will help to establish the diagnosis because of the higher sensitivity of these imaging modalities to inhomogeneity. On an IVP, the difference between a multicystic kidney and polycystic kidneys is that mild forms of autosomal recessive polycystic kidney disease show functioning kidneys with typical radial streaking (nephrogram). A liver biopsy will also confirm the diagnosis by demonstrating biliary ectasia and periportal fibrosis.

### 14.2.2.2
### Treatment

There is no effective treatment of autosomal recessive polycystic kidney disease. In mild forms, salt losing may be present and its replacement is of importance. The multiorgan involvement of kidney, liver, and lung (pulmonary hypoplasia) may be treated symptomatically but none of these children will survive the complications of their disease.

### 14.2.3
### Polycystic Kidney (Type III Potter)

*Synonyms*: Potter III (genetic form) – autosomal dominant; "adult" type of polycystic kidney disease

This autosomal dominant form of polycystic kidney disease is far more frequent than the recessive form and accounts for 10% of all the patients in Europe and the United States who are receiving chronic hemodialysis (European Dialysis and Transplant Association, 1978). The gene responsible for this disease has been localized on chromosome 16 (BREUNING et al. 1986). The disease affects both kidneys and can be recognized at birth. However, before the era of ultrasound, most patients were diagnosed late, when they became symptomatic between the age of 30 and 50 years. If neonates are symptomatic with the disease, the degree of significant respiratory distress and renal failure will predict the prognosis of these children. There will most often be no effect on the renal function before the age of 40 years. Other organs, such as liver, pancreas, spleen, and lungs may also present with cysts.

### 14.2.3.1
### Staging

Neonates with the disease may present clinically with enlarged kidneys. However, in some cases renal failure will have caused prenatal pulmonary hypoplasia, and the prognosis is then bad. Routine use of ultra-

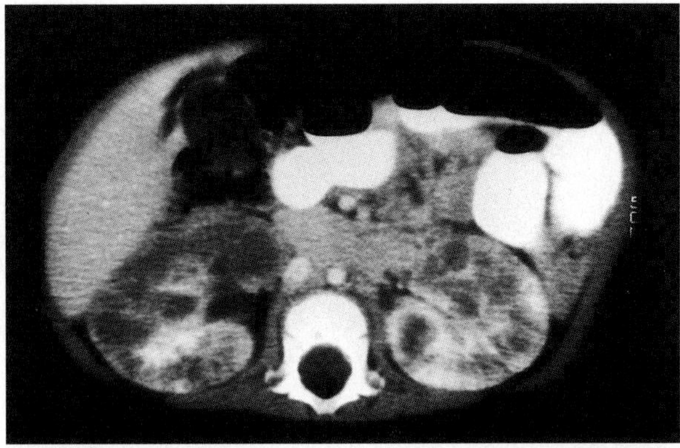

a

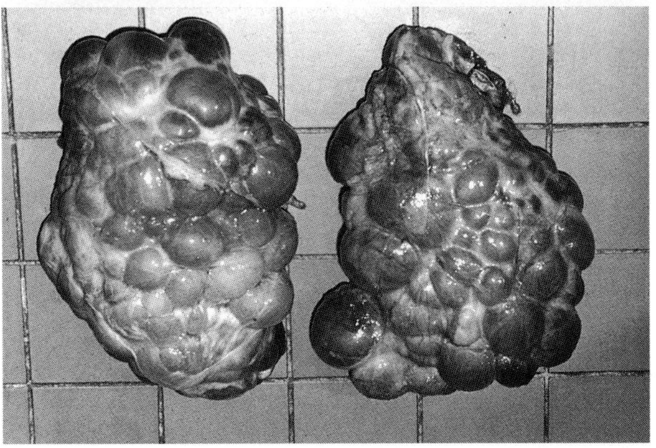

b

**Fig. 14.2. a** CT image of a 13-year-old girl with the autosomal dominant form of polycystic kidney disease. **b** Macroscopic appearance after surgical removal of enormous kidneys from an adult patient with the autosomal dominant form of polycystic kidney disease

sound in children of families at risk can detect the disease early (Fig. 14.2a). However, an in-depth family history of two or three generations will provide the most valuable information. If this history is inconclusive, both parents should undergo an ultrasound examination of the abdomen.

On a nuclear renal scan, a typical "Swiss cheese" effect is present. In addition, the diagnosis of autosomal dominant polycystic kidney can be made within a family by chromosomal analysis looking for the abnormality of chromosome 16.

### 14.2.3.2
### Treatment

As with multicystic kidney disease, there is no cure for polycystic kidney disease itself. Therefore, management of these patients is focused on treating secondary problems such as urinary infections, urinary stone formation, hypertension, and renal failure.

Better medical treatment of hypertension, extracorporeal shock wave treatment, and the use of prophylactic antibiotics have improved the outcome in these patients.

Surgery may consist in unroofing cysts or removing the enormous kidneys (Fig. 14.2b). Surgery is only indicated if pain becomes significant or if hypertension is difficult to control with medical therapy. Percutaneous aspiration of cysts is not helpful because the cysts do not collapse and hypertension cannot be controlled (BENNETT et al. 1987).

Kidney transplantation is often necessary. However, until recently living donor transplantation from siblings was not indicated because of the high risk of autosomal dominant polycystic kidney disease in the donors. Now genetic screening tests can be used to effectively screen potential donors.

## 14.2.4
## Pseudotumor

*Synonym*: Anomalous calyx

### 14.2.4.1
### Staging

If a localized renal mass is seen between the infundibulum of the upper and middle calyces, it might be a hypertrophied column of Bertin. Ultrasound examination will show a normal echogenic pattern of the renal parenchyma and a nuclear renal scan will show normal uptake and drainage in this area (PARKER et al. 1976).

### 14.2.4.2
### Treatment

No treatment is necessary.

## 14.2.5
## Hydronephrosis and Urinoma

Hydronephrosis is easily detected by ultrasound. However, dilated calyces might be mistaken for renal cysts. Hydronephrosis is usually due to an inefficient drainage of urine out of the kidney. If unilateral, a UPJ or ureterovesical junction obstruction will be the most common underlying cause. If bilateral hydronephrosis is present, the obstruction will be subvesical and vesicorenal reflux will commonly be seen.

Nonobstructive hydronephrosis may be due to megacalycosis, megaureter, and hydrocalycosis or the prune-belly syndrome.

A urinoma is a urine-containing pseudocyst around the kidney due to acute high hydrostatic intrarenal pressure resulting in rupture of a fornix. It is mostly seen in children with an intravesical obstruction.

### 14.2.5.1
### Staging

Differential diagnosis between cysts, dilated calyces, and tumor is essential. A combination of family history, physical findings, ultrasound examination, renal scan, and CT scan or MRI will help to make an accurate diagnosis. An impression of urinary drainage (degree of obstruction) is obtained by performing a renal isotope scan using mercaptoacetyltriglycine and furosemide.

A urinoma is visualized by ultrasound as a fluid collection adjacent to the kidney. Usually a certain degree of calyceal dilatation is seen. If the obstruction was released by the rupture of a calyx, the calyceal dilatation may not be a predominant feature.

### 14.2.5.2
### Treatment

The treatment of hydronephrosis and urinoma will depend on the symptoms and must be specific to the etiology.

## 14.2.6
## Mesoblastic Nephroma

*Synonym*: Congenital mesoblastic nephroma

Mesoblastic nephroma is usually unilateral and is more common in boys. These children will present in the neonatal period with an asymptomatic renal tumor. Mesoblastic nephroma is often associated with a history of polyhydramnios. Clinical findings are similar to those in Wilms' tumor and the only difference is the age of the patients.

When congenital mesoblastic nephroma is completely excised, the prognosis is good (SNYDER et al. 1981).

### 14.2.6.1
### *Staging*

Diagnosis and staging are achieved using classical imaging techniques, ultrasound, and three-dimensional imaging with CT scan or MRI.

### 14.2.6.2
### Treatment

Complete surgical removal must be performed because the tumor tends to be infiltrating. If the kidney is completely removed, no other therapy is necessary. When treated as a Wilms' tumor with radiation and chemotherapy, the treatment morbidity found in these children was significantly worse (WIGGER 1969; WIGGER and BAERT 1970). Hence an accurate preoperative diagnosis is essential.

### 14.2.7
### Nephroblastomatosis

Nephroblastomatosis is a bilateral renal disease with a genetic predisposition and a high potential for development of a malignant Wilms' tumor. Nephroblastomatosis is defined as the diffuse or multifocal presence of nephrogenic rests or their recognized derivatives. Because of the similarity on ultrasound and CT scan, differentiation from autosomal recessive polycystic kidney disease and bilateral Wilms' tumor can be difficult.

It is now widely accepted that nephro-blastomatosis is a precursor of Wilms' tumor, and the recognition of this disease has tremen-dously improved the understanding of the patho-genesis of the Wilms' tumor (BOVE and McADAMS 1976). More recently, Beckwith et al. have reexamined this pathogenesis and speculated that in the development of a Wilms' tumor, the lesions of nephroblastomatosis are the precursors that undergo a second "hit" in the two-step process of oncologic induction (BRESLOW et al. 1988; BECKWITH et al. 1990).

### 14.2.7.1
### *Staging*

Complete three-dimensional imaging of the abdomen and thorax is necessary for staging.

### 14.2.7.2
### Treatment

Nephroblastomatosis does not require treatment. If there is no effect on renal function, observation is sufficient. This condition may mature to normal kidney, but if massive it can develop into a Wilms' tumor. After chemotherapy it usually regresses and no radiation therapy is necessary.

### 14.2.8
### Renal Vein Thrombosis

Renal vein thrombosis occurs most frequently in the neonatal period (65% of cases occur in the first 2 weeks of life) (LLOYD 1986). Although renal vein thrombosis may be seen in otherwise healthy neonates, it is most often secondary to a severe illness. These neonates with secondary renal vein thrombosis usually have sepsis, dehydration, and/or maternal diabetes. They will present with an abdominal mass, severe hematuria, proteinuria, and hypertension (PARROTT and WOODARD 1976). Renal vein thrombosis is most often unilateral, but also can be bilateral (20%).

### 14.2.8.1
### *Staging*

These children either will present with a renal mass, severe hematuria, proteinuria, and hypertension or will develop these symptoms as a complication of a previous serious illness.

The kidney on ultrasound is enlarged and shows regions of low and high echogenicity as a result of the hemorrhagic areas. The thrombus in the renal vein is usually well demonstrated. CT scan and/or MRI may help to evaluate the extent of the thrombus, but usually do not affect the treatment or prognosis.

### 14.2.8.2
### *Treatment*

Unilateral renal vein thrombosis is treated with immediate hydration, correction of the electrolyte imbalance, and systemic antibiotics. Two management alternatives are currently available. First, selective intravenous thrombolytic therapy with tissue plasminogen activator (TPA) or low-dose streptokinase (50 U/kg per hour) (LeBLANC et al. 1986). Potential complications of this treatment are bleeding and allergic reactions; however, the low-dose treatment regimen in children has shown an acceptable morbidity. The second alternative is anticoagulant therapy with high-dose heparin (100 U/4 h) maintained for 2 weeks (BELMAN et al. 1970).

In bilateral renal vein thrombosis the treatment may be the same, if the clinical course allows sufficient time. Renal failure, pulmonary embolism, and death are the threatening complications. If the caval thrombus is large, surgical removal may be the best choice. Clinical experience has demonstrated that even with little back bleeding from the renal veins at the time of removal of the thrombus, the kidneys can be preserved (BROMBERG and FIRLIT 1990).

## 14.2.9
## Wilms' Tumor

*Synonyms*: Renal embryoma; nephroblastoma

Wilms' tumor is a solid malignant tumor of embryonic renal tissue. It is the most common malignant neoplasm of the urinary tract in children and accounts for 6% of all childhood tumors. In 75% of cases, the diagnosis is made between 1 and 5 years of age, with a peak incidence between 3 and 4 years. The male to female ratio is 1:1.

Two forms of the disease are recognized: hereditary and nonhereditary. Genetic research has discovered that loci on chromosome 11 are important in association with the Beckwith-Wiedemann syndrome and the Wilms' tumor–aniridia–genitourinary abnormalities–mental retardation (= WAGR) syndrome (RICCARDI et al. 1978; YUNIS and RAMSAY 1980; KOUFOS et al. 1984). It has been suggested that on the short arm of chromosome 11 is a recessive tumor suppressor gene. Other associations have been found with the insulin growth factor II gene and the tumor suppressor gene p53 (JUNIEN and HENRY 1994).

Approximately 15% of the children with a Wilms' tumor have associated anomalies listed below (PENDERGRASS 1976):

- WAGR syndrome
- Denys-Drash syndrome (nephropathy and pseudohermaphroditism)
- Beckwith-Wiedemann syndrome (visceromegaly, omphalocele, hemihypertrophy, microcephaly, and mental retardation)
- Aniridia (Wilms' tumor occurs in 33% of children with aniridia)

- Hemihypertrophy (2.9% of the patients with Wilms' tumor)
- Musculoskeletal anomalies (2.9% of the patients with Wilms' tumor)
- Genitourinary abnormalities (4.4% of the patients with Wilms' tumor): renal hypoplasia, ectopia, hypospadias, cryptorchidism
- Second malignant neoplasm (15% of the patients with Wilms' tumor)

### 14.2.9.1
### Staging

In most of the cases, the children are asymptomatic. An abdominal mass is a common finding and one-third of the children will present with abdominal pain. Gross hematuria may be observed, and it is usually a sign that the tumor has invaded the collecting system.

On clinical examination 25% of the children will have hypertension. Also, if a renal tumor is suspected, one should look for associated anomalies such as aniridia, hemihypertrophy, and other genitourinary abnormalities.

As usual, ultrasound will be the first study that will help to make the diagnosis of a renal tumor (Fig. 14.3a). It may also be the first step in staging by visualizing and allowing evaluation of the vena cava and the renal vein. However, CT and MRI will provide the surgeon with accurate delineation of the tumor. These imaging studies will help to examine the large vessels, the contralateral kidney, and the lungs (Fig. 14.3b–d). If the radiographic studies cannot rule out the possibility of a neuroblastoma, urinary catecholamines should be determined.

The most commonly used staging systems are those of the American National Wilms' Tumor Study Group and the classic TNM classification:

1. *National Wilms' Tumor Study Group staging system* (D'ANGIO et al. 1989):
- Stage I: Tumor limited to the kidney and completely excised. The capsule is intact. There is no spillage of tumor during removal.
- Stage II: Tumor extends beyond the kidney but is completely removed and/or vessels contain tumor thrombus, and/or there is local spillage confined to the flank or if a biopsy is performed.
- Stage III: Residual tumor confined to the abdomen exists after resection. Lymph nodes are involved, diffuse contamination has occurred, peritoneal implants are found, tumor extends beyond surgi-

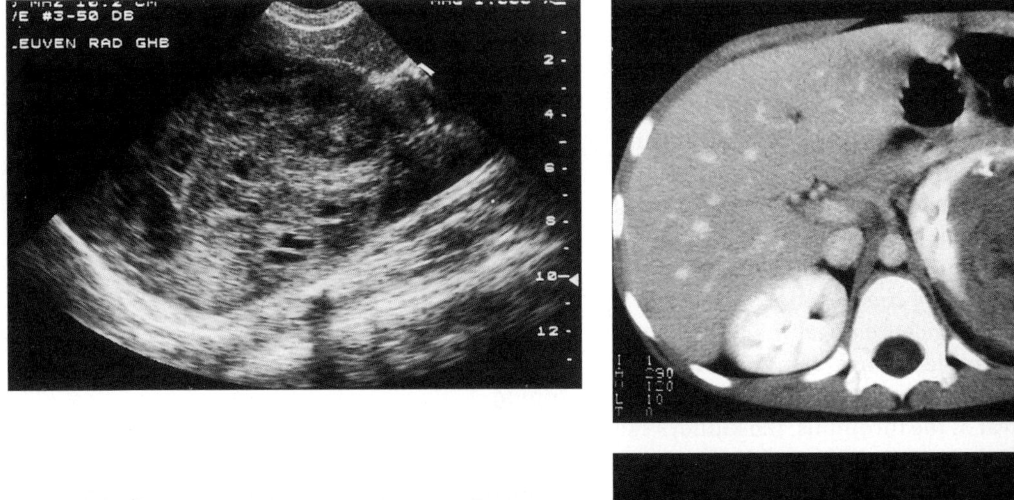

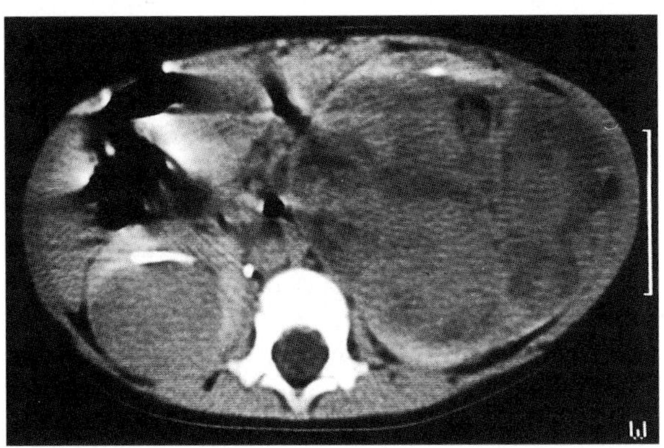

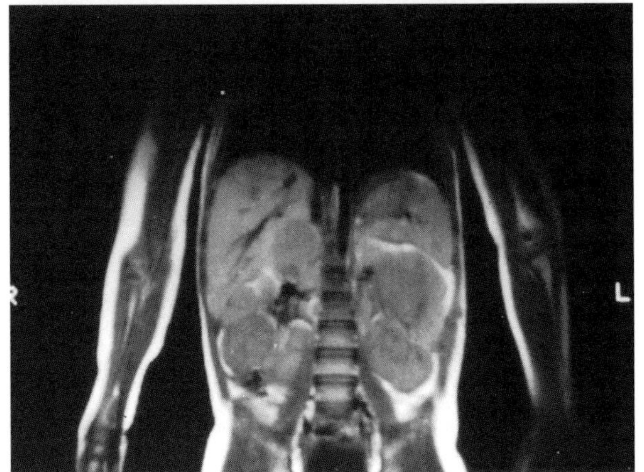

**Fig. 14.3. a** Sonogram of a Wilms' tumor in the left kidney. **b** CT image of a Wilms' tumor in the left kidney. **c** CT image of a bilateral Wilms' tumor. **d** MR image of the same child as in **c**

cal margins, and/or the tumor is not completely resected.

- Stage IV: Hematogenous metastases are found such as lung metastases.
- Stage V: Bilateral renal involvement is found at diagnosis.

2. *TNM classification*
- T1: Tumor limited to one kidney; surface of the kidney and the tumor <80 cm$^2$
- T2: Tumor limited to one kidney; surface of the kidney and the tumor >80 cm$^2$
- T3: Rupture of the tumor before treatment and/or involvement of adjacent abdominal organs
- T4: Bilateral tumors
- N0: No involvement of the regional lymph nodes
- N1: Involvement of one positive lymph node
- M0: No evidence of metastasis
- M1: Evidence of distant metastasis

### 14.2.9.2
### Treatment

The treatment of a Wilms' tumor is coordinated by national or international multicenter studies. The largest groups are: NWTS (National Wilms' Tumor Study, U.S.) and the SIOP (Societe International d'Oncologie Pediatrique).

In the United States the current treatment protocol consists of a combination of surgery and subsequent chemotherapy. In Europe, the treatment protocols rely first on chemotherapy to decrease the size of the tumor, with secondary surgical tumor removal.

The treatment recommendations of the U.S. National Wilms' Study Group are as follows (BRESLOW et al. 1991):

- *Stage I favorable histology*: Age <24 months and tumor less than 550 g. The treatment consists of nephrectomy with abdominal ultrasound and chest x-rays every 3 months for the first 2 years.

- *Stage II favorable histology*: Age >24 months or tumor greater than 550 g; this can be a stage I with focal or diffuse anaplasia and stage II with favorable histology. The treatment consists of nephrectomy followed by two-drug chemotherapy using dactinomycin and vincristine.
- *Stage III favorable histology and stages II and III with focal anaplasia*: The treatment consists of nephrectomy followed by abdominal irradiation, and three-drug chemotherapy using dactinomycin, vincristine, and doxorubicin.
- *Stage IV with favorable histology and focal anaplasia*: The treatment consists of nephrectomy followed by abdominal irradiation, pulmonary irradiation, and three-drug chemotherapy as in stage III.
- *Stage V*: The initial treatment is bilateral tumor biopsy and treatment with chemotherapy. This is followed if possible by renal parenchyma-sparing surgery.

If the vena cava is involved, it is recommended that chemotherapy be administered first, to shrink the intracaval tumor followed by nephrectomy and removal of the thrombus.

The treatment of metastatic and recurrent tumor is challenging. The lungs are the most common location for hematogenous metastases. If there are any such manifestations of the disease, both lungs should be irradiated and a dose of 1200 cGy is recommended. If the liver is involved, a dose of 2000–3000 cGy is delivered to the liver over a 2- to 4-week period. Several patients with lung and liver metastases have been reported to have been cured by a combination of radiotherapy, chemotherapy, and surgery. If a local recurrence or metastasis occurs, chemotherapy will depend on the drugs that have been administered previously. There is no simple strategy and each case should be discussed individually.

### 14.2.9.3
### *Treatment Complications and Prognosis*

The most important prognostic aspect of the tumor is its histology (SNYDER et al. 1992). There is a considerable acute and chronic morbidity during and after each treatment regardless of whether it is surgery, chemotherapy, or radiation. There is a 2%–15% mortality due to the treatment-associated

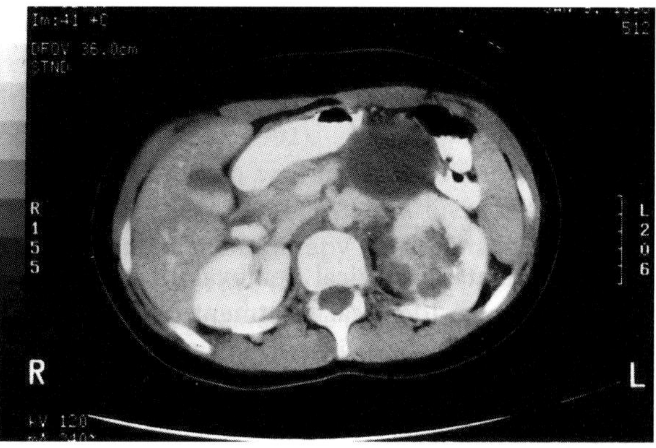

**Fig. 14.4.** CT image of a renal cell carcinoma of the left kidney in a 12-year-old girl

problems. These problems are acute hematologic toxicity (chemotherapy), hepatic toxicity (chemotherapy), orthopedic damage (late after radiation), renal damage (radiation), pulmonary damage (radiation), and myocardial damage (chemotherapy). It is also known that treatment for Wilms' tumor results in a higher rate of secondary malignancy such as osteochondroma, acute leukemia, hepatoma, thyroid carcinoma, and colon cancer.

The prognosis for children with Wilms' tumor has been drastically improved over the years (15% 5-year survival rate in 1942 vs 85% in 1990) and further advances are likely. Today, the 2-year survival rate for stage I disease with favorable histology is 97%. Survival rates for stages IV and V are 81% at 2 years and 70% at 10 years.

### 14.2.10
### Renal Cell Carcinoma

*Synonym*: Hypernephroma

Renal cell carcinoma is very uncommon in children and occurs only in those over 10 years of age (median 12 years). Most of the patients seem to be sporadic cases, but some families with an increased incidence have been reported (COHEN et al. 1979; SNYDER et al. 1992).

### 14.2.10.1
### *Staging*

The diagnosis and clinical presentation are very variable. A palpable mass or abdominal discomfort is usually the first symptom. Staging will be based

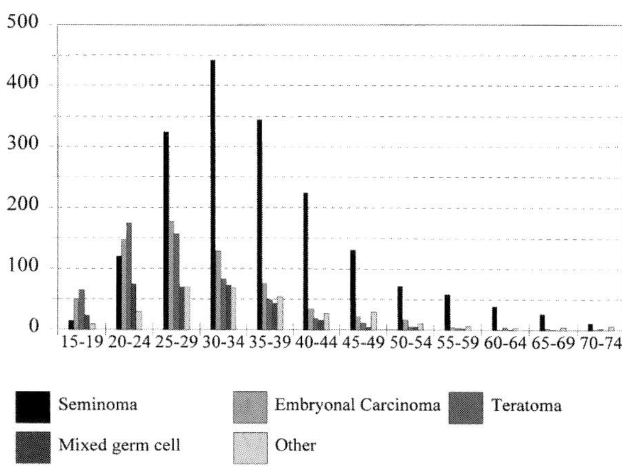



**Fig. 15.1.** Number of testicular germ cell neoplasms in Los Angeles County from 1972 to 1995 by age

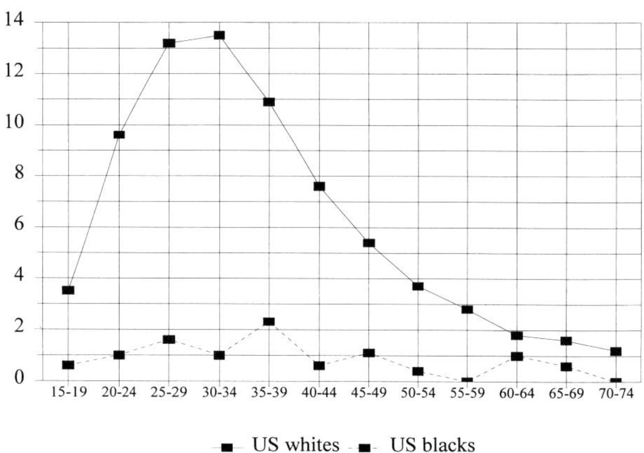



**Fig. 15.3.** 1983–1987 age-specific testicular cancer incidence per 100 000 in the United States by race (Cancer Incidence in Five Continents, vol VI)

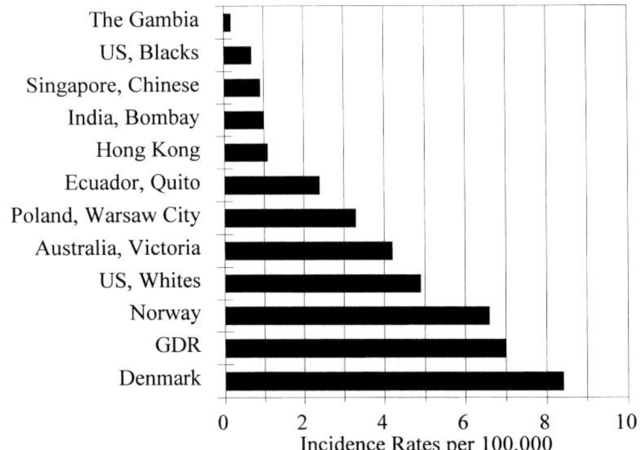



**Fig. 15.2.** Age-adjusted testicular cancer incidence rates per 100 000 (world standard population) for selected countries (Cancer Incidence in Five Continents, vol VI)

### 15.2.2
### United States Patterns

Testicular cancer accounts for less than 1% of all cancers in the United States (PARKIN et al. 1992). Incidence rates are highest in whites, as is found internationally. The disparity in incidence between blacks and white is quite evident in the United States. Unlike (in the case of) prostate cancer, whites in the United States have at least a fourfold higher incidence of testicular cancer compared with blacks (Fig. 15.3). This difference in incidence is apparent in all age groups, but is most striking in 15- to 44-year-olds. In the years 1983–1987, testicular cancer accounted for 1.4% of all cancers in whites, but only 0.3% of all cancers in blacks. During the period 1983–1987 there were 49 incident cases of testicular cancer in blacks and 2640 cases in whites (PARKIN

et al. 1992). The reason for this disparity in incidence is thus far undetermined.

The age-specific incidence rates are quite different from the overall age-adjusted testicular cancer rates. Cancer of the testes is the most common cancer in whites in the 20- to 34-year age range (Table 15.1) according to 1983–1987 SEER data (PARKIN et al. 1992). The latter data showed that the annual incidence of this cancer peaks at 13.5/100 000 population in the 30- to 34-year age group in whites and at 2.3/100 000 population in the 35- to 39-year age range in blacks (PARKIN et al. 1992). Testicular cancer follows a reverse pattern to most cancers, with decreasing incidence rates with increasing age. The pattern suggests that early exposures play a large role in risk for this cancer.

### 15.3
### Risk Factors

### 15.3.1
### Cryptorchidism

The single strongest risk factor for testicular cancer identified to date is cryptorchidism or undescended testis. Various studies have reported between a 3.6- and 9-fold increased risk associated with this condition (STRADER et al. 1988b; GIWERCMAN et al. 1987; PINCZOWSKI et al. 1991; United Kingdom Testicular Cancer Study Group 1994a; SWERDLOW et al. 1997b; POTTERN et al. 1985; DEPUE et al. 1983).

A persistently undescended testis is accompanied by considerable structural abnormalities. The testis is smaller and, histologically, tubule development

**Table 15.1.** 1983–1987 age-specific annual incidence rates per 100 000 for whites and blacks in the United States for the most common cancers (SEER data)

| Age 15–19 years | Rate | Age 20–24 year | Rate | Age 25–29 years | Rate | Age 30–34 years | Rate | Age 35–39 years | Rate |
|---|---|---|---|---|---|---|---|---|---|
| Cancer site | Rate | Cancer site | Rate | Cancer site | Rate | Cancer site | Rate | Cancer site | Rate |
| *a) Whites* | | | | | | | | | |
| Hodgkin's lymphoma | 4.4 | Testes | 9.6 | Testes | 13.2 | Testes | 13.5 | Melanoma | 13.7 |
| Testes | 3.5 | Hodgkin's lymphoma | 5.7 | Melanoma of the skin | 5.1 | Melanoma of the skin | 8.9 | Testes | 10.9 |
| Brain/nervous system | 2.4 | Melanoma of the skin | 2.7 | Hodgkin's lymphoma | 5.0 | Non-Hodgkin's lymphoma | 6.2 | Non-Hodgkin's lymphoma | 10.0 |
| Non-Hodgkin's | 2.1 | Brain/nervous system | 2.4 | Non-Hodgkin's lymphoma | 3.3 | Hodgkin's lymphoma | 4.5 | Lung lymphoma | 5.6 |
| *b) Blacks* | | | | | | | | | |
| Brain/nervous system | 2.4 | Hodgkin's lymphoma | 3.4 | Non-Hodgkin's lymphoma | 4.0 | Non-Hodgkin's lymphoma | 4.2 | Lung | 10.4 |
| Bone | 2.0 | Non-Hodgkin's lymphoma | 1.6 | Hodgkin's lymphoma | 2.1 | Hodgkin's lymphoma | 2.7 | Non-Hodgkin's lymphoma | 7.0 |
| Hodgkin's lymphoma | 1.7 | Myeloid leukemia | 1.6 | Testes | 1.6 | Lung | 2.2 | Colon | 4.9 |
| Myeloid leukemia | 1.4 | Brain/nervous system | 1.5 | Connective tissue | 1.1 | Brain/nervous system | 1.8 | Kidney | 3.8 |
| | | | | Myeloid leukemia | 1.1 | | | | |
| | | | | Colon | 1.1 | | | | |

and spermatogenesis are retarded. Sertoli cell development is delayed and there are abnormalities of the Leydig cells (LIPSHULTZ et al. 1976). Generally, however, individuals born with maldescended testis receive intervention, either orchidopexy or hormonal therapy, to bring the testis into the scrotum.

The risk of testicular cancer associated with cryptorchidism is clearly not solely related to the abnormality, however. If this were the case, individuals who have undergone treatment would no longer be at increased risk for the disease. Further, the contralateral testis would also not be at risk. Several studies have examined the association between correction of the undescended testis and risk of testicular cancer. PRENER et al. (1996) found no decrease in risk associated with correction of the undescended testicle, although the United Kingdom Testicular Cancer Study Group (1994a) reported in their case-control study that boys who underwent orchidopexy before the age of 10 years were not at increased risk for the disease. It is not clear whether age at correction of the undescended testicle is important. SWERDLOW et al. (1997b) found no decrease in risk with age at orchidopexy, whereas MOLLER et al. (1996) found that the relative risk of testicular cancer increased with age at treatment for an undescended testicle.

The view that the pathogenic nature of the cryptorchid testis is not solely related to the intra-abdominal location is further supported by the risk of cancer in the normally descended testis. STRADER and colleagues examined this association and found that cancer in the contralateral testicle does occur with an associated odds ratio of 1.6, but this result was not statistically significant (STRADER et al. 1988a). The United Kingdom Testicular Cancer Study Group (1994a) also found an increased risk of cancer in the normally descended testis (OR = 1.42).

Normal descent of the testes is under hormonal control (GOODMAN and GILMAN 1970). Animal experiments have shown that nonsteroidal estrogen treatment of pregnant mice can lead to undescended and hypogenetic testes (NOMURA and KANZAKI 1977). Similar abnormalities have been reported in male offspring of women exposed to diethylstilbestrol (COSGROVE et al. 1977) and to oral contraceptives during pregnancy (ROTHMAN and LOUIK 1978). In the study by Depue and co-workers, gestational exposure to exogenous estrogens increased the risk of cryptorchidism (OR = 3.3, $P = 0.04$) (DEPUE et al. 1984). Bernstein and colleagues also found statistically significant higher levels of maternal albumin-bound and free estradiol in early gestation of cryptorchid boys (BERNSTEIN et al. 1988). Furthermore Key and co-workers found slightly elevated geometric mean estradiol levels during gestational weeks 6–20 in the mothers of males born with cryptorchidism (KEY et al. 1996).

As testicular cancer rates have increased, there is evidence that cryptorchidism has also increased. An increase in cryptorchidism in army recruits during the past 50 years has been reported (CAMPBELL 1959), as well as an increase in incidence in white infant males in Atlanta, Georgia during the period 1968–1977 (Center of Disease Control 1979). Further, reports from England suggest a doubling of the frequency of undescended testis between 1962 and 1981 (CHILVERS et al. 1984). There is also evidence that the incidence of cryptorchidism in blacks is lower than in whites, which mirrors the excess risk of testicular cancer found in whites (SPITZ et al. 1986; HEINONEN et al. 1977).

## 15.3.2
## Hormones

The clear relationship between testicular descent and hormones begs the question of whether endogenous and/or exogenous hormones play a large role in testicular cancer in addition to cryptorchidism. The use of estrogens for threatened abortion and other complications of pregnancy was a common practice between 1940 and 1970 in the United States (SHAPIRO and SLONE 1979; MARSELOS and TOMATIS 1992; BIBBO et al. 1977). Women have also taken estrogens (and progestins) as a test for pregnancy and birth control (SHAPIRO and SLONE 1979). The association between prenatal DES exposure during pregnancy and testicular cancer has been explored in a number of studies (LEARY et al. 1984). Although an association has been demonstrated in animal models, the results in humans are mixed (GIUSTI et al. 1995). Several human studies have shown an increased risk of testicular cancer associated with the mother taking hormones during pregnancy (DEPUE et al. 1983; SCHOTTENFELD et al. 1980; HENDERSON et al. 1979). However, neither Moss et al. (1986) nor BROWN et al. (1986) found an association between testicular cancer and hormones during pregnancy. It should be pointed out that this relationship is not easy to examine due to difficulties of recall by the mother.

Studies by HENDERSON et al. (1979), DEPUE et al. (1983), and PETRIDOU et al. (1997) provide further evidence that hormonal levels during pregnancy are risk factors for testicular cancer. These three studies have shown that pregnancies accompanied by severe nausea increased the odds of the offspring having testicular cancer. In so far as nausea during pregnancy is associated with higher levels of estrogen, a relationship between prenatal estrogen levels and testicular cancer is possible. We have previously suggested that the increasing rates of testicular cancer may be associated with decreasing age at first full-term pregnancy (FFTP) (HENDERSON et al. 1997). Women at highest risk for hyperemesis gravidarum are young and nulliparous and have high body weight (DEPUE et al. 1987). The relationship between decreasing age at FFTP, risk of severe nausea, and increasing testicular cancer rates supports maternal hormonal levels as a risk factor for testicular cancer. SWERDLOW and colleagues have also shown that dizygotic twins are at increased risk for testicular cancer compared with monozygotic twins (SWERDLOW et al. 1997a). It is believed that there is higher in utero estrogen during dizygotic pregnancies, again suggesting that prenatal estrogen levels are related to testicular cancer risk.

Early age at puberty has been found to be associated with testicular cancer as well. This finding is similar to the increased breast cancer risk found in women who had an early age at menarche. The United Kingdom Testicular Cancer Study Group (1994a) found a statistically significant protective trend for testicular cancer and later age at voice breaking ($P = 0.01$), age at starting to shave ($P = 0.007$), and age at first nocturnal emission ($P = 0.031$). A second study found increased risks associated with early age at puberty as measured by first pubic hair growth (OR = 2.3) (Moss et al. 1986). The apparent association between age at puberty and testicular cancer lends additional support to the role of hormones in testicular cancer.

## 15.3.3
## Familial Predisposition

A number of studies have suggested that testicular cancer tends to cluster in families (HEIMDAL et al. 1997; FULLER and PLENK 1986; TOLLERUD et al. 1985; DIECKMANN and PICHLMEIER 1997). There is increased risk for individuals with an affected first-degree relative, with some studies suggesting the relative risk to brothers to be between 3 and 6 (TOLLERUD et al. 1985; DIECKMANN and PICHLMEIER 1997). A recent segregation analysis by HEIMDAL and colleagues using both Norwegian and Swedish families suggested that this cancer follows a recessive major gene model of inheritance (HEIMDAL et al. 1997). Although these results need to be independently confirmed, this information does provide some of the first guidance toward understanding the genetic component of testicular cancer. This analysis did show, however, that the penetrance of a testicular cancer gene is low, which suggests that most disease is probably caused by environmental factors, including in utero endogenous and exogenous estrogen exposure. Additional studies have attempted to identify specific genetic characteristics which may predispose families to testicular cancer. The number of $(CAG)_n$ repeat tracts in particular genes has been identified as important in several genetic diseases (KING et al. 1997). King and co-workers have also found nonspecific evidence that this genetic characteristic may play a role in familial testicular cancer risk (KING et al. 1997). There is also increased risk of testicular cancer in twins, which lends support to both genetic and prenatal disease etiology (SWERDLOW et al. 1997a).

## 15.3.4
## Other Risk Factors

A number of additional risk factors for testicular cancer have been examined. These factors include vasectomy, socioecomonic status, occupational exposures, extreme temperatures, and immune suppression.

### 15.3.4.1
### Vasectomy

The role of vasectomy as a risk factor for testicular cancer has been examined by many investigators (STRADER et al. 1988a; HEWITT et al. 1993; WEST 1992; ROSENBERG et al. 1994; MOLLER et al. 1994; SKEGG 1993). It was suggested that the increase in testicular cancer incidence could be explained in part by the increase in number of men undergoing vasectomy during the same period. This association has not been borne out. STRADER and colleagues found no association between vasectomy and testicular cancer with the exception of Catholic men (STRADER et al. 1988a). This relationship is attributed to response biases associated with contraception and Catholicism. A number of other studies have found no association between vasectomy and testicular cancer risk (HEWITT et al. 1993; ROSENBERG et al. 1994; MOLLER et al. 1994).

### 15.3.4.2
### Temperature

The position of the testicles in the scrotum, but outside of the abdomen, serves as a protective mea-

sure against high temperature. High temperature has been associated with decreased sperm production, and it was further hypothesized that exposure to extreme temperatures may be associated with testicular cancer. In 1980 LOUGHLIN et al. published a study describing an association with jockey-type underwear and occupations involving exposure to heat and cancer of the testes. Since that time, additional studies have investigated this relationship with varying results. SWERDLOW and colleagues in 1988 found no association with occupational exposure to heat or wearing jockey shorts (SWERDLOW et al. 1988). Similarly, BROWN et al. (1987) and the United Kingdom Testicular Cancer Study Group (1994b) found that neither type of underwear worn nor bathing habits (bath versus shower) was related to testicular cancer risk. On the other hand, ZHANG and colleagues did find a statistically significant association between exposure to extreme temperatures and testicular cancer (OR = 1.71, 95% CI 1.13–2.60) (ZHANG et al. 1995). The importance of this exposure and the mechanism through which it may act remains unclear.

### 15.3.4.3
### Immune Suppression

The relationship between immunosuppression and testicular cancer is unclear. Some studies have suggested a relationship between HIV-positive status and an increase in this cancer, but this association has not been confirmed epidemiologically. Testicular cancer does not meet the CDC definition of AIDS currently (Center for Disease Control 1992). The frequency of bilateral disease is more common in HIV-infected individuals, however (KRISTIANSLUND et al. 1986; SCHEIBER et al. 1987).

There does appear to be a relationship between immune-suppressed organ transplant patients and frequency of testicular cancer (LEIBOVITCH et al. 1996). The frequency of seminoma versus nonseminoma appears to be fairly equal in this patient population, however.

### 15.3.4.4
### Occupation and Socioeconomic Status

Several studies have explored the relationship between occupation, socioeconomic status (SES), and testicular cancer risk (VAN DEN EEDEN et al. 1991; SWERDLOW et al. 1991; KNIGHT et al. 1996; RIMPELA and PUKKALA 1987; PEARCE et al. 1987;

STENLUND and FLODERUS 1997; MILLS et al. 1984; BROWN and POTTERN 1984; McDOWALL and BALARAJAN 1984; SEWELL et al. 1986). High SES has been associated with increased risk of testicular cancer (SWERDLOW et al. 1991; RIMPELA and PUKKALA 1987) The available data on occupation are less clear, as the comparability of studies has been limited by the categorization of occupations, as well as the methods of data collection. In some cases, information on occupation has been gathered retrospectively through medical record review in some cases and via interview in others. Also, some studies have categorized various job types into ever/never having worked in that occupation versus an alternate approach of the job held longest in the years preceding disease development. Several studies have found associations between both white and blue collar occupations, although the United Kingdom Testicular Cancer Study Group (1994b) found no relationship between occupation and risk of testicular cancer in their 1994 study.

A fairly consistent association between employment in white collar occupations and increased odds of testicular cancer has been found (VAN DEN EEDEN et al. 1991; PEARCE et al. 1987). VAN DEN EEDEN and colleagues found an odds ratio of 1.5 (95% CI 1.1, 2.2) for ever having worked as an administrator or manager (VAN DEN EEDEN et al. 1991). Also, ever having worked as a physician or other health-diagnosing profession was found to carry more than a fivefold increased risk of having the disease. This result is similar to findings by PEARCE and colleagues (1987) as well as a second study in which podiatrists were found to be at increased risk (ROSE et al. 1983). These findings are consistent with those observed between high socioeconomic status and disease risk. SWERDLOW et al. (1991) found that high social class based on occupation of both the father and the patient was positively associated with testicular cancer. Further, this study found that attendance at more selective schools, as a measure of high SES, increased a man's risk of testicular cancer.

VAN DEN EEDEN and others have also found associations between occupation in blue collar jobs and testicular cancer (VAN DEN EEDEN et al. 1991; KNIGHT et al. 1996). VAN DEN EEDEN and co-workers found that electricians were 2.8 times (95% CI 1.2,6.4) more likely to have testicular cancer and that sailors, deckhands, pilots, and fisherman have a threefold increased risk (95% CI 1.2,7.9) (VAN DEN EEDEN et al. 1991). KNIGHT and colleagues found no overall association between occupation and testicu-

lar cancer, but did find individuals in blue collar occupations to be at increased risk for nonseminoma testicular cancer (KNIGHT et al. 1996). In their 1996 study, these investigators found statistically significant increased odds associated with employment as miners (OR = 12.39) and food and beverage processors (OR = 3.20), as well as in the utilities industry (OR = 3.15). An odds ratio of 4.6 (not significant) was found for employment in the leather products industry, which supports previous findings of increased risk for leather workers. Clusters of testicular cancer in workers in a leather tannery have been reported (LEVIN et al. 1987).

Occupational exposure to magnetic fields (MF) was found to increase disease odds of nonseminoma testicular cancer in men aged 40 and younger in a study conducted by STENLUND and FLODERUS (1997). Several studies have also examined the association between agricultural employment and testicular cancer risk, but there are conflicting results, with odds ratios ranging from 0.6 to 6.27 (VAN DEN EEDEN et al. 1991; MILLS et al. 1984; BROWN and POTTERN 1984; McDOWALL and BALARAJAN 1984; SEWELL et al. 1986). This relationship remains unclear.

## 15.4
## Conclusions

Testicular cancer incidence has been increasing for the last 50 years, although it appears there may have been a leveling off or even a decrease in this trend (Los Angeles 1972–1995 SEER Registry) (HENDERSON et al. 1997). The reason for the previous increase is unknown, but it does appear to be a birth cohort, rather than calendar year, phenomenon (BERGSTROM et al. 1996). Current evidence suggests that hormonal factors are strongly influential during the prenatal period. The age-specific incidence rates support either a prenatal or young-age exposure in the risk of testicular cancer. The familial clustering and racial risk difference provide important avenues of study in attempting to determine further the etiology of testicular cancer. It is likely that future research on this disease will refine the existing hormonal etiologic hypothesis, explore issues of male reproductive health, and generate genetic models of disease susceptibility to further the understanding of determinants of risk and the causes of testicular cancer.

# References

Bergstrom R, Adami HO, Mohner M, et al. (1996) Increase in testicular cancer incidence in six European countries: a birth cohort phenomenon. J Natl Cancer Inst 88:727–733

Bernstein L, Pike MC, Depue RH, Ross RK, Moore JW, Henderson BE (1988) Maternal hormone levels in early gestation of cryptorchid males: a case-control study. Br J Cancer 58:379–381

Bibbo M, Gill WB, Azizi F, et al. (1977) Follow-up study of male and female offspring of DES-exposed mothers. Obstet Gynecol 49:1–8

Brown LM, Pottern LM (1984) Testicular cancer and farming. Lancet I:1356

Brown LM, Pottern LM, Hoover LM (1986) Prenatal and perinatal risk factors for testicular cancer. Cancer Res 46:4812–4816

Brown LM, Pottern LM, Hoover RN (1987) Testicular cancer in young men: the search for causes of the epidemic increase in the United States. J Epidemiol Community Health 41:349–354

Campbell HE (1959) The incidence of malignant growth of the undescended testicle: a reply and re-evaluation. J Urol 81:663–668

Center of Disease Control (1979) Congenital malformation surveillance report, January-December 1978. Atlanta Ga., September DHEW publ no. [CDC]80-8262

Center for Disease Control (1992) 1993 revised classification system for HIV infection and expanded surveillance case definition for AIDS among adolescents and adults. MMWR Morb Mortal Wkly Rep 41:1–19

Chilvers C, Forman D, Pike MC, et al. (1984) Apparent doubling of frequency of undescended testis in England and Wales in 1962–1981. Lancet II:330–332

Cosgrove MD, Benton B, Henderson BE (1977) Male genitourinary abnormalities and maternal diethylstilbestrol. J Urol 117:220–222

Depue RH (1984) Maternal and gestational factors affecting the risk of cryptorchidism and inguinal hernia. Int J Epidemiol 13:311–318

Depue RH, Pike MC, Henderson BE (1983) Estrogen exposure during gestation and risk of testicular cancer. J Natl Cancer Inst 71:1151–1155

Depue RH, Bernstein L, Ross RK, Judd HL, Henderson BE (1987) Hyperemesis gravidarum in relation to estradiol levels, pregnancy outcome, and other maternal factors: a seroepidemiologic study. Am J Obstet Gynecol 156:1137–1141

Dieckmann KP, Pichlmeier U (1997) The prevalence of familial testicular cancer – an analysis of two patient populations and a review of the literature. Cancer 80:1954–1960

Fuller DB, Plenk HP (1986) Malignant testicular germ cell tumors in a father and two sons – case report and literature review. Cancer 58:955–958

Giusti RM, Iwamoto K, Hatch EE (1995) Diethylstilbestrol revisited: a review of the long-term health effects. Ann Intern Med 122:778–788

Giwercman A, Grindsted J, Hansen B, Jensen OM, Skakkebaek NE (1987) Testicular cancer risk in boys with mal-descended testis: a cohort study. J Urol 138:1214–1216.

Goodman LS, Gilman A (eds) (1970) The pharmacological basis of therapeutics. Macmillan, London, p 1528

Heimdal K, Olsson H, Tretli S, Fossa SD, Borresen AL, Bishop DT (1997) A segregation analysis of testicular cancer based on Norwegian and Swedish families. Br J Cancer 75:1084–1087

Heinonen OP, Slone D, Shapiro S (1977) Malformation of the genitourinary system. In: Kaufman DW (ed) Birth defects and drugs in pregnancy. Publishing Sciences Group, Littleton, Mass., pp 176–199

Henderson BE, Benton B, Jing J, Yu MC, Pike MC (1979) Risk factors for cancer of the testis in young men. Int J Cancer 23:598–602

Henderson BE, Ross RK, Yu MC, Bernstein L (1997) An explanation for the increasing incidence of testis cancer: decreasing age at first full-term pregnancy. J Natl Cancer Inst 89:818–819

Hewitt G, Logan CJH, Curry RC (1993) Does vasectomy cause testicular cancer? Br J Urol 71:607–608

Key TJA, Bull D, Ansell P, et al. (1996) A case-control study of cryptorchidism and maternal hormone concentrations in early pregnancy. Br J Cancer 73:698–701

King BL, Peng HQ, Goss P, Huan S, Bronson D, Kacinski BM, Hogg D (1997) Repeat expansion detection analysis (CAG)$_n$ tracts in tumor cell lines, testicular tumors, and testicular cancer families. Cancer Res 57:209–214

Knight JA, Marett LD, Weir HK (1996) Occupation and risk of germ cell testicular cancer by histologic type in Ontario. J Occup Environ Med 38:884–890

Kristianslund S, fossa SD, KjellevoldK (1986) Bilateral malignant testicular germ cell cancer. Br J Urol 58:60–63

Leary FJ, Ressenguie LJ, Kurland LT, O'Brien PC, Emslander RF, Noller KL (1984) Males exposed in utero to diethylstilbestrol. JAMA 252:2984–2989

Leibovitch I, Baniel J, Rowland RG, Smith ER, Ludlow JK, Konohue JP (1996) Malignant testicular neoplasms in immunosuppressed patients. J Urol 155:1938–1942

Levin SM, Baker DB, Landrigan PJ, et al. (1987) Testicular cancer in leather tanners exposed to dimethylformamide. Lancet II:1153

Lipshultz LI, Caminos-Torres R, Greenspan CS, et al. (1976) Testicular function after orchiopexy for unilaterally undescended testis. N Engl J Med 295:15–18

Loughlin JE, Robboy SJ, Morrison AS (1980) Risk factors for cancer of the testis. N Engl J Med 303:112–113

Marselos M, Tomatis L (1992) Diethylstilboestrol: I. pharmacology, toxicology and carcinogenicity in humans. Eur J Cancer 28A:1182–1189

McDowall M, Balarajan R (1984) Testicular cancer and employment in agriculture. Lancet I:510–511

Mills PK, Newell GR, Johnson DE (1984) Testicular cancer associated with employment in agriculture and oil and natural gas extraction. Lancet I:207–210

Moller H, Knudsen LB, Lynge E (1994) Risk of testicular cancer after vasectomy: cohort study of over 73 000 men. BMJ 309:295–299

Moller H, Prener A, Skakkebaek NE (1996) Testicular cancer, cryptorchidism, inguinal hernia, testicular atrophy, and genital malformations: case-control studies in Denmark. Cancer Causes Controls 7:264–274

Moss AR, Osmond D, Bacchetti P, Torti FM, Gurgin V (1986) Hormonal risk factors in testicular cancer – a case-control study. Am J Epidemiol 124:39–52

Nomura T, Kanzaki T (1977) Induction of urogenital anomalies and some tumors in the progeny of mice receiving diethylstilbestrol during pregnancy. Cancer Res 37:1099–1104

Parkin DM, Muir CS, Whelan SL, Gao YT, Ferlay J, Powell J (eds) (1992) Cancer incidence in five continents, vol VI. IARC scientific publications No. 120. Lyon, International Agency for Research on Cancer

Pearce N, Sheppard RA, Howard JK, Fraser J, Lilley BM (1987) Time trends and occupational differences in cancer of the testis in New Zealand. Cancer 59:1677–1682

Petridou E, Roukas KI, Dessypris N, et al. (1997) Baldness and other correlates of sex hormones in relation to testicular cancer. Int J Cancer 71:982–985

Pinczowski D, McLaughlin JK, Lackgren G, Adami HO, Persson I (1991) Occurrence of testicular cancer in patients operated on for cryptorchdism and inguinal hernia. J Urol 146:1291–1294

Pottern LM, Brown LM, Hoover RN, Javadpour N, O'Connell KJ, Stutzman RE, Blattner WA (1985) Testicular cancer risk among young men: role of cryptorchidism and inguinal hernia. J Natl Cancer Inst 74:377–381

Prener A, Engholm G, Jensen OM (1996) Genital anomalies and risk for testicular cancer in Danish men. Epidemiology 7:14–19

Rimpela AH, Pukkala EI (1987) Cancers of affluence: positive social class gradient and risking incidence trend in some cancer forms. Soc Sci Med 24:601–606

Rose LI, Weiss W, Gibley CW Jr, Borowski G, Levy RA (1983) Carcinoma of the testis in podiatrists. Ann Intern Med 99:636–637

Rosenberg L, Palmer JR, Zauber AG, Warshauer ME, Strom BL, Harlap S, Shapiro S (1994) The relationship of vasectomy to the risk of cancer. Am J Epidemiol 140:431–438

Rothman KJ, Louik C (1978) Oral contraceptives and birth defects. N Engl J Med 299:522–524

Scheiber K, Ackermann D, Studer UE (1987) Bilateral testicular germ cell tumors: a report of 2 cases. J Urol 138:73–76

Schottenfeld D (1996) Testicular cancer. In: Schottenfeld D, Fraumeni JF Jr (eds). Cancer epidemiology and prevention, 2nd edn. Oxford University Press, New York, pp 1207–1219

Schottenfeld D, Warshauer ME, Sherlock S, et al. (1980) The epidemiology of testicular cancer in young adults. Am J Epidemiol 112:232–246

Sewell CM, Castle SP, Hull HF, Wiggins C (1986) Testicular cancer and employment in agriculture and oil and natural gas extraction. Lancet I:553

Shapiro S, Slone D (1979) The effects of exogenous female hormones on the fetus. Epidemiol Rev 1:110–123

Skegg DCG (1993) Vasectomy and risk of cancers of prostate and testis. Eur J Cancer 29A:935–936

Spitz MR, Sider JG, Pollack ES, Lynch HK, Newell GR (1986) Incidence and descriptive features of testicular cancer among United States white, blacks and Hispanics, 1973–1982. Cancer 58:1785–1790

Stenlund C, Floderus B (1997) Occupational exposure to magnetic fields in relation to male breast cancer and testicular cancer: a Swedish case-control study. Cancer Causes Controls 8:184–191

Strader CH, Weiss NS, Daling JR (1988a) Vasectomy and the incidence of testicular cancer. Am J Epidemiol 128:56–63

Strader CH, Weiss NS, Daling JR, Karagas MR, McKnight B (1988b) Cryptorchism, orchiopexy, and the risk of testicular cancer. Am J Epidemiol 127:1013–1018

Swerdlow AJ, Huttly SRA, Smith PG (1988) Is the incidence of testis cancer related to trauma or temperature? Br J Urol 61:518–521

Swerdlow AJ, Douglas AJ, Huttly SRA, Smith PG (1991) Cancer of the testis, socioeconomic status, and occupation. Br J Ind Med 48:670–674

Swerdlow AJ, De Stavola BL, Swanwick MA, Maconochie NES (1997a) Risks of breast and testicular cancers in young adult twins in England and Wales: evidence on prenatal and genetic aetiology. Lancet 350:1723–1728

Swerdlow AJ, Higgins CD, Pike MC (1997b) Risk of testicular cancer in cohort of boys with cryptorchidism. BMJ 314:1507–1511

Tollerud DJ, Blattner WA, Fraser MC, et al. (1985) Familial testicular cancer and urogenital developmental anomalies. Cancer 55:1849–1854

United Kingdom Testicular Cancer Study Group (1994a) Aetiology of testicular cancer: association with congenital abnormalities, age at puberty, infertility, and exercise. BMJ 308:1393–1399

United Kingdom Testicular Cancer Study Group (1994b) Social, behavioural and medical factors in the aetiology of testicular cancer: results from the UK study. Br J Cancer 70:513–520

Van Den Eeden SK, Weiss NS, Strader CH, Daling JR (1991) Occupation and the occurrence of testicular cancer. Am J Ind Med 19:327–337

West RR (1992) Vasectomy and testicular cancer. BMJ 304:79–80

Zhang ZF, Vena JE, Zielezny M, Graham S, Haughey BP, Brasure J, Marshall JR (1995) Occupational exposure to extreme temperature and risk of testicular cancer. Arch of Environ Health 50:13–18

# 16 Carcinoma of the Testis: Pathology

P.W. NICHOLS

CONTENTS



---

P.W. NICHOLS, MD, Professor of Pathology, Director of Laboratories, Kenneth Norris Jr Cancer Hospital and Research Institute, USC School of Medicine, 1441 Eastlake Avenue, Los Angeles, CA 90033, USA

## 16.1
## Introduction

The basis of the current classification of testicular germ cell tumors was established by the work of FRIEDMAN and MOORE, who reviewed almost 1000 cases of testicular cancer and published their findings in 1946 (FRIEDMAN and MOORE 1946). Refinements to their classification were based on observations of many but by Teilum in particular. MOSTOFI and SOBIN, with the assistance of a distinguished group of pathologists, created the World Health Organization classification in the 1970s, the preferred classification in the United States. PUGH and his colleagues established a somewhat comparable classification, the British Testicular Tumor Panel classification. SKAKKEBAEK and colleagues, through numerous publications, have demonstrated the importance of carcinoma in situ, or intratubular germ cell neoplasia, defining the pathogenesis of germ cell tumors. The classification of germ cell tumors created a framework to evaluate therapeutic strategies, leading to a dramatic decrease in the mortality among patients with a highly lethal tumor. Additionally, the work has led to a histogenetic scheme that has provided the framework to formulate hypotheses that can answer the many remaining questions concerning testicular cancer (LEAHY 1992; GINSBURG 1997).

## 16.2
## Anatomy

The testes lie obliquely oriented in the scrotum, each supported by its spermatic cord and separated by a septum. Normally the left testis, although slightly smaller, descends further than the right. The scrotum is composed of a layer of thin skin and an associated layer of fascia and smooth muscle known as dartos tunic. Dartos tunic separates the scrotum into two compartments. The scrotum has an independent blood supply, innervation and lymphatic drainage from that of the spermatic cord, the testis, and its coverings.

The testis in the adult is about 4 cm in length, 2.5 cm in width and 3 cm in anterior-posterior dimension. It has a thick, smooth white outer covering known as the tunica albuginea. Loosely attached to the entire dorsomedial portion of the testis is the epididymis, a structure composed of tightly coiled tubules. Its most superior end is the head, its middle region is the body, and its most inferior region, the tail. On the superior part of the posterolateral side of the testis is the mediastinum, a rough thickening 8–10 mm in dimension. Septa radiate from the mediastinum to the opposite internal walls of the tunica albuginea. These septa enclose cone-shaped lobules with apices oriented toward the mediastinum of the testis. Each testis has 250–400 lobules. Within each lobule are one to three convoluted seminiferous tubules, each measuring up to 80 cm when uncoiled. The space around the seminiferous tubules is known as the interstitium; it accounts for 25%–35% of the testicular parenchyma. As the seminiferous tubules approach the mediastinum, they straighten and merge into 15–20 larger ducts known as the tubuli recti. These tubules then develop an anastomotic network within the dense connective tissue of the mediastinum known as the rete testis. The tubules of the rete testis terminate to form approximately 20 ducts that penetrate the tunica albuginea at the mediastinum, at which point they become the ductuli efferentes. These ductuli travel in a straight course to the head of the epididymis, where they converge into a highly convoluted single duct that forms the head, body, and tail of the epididymis. At this point the duct becomes the ductus deferens, the major excurrent duct of the testis. It enters the spermatic cord at the inferior pole of the testis.

The testis and the spermatic cord are surrounded by an outpouching of the fascial and muscular layers of the abdominal wall, formed as the testis descends into the scrotum. Each outpouching surrounds the cord in a tubular fashion, extending into the scrotum and forming a blind sac that surrounds the testis within the scrotum. These coverings are a continuation of the abdominal wall and are called the external spermatic fascia, cremasteric layer, and internal spermatic fascia. A partial covering of the testis known as the tunica vaginalis lines each pouch. This layer is a serous membrane derived from the peritoneum that preceded the descent of the testis into the scrotum. Although other coverings of the testis are continuous with the abdominal wall, the tunica vaginalis is discontinuous as the connection with the peritoneum is obliterated during development. The cremasteric layer comprises smooth muscle within the spermatic cord. The smooth muscle of the cremasteric layer is often lost as it surrounds the testis.

## 16.2.1
## Blood Supply

The main arterial blood supply to the testes is via the testicular arteries which originate from the aorta, travel retroperitoneally, and course through the deep inguinal ring, the inguinal canal, and the superficial inguinal canal where it enters the scrotum and the spermatic cord. Minor arterial blood supply is derived from the cremasteric artery, a branch of the inferior epigastric artery and the artery of the ductus deferens, a branch of the superior vesical artery. Each of the last two arteries supplies blood by anastomotic branches in the area of the cord as well as the testis. These more minor vessels provide adequate flow to prevent infarction but not atrophy if the testicular artery is severed before it enters the scrotum. The inner two-thirds of the testicular parenchyma is drained by the centripetal veins, which follow the septal support structure. The outer one-third is drained by veins of the tunica vasculosa, which forms the inner layer of the tunica albuginea. Both sets of veins leave the testis at the mediastinum, where they join the venous drainage of the epididymis to form a complex of veins known as the plexus pampiniformis. This venous plexus makes up a significant portion of the spermatic cord and appears to help regulate the testicular temperature, usually 2°C less than the core body temperature. This plexus progressively diminishes in number of channels, and, in the abdomen, it becomes a single channel. On the right, the testicular vein then travels retroperitoneally to empty into the vena cava at an oblique angle and on the left, into the renal vein at a right angle.

## 16.2.2
## Lymphatics

The lymphatics from the testis and its immediate coverings travel in multiple channels parallel to the testicular veins anterior to the psoas muscle. From the area of the testicular vein, they cross the ureter to where they enter lymph nodes in the retroperitoneum at about the level that the testicular veins terminate. The lymphatics of the scrotum drain to inguinal lymph nodes.

The supportive structures of the testes originate from the urogenital ridge, which is of endodermal origin. The germ cells are segregated early in development in the yolk sac. During fetal development, they migrate into the developing gonad, in the gonadal ridge. Subsequently the testis passes caudally behind the peritoneum and descends into the inguinal region, guided by the genital inguinal ligament to the inguinal bursa, an outpouching of the abdominal wall. The deepest portion of the inguinal bursa has a structure called the gubernaculum testis, which is the terminal portion of the genital femoral ligament in the fetus. These structures then migrate into the scrotum with the components of the abdominal wall forming the tunics already mentioned. Descent of the testes has occurred by the time of birth in most newborns, but full descent fails to occur in as many as 14% of infants 1 year of age. However, most of these testes are fully descended by the age of 5 years.

### 16.2.3
### Histology

Histologically, the parenchyma of the testis is composed primarily of seminiferous tubules and the interstitium, which occupy approximately 25%–35% of the total space. The seminiferous tubules in a young adult are approximately 250 µm in diameter. Within the seminiferous tubules are two cell types. The Sertoli cell, a nondividing cell in adults, accounts for about 10% of the cellular elements of the seminiferous tubules. The Sertoli cell, through its cytoplasmic processes, creates ill-defined compartments, one basal and the other adluminal. Early phases of spermatogenesis appear to occur in the basal compartment and later stages of development in the adluminal compartment. The Sertoli cell's function appears to be the production of estrogen, the production of proteins necessary for spermatogenesis, and the phagocytosis of shed cytoplasm of mature germ cells and maldeveloped spermatogonia.

The germ cells that migrated from the yolk sac to the gonadal ridge constitute the remaining cells within the seminiferous tubules. Germ cells undergo continuous maturation, maturing in a spiral fashion through the seminiferous tubules. The germ cells account for almost all carcinomas that arise in the testis. The migration during embryogenesis accounts for the extragonadal location of germ cell

tumors. The interstitium, which accounts for up to a third of the testicular parenchyma, is composed of blood and lymphatic vessels, nerves, macrophages, and mast cells. In addition, an important endocrine cell, the Leydig cell, is present within the interstitium. Leydig cells can also be seen in the tunica albuginea, spermatic cord, epididymis, and mediastinum of the testis, accounting for extragonadal locations of rare tumors that arise from these cells. These cells produce testosterone and are found singly and in clusters often in association with nerves, particularly in extratesticular locations. A characteristic inclusion known as the crystalloid of Reinke may be found in the cytoplasm of the Leydig cell.

## 16.3
## Classification and Staging

Two classifications of testicular tumors are currently used worldwide, the World Health Organization (WHO) and the British Testicular Tumor Panel (BTTP), largely created by Pugh. In the United States, the WHO system is clearly preferred (Table 16.1).

### 16.3.1
### WHO Classification

The WHO system has six broad categories: germ cell tumors, sex-cord stromal tumors, mixed germ cell stromal tumors, tumors of the rete testis, tumors of hematopoietic origin, and miscellaneous tumors. The germ cell tumors account for approximately 95% of all testis tumors. The WHO classification had its inception in the 1940s with the classification of Friedman and Moore. The germ cell category recognizes tumors of one histologic type that include seminomas, spermatocytic seminomas, embryonal carcinomas, yolk sac tumors, polyembryomas, choriocarcinomas, and teratomas. Germ cell tumors of more than one histologic type are referred to as mixed germ cell tumors. These categories of germ cell tumors of the WHO classification will be discussed in greater detail.

### 16.3.2
### British Classification

The British system recognizes similar groups of nongerm cell tumors but has significant differences

**Table 16.1.** WHO classification of testicular tumours

I.   Germ cell tumors
A.   Tumors of one histologic type
     1. Seminoma
     2. Spermatocytic seminoma
     3. Embryonal carcinoma
     4. Yolk sac tumor (embryonal carcinoma, infantile
        type; endodermal sinus tumor)
     5. Polyembryoma
     6. Choriocarcinoma
     7. Teratomas
        (a) Mature
        (b) Immature
        (c) With malignant transformation
B.   Tumors of more than one histologic type
     1. Embryonal carcinoma and teratoma
        (teratocarcinoma)
     2. Choriocarcinoma and any other types (specify type)
     3. Other combinations (specify)

II.  Sex cord/stromal tumors
A.   Well-differentiated forms
     1. Leydig cell tumor
     2. Sertoli cell tumor
     3. Granulosa cell tumor
B.   Mixed forms (specify)
C.   Incompletely differentiated forms

III. Tumors and tumor-like lesions containing both germ
     cell and sex cord/stromal elements
A.   Gonadoblastoma
B.   Others

IV.  Miscellaneous tumors
A.   Carcinoid

V.   Lymphoid and hematopoietic tumors

VI.  Secondary tumors

VII. Tumors of collecting ducts, rete, epididymis, spermatic
     cord, capsule, supporting structures, and appendices
A.   Adenomatoid tumor
B.   Mesothelioma
C.   Adenoma
D.   Carcinoma
E.   Melanotic neuro-ectodermal tumor
F.   Brenner tumor
G.   Soft tissue tumors
     1. Embryonal rhabdomyosarcoma
     2. Others

IX.  Tumor-like lesions
A.   Epidermal (epidermoid) cyst
B.   Nonspecific orchitis
C.   Nonspecific granulomatous orchitis
D.   Specific orchitis
E.   Malakoplakia
F.   Fibromatous periorchitis
G.   Sperm granuloma
H.   Lipogranuloma
I.   Adrenal rests
J.   Others

from the WHO classification in the germ cell tumor category. It recognizes seminomas but places all nonseminomatous tumors within subgroups of a teratoma category (Table 16.2).

In testicular cancer, there is no universally accepted staging system despite the existence of many; however, most authorities agree on broad concepts of staging. The widely accepted stages include confinement to the testes, extension to extragonadal structures, regional (retroperitoneal) lymph node involvement, supradiaphragmatic lymph node involvement, and distant metastases. The greatest variation among the many staging systems lies in the separation of patients whose retroperitoneal lymph nodes are involved. The divisions in this group of retroperitoneal (regional) lymph nodes have evolved because of variations in chemotherapeutic treatment protocols.

### 16.3.3
### The USC Staging System

At the USC, the Skinner system is used to make therapeutic decisions (Table 16.3). The American Joint Committee on Cancer (AJCC) staging also is used, and is also presented here (Table 16.4). For purposes of staging, regional lymph nodes are the

**Table 16.2.** BTTP classification of testicular tumors

Seminoma
Spermatocytic seminoma
Malignant teratoma, undifferentiated (MTU)
Yolk sac tumor
Teratoma, differentiated (TD)
Malignant teratoma, intermediate (MTI)
Seminoma and TD
Seminoma and MTU
Malignant teratoma, trophoblastic (MTT)
MTT and seminoma

**Table 16.3.** Skinner staging

A.   Confined to testis; no clinical or x-ray evidence of
     spread; no positive nodes on lymph node dissection
B.   Disease below diaphragm, normal mediastinum, normal
     chest x-ray
     $B_1$: <6 positive nodes that are well encapsulated and
           show no extension into retroperitoneal fat
     $B_2$: >6 positive nodes that are capsular and may or may
           not show extension into retroperitoneal fat; any
           node >2 cm
     $B_3$: Bulky, palpable abdominal mass (>5 cm)
C.   Metastases above diaphragm or liver involvement

**Table 16.4.** AJCC staging

*Primary tumor (pT)*
The extent of primary tumor is classified after radical orchiectomy.

pTX  Primary tumor cannot be assessed. (If no radical orchictectomy has been performed, TX is used.)
pT0  No evidence of primary tumor (e.g., histologic scar in testis)
pTis  Intratubular germ cell neoplasia (carcinoma in situ)
pT1  Tumor limited to the testis and epididymis without vascular/lymphatic invasion. Tumor may invade into the tunica albuginea but not the tunica vaginalis
pT2  Tumor limited to the testis and epididymis with vascular/lymphatic invasion, or tumor extending through the tunica albuginea with involvement of the tunica vaginalis
pT3  Tumor invades the spermatic cord with or without vascular/lymphatic invasion
pT4  Tumor invades the scrotum with or without vascular/lymphatic invasion

*Regional Lymph nodes (N)*
*Clinical*
NX  Regional lymph nodes cannot be assessed
N0  No regional lymph node metastasis
N1  Metastasis with a lymph node mass 2 cm or less in greatest dimension; or multiple lymph nodes, none more than 2 cm in greatest dimension
N2  Metastasis with a lymph node mass more than 2 cm but not more than 5 cm in greatest dimension
N3  Metastasis with a lymph node mass more than 5 cm in greatest dimension

*Pathologic (pN)*
pNX  Regional lymph nodes cannot be assessed
pN0  No regional lymph node metastasis
pN1  Metastasis with a lymph node mass 2 cm or less in greatest dimension and less than or equal to 5 nodes positive, none more than 2 cm in greatest dimension
pN2  Metastasis with a lymph node mass, more than 2 cm but not more than 5 cm in greatest dimension; or more than 5 nodes positive, none more than 5 cm; or evidence of extranodal extension of tumor
pN3  Metastasis with a lymph node mass more than 5 cm in greatest dimension

*Distant metastasis (M)*
MX  Distant metastasis cannot be assessed
M0  No distant metastasis
M1  Distant metastasis
  M1a  Nonregional nodal or pulmonary metastasis
  M1b  Distant metastasis other than to nonregional lymph nodes and lungs

*Serum tumor markers (S)*
SX  Marker studies not available or not performed
S0  Marker study levels within normal limits
S1  LDH           $<1.5 \times N$ and
    hCG (mlu/ml)  $<5000$ and
    AFP (ng/ml)   $<1000$
S2  LDH           $1.5{-}10 \times N$ or
    hCG (mlu/ml)  $5000{-}50\,000$ or
    AFP (ng/ml)   $1000{-}10\,000$
S3  LDH           $>10 \times N$ or
    hCG (mlu/ml)  $>50\,000$ or
    AFP (ng/ml)   $>10\,000$

N indicates the upper limit of normal for the LDH assay.

*Stage grouping*

| Stage | pT | N | M | S |
|---|---|---|---|---|
| 0 | pTis | N0 | M0 | S0 |
| I | pT1–4 | N0 | M0 | SX |
| IA | pT1 | N0 | M0 | S0 |
| IB | pT2 | N0 | M0 | S0 |
|  | pT3 | N0 | M0 | S0 |
|  | pT4 | N0 | M0 | S0 |
| IS | Any pT/Tx | N0 | M0 | S1–3 |
| II | Any pT/Tx | N1–3 | M0 | SX |
| IIA | Any pT/Tx | N1 | M0 | S0 |
|  | Any pT/Tx | N1 | M0 | S1 |
| IIB | Any pT/Tx | N2 | M0 | S0 |
|  | Any pT/Tx | N2 | M0 | S0 |
| IIC | Any pT/Tx | N3 | M0 | S0 |
|  | Any pT/Tx | N3 | M0 | S1 |
| III | Any pT/Tx | Any N | M1 | SX |
| IIIA | Any pT/Tx | Any N | M1a | S0 |
|  | Any pT/Tx | Any N | M1a | S1 |
| IIIB | Any pT/Tx | N1–3 | M0 | S2 |
|  | Any pT/Tx | Any N | M1a | S2 |
| IIIC | Any pT/Tx | N1–3 | M0 | S3 |
|  | Any pT/Tx | Any N | M1a | S3 |
|  | Any pT/Tx | Any N | M1b | Any S |

interaortocaval, para-aortic, paracaval, preaortic, precaval, retroaortic, and retrocaval. If the patient has had scrotal or inguinal surgery, the intrapelvic, external iliac, and inguinal lymph nodes also are considered regional.

## 16.4
## Pathologic Evaluation of a Testis

Proper staging and classification of testicular tumors depends on a careful gross and microscopic examination of the specimen containing the tumor. Almost all testicular tumors received in a surgical pathology laboratory are the result of a radical or inguinal orchiectomy, done to prevent contamination of the scrotum (particularly the tunica vaginalis) should a mass within the testis prove to be a neoplasm.

### 16.4.1
### Gross Pathologic Examination

Ideally, the radical orchiectomy specimen is examined fresh, as soon after removal as possible. After opening the tunica vaginalis, the specimen is weighed and measurements of the testis and cord recorded. Careful gross examination must include the tunica albuginea, mediastinum, and epididymis, to look for distortion of the tunica or other evidence of extension into the tunica, or involvement of the mediastinum or epididymis. The spermatic cord is examined closely for areas of distortion or nodularity. Next, the testis is bivalved, cutting sagittally across the tunica albuginea through the widest area of the tumor and towards the mediastinum. The size of the tumor in three dimensions should be recorded. Depending on the size of the tumor or distortion of the testis, an occasional variation in the cut may be necessary. Make additional cuts parallel to the first at approximately 3-mm intervals. The objective is to document the relationship of tumor to adjacent structures and to demonstrate all variations of the tumor's appearance. The cut surface of the tumor should be carefully measured in three dimensions. Careful observation of the tumor's relationship to the rete testis and epididymis is particularly important in staging. The cut surface of a testicular tumor can be highly predictive of its histologic type. For this reason, it is important to record the gross appearance of the tumor, and it is critical to sample all variants observed grossly. If the tumor is small, we submit the whole tumor. If the tumor is large, we submit a section of all distinct gross appearances and at least one additional cassette of tissue for each centimeter of the tumor's greatest dimension. Other essential sections include the interface of tumor and noninvolved testis, noninvolved testis, epididymis, and spermatic cord in several locations including the proximal margin (resected end). The uninvolved testis is examined for fibrosis or atrophy, and representative areas sampled. It is important to sample nontumorous areas with a new surgical blade or a carefully cleaned blade because many testis tumors can be carried over to nontumorous areas in the cutting room.

### 16.4.2
### Pathology Report

A surgical pathology report should include the size of the testis and the size of the tumor, and a histologic classification of all elements present; when more than one histologic type of tumor is present, an estimate of the amount of each type should be recorded. As well, there should be a comment on the presence or absence of vascular and/or lymphatic invasion. Last, a comment as to involvement or noninvolvement of the tunica albuginea, rete testis, epididymis, tunica vaginalis, and spermatic cord including the cord's resection margin should be present (Ro et al. 1996).

## 16.5
## Intratubular Germ Cell Neoplasia

### 16.5.1
### Clinical Features

Intratubular germ cell neoplasia is defined as the presence of cytologically malignant germ cells similar to seminoma cells present within the seminiferous tubules. They line the atrophic seminiferous tubules in a continuous rim, pushing normal tubular cells centrally. The tubule has a thickened basement membrane and there is usually peritubular fibrosis. Although Wilms recognized these cells in association with testicular germ cell tumors over 100 years ago, Skakkebaek refocused attention on them in 1972, when he proposed their role as a precursor cell to both seminomas and nonseminomatous germ cell tumors in the testes. The preponderance of evidence now supports his hypothesis (VAN ECHTEN et al.

1995; LOOIJENGA 1995; DAUGAARD et al. 1996; DIECKMANN and LOY 1996; LEAHY 1992). In the European literature, this lesion is referred to as carcinoma in situ, which should be considered a synonymous term to intratubular germ cell neoplasia (ITGCN). Certain American authors argue against carcinoma in situ because they point out the precursor cells are not epithelial and some tumors that arise from them are not carcinomas (YOUNG and SCULLY 1990).

The intratubular and morphologically malignant germ cells are found adjacent to most germ cell tumors with the exception of pure mature teratomas, pure yolk sac tumors, and spermatocytic serminomas. In addition, they are found in the contralateral testis of patients with testicular germ cell tumors 5% of the time (DAUGAARD et al. 1996; HARLAND et al. 1996). SKAKKEBAEK first pointed out in 1972 their existence in the testes of infertile men. When found on biopsy, these men often developed malignant germ cell tumors including seminoma, embryonal carcinoma, teratoma, and mixed germ cell tumors. Not all agree with an approach on how to manage this clinical problem (LEAHY 1992), with some advocating contralateral testicular biopsy with treatment if ITGCN is found (DE LA TAILLE et al. 1997; HOULGATTE et al. 1995), and others recommending close clinical follow up (HERR and SHEINFELD 1997).

Cryptorchid testes, even after correction, have been found to have ITGCN. Patients with gonadal dysgenesis and androgen insensitivity syndrome also have these lesions. Last, patients without primary testicular tumors but extragonadal germ cell tumors often have ITGCN in their testes.

## 16.5.2
## Pathologic Features

The testis of patients with intratubular germ cell neoplasia and no infiltrating tumor is generally small. There is often loss of seminiferous tubules with replacement by fibrosis. Histologically, the neoplastic cells are located on the basement membrane of the seminiferous tubules, which usually are thickened. The critical cell is enlarged with clear cytoplasm that contains glycogen like a seminoma cell. The nuclei are spherical to ovoid and measure 9.7 µm in average diameter as opposed to the 6.5 µm of a normal primary spermatogonia (GIWEZCMAN et al. 1989). The cellularity varies from just a few cells abutting the basement membrane to complete occlu-

sion of the lumen of the seminiferous tubule (Fig. 16.1). Normal spermatogenesis is at least greatly decreased in affected tubules and is usually completely absent. Sertoli cells are generally diminished as well. If normal cells of the seminiferous tubule are present, they are pushed centrally within the lumen. Mitoses are often present. When clusters of neoplastic cells are present, they may be associated with lymphocytes.

The lesions are often patchy and associated with thickening of the basement membrane, fibrosis, and Leydig cell hyperplasia. The neoplastic cells can extend into the rete testis in a pagetoid fashion (Fig. 16.2). Most often, these lesions resemble seminoma; however, syncytiotrophoblasts have been seen in association with these lesions and intratubular foci resembling embryonal carcinoma are also reported (Figs. 16.3, 16.4). Intratubular germ cell spermatocytic seminoma is often observed. Scully described a pure intratubular spermatocytic seminoma. Intratubular spermatocytic seminoma

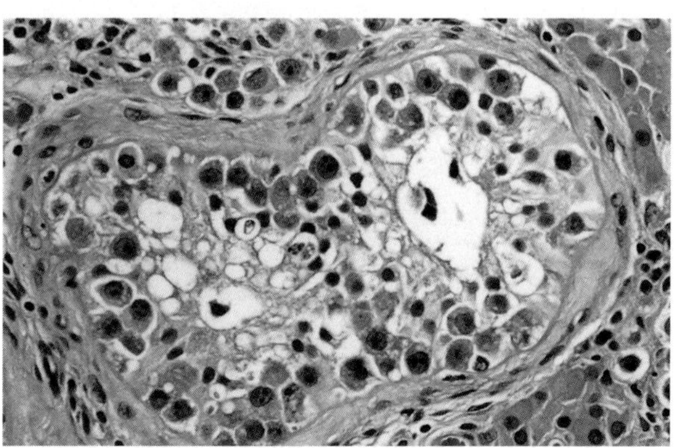

**Fig. 16.1.** Intratubular germ cell neoplasia

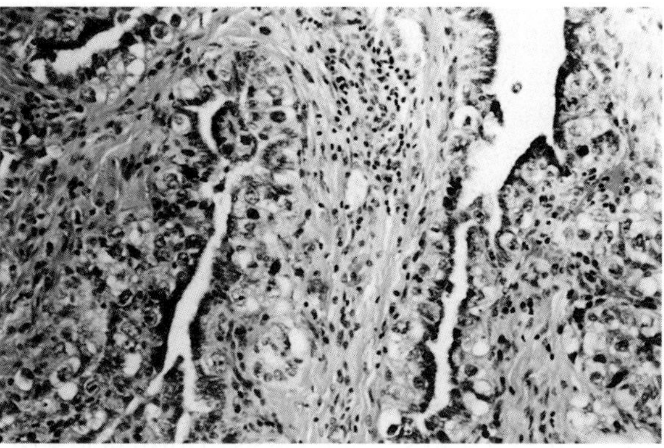

**Fig. 16.2.** Pagetoid spread of seminoma cells into rete testis

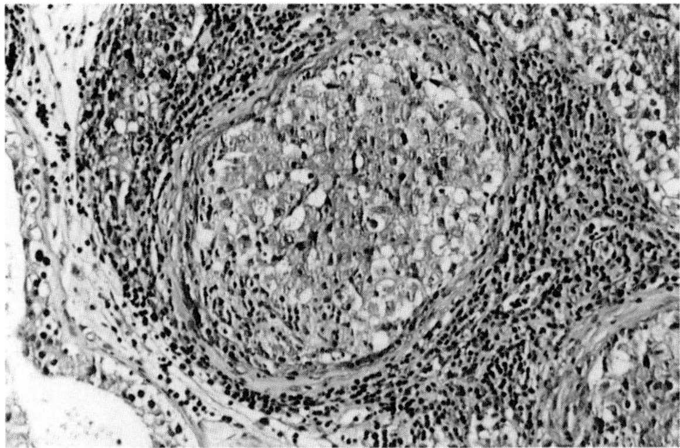

**Fig. 16.3.** Seminoma in situ

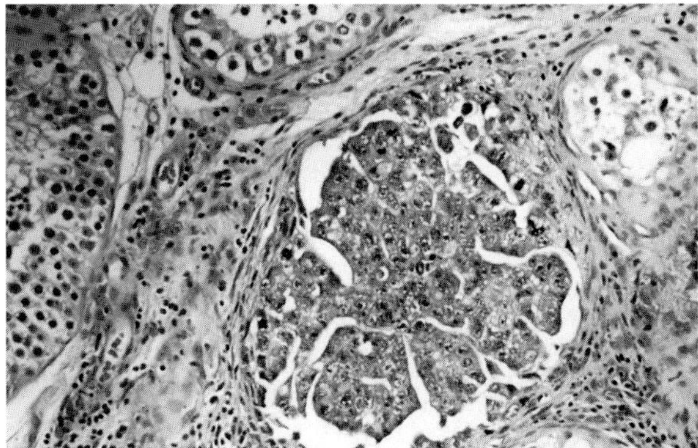

**Fig. 16.4.** Embryonal carcinoma in situ

has not been described with other germ cell tumors. I could not find a report of an intratubular germ cell teratoma.

Immunohistochemical stains are not of great value. Ferritin staining of the critical cells has been reported. Placental alkaline phosphatase staining is positive in most cases with a pattern of staining similar to seminoma. There are investigators who have developed antibodies to germinal epithelium or used them to study tumorigenesis (HIRAOKA et al. 1997; JORGENSEN et al. 1995b).

## 16.6
## Seminoma

### 16.6.1
### Clinical Features

Seminoma is the most common pure form of testicular germ cell tumor, accounting for between 40% and 50% of all germ cell tumors. It is a tumor of adults with only rare reports of its occurrence prior to puberty. A case report from the Armed Forces Institute of Pathology described a 10-year-old child with seminoma. The average patient is in the fourth decade, approximately 10 years later than the onset of nonseminomatous germ cell tumors. The typical presentation is that of an enlarged testis with heaviness and rarely dull pain. As well, some patients present with a hydrocele. Rarely, patients can present with gynecomastia which normally correlates with human chorionic gonadotropin (hCG) production. Some 2%–3% of patients present with symptoms due to metastases in retroperitoneal lymph nodes, bone, or lung. These symptoms may be bone pain or lung metastasis, but are more commonly back pain related to retroperitoneal lymph node metastases. Thirty percent of patients with seminoma are found to have metastases at the time of presentation. This tumor is most common in patients with maldescent of the testis. It is important to recognize that such patients with this developmental abnormality also may have a germ cell tumor presenting in the normally descended testis.

Seminomas almost always spread by lymphatics to the para-aortic, para-iliac, mediastinal, and supraclavicular lymph nodes. Later in the course of the disease, hematogenous spread can occur with the usual sites of metastases being liver, lung, and bones. If seminomas recur, they usually do so within 2 years of therapy; however, there are reports of recurrences 10–20 years after successful treatment.

### 16.6.2
### Tumor Markers

Elevated serum lactate dehydrogenase, placental alkaline phosphatase, and neuron-specific enolase may be found in patients with seminoma. These enzymes are most useful in monitoring patients with known disease, because they lack both specificity and sensitivity. Both placental alkaline phosphatase and the LD1 isoenzyme of lactate dehydrogenase can be used as indicators of the tumor burden as well as tumor response to chemotherapy. In 8%–10% of patients, hCG is found, usually correlated with the presence of syncytiotrophoblasts within the tumor. This pathologic finding does not alter the prognosis of these patients (BUTCHER et al. 1985). It is of interest that when blood from the testicular vein is sampled, the hCG level is elevated more often than when peripheral blood is sampled (FIET et al. 1985).

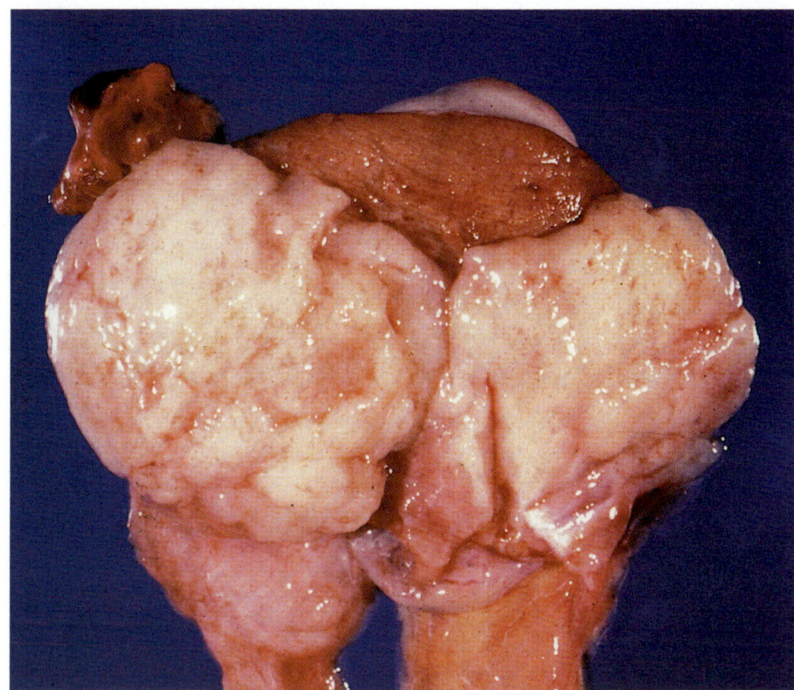

**Fig. 16.5.** Gross appearance of seminoma

α-Fetoprotein is virtually never present in seminoma and its presence in a patient with seminoma is an indication of nonseminomatous elements present in a patient's tumor. Therefore, knowledge of either α-fetoprotein or hCG elevations is important for a surgical pathologist so that a diligent search can be made for the histologic elements producing these substances.

## 16.6.3
## Pathologic Features

Generally the testis is diffusely and uniformly enlarged, although in 15% of patients the size of the testis is normal or slightly decreased (Figs. 16.5–16.9). On cut surface, the tumor is usually multinodular and has a cream to yellow color. When the tumors are unusually large (up to 10 times the size of a normal testis), areas of necrosis may be present grossly; otherwise, necrosis is an unusual gross feature. The cut surface should be carefully examined for petechial hemorrhages as these generally correlate with areas containing syncytiotrophoblasts. The consistency of the tumor varies depending on the amount of fibrous tissue present within fibrous septa of the tumor. Those with scanty fibrous septa are soft whereas those with more extensive fibrosis are firmer.

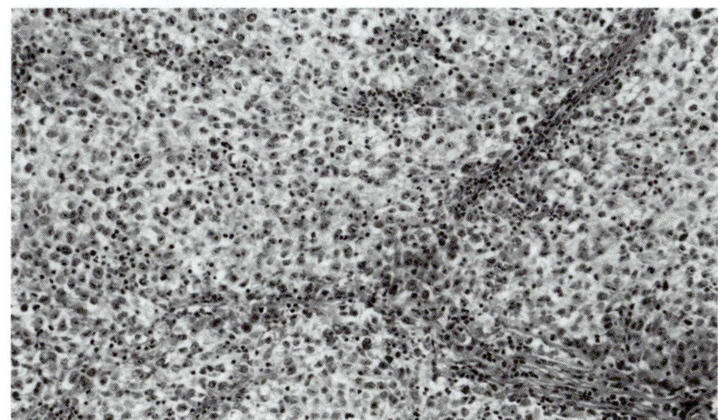

**Fig. 16.6.** Seminoma with lymphoid stroma

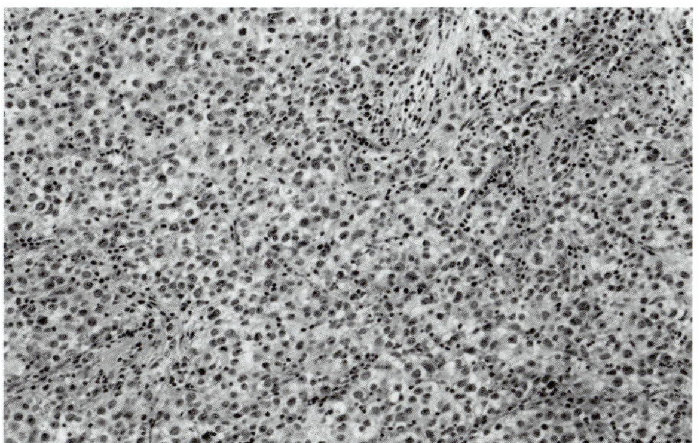

**Fig. 16.7.** Seminoma with scant stroma

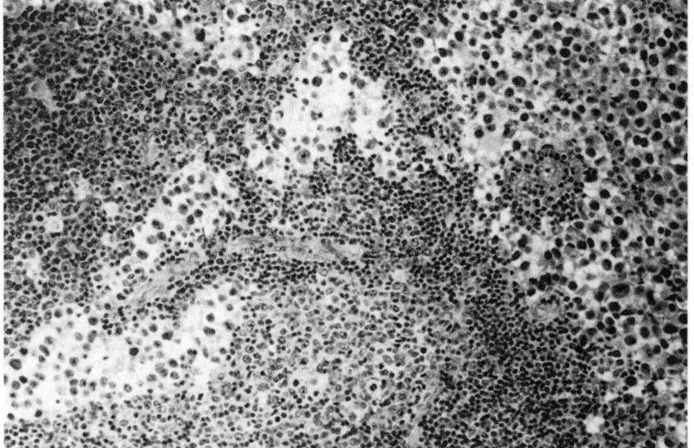

**Fig. 16.8.** Seminoma with abundant lymphoid stroma

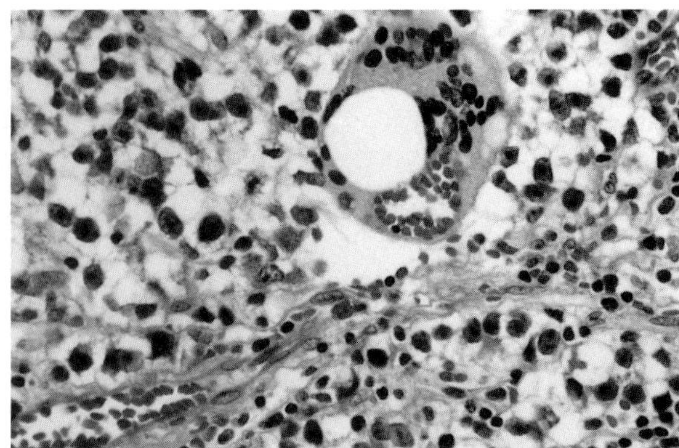

**Fig. 16.10.** Seminoma with syncytiotrophoblast

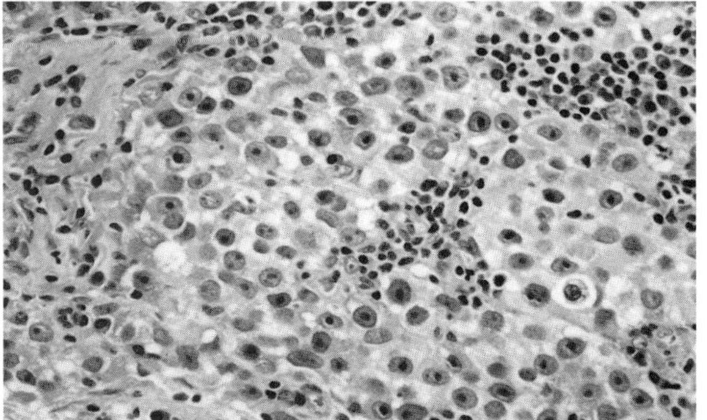

**Fig. 16.9.** Cytologic detail of seminoma

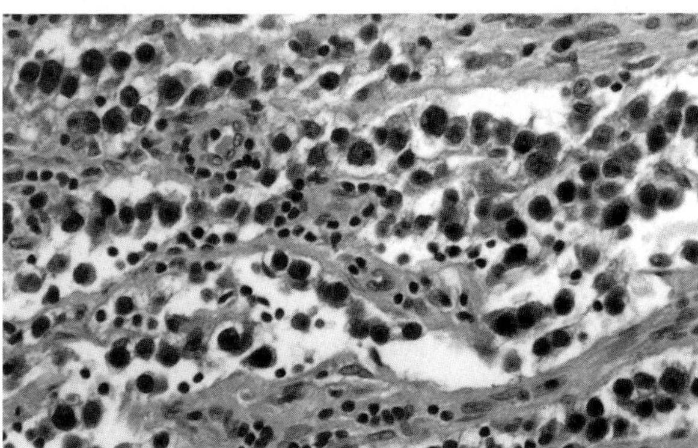

**Fig. 16.11.** Infiltrative cord-like pattern produced by seminoma

### 16.6.3.1
### *Microscopic Appearance*

Microscopically, the tumors are composed of sheets of uniformly sized neoplastic cells divided by septa. The neoplastic cells are generally 15–25 μm in diameter and have well-delineated cytoplasmic borders and spherical to ovoid nuclei with sharply defined nuclear membranes. The cytoplasm generally is clear due to the accumulation of glycogen. The nuclear chromatin is generally vesicular and prominent nucleoli are seen. Associated with the fibrous septa are abundant lymphocytes in approximately 80% of cases; these lymphocytes mark as T cells. At the microscopic level, necrosis is common as well as apoptosis.

Variations in microscopic appearance do occur. A granulomatous reaction composed of small lymphocytes as well as histiocytes with abundant cytoplasm but without necrosis is seen in as many as 50% of cases; this response is marked in 20% of cases. The

granulomatous reaction can be of such a degree that tumor cells are difficult to identify and the diagnosis missed on small biopsies. In some tumors, prominent intercellular edema produces a microcystic pattern. This pattern is important to recognize because it can often be confused with a yolk sac tumor. In 8% of cases syncytiotrophoblasts are present (Fig. 16.10). These generally appear as single or small clusters of multinucleated giant cells appearing similar to the syncytiotrophoblasts found in the placenta. When stained immunohistochemically for hCG, these cells usually are positive. Because choriocarcinoma does still impart a poor prognosis, it is important to search carefully in tumors with syncytiotrophoblasts to be certain that there are no areas of choriocarcinoma. Rarely, seminoma can produce a cord-like or trabecular pattern reminiscent of the Indian-file pattern of lobular breast cancer (Fig. 16.11). Occasionally, the tumor infiltrates around seminiferous tubules, usually at the interface of the tumor and noninvolved testis.

A now somewhat controversial variation referred to as anaplastic seminoma may also be present. MOSTOFI and PRICE identified a group of patients with a higher mitotic rate (greater than three mitoses per high power field) that they believe imparted a worse prognosis. It is true that the numbers of mitoses vary considerably in seminoma, which is a tumor generally of high proliferative rate. More recent studies, however, do not seem to support the concept of anaplastic seminoma as a distinct and separate entity (PERCARPIO et al. 1997; ZUCKMAN et al. 1988). This loss of distinction may be due to the more successful modern-day therapy with all germ cell tumors.

### 16.6.3.2
### *Special Stains*

A number of histochemical and immunohistochemical stains are available to the surgical pathologist to aid in the diagnosis of this tumor. The presence of glycogen within the cytoplasm is a hallmark of this tumor and can be quite helpful in characterizing it. It is important to recognize that glycogen can be easily removed in tissue processing and therefore accurate interpretation of periodic acid-Schiff stains for glycogen requires information on how the tissue was processed. Seminoma does express on its membranes a distinct marker, placental alkaline phosphatase, and given the proper pattern, this immunohistochemical stain is quite specific for seminoma. Keratins are generally not expressed extensively in seminoma cells; however, some low molecular weight keratins can be demonstrated using frozen sections. Higher molecular weight keratins and epithelial membrane antigen are not expressed in seminomas. A useful immunohistochemical panel of stains for seminoma includes placental alkaline phosphatase (positive), epithelial membrane antigen (negative) and combination of AE-1/AE-3 keratin staining (negative) (NIEHANS et al. 1988; WICK et al. 1987).

## 16.7
## Spermatocytic Seminoma

### 16.7.1
### Clinical Features

In 1946, MASSON described a group of testicular tumors that he referred to as "spermatocytic seminoma," suggesting they were a subset of seminoma. It is now generally accepted that spermatocytic seminoma is a separate and unique tumor and should not be considered a subtype of seminoma.

This tumor represents approximately 2% of all testicular germ cell tumors. The average age of patients with this tumor is 54 years. TALERMAN has reported his experience of 22 patients with spermatocytic seminoma over a period of approximately 30 years and found it accounted for 4.4% of all seminomas seen during the same period. The tumor has not been reported in children. At presentation, the patients generally describe painless insidious enlargement of the testis. The tumor is often bilateral, with 6%–10% of patients having both testes involved. Only 2% of typical seminomas have bilateral testicular involvement. Spermatocytic seminoma does not seem to occur in patients with undescended testes. It is of interest that this tumor does not occur in extragonadal sites as other germ cell tumors do. TALERMAN's series of spermatocytic seminoma did include two cases in which the contralateral testis was undescended.

Spermatocytic seminoma rarely metastasizes, and only a few cases that may represent true metastasis have been reported. Early reports of metastases were recorded but it is now generally thought that these represent examples of lymphoma mimicking spermatocytic seminoma. Because of the low incidence of metastases, the prognosis of spermatocytic seminomas is excellent and most patients are cured with orchiectomy alone. It is important to recognize that spermatocytic seminomas can be associated with a sarcoma and when present this combination has a much worse prognosis (TRUE et al. 1988; FLOYD et al. 1988). In contrast to spermatocytic seminoma, the small subset of patients with an associated sarcoma have a poor prognosis even with modern-day chemotherapy. Serum markers are of no benefit in evaluating patients with spermatocytic seminoma.

### 16.7.2
### Pathologic Features

The gross appearance of spermatocytic seminoma is distinctive. The tumor is usually large, many being greater than 5 cm, and the testis usually is expanded uniformly. The cut surface is homogeneous, soft, pale gray, friable, and edematous. Despite the large size of these tumors, necrosis is generally not a feature. As well, the tumors have a gelatinous or mucoid cut surface. The tunica is not usually involved but some of the largest tumors have destroyed the epididymis.

### 16.7.2.1
### *Microscopic Appearance*

The microscopic appearance reveals diffuse sheets of polymorphic neoplastic cells that lack the fibrous stroma of the typical seminoma. Frequently, there is intracellular edema, with lakes of eosinophilic precipitate. The tumor appears to involve both the intratubular and the interstitial compartments of the testis, and the tubules are greatly expanded, often by the intratubular component. The polymorphous population of cells is made up of three types. The most common type is a medium-size cell of 15–18 μm with a spherical nucleus and abundant eosinophilic cytoplasm. The chromatin has a unique granular appearance that is important in recognizing this tumor. In addition, a smaller cell is present in significant numbers. It is about 6–8 μm and appears similar to a small lymphocyte. These cells have a rim of cytoplasm and resemble secondary spermatocytes but are not haploid. The third cell type is uncommon but is distinctive, measuring 50–100 μm in diameter. It has an ovoid nucleus with clumped, filamentous chromatin and rather abundant cytoplasm. This chromatin pattern is unique and is often referred to as a spireme pattern. Intratubular involvement is common, having the same morphologic appearance as the infiltrative component (SOOSAY et al. 1991). Mitoses are rare in all these cell types. The variations in tumor morphology seen in seminoma, such a granulomatous reaction and presence of syncytiotrophoblasts, are not present in this tumor. The amount of cytoplasmic glycogen present is scant and, as opposed to seminoma, the cells are only focally positive for placental alkaline phosphatase. Low molecular weight keratin is usually negative with some staining with dot-like positivity to CK18. It is of interest that these tumors display moderate degrees of aneuploidy when examined by flow cytometry.

## 16.8
## Embryonal Carcinoma

### 16.8.1
### Clinical Features

Embryonal carcinoma is a testicular tumor that occurs on average a full decade earlier than seminoma, the usual age ranging from 20 to 33. The tumor rarely occurs in infants and children. Confusion is caused by the term "infantile embryonal carcinoma," which is a distinct and separate tumor from pure embryonal carcinoma. A preferable name for the so-called infantile embryonal carcinoma is yolk sac tumor (see Sect. 16.9). There is considerable variation in the reporting of the incidence of embryonal carcinoma, with some figures as low as 2%–3% and others as high as 35%–40%. This probably is due to variation in recognition and recording of the yolk sac elements in embryonal carcinoma. It is important to differentiate between embryonal carcinomas and yolk sac tumors. When this is done, the incidence of pure embryonal carcinomas is in the range of 2%–5% (MOSTOFI et al. 1987).

The clinical presentation of embryonal carcinoma is one of gradual swelling of the testis with or without pain. Pain does, however, occur more commonly in embryonal carcinoma. Gynecomastia usually correlates with the presence of syncytiotrophoblasts producing hCG in the primary tumor. These tumors also occur in maldescended testis but appear to occur less frequently than seminomas.

At presentation, a third to a half of patients with embryonal carcinoma have metastases. The usual site is the retroperitoneal lymph nodes. When the right testis is involved by the tumor, it is generally the interaortocaval lymph nodes at the level of the 2nd lumbar vertebra that are involved first. When the left testis is involved, the nodes first involved usually are the left para-aortic lymph nodes below the renal vein and preaortic nodes (DONOHUE 1983). An autopsy study of metastatic sites revealed a distribution given in descending order as follows: para-aortic lymph nodes, iliac lymph nodes, lung, liver, pleura, bones, and gastrointestinal tract. This study demonstrated that 96% of metastases were embryonal carcinoma with 8% containing teratoma and 5% revealing choriocarcinoma. These elements were found in metastases despite their absence in the primary tumor.

Serum tumor markers, when present, can be of benefit by monitoring a patient's response to therapy. Lactate dehydrogenase, placental alkaline phosphatase, and hCG can all be elevated, with hCG being reported in as many as 60% of these tumors. If elevated at all, α-fetoprotein in pure embryonal carcinomas is only minimally elevated and when marked elevation is identified, it usually indicates the presence of yolk sac elements (TALERMAN et al. 1980; MOSTOFI et al. 1987).

## 16.8.2
## Pathologic Features

Embryonal carcinomas at presentation in the testis are generally the smallest of the common germ cell tumors, being considerably smaller than seminomas. They frequently distort the tunica and often replace all or most of the testis (Figs. 16.12–16.15). In 10%–20% of cases the epididymis is involved. The cut surface of the tumor is usually variegated with gray-white areas of tumor separated by foci of hemorrhage and necrosis. The variegated appearance of these tumors with hemorrhage and necrosis within even small tumors is distinctive.

## 16.8.2.1
## *Microscopic Appearance*

Microscopically, these tumors appear as epithelial neoplasms with clear-cut features of malignancy. Histologically, they grow in three basic patterns: solid, papillary, and tubular or glandular. These tumors also can be found in intratubular sites. Cytologically, the cells are anaplastic in appearance but are distinctly epithelial. The cells are varied in size and shape, but are generally large and may have a cuboidal, flattened, columnar, or even polyhedral appearance. The cell borders are generally indistinct, giving a syncytial growth pattern. The cytoplasm is

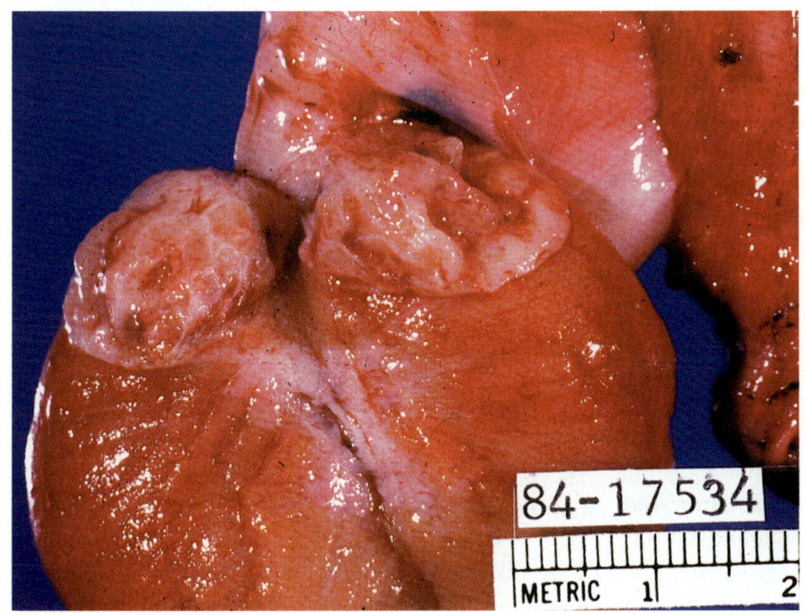


**Fig. 16.12.** Gross appearance of embryonal carcinoma

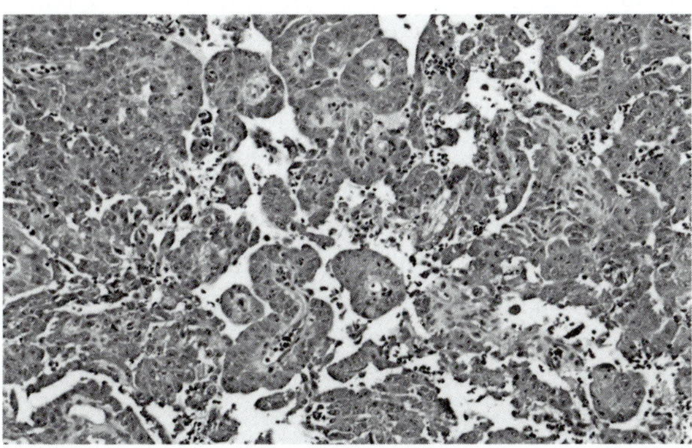

**Fig. 16.13.** Embryonal carcinoma, papillary pattern

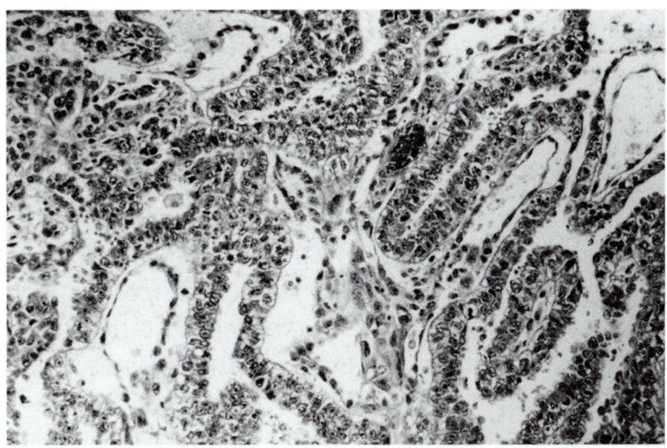

**Fig. 16.14.** Embryonal carcinoma with a double cell layered glandular pattern

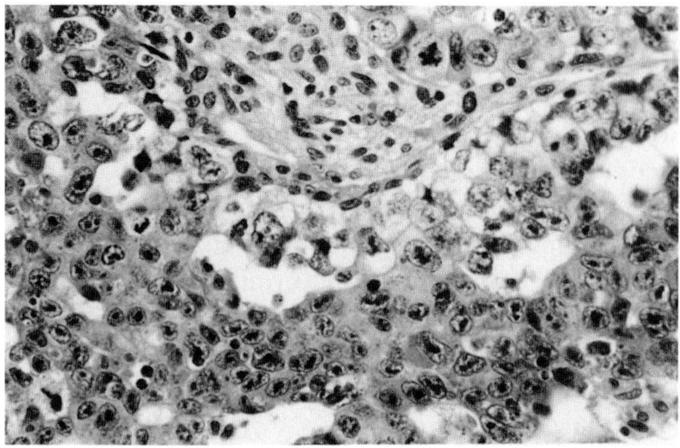

**Fig. 16.15.** Cytologic features of embryonal carcinoma, glandular pattern

generally eosinophilic, and occasionally cleared. The nuclei are usually round to oval with coarse nuclear membranes and often coarse chromatin. Generally, lymphocytes and granulomas are absent, but in a few cases can be seen. As well, there is often a delicate fibrovascular stroma with a primitive mesenchymal appearance. It is important to search diligently for syncytiotrophoblasts to assure that a focus of choriocarcinoma is not present. The papillary pattern of embryonal carcinoma can produce structures mimicking the Schiller-Duvall bodies seen in yolk sac tumors. In addition, embryonal carcinomas can focally produce a distinct structure consisting of an ectodermal bilaminar layer of cells with an amniotic cavity on one side and yolk sac elements on the other. These structures are referred to as embryoid bodies and they have a striking resemblance to a 13-day embryo (JACOBSEN and TALERMAN 1989).

### 16.8.2.2
### Special Stains

Immunohistochemical stains in the diagnosis of these tumors can be helpful. The combination of placental alkaline phosphatase, cytokeratin, and epithelial membrane antigen is an effective battery of stains (JACOBSEN et al. 1981). Placental alkaline phosphatase is present in cytoplasmic borders of approximately 90% of cases but it has a different pattern than seminoma in that it is weaker in staining and is usually patchy. In embryonal carcinoma the cytokeratins are typically more positive but they are similar to the range of positive cytokeratins in seminoma in that keratins 8, 18, 19, and even 4 and 17 can be positive. One expects the epithelial mem-

brane antigen to be negative in embryonal carcinoma. α-Fetoprotein staining is a marker of yolk sac elements and can assist in identifying the subtle presence of yolk sac elements in an otherwise pure embryonal carcinoma (TALERMAN et al. 1980; MOSTOFI et al. 1987).

### 16.9
### Polyembryoma

A special designation in the WHO classification is made for polyembryoma, a rare morphologic pattern that almost never appears as a pure tumor. Grossly, these tumors are described as solid but soft and edematous. Their unique feature is the presence of numerous organoid structures that resemble embryonic structures of 1–2 weeks' gestation. These structures generally have a central embryonic disc with a cavity that resembles the amniotic cavity on one surface and tissues resembling the yolk sac endoderm on the other. These embryoid bodies are usually separated by primitive mesenchyme. Because only a few cases of this rare but distinct morphologic entity have been reported, it is difficult to predict the prognosis and behavior of patients with this tumor.

### 16.10
### Yolk Sac Tumor

### 16.10.1
### Clinical Features

The yolk sac tumor is the most recently recognized testicular germ cell tumor. Its recognition occurred as the result of Teilum's work in recognizing the resemblance of the yolk sac tumor patterns to the endodermal sinuses of Duvall seen in the rat placenta (TEILUM 1959, 1976). This tumor distinguishes itself in that it is the most common testicular germ cell tumor in children, accounting for 82% of prepubertal germ cell tumors. In its pure form, the tumor usually occurs in children less than 3 years, but may occur as late as 9 years. The tumor is rare in adults in the pure form but is a common component of mixed germ cell tumors. Children with this tumor present with a testicular mass or gradual testicular enlargement and around 12% (range 6%–16%) have metastases at presentation. This tumor is not associated with maldescended testes. The pattern of metastasis is through both the lymphatic and hematogenous routes. In adults its presence in a mixed germ cell tumor predicts for a lower stage at presentation. Prior to modern-day chemotherapy, this tumor had a poor prognosis but its prognosis now is good (KAY 1993).

## 16.10.2
## Tumor Markers

The serum tumor marker α-fetoprotein is produced by these tumors and is very helpful in the initial evaluation of these patients as well as in their follow-up. Patients with this tumor often present with α-fetoprotein levels in the range of thousands (TALERMAN et al. 1980). Because of the high levels of α-fetoprotein and the lack of other clinical conditions raising the α-fetoprotein to this level, this marker is a good diagnostic tool. In addition, it is an effective means of monitoring the patient's disease.

## 16.10.3
## Pathologic Features

In children, this tumor is generally confined to the testis and often almost completely replaces it. The tumor is generally well-circumscribed but does not appear to have a capsule. The cut surface of the tumor is generally solid, soft, and gray-white to yellow-tan; it is usually homogeneous and often has a gelatinous appearance. Areas of hemorrhage are common, and necrosis may be present if the tumor is large.

### 16.10.3.1
### Microscopic Appearance

The microscopic appearance of this tumor is extremely varied, accounting for the difficulty in recognizing it in adult mixed germ cell tumors (Figs. 16.16–16.20). The neoplastic cells have an endothelial appearance and may be columnar, cuboidal, or flattened, with indistinct borders. The nuclei are spherical to ovoid with distinct nucleoli. The cytoplasm is vacuolated or clear, often with pale eosinophilic material. JACOBSEN and TALERMAN described ten histologic patterns: microcystic or reticular, macrocystic, solid, glandular-alveolar, endodermal sinus, papillary, myxomatous, polyvesicular vitelline, hepatoid, and primitive intestinal (enteric). The most common pattern in the adult testis is the microcystic. It produces a honeycomb pattern due to

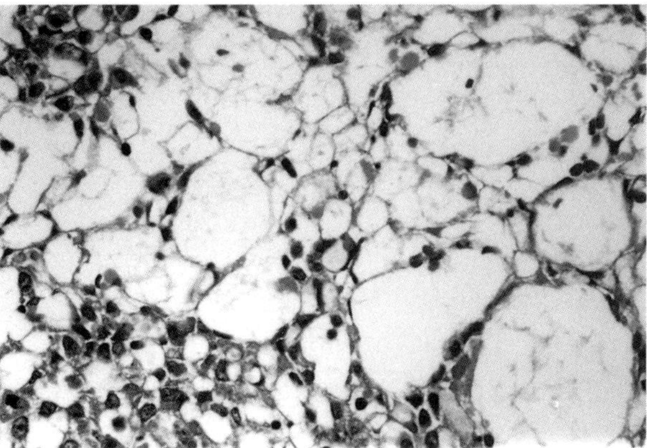

Fig. 16.16. Yolk sac tumor with a macro- and microcystic pattern

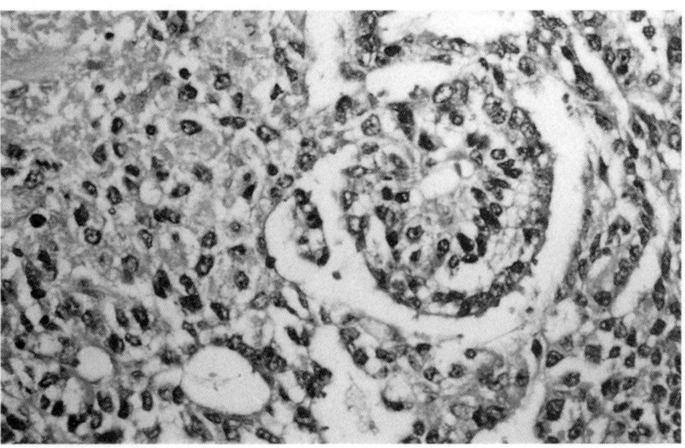

Fig. 16.17. Schiller-Duvall body

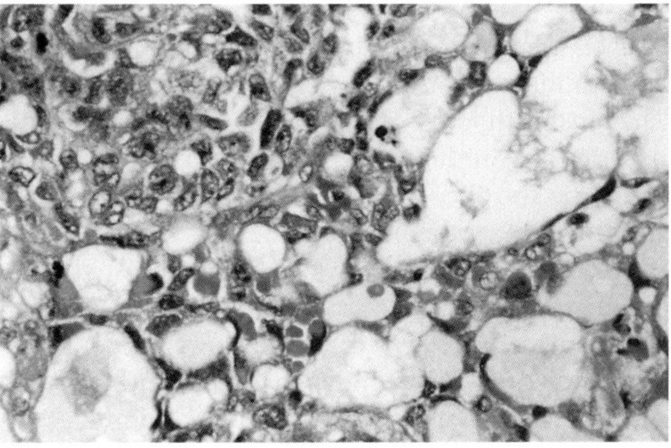

Fig. 16.18. Eosinophilic globules in yolk sac tumor

intracellular and extracellular vacuoles that often contain α-fetoprotein-positive eosinophilic material. The macrocystic pattern is more common in infantile yolk sac tumors. The larger cysts are lined by flattened cells that are also α-fetoprotein positive.

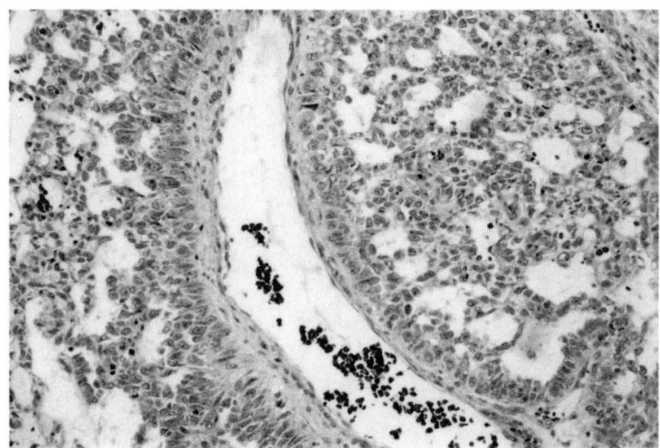

**Fig. 16.19.** Yolk sac tumor with endodermal sinus pattern

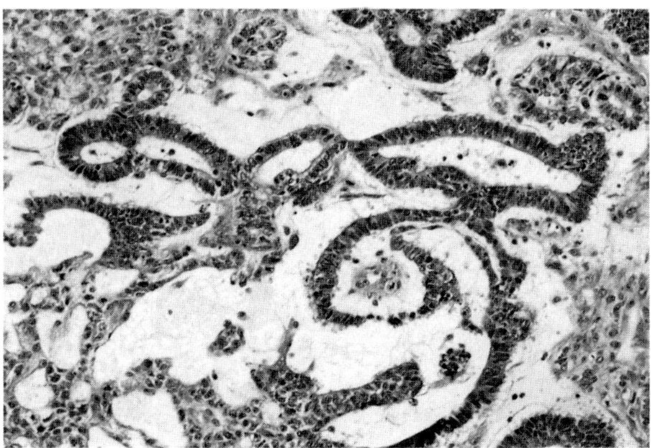

**Fig. 16.20.** Yolk sac tumor with glandular alveolar pattern

As well, there is a solid pattern resembling embryonal carcinoma in as many as a quarter of patients. The most distinctive pattern is the endodermal sinus pattern that produces distinctive microscopic structures, the so-called Schiller-Duvall bodies. It is these structures that resemble endodermal sinuses of the rat placenta and although not always present, they are diagnostic of yolk sac carcinoma. Schiller-Duvall bodies are characterized by a central vessel that is surrounded by loose mesenchymal tissues that are then, in turn, capped by cuboidal to columnar cells. This vascular structure sits in a cystic space lined by flattened neoplastic cells.

Often eosinophilic globules are found in the cytoplasm of these tumors and these are usually $\alpha$-fetoprotein positive. In addition, these globules stain with $\alpha_1$-antitrypsin, a marker that is commonly present in tumors with an endodermal sinus pattern. In addition, cytokeratins are present in almost all endodermal sinus tumors and epithelial membrane antigen (EMA) is usually absent (NIEHANS et al. 1988). Placental alkaline phosphatase is usually patchy. This can be particularly problematic in distinguishing solid areas of endodermal sinus tumor from seminoma or embryonal carcinoma.

## 16.11
## Teratoma

### 16.11.1
### Clinical Features

Teratoma is a germ cell tumor usually of more than one of the three germ cell layers, ectoderm, endoderm, and mesoderm. In the WHO classification, the teratomas are divided into mature teratoma, immature teratoma, and teratoma with malignant transformation. It should be recognized that the morphology and behavior of the teratomas are quite varied and, in adults, all must be considered capable of metastases. The category of teratoma with malignant transformation is a tumor which has an overtly malignant histologic component. These tumors are always malignant whereas the mature and immature teratomas may or may not be malignant. Within the category of teratoma is a group of rare tumors containing elements apparently derived from only one germ cell layer. I prefer to consider these tumors as monodermal variants of teratomas. The group includes the carcinoid tumor, the dermoid, the primitive neuroectodermal tumor, and, perhaps, the epidermoid cyst (HEIDENREICH et al. 1995, 1996).

Teratomas in the pure state represent approximately 2%–9% of testicular nonseminomatous germ cell tumors and have a bimodal age distribution (SIMMONDS et al. 1996; HEIDENREICH et al. 1997). This is the second most common tumor in children, with the mean age being approximately 20 months. In adults most teratomas are seen in the first three decades of life. Teratoma is a common component of mixed germ cell tumors, with approximately 50% having teratomatous components. Most childhood teratomas occur in the first 4 years, with very few teratomas being seen between age 4 and 12 (or the age of puberty). Childhood teratoma can be associated with such congenital anomalies as spina bifida and hemihypertrophy. The patients generally present with a slightly enlarged testis creating a palpable mass. The second most common complaint is pain. The childhood teratomas are generally found on routine physical examination or by a parent.

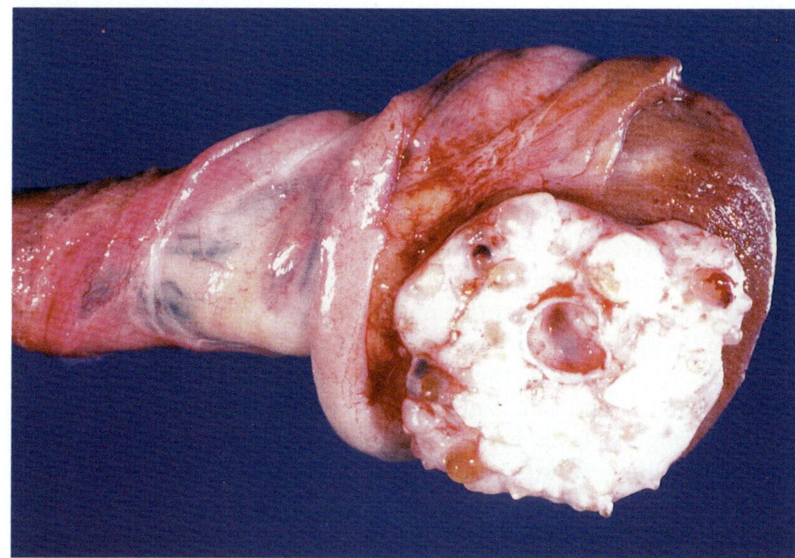

**Fig. 16.21.** Gross appearance of teratoma

The pattern of metastases varies with the age group. Children less than 4 years of age almost never have metastatic disease, and children between the age of 4 and 12 rarely have metastases. In adults with pure teratomas, up to 25% have metastatic disease. Patients with pure teratomas have presented with metastasis of embryonal carcinoma. It is of interest that those pure teratomas that do metastasize usually have an intratubular germ cell tumor present in the resected testis. Serum markers used for germ cell tumors are helpful in screening these patients, but usually identify a group of patients who have an undetected nonteratomatous component.

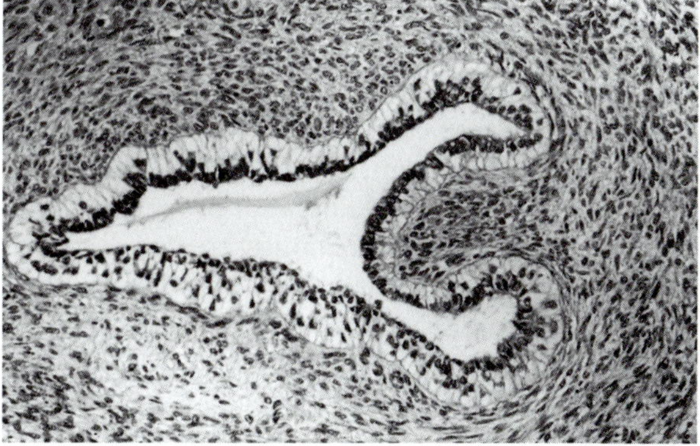

**Fig. 16.22.** Epithelial and mesenchymal area of a teratoma

## 16.11.2
## Pathologic Features

The testis involved by a teratoma generally has an irregular tunica deformed by the underlying tumor (Figs. 16.21, 16.22). On cut surface, the tumor is a well-circumscribed and often encapsulated mass. Multiple cyst-like structures up to 1 cm containing watery or mucoid material may be present; they are separated by fibromuscular tissue. Other areas of the tumor may be solid, and contain grossly obvious cartilage. Sometimes the solid areas are more hemorrhagic, fleshy, and even encephaloid in appearance; such areas generally reflect areas of immaturity. It is important to sample all areas generously to exclude the presence of nonteratomatous elements.

### 16.11.2.1
### *Microscopic Appearance*

The microscopic appearance of teratomas is highly complex, with many of the mature tumors displaying areas of cartilage, smooth and striated muscle, neuroglia, enteric glands, respiratory epithelium, squamous epithelium, and urothelial islands. Less commonly bone, choroid, and even kidney, liver, and pancreas can be seen. All of these elements can be mature or immature, resulting in subcategories of some authors' classifications. Atypia can be present in either the childhood or the adult forms and these atypia are often associated with aneuploidy. However, the atypia and aneuploidy do not appear to correlate with outcome, which is correlated best with the age of the patient. As mentioned above, children less than 4 years old virtually never have metastases even though they have significant areas of immaturity associated with atypia and aneuploidy. The teratomas in adults have associated intratubular germ cell neoplasia whereas the tumors in children less than 4 years old lack this feature. Although as yet unproven, it may be that the presence of intratubular germ cell neoplasia helps to distinguish the teratoma that can metastasize from one that cannot in the age range of 4–12 years (JORGENSEN et al. 1995a).

Teratoma with malignant transformation can occur with either the mature or the immature component. In addition to the teratomatous elements, this variant has a component that is cytologically malignant, destructive, and invasive. This so-called malignant transformed component can be an adenocarcinoma, squamous carcinoma, or even an undifferentiated carcinoma. As well, sarcomas and even lymphomas can occur in teratomas but these are difficult to distinguish from the immature mesenchyme that may be present in an immature teratoma. Generally, sarcomatous or lymphomatous malignant transformation is recognized by an overgrowth of one particular pattern. Its presence in a teratoma prior to treatment or confined to the testis does not necessarily result in a poor prognosis. However, its occurrence in a previously treated germ cell tumor or a distant metastatic site does confer a much poorer prognosis (AHMED et al. 1985; AMSTERDAM et al. 1996).

### 16.11.2.2
### Special Stains

Immunohistochemical stains on this particular group of tumor are not of much benefit because most of the patterns of staining in other germ cell tumors can be present in teratoma, with α-fetoprotein being seen in enteric epithelium or liver (NIEHANS et al. 1988). In addition, $\alpha_1$-antitrypsin, carcinoembryonic antigen, and ferritin immunostaining has been reported in teratomatous epithelium (JACOBSEN et al. 1981).

### 16.11.2.3
### Monodermal Variants

The two testicular tumors that are most likely candidates for monodermal variants of teratoma are the carcinoid tumor and the primitive neuroectodermal tumor. As well, the dermoid cyst and the epidermoid cyst may be examples of monodermal variants of teratoma. Only a few cases of pure carcinoid tumor that appears to be primary in the testis have been reported. However, carcinoid tumor can be a component of a teratoma. Up to a quarter of tumors with a large carcinoid component also have teratomatous elements. The pure tumor occurs in an older age group, with a median age range of 50. Grossly, these tumors have the same appearance as carcinoids elsewhere: they are generally well circumscribed, yellow to tan, and solid. Primary carcinoid tumor of the testis has a good prognosis. One of the difficulties with this tumor is distinguishing origin in the testis versus metastasis. This distinction is difficult on a pathologic basis and generally requires close clinical correlation.

A second, rare monodermal variant of teratoma is the primitive neuroectodermal tumor, a neoplasm with distinct neuroepithelial features, occurring most often in young or middle-aged adults. Most patients have had an aggressive clinical course. A dermoid cyst can also rarely occur in the testis. It appears to be the homologue of the more common dermoid cyst of the ovary. These tumors are composed of skin with its appendages, including hair and sebaceous glands; sloughed keratohyaline material is found in the cystic spaces. Teeth, bone, and cartilage also can be present. Rare examples of dermoid cyst with thyroid and pancreatic tissue have been reported. These tumors generally do not metastasize. The epidermoid cyst is a slightly more common monodermal variant of teratoma (HEIDENREICH et al. 1995, 1996). It has the squamous epithelial components of a dermoid cyst but lacks skin appendages as well as all other elements in a dermoid cyst. This tumor also is not known to metastasize. It is important to examine these cases for the presence of intratubular germ cell neoplasia in the seminiferous tubules of the uninvolved testis. It has been suggested that when intratubular germ cell neoplasia is present, these tumors behave as an adult teratoma.

The tumor described as polyembryoma is one of interest in that it may be considered as the most immature teratoma by some but we prefer to include this tumor in a separate category.

## 16.12
## Choriocarcinoma

### 16.12.1
### Clinical Features

Choriocarcinoma in its pure form is a tumor occurring in only 18 of 6000 cases reported from the Armed Forces Institute of Pathology (MOSTOFI 1977) and absent in 2739 cases in the report of the British Testicular Tumor Panel (PUGH 1976). The Danish Testicular Carcinoma Project reported two cases in a group of 1053 patients with testicular germ cell tumors (JACOBSEN et al. 1984). The usual age range is 18–35 years, but the tumor has been reported in prepubertal children. About 10% of patients present with gynecomastia. Often, patients present with metastases and a primary tumor that is small and rarely enlarges the testis. They usually do not have pain. On occasion, this tumor can present with metastatic disease and no primary tumor is identified clinically. However, an area of scar associated with hemosiderin-laden macrophages, presumed to be the primary, is found in the testis. These testes also have areas of intratubular germ cell neoplasia.

The pattern of metastasis is one in which both the lymphatic and hematogenous routes appear to be involved. The most common site of distant metastasis is the lung, with almost all reported cases of pure choriocarcinoma having had pulmonary metastases. In addition to lymphatic sites within the retroperitoneum, the intestine, spleen, adrenals, brain, and skin (SHIMIZU et al. 1996) may be involved.

This tumor has the worst prognosis of all testicular tumors, which may be due to the advanced nature of the disease when patients first present. Prior to the modern era of chemotherapy, most patients with this tumor were dead within 9 months. It is significant, however, that with modern-day approaches to chemotherapy, significant tumor-free survival is now being achieved.

### 16.12.2
### Pathologic Features

The gross examination of the testis involved by choriocarcinoma reveals an undistorted tunica. The testicular parenchyma usually has a small, grossly hemorrhagic lesion, often surrounded by a gray-white peripheral zone. The central area usually has the greatest degree of necrosis and the whole lesion is usually soft.

### 16.12.2.1
### Microscopic Appearance

Microscopically, hemorrhage dominates the picture. Two distinct cell components can be identified: cytotrophoblast and syncytiotrophoblast, resembling the cells of immature placental villi (Figs. 16.23, 16.24). The cytotrophoblastic component is generally composed of a uniform population of small to medium-sized cells with distinct borders, polyhedral shapes, clear cytoplasm, and a single vesicular nucleus. Syncytiotrophoblasts, large multinucleated giant cells that occur in a variety of sizes, often cap nests of cytotrophoblasts. The cytoplasm of the syncytiotrophoblasts is frequently vacuolated and the vacuoles often contain red cells or precipitated eosinophilic protein. In addition, the syncytiotrophoblasts often appear to line blood-filled spaces in a highly distinctive fashion. Immunohistochemical stains for human placental lactogen and hCG are positive. As well, about 25% of cases will have carcinoembryonic antigen and 50% show focal placental alkaline phosphatase (NIEHANS et al. 1988). These tumor cells also produce cytokeratin, and stains for cytokeratin 7, 8, 18, and 19 are usually positive (CLARK and DAMJANOV 1985).

Virtually all these tumors produce hCG, although in some patients the protein has an aberrant structure. Serum markers for hCG are of great clinical importance in following a patient's response to therapy and monitoring for recurrence.

## 16.13
## Mixed Germ Cell Tumors

### 16.13.1
### Clinical Features

Approximately a third of germ cell tumors present as mixtures of several types. When one excludes pure seminomas, approximately 70% of testicular tumors are mixed. This type is placed in the category of nonseminomatous germ cell tumors, even though seminoma may be a component in about 30% of them. They present as a testicular mass, often with metastases, and pain is a frequent finding. These tumors are extremely unusual in prepubertal children, with an age range similar to that of embryonal carci-

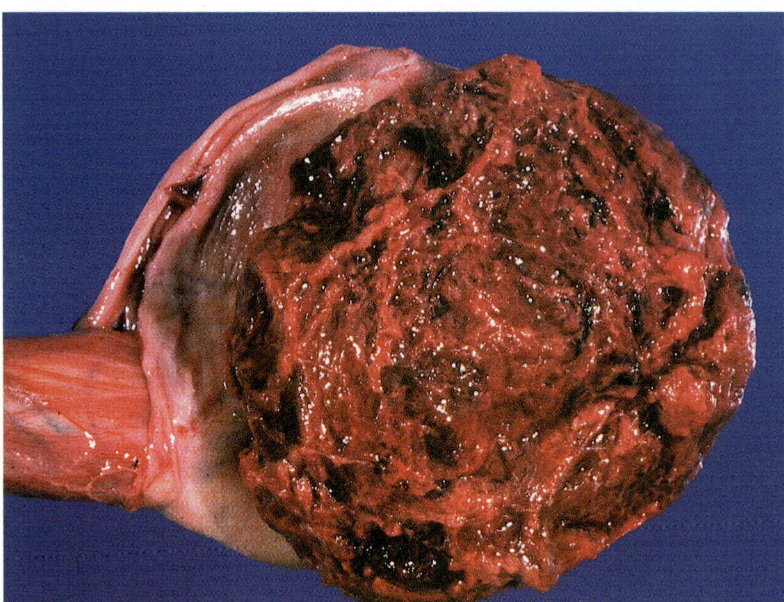

Fig. 16.23. Gross appearance of choriocarcinoma

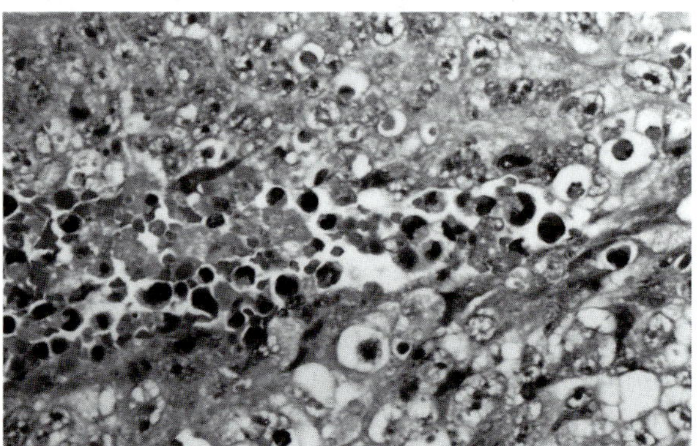

Fig. 16.24. Choriocarcinoma showing syncytiotrophoblasts capping clear-celled cytotrophoblasts

noma. Interestingly, if one looks at the group of mixed germ cell tumors in which seminoma is a dominant component, the median age is about 5 years older than in those with embryonal carcinoma as the dominant component. When chorio-carcinoma is a significant component these tumors may metastasize through a hematogenous route; otherwise they spread via lymphatics. With combined chemotherapy, the prognosis of this group of tumors is excellent. Some authors still suggest that tumors with a significant component of choriocarcinoma have a slightly worse prognosis. Serum markers are helpful in that as many as 90% of the patients have elevations of $\alpha$-fetoprotein or hCG.

## 16.13.2
## Pathologic Features

The testis containing a mixed germ cell tumor is usually enlarged and the tunica may be distorted, particularly if elements of teratoma or embryonal carcinoma are present. The cut surface of these tumors is complex, with the areas of seminoma and mature teratoma being the most easily recognized. The variegated appearance is the most telling predictor of a mixed germ cell tumor. It is important to sample all areas of these tumors to look for each component.

### 16.13.2.1
### *Micrscopic Appearance*

Microscopically, this is an extremely variable group, in that almost all combinations of the various types of single germ cell tumors can be found. The most common combination appears to be the presence of embryonal carcinoma and teratoma, accounting for about 25% of mixed testicular germ cell tumors (Figs. 16.25, 16.26). Studies over time tend to vary in descriptions of the varying proportions of tumor types present. This is at least partly due to the more recent emergence of yolk sac tumor as a distinct type. The tumors are best reported by including all elements present in the order of frequency in which they occur. We also try to designate a rough percent-

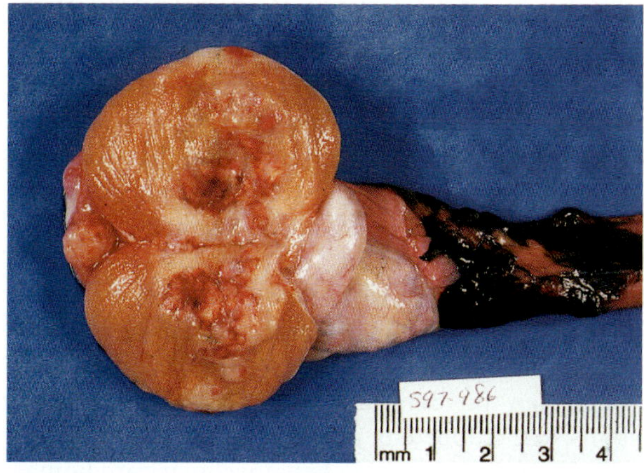

**Fig. 16.25.** Gross appearance of mixed germ cell tumor

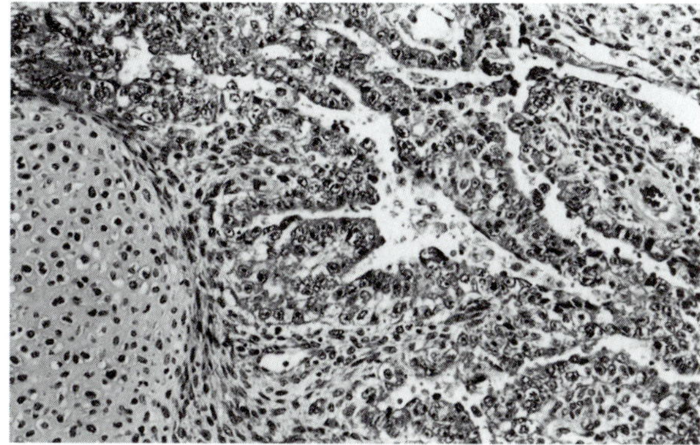

**Fig. 16.26.** Mixed germ cell tumor. Teratoma with embryonal carcinoma

age of each tumor element present. The tumor must be generously sampled with all gross patterns represented or these percentages can be misrepresented. The most common component that occurs in mixed germ cell tumors clearly is embryonal carcinoma and the least common component is choriocarcinoma.

### 16.13.2.2
### *Special Stains*

Immunohistochemical stains can be helpful in recognizing and defining some of these components, especially the yolk sac tumor. Yolk sac tumor is generally most difficult to recognize when it is present in conjunction with embryonal carcinoma or with edematous areas of seminoma. hCG can be helpful in delineating areas of choriocarcinoma. It should be

remembered that seminoma with syncytiotrophoblasts is not considered a mixed germ cell tumor. This is because seminoma with just syncytiotrophoblasts has a clinical behavior and age range similar to that of a seminoma (BUTCHER et al. 1985).

## 16.14
## Extragonadal Presentations of Germ Cell Tumors

In about 5% of patients, the presentation of a germ cell tumor is extragonadal (ASIF and UEHLING 1968). In many such patients metastases are recognized first and the testicular mass is found by a physician. In other patients, the primary is truly extragonadal.

True extragonadal tumors are found along the path of germ cell migration during embryogenesis. The most common reported sites are the pineal, the anterior mediastinum, and the retroperitoneum. The retroperitoneum is also the first and most common site of metastasis from a primary in the gonad. It appears that some retroperitoneal presentations thought to be extragonadal primaries in fact are instances in which the testicular primary has undergone regression following metastasis. Testis may contain a microscopic or occult primary germ cell tumor, or in some patients, a small scar within the testicle associated with histiocytes, fibroblasts, and hemosiderin (MEARES and BRIGGS 1972). Choriocarcinoma is the tumor most likely to present with metastases and a testicular scar most likely representing the testicular primary.

Some patients who present with extensive metastasis and a testicular mass undergo combination chemotherapy before an orchiectomy. SIMMONDS et al. (1995) reported their clinical and pathologic findings in 24 patients whose orchiectomy followed initiation of chemotherapy. It is interesting that even after chemotherapy, ten (39%) of these patients had persistent disease in the testis. Of these ten, two had invasive nonseminomatous germ cell tumors, one had seminoma, six had mature teratoma, and one had carcinoma in situ. The two patients with invasive nonseminomatous germ cell tumor died of disease, and the one with seminoma has relapsed with an elevated α-fetoprotein. That patient was undergoing salvage chemotherapy at the time of publication of Simmond's paper. It seems that chemotherapy in patients with advanced disease does not effectively treat disease within the testis. Therefore, orchiectomy is required at some time in treating patients with gonadal primaries and extensive disease.

## 16.15
## Tumor Markers in Germ Cell Tumors

Three specific tumor markers play an important role in patients with testicular carcinomas: α-fetoprotein, hCG, and placental alkaline phosphatase. All three can be identified in both tissue and serum, allowing for tissue localization by immunohistochemistry and quantitation within the serum. Tissue localization of hCG, α-fetoprotein, and placental alkaline phosphatase plus others is used in the diagnosis of specific tumor types. Quantitation within the serum assists in clinical diagnosis, staging, and monitoring response to therapy and recurrence (BURTIS and ASHWOOD 1994; JAVADPOUR 1980).

Human chorionic gonadotropin is a glycoprotein composed of two dissimilar α- and β-subunits. The α-subunit is also common to luteinizing hormone, follicle-stimulating hormone, and thyroid-stimulating hormone. The β-subunit is unique, with the 30 or so amino acids on the carboxyl terminal end being distinctive. The hormone has a molecular weight of roughly 45 000 daltons and it is produced normally in syncytiotrophoblastic cells of the human placenta (BURTIS and ASHWOOD 1994).

Immunohistochemical techniques using antibodies to the antigenically distinct carboxyl end of the β-chain allow for localization within neoplastic cells. Virtually all choriocarcinomas have hCG within the syncytiotrophoblasts. In addition, one-half to three-quarters of embryonal carcinomas have hCG localized to giant cells within them. About 10% of patients with seminoma have giant cells that stain with hCG (JAVADPOUR 1980).

Serum hCG is elevated in roughly 70% of patients with nonseminatomatous testicular tumors. This hormone is most useful in monitoring response to treatment and recurrence of tumors. The use of hCG in tissue diagnosis of testicular tumors is of interest in characterizing giant cells within seminoma.

The second tumor marker, α-fetoprotein, is an oncofetal antigen composed of a single polypeptide that has a molecular weight of 70 000 daltons and comprises approximately 4% carbohydrate. α-Fetoprotein is closely related structurally to albumin and has a number of homologies in amino acid sequence. Genes for both proteins are located in a similar region of the human genome. α-Fetoprotein is normally produced in large quantities by the fetal

yolk sac and liver and can be found in newborns until approximately 18 months after birth, at which time it reaches the low levels found in normal adults (BURTIS and ASHWOOD 1994).

Careful studies using α-fetoprotein have demonstrated the presence of this tumor marker primarily in endodermal sinus or yolk sac tumors. It can be helpful in demonstrating the yolk sac component, which, in some cases of embryonal carcinoma, can be subtle. Tumors containing α-fetoprotein often have eosinophilic globules within the cytoplasm which can be detected by immunohistochemical stains. α-Fetoprotein is not a specific marker because it is also present in hepatocellular carcinomas. However, it is of great benefit in monitoring patients for response to chemotherapy and monitoring for relapse following orchiectomy and retroperitoneal node dissection. α-Fetoprotein also can be useful in identifying occult yolk sac tumor elements in patients with otherwise pure seminomas or teratomas.

Either α-fetoprotein or hCG is elevated in 90% of patients with nonseminomatous testicular tumors (JAVADPOUR 1980). The elevations do correlate with tumor volume. Although once indicative of prognosis, with modern-day chemotherapy they are no longer good predictors of prognosis. The exception to this is the very high hCG level in patients with choriocarcinoma, a rare event.

Placental alkaline phosphatase is an isoenzyme of alkaline phosphatase, also known as the "Regan" isoenzyme. It appears to be synthesized by the trophoblast and was first identified in 1968 by FISHMAN et al. This enzyme is found in a number of neoplasms, including tumors of ovary, lung, trophoblast, and gastrointestinal tract and Hodgkin's disease.

Immunohistochemical studies have revealed that placental alkaline phosphatase is found in up to 98% of patients with seminoma, 97% of those with embryonal carcinomas, and 85% of those with endodermal sinus tumors (MANIVEL et al. 1987). In addition, cytotrophoblastic cells focally have stained positively in patients with choriocarcinoma. The staining for placental alkaline phosphatase is most characteristic in seminoma, where it stains the cell membranes distinctly and uniformly, and may stain the cytoplasm as well. Embryonal carcinomas can have similar patterns of staining; however, it is focal rather than the uniform staining seen in seminomas. In endodermal sinus tumors, the staining is even more focal than in either seminoma or embryonal carcinoma. It is of interest that placental alkaline phosphatase staining has also been identified in areas of intratubular germ cell neoplasia.

Placental alkaline phosphatase can also be found in the serum and it is used as a marker in patients with testicular germ cell tumors. However, its role in monitoring patients with these tumors has largely been usurped by α-fetoprotein and hCG. Germ cell tumors do produce the LD-1 isoenzyme of lactate dehydrogenase. Therefore lactate dehydrogenase, an enzyme in the glycolytic pathway, can be of benefit in assessing prognosis and monitoring therapy (LIESKOVSKY and SKINNER 1979). A variety of other markers are identified in patients with testicular tumors. These markers, which include neuron-specific enolase, ferritin, placental lactogen, carcinoembryonic antigen, and $\alpha_1$-antitrypsin, have not found great clinical utility. Recently, CA19-9 has been added by TSURUTA et al. (1997) to the list of tumor markers used in the diagnosis and monitoring of patients with embryonal carcinoma. This marker is routinely available in clinical laboratories and could perhaps become more useful in testicular neoplasia.

## 16.16
## Pathologic Features Influencing Prognosis in Germ Cell Tumors

The last 30 years have seen a dramatic change in the prognosis of testicular tumors. The survival rate of patients with carcinoma of the testis in the early 1960s was 63% whereas this figure has risen to 95% in the United States between 1986 and 1993 (*CA, a Cancer Journal for Clinicians*). The most dramatic improvement occurred with the introduction of cisplatin therapy in the late 1970s and early 1980s. This led to a careful reassessment of pathologic data to identify those patients who could benefit from less intensive surgery and chemotherapy.

### 16.16.1
### Tumor Stage

Cumulative data published by SOGANI and FAIR in 1988 indicate that patients with stage 1 or stage A testis cancer followed for 3–97 months had relapse rates ranging from 20% to 40% with a mean of 27.7%. Five hundred and fifty-four, or 99%, of these patients were currently alive and free of disease. Four hundred and five of these patients, or 72.3%, required only orchiectomy. One hundred and forty-nine of

the 560 patients required chemotherapy and/or a radical retroperitoneal lymph node dissection. These data led to a change in management of the patient with testicular cancer limited to the testis and the standard became careful surveillance. Clearly, the strategy of surveillance only for patients was beneficial to those patients who had no disease (PECKHAM et al. 1982). However, those patients who were undergoing surveillance and still had clinically undetectable disease had eventual higher stage presentations. It is of interest that this higher stage presentation did not lead to a greatly diminished survival; however, more aggressive therapy was required (MOUL et al. 1990).

### 16.16.2
### Vascular Invasion

Because of this change in treatment strategy, careful and detailed analysis of pathologic findings influencing patient relapse was performed in the 1980s. These studies all showed that the presence of vascular space invasion by tumor clearly predicted relapse as well as involvement of retroperitoneal lymph nodes (Figs. 16.27, 16.28). The finding of vascular space invasion appears to be the most consistent pathologic finding for predicting retroperitoneal lymph node involvement (MORIYAMA et al. 1985; FUGIME et al. 1984). Criteria for diagnosing tumor within vessels include clear presence within an endothelial lined space (LITTLE et al. 1986), usually with either demonstrated invasion through a vessel wall or adherence of tumor cells to a vessel wall. Additionally, incorporation of tumor cells into thrombus and molding of the tumor to the shape of the vessel are helpful criteria when present. The dis-

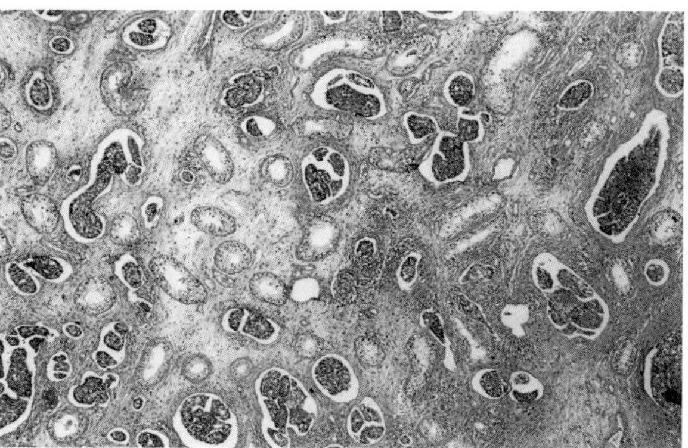

**Fig. 16.27.** Lymphovascular invasion by embryonal carcinoma

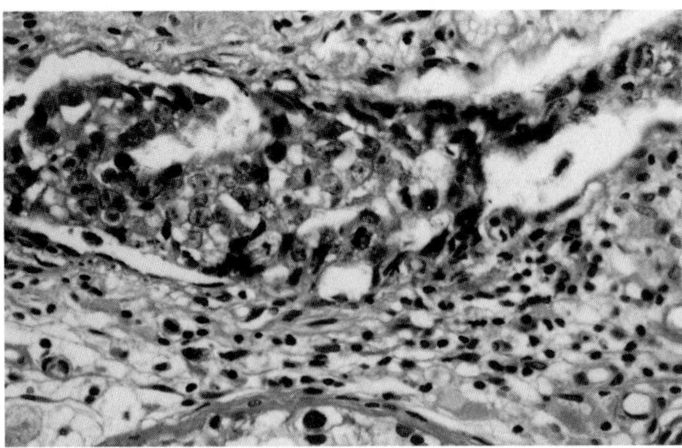

**Fig. 16.28.** Intravascular invasion with adherence to vascular wall

tinction between small blood vessels and lymphatics is not usually possible on H&E sections unless the vessel has a substantial smooth muscle wall identifying it as a blood vessel. Vascular space invasion is usually identified within the tumor itself. However, RODRIGUEZ et al. (1986) point out the tumor is often found in the tunica vasculosa. A number of other important pathologic findings predicting the relapse of stage A testicular cancer include the proportions of different morphologic types of nonseminatous tumor, the substaging of the testicular tumor, the microvessel density, the degree of aneuploidy, and high S-phase fractions as measured by flow cytometry (DIXON and MOORE 1953; DUNPHY et al. 1988; FRALEY et al. 1980; FREEDMAN et al. 1987; FUNG and GARNICE 1988; FUNG et al. 1988; HOSKIN et al. 1986; JAVADPOUR et al. 1986; RAGHAVAN et al. 1982).

Most studies with enough cases to evaluate critically the proportion of various histologic types present in the tumor have found a correlation with relapse or occult retroperitoneal metastases. It appears that a pure embryonal carcinoma, or a mixed germ cell tumor with more than 80% embryonal carcinoma, is more likely to have clinically undetected metastases in the retroperitoneum. As well, it appears that tumors comprising more than 50% teratoma are less likely to involve retroperitoneal lymph nodes. However, when teratoma does metastasize to retroperitoneal lymph nodes, it is less likely to respond to chemotherapy (RABBANI et al. 1996). Another interesting observation has been that yolk sac elements in significant amounts suggest a less likely chance for retroperitoneal lymph node involvement. Not all studies examined the proportions of yolk sac tumor in the same way because of the variations in definition of yolk sac tumor that existed

in the 1980s. Not many studies had patients with significant amounts of choriocarcinoma. However, when they did, the presence of choriocarcinoma seemed to predict a worse prognosis. Several studies indicated that a high α-fetoprotein level predicted a greater chance of retroperitoneal disease, although one study indicated the opposite.

The presence of neovascularity within the tumor appears to predict for a greater chance of metastasis in germ cell tumors of the testis. A study by OLIVAREZ et al. (1994) indicated that high levels of microvessel density in focal areas of the tumor predicted for a greater chance of retroperitoneal involvement. This study also pointed out that when microvessel density counts were low, there was an inability to predict patients who had retroperitoneal lymph node involvement. In other words, the finding was of benefit only when levels of microvessel density were high.

A number of studies found that involvement of capsule, the rete testis, and the cord were important in evaluation of the orchiectomy specimen. It was interesting that tumor size and grade were not important in predicting occurrence of retroperitoneal node involvement. In cases of pure teratoma, patients with intratubular germ cell neoplasia were more likely to have metastases than those without it (JORGENSEN et al. 1995a).

Recently, studies have begun to analyze the S-phase fraction with particular focus on the degree of aneuploidy within the nonseminomatous component as well as the percent of aneuploid tumor cells in S-phase. Highly aneuploid or multiple aneuploid stemlines correlate with more malignant behavior. The percent of aneuploid tumor cells in S-phase predicts for pathologic stage (ALLHOFF et al. 1990; DE GRAAFF et al. 1993; DE RIESE et al. 1994; SUZUKI et al. 1996). Studies of the p53 gene (CHRESTA et al. 1996) have revealed p53 mutations in intratubular germ cell neoplasia (KUCZYK et al. 1996). As well, seminoma and embryonal carcinoma are the most likely tumors to show p53 nuclear expression immunohistochemically. Patients with high levels of p53 expression appeared to have the most sensitive tumors to chemotherapy (EID et al. 1997b; HANNA et al. 1996). Studies have differed, however, concerning correlation of stage with p53 expression (EID et al. 1997b; HANNA et al. 1996). Additional markers under active investigation include metallothionein, P-glycoprotein, vascular endothelial growth factor, chromosome 12p, and glutathione-related enzymes (EID et al. 1996, 1997a; VIGLIETTO et al. 1996; BLOUGH 1995; INSTITORIS et al. 1995).

Unfortunately, none of the pathologic observations have proven to be so precise that prediction of metastases is both sensitive and specific. At this point, it is only possible to predict patients at high risk of relapse. Until more accurate prediction of tumor behavior is possible, the possibility of surgery without certainty of benefit will still be with us. Fortunately, the surgical complications are not severe. The most common complication is the loss of ejaculatory function due to the interruption of the sympathetic ganglia, occurring at a young age. The rate of this complication can be as high as 70%; however, modification of the retroperitoneal node dissection has reduced it to <5% (SKINNER D, personal communication). Other complications of chemotherapy and radiation include leukemia, myelodysplasia, and radiation-induced neoplasms, but these are far less common. The complication of infertility related to chemotherapy is alleviated by sperm banking. The complication of bone marrow damage is less common today, especially at the levels of irradiation used in the treatment of most of these tumors.

# References


Ahmed T, Bosl GJ, Hajdu SI (1985) Teratoma with malignant transformation in germ cell tumors in men. Cancer 56:860–863

Allhoff EP, Liedkes S, Wittekind C, de Riese W, Lenis G, Tanke H, Jonas U (1990) DNA content in NSGC T/CSI: a new prognosticator for biologic behaviour. J Cancer Res Clin Oncol 1(Suppl):592

Amsterdam A, Prieto V, Mazumdar M, Bosl GJ, Vlamis V, Reuter V, Motzer RJ (1996) Teratoma with malignant transformation (TMT): histologic and clinical correlations (meeting abstract). Proc Annu Meet Am Soc Clin Oncol 15:A639

Asif S, Uehling DT (1968) Microscopic tumor foci in testes. J Urol 99:776–779

Blough RI (1995) Cytogenetic and molecular cytogenetic studies of residual male germ cell tumors, and comparison with established cell lines and archival tissue specimens. Diss Abstr Int [B] 56:2437

Burtis CA, Ashwood ER (eds) (1994) Tietz textbook of clinical chemistry, 2nd edn. W.B. Saunders, Philadelphia

Butcher DB, Gregory WM, Gunter PA, Masters JRW, Parkinson MC (1985) The biological and clinical significance of HCG-containing cells in seminoma. Br J Cancer 51:573–478

Chresta CM, Arriola EL, Hickman JA (1996) Characterization of the genetic determinants of chemosensitivity in human testicular cancer (meeting abstract). Proc Annu Meet Am Assoc Cancer Res 37:A2819

Clark RK, Damjanov I (1985) Intermediate filaments of human trophoblast and choriocarcinoma cell lines. Arch Pathol Anat 407:203–208

Daugaard G, Giwercman A, Skakkebaek NE (1996) Should the other testis be biopsied? Semin Urol Oncol 14:8–12

de Graaff WE, Slieffer DT, de Jong B, Dam A, Schraffordt Koops H, Oosterhuis JW (1993) Significance of aneuploid stemlines in testicular nonseminomatous germ cell tumors. Cancer 72:1300–1304

de la Taille A, Houlgatte A, Houdelette P, et al. (1997) Role of testicular biopsy in the investigation of a carcinoma in situ. Prog Urol 7:209–214

de Riese WT, Albers P, Walker EB, et al. (1994) Predictive parameters of biologic behavior of early stage nonseminomatous testicular germ cell tumors. Cancer 74:1335–1341

Dieckmann KP, Loy V (1996) Prevalence of contralateral testicular intraepithelial neoplasia in patients with testicular germ cell neoplasms. J Clin Oncol 14:3126–3132

Dixon F, Moore RA (1953) Testicular tumors. A clinicopathological study. Cancer 6:427–454

Donohue JP (ed) (1983) Testis tumors. International perspectives in urology, vol. 7. Williams & Wilkins, Baltimore

Donohue JP (1984) Metastatic pathways of nonseminomatous germ cell tumors. Semin Urol 2:217–229

Dunphy CH, Ayala AG, Swanson DA, Ro JY, Logothetis C (1988) Clinical stage I nonseminomatous and mixed germ cell tumors of the testis. A clinicopathologic study of 93 patients on a surveillance protocol after orchiectomy alone. Cancer 62:1202–1206

Eid H, Bodrogi I, Csokay B, Olah E, Bak M (1996) Multidrug resistance of testis cancers: the study of clinical relevance of P-glycoprotein expression. Anticancer Res 16:3447–3452

Eid H, Institoris E, Bodrogi I, Bak M (1997a) Metallothionein expression as a marker of therapeutic sensitivity in the early stages of testicular cancer. Orv Hetil 138:135–139

Eid H, Van der Looij M, Institoris E, Geczi L, Bodrogi I, Olah E, Bak M (1997b) Is p53 expression, detected by immunohistochemistry, an important parameter of response to treatment in testis cancer? Anticancer Res 17:2663–2669

Fiet J, Jardin A, Gourmel B, Villette JM, Guechot, Gueux B (1985) Spermatic blood βHCG levels in testicular tumors and in varicocele. In: Khoury S, Kuss R, Murphy GP, Chatelain C, Karr JP (eds) Testicular cancer. Alan R. Liss, New York, pp 117–120

Fishman WH, Inglis NR, Stolbach LL, Krant MJ (1968) A serum alkaline phosphatase isoenzyme of human neoplastic cell origin. Cancer Res 28:150–154

Floyd C, Ayala AG, Logothetis CJ, Silva EG (1988) Spermatocytic seminoma with associated sarcoma of the testis. Cancer 61:409–414

Fraley EE, Lange PH, Williams RD, Ortlip SA (1980) Staging of early nonseminomatous germ-cell testicular cancer. Cancer 45:1762–1767

Freedman LS, Parkinson MC, Jones WG, et al. (1987) Histopathology in the prediction of relapse of patients with stage I testicular teratoma treated by orchidectomy alone. Lancet II:294–297

Friedman NB, Moore RA (1946) Tumors of the testis: a report on 922 cases. Mil Surg 99:573–593

Fugime M, Chang H, Lin C-W, Prout GR Jr (1984) Correlation of vascular invasion and metastasis in germ cell tumors of testis – a preliminary report. J Urol 131:1237–1241

Fung CY, Garnice MB (1988) Clinical stage I carcinoma of the testis: a review. J Clin Oncol 6:734–750

Fung CY, Kalish LA, Brodsky GL, Richie JP, Garnick MB (1988) Stage I nonseminomatous germ cell testicular tumor: prediction of metastatic potential by primary histopathology. J Clin Oncol 6:1467–1473

Ginsburg J (1997) Unanswered questions in carcinoma of the testis. Lancet 349:1785–1786

Giwercman A, Skakkebaek NE (1989) Carcinoma-in-situ (gonocytoma-in-situ) of the testis. In: Burger H, de Kretser D (eds) The testis, 2nd ed. Raven Press, New York

Hanna E, Bodrogi I, Institoris E, Bak M (1996) Correlation between p-53 expression and clinical resistance in testicular cancer. Orv Hetil 137:59–64

Harland SJ, Cook PA, Fossa SD, et al. (1996) Quantitating risk of contralateral testicular carcinoma in situ (CIS) in patients with testicular cancer: an MRC study (meeting abstract). Proc Annu Meet Am Soc Clin Oncol 15:A592

Heidenreich A, Engelmann UH, Vietsch HV, Derschum W (1995) Organ preserving surgery in testicular epidermoid cysts. J Urol 153:1147–1150

Heidenreich A, Zumbe J, Vorreuther R, Klotz T, Vietsch H, Engelmann UH (1996) [Testicular epidermoid cyst: orchiectomy or enucleation resection?] Urologe A 35:1–5

Heidenreich A, Moul JW, McLeod DG, Mostofi FK, Engelmann UH (1997) The role of retroperitoneal lymphadenectomy in mature teratoma of the testis. J Urol 157:160–163

Herr HW, Sheinfeld J (1997) Is biopsy of the contralateral testis necessary in patients with germ cell tumors? J Urol 158:1331–1334

Hiraoka N, Yamada T, Abe H, Hata J (1997) Establishment of three monoclonal antibodies specific for prespermatogonia and intratubular malignant germ cells in humans. Lab Invest 76:427–438

Hollinshead WH (1962) Textbook of anatomy: Harper & Row, New York, 20:620–623, 22:790–794

Hoskin P, Dilly S, Easton D, Horwich A, Hendry W, Peckham MJ (1986) Prognostic factors in stage I non-seminomatous germ-cell testicular tumors managed by orchiectomy and surveillance: implications for adjuvant chemotherapy. J Clin Oncol 4:1031–1036

Houlgatte A, Houdelette P, Berlizot P, Fournier R, Bernard O, Schill H (1995) Bilateral tumors of the testis: the role of the diagnosis of carcinoma in situ in early detection. Prog Urol 5:540–543

Institoris E, Eid H, Bodrogi I, Bak M (1995) Glutathione related enzymes in human testicular germ cell tumors and normal testes. Anticancer Res 15:1371–1374

Jacobsen GK, Talerman A (1989) Atlas of germ cell tumours. Munksgaard, Copenhagen

Jacobsen GK, Jacobsen M, Clausen PP (1981) Distribution of tumor-associated antigens in various histologic components of germ cell tumors. Am J Surg Pathol 5:257

Jacobsen GK, Barlebo H, Olsen J, Schultz HP, Starklint H, Sogaard H, Vaeth M (1984) Testicular germ cell tumours in Denmark 1976–1980. Pathology of 1958 consecutive cases. Acta Radiol 23:239

Javadpour N (1980) The role of biologic tumor markers in testicular cancer. Cancer 45:1755–1761

Javadpour N, Canning DA, O'Connell KJ, Young JD (1986) Predictors of recurrent clinical stage I nonseminomatous testicular cancer. A prospective clinicopathologic study. Urology 27:508–511

Javadpour N, Young Jr JD (1986) Prognostic factors in nonseminomatous testicular cancer. J Urol 135:497–499

Jorgensen N, Muller J, Giwercman A, Visfeldt J, Moller H, Skakkebaek NE (1995a) DNA content and expression of tumour markers in germ cells adjacent to germ cell tumours in childhood: probably a different origin for infantile and adolescent germ cell tumours. J Pathol 176:269–278

Jorgensen N, Rajpert-De Meyts E, Graem N, Muller J, Giwercman A, Skakkebaek NE (1995b) Expression of immunohistochemical markers for testicular carcinoma in situ by normal human fetal germ cells. Lab Invest 72:223–231

Kay R (1993) Prepubertal testicular tumor registry. J Urol 150:671–674

Kuczyk MA, Serth J, Bokemeyer C, Jonassen J, Machtens S, Werner M, Jonas U (1996) Alterations of the p53 tumor suppressor gene in carcinoma in situ of the testis. Cancer 78:1958–1966

Landis SH, Murray T, Bolden S, Wingo PA (1998) Cancer statistics 1998. CA Cancer J Clin 48:6–29

Leahy M (1992) Cancer of testis. Lancet 340:1281–1282

Lieskovsky G, Skinner DG (1979) Significance of serum lactic dehydrogenase in stages B and C non-seminomatous testis tumors. J Urol 123:516–517

Little D, Said JW, Siegel RJ, Fealy M, Fishbein MC (1986) Endothelial cell markers in vascular neoplasms: an immunohistochemical study comparing factor VIII-related antigen, blood group specific antigens, 6-keto-PGF1 alpha, and *Ulex europaeus* 1 lectin. J Pathol 149:89–95

Looijenga LH (1995) Pathobiology of germ cell tumors of the adult testis: views and news. Diss Abstr Int 55:5182

Manivel JC, Jessurun J, Wick MR, Dehner LP (1987) Placental alkaline phosphatase immunoreactivity in testicular germ-cell neoplasms. Am J Surg Pathol 11:21–29

Masson P (1946) Etude sur le seminome. Rev Canad Biol 5:381–387

Meares Jr. EM, Briggs EM (1972) Occult seminoma of the testis masquerading as primary extragonadal germinal neoplasms. Cancer 30:300–306

Moriyama N, Daly JJ, Keating MA, Lin C-W, Prout GR (1985) Vascular invasion as a prognosticator of metastatic disease in nonseminomatous germ cell tumors of the testis. Importance in "surveillance only" protocols. Cancer 56:2492–2498

Mostofi FK (1977) Histological typing of testis tumours. In: WHO, International Histological Classification of Tumours 16

Mostofi FK, Price EB Jr (1973) Tumors of the male genital system. Atlas of tumor pathology, 2nd series, Fasc 8. Armed Forces Institute of Pathology, Washington, D.C.

Mostofi FK, Sesterhenn IA, Davis CJ Jr (1987) Immunopathology of germ cell tumors of the testis. Semin Diagn Pathol 4:320–341

Moul JW, Paulson DF, Dodge RK, Walther PJ (1990) Delay in diagnosis and survival in testicular cancer: impact of effective therapy and changes during 18 years. J Urol 143:520–523

Moul JW, Foley JP, Hitchcock CL, McCarthy WF, Sesterhenn IA, Becker RL, Griffin JL (1993) Flow cytometric and quantitative histological parameters to predict occult disease in clinical stage I nonseminomatous testicular germ cell tumors. J Urol 150:879–883

Moul JW, McCarthy WF, Fernandez EB, Sesterhenn IA (1994) Percentage of embryonal carcinoma and of vascular invasion predicts pathologic stage in clinical stage I nonseminomatous testicular cancer. Cancer Res 54:362–364

Niehans GA, Manivel JC, Copland GT, Scheithauer BW, Wick MR (1988) Immunohisto- chemistry of germ cell and trophoblastic neoplasms. Cancer 62:1113–1123

Olivarez D, Ulbright T, DeRiese W, Foster R, Reister T, Einhorn L, Sledge G (1994) Neovascularization in clinical stage A testicular germ cell tumor: prediction of metastatic disease. Cancer Res 54:2800–2802

Peckham MJ, Barrett A, Husband JE, Hendry WF (1982) Orchidectomy alone in testicular stage I nonseminomatous germ-cell tumours. Lancet II:678–680

Percarpio B, Clements JC, McLeod DG, Sorgen SD, Cardinale FS (1979) Anaplastic seminoma. An analysis of 77 patients. Cancer 43:2510–2513

Petersen PM, Lenz SC, Giwercman AJ, Sommer P, Skakkebaek NE (1997) Testicular carcinoma in situ detected by ultrasound in infertile men. Ugeskr Laeger 159:3962–3963

Pugh RCB (ed) (1976) Pathology of the testis, 6. Blackwell Scientific, Oxford

Rabbani F, Gleave ME, Coppin CM, Murray N, Sullivan LD (1996) Teratoma in primary testis tumor reduces complete response rates in the retroperitoneum after primary chemotherapy. The case for primary retroperitoneal lymph node dissection of stage IIb germ cell tumors with teratomatous elements. Cancer 78:480–486

Raghavan D, Vogelzang NJ, Bosl GJ, et al. (1982) Tumor classification and size in germ-cell testicular cancer. Influence on the occurrence of metastases. Cancer 50:1591–1595

Ro JY, Amato RJ, Ayala AG (1996) What does the pathology report really mean? Semin Urol Oncol 14:2–7

Rodriguez PN, Hafez GR, Messing EM (1986) Nonseminomatous germ cell tumor of the testicle: Does extensive staging of the primary tumor predict the likelihood of metastatic disease? J Urol 136:604–608

Shimizu S, Nagata Y, Han-yaku H (1996) Metastatic testicular choriocarcinoma of the skin. Report and review of the literature. Am J Dermatopathol 18:633–636

Simmonds PD, Mead GM, Lee AHS, Theaker JM, Dewbury K, Smart CJ (1995) Orchiectomy after chemotherapy in patients with metastatic testicular cancer. Is it indicated? Cancer 75:1018–1024

Simmonds PD, Lee AH, Theaker JM, Tung K, Smart CJ, Mead GM (1996) Primary pure teratoma of the testis. J Urol 155:939–942

Skakkebaek NE (1972) Possible carcinoma-in-situ of the undescended testis. Lancet 2:516–517

Skakkebaek NE, Berthelsen JG, Grigor KM, Visfeldt J (1981) Early detection of testicular cancer. Scriptor, Copenhagen

Skinner DG (1969) Non-seminomatous testis tumors: a plan of management based on 96 patients to improve survival in all stages by combined therapeutic modalities. J Urol 115:65–69

Sogani PC, Fair WR (1988) Surveillance alone in the treatment of clinical stage I nonseminomatous germ cell tumor of the testis (NSGCT). Semin Urol 6:53–56

Soosay GN, Bobrow L, Happerfield L, Parkinson MC (1991) Morphology and immunohistochemistry of carcinoma in situ adjacent to testicular germ cell tumours in adults and children: implications for histogenesis. Histopathology 19:537–544

Sturgeon JFG, Jewett MAS, Alison RE, et al. (1992) Surveillance after orchidectomy for patients with clinical stage I nonseminomatous testis tumors. J Clin Oncol 10:564–568

Suzuki M, Hosaka Y, Matsushima H, Mizutani T, Kawabe K (1996) Nuclear deoxyribonucleic acid ploidy of testicular tumors: peculiar features and clinical significance. Urol Int 57:203–208

Talerman A (1980) Spermatocytic seminoma. Clinicopathological study of 22 cases. Cancer 45:2169–2176

Talerman A, Haije WG, Baggerman L (1980) Serum alphafetoprotein (AFP) in patients with germ cell tumors of the gonads and extragonadal sites. Correlation between endodermal sinus (yolk sac) tumor and raised serum AFP. Cancer 46:380–385

Tauseef A, Bosl GJ, Hajdu SI (1985) Teratoma with malignant transformation in germ cell tumors in men. Cancer 56:860–863

Teilum G (1959) Endodermal sinus tumors of the ovary and testis. Comparative morphogenesis of the so-called mesonephroma ovarii (Schiller) and extraembryonic (yolk sac-allantoic) structures of the rat's placenta. Cancer 12:1092

Teilum G (1976) Special tumors of the ovary and testis and related extragonadal lesions. Comparative pathology and histologic identification, 2nd edn. Munksgaard, Cophenhagen

Thompson J, Williams CJ, Whitehouse JMA, Mead GM (1988) Bilateral testicular germ cell tumours: an increasing incidence and prevention by chemotherapy. Br J Urol 62:374–376

Trainer TD (1997) Testis and excretory duct system. In: Sternberg SS (ed) Histology for pathologists, 2nd edn. Lippincott-Raven, Philadelphia, pp 1019–1039

True LD, Otis CN, Delprado W, Scully RE, Rosai J (1988) Spermatocytic seminoma of testis with sarcomatous transformation. A report of five cases. Am J Surg Pathol 12:75–82

Tsuruta T, Ogawa A, Ishii K, Ikado S (1997) CA19-9: a possible serum marker for embryonal carcinoma. Urol Int 58:20–24

van Echten J, van Gurp RJ, Stoepker M, Looijenga LH, de Jong J, Oosterhuis W (1995) Cytogenetic evidence that carcinoma in situ is the precursor lesion for invasive testicular germ cell tumors. Cancer Genet Cytogenet 85:133–137

Viglietto G, Romano A, Maglione D, et al. (1996) Neovascularization in human germ cell tumors correlates with a marked increase in the expression of the vascular endothelial growth factor but not the placenta-derived growth factor. Oncogene 13:577–587

Wick MR, Swanson PE, Manivel JC (1987) Placental-like alkaline phosphatase reactivity in human tumors: an immunohistochemical study of 520 cases. Hum Pathol 18:946–954

Wishnow KI, Dunphy CH, Johnson DE, et al. (1989) Identifying patients with low-risk clinical stage I nonseminomatous testicular tumors who should be treated by surveillance. Urology 34:339–343

Young RH, Scully RE (1990) Testicular tumors. ASCP Press, Chicago

Zuckman MH, Williams G, Levin HS (1988) Mitosis counting in seminoma: an exercise of questionable significance. Hum Pathol 19:329–335

# 17 Imaging of Testicular Neoplasms

R.H. Oyen, B.M. Verbist, and G.A. Verswijvel

CONTENTS



R.H. Oyen, MD, PhD, Adjunct Clinic Head, Department of
Radiology, University Hospitals Gasthuisberg, Catholic University of Leuven, Herestraat 49, B-3000 Leuven, Belgium
B.M. Verbist, MD, Department of Radiology, University
Hospitals Gasthuisberg, Catholic University of Leuven,
Herestraat 49, B-3000 Leuven, Belgium
G.A. Verswijvel, MD, Department of Radiology, University
Hospitals Gasthuisberg, Catholic University of Leuven,
Herestraat 49, B-3000 Leuven, Belgium

## 17.1 Examination Techniques

### 17.1.1 Ultrasonography

The scrotum and its contents are examined with a linear or curvilinear high-resolution, high-frequency (7.5–10 MHz) dedicated small parts transducer with color and duplex Doppler capability. Sagittal and transverse images of both testes and epididymis are obtained. If there is a palpable abnormality on physical examination, it is often helpful to perform targeted scanning during palpation to correlate potential ultrasonographic (US) abnormalities with physical examination (Hamm 1997).

Color Doppler settings are optimized to detect slow flow: the highest color gain setting allowing an acceptable signal-to-noise ratio, the lowest wall filter, and the lowest velocity scale.

Ultrasonography is the modality of choice for primary tumor detection. Nevertheless, the findings are nonspecific. In general, in adulthood, any painless solid testicular mass must be considered malignant until proven otherwise. Furthermore, results for local staging (T-staging) are disappointing. US is infrequently used for the staging of the retroperitoneal area. In selected cases, as in very thin patients, US nevertheless can be helpful for distinguishing vascular structures from lymph nodes.

### 17.1.2 Magnetic Resonance Imaging

The patient is usually positioned supine and a surface coil is employed to increase the signal-to-noise ratio. Both T1- and T2-weighted images are obtained with a slice thickness of 3–5 mm. Fast spin-echo images are now routinely used. Additional sequences (e.g., fat saturation) may be helpful in selected cases. The coronal plane is generally preferred for imaging the scrotum because it allows comparison of both parts of the scrotum, with good visualization of the relation of the testis to the epididymis and to the spermatic cord (OYEN et al. 1993; HAMM et al. 1995). Furthermore, signal intensity variability is minimized because the coil is parallel to the coronal imaging plane. The administration of intravenous gadolinium may provide further information on the integrity of the blood–testis barrier, and may improve diagnostic yield in cases of infection and torsion (HAMM et al. 1995).

Virtually all neoplasms of the testis present as decreased signal intensity on T2-weighted images when compared with the normal testis. In most cases, a rim of normal testicular parenchyma is preserved, thus allowing a relative comparison of normal and abnormal tissue characteristics. Discontinuity of the dark, hypointense tunica albuginea is suggestive of extratesticular invasion.

Differentiation and specification of tumors cannot be achieved by magnetic resonance imaging (MRI), nor does it allow accurate evaluation of subacute torsion of the testis. In such cases, dynamic MRI following intravenous administration of gadolinium may improve the diagnostic accuracy (OYEN et al. 1993; HAMM et al. 1995; NAGLER-REUS et al. 1995).

In a comparative study of 75 patients, MRI showed diagnostic advantages in the detection and characterization of malignant tumors and in the detection of nontumorous testicular pathology (missed torsion, periorchitis, old hematoma) (DEROUET et al. 1993). MRI may be useful when US is inconclusive or equivocal, or fails to demonstrate a clinically suspected lesion.

Staging accuracy of retroperitoneal disease is comparable to that of computed tomography (CT). Like CT, lymph node enlargement is the main assessed criterion. Overall signal characteristics have been unreliable for differentiating benign and malignant enlarged lymph nodes or residual masses.

### 17.1.3
### Computed Tomography

Computed tomography is presently the modality of choice for evaluating retroperitoneal tumor spread. CT detection of retroperitoneal involvement is based on metastases causing lymph node enlargement. Any number of lymph nodes, regardless of size, in the expected primary retroperitoneal drainage area must be suspected of having a high risk of harboring occult nodal disease.

Computed tomography has the advantage of being able to evaluate for abdominal, thoracic, brain, and osseous extranodal metastases.

### 17.1.4
### Lymphangiography

Lymphangiography is still utilized at some centers to evaluate equivocal CT findings in patients with elevated serum markers and normal CT, as well as in some surveillance protocols and radiation treatment planning.

## 17.2
## Malignant Testicular Tumors

### 17.2.1
### Germ Cell Tumors

#### *17.2.1.1*
#### *Seminomatous Germ Cell Tumors*

Seminomas constitute 40% of germ cell neoplasms. The incidence of bilateral seminoma is about 4%. In approximately 10% of cases, metastases are detected in the retroperitoneal lymph nodes at the time of presentation.

Sonographically seminoma presents as a focal nodular or multinodular, well-circumscribed hypoechoic mass in the majority of cases (Figs. 17.1, 17.2a). Multifocal hypoechoic areas may be seen as well

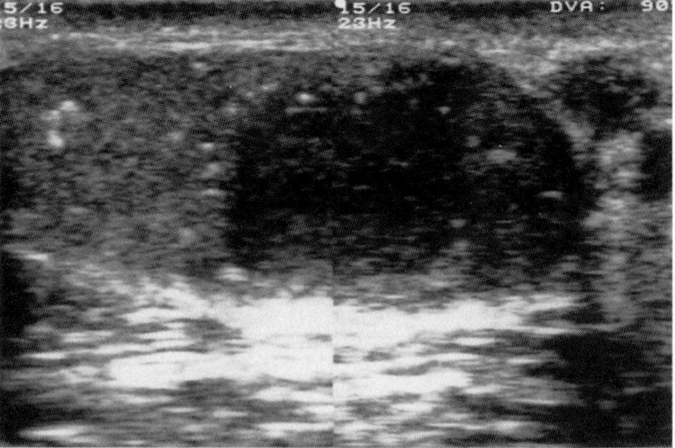

Fig. 17.1. Seminoma. Longitudinal US. Hypoechoic mass lesion in the lower pole of the testis, indiscernible from the tunica albuginea: seminoma. Note the hyperechoic spots throughout the testicular parenchyma, consistent with testicular microlithiasis ("snowstorm" appearance)

(Fig. 17.3a). Occasionally, diffuse involvement of the entire testis and heterogeneous echotexture is seen. Microcalcifications are seen in about one-third of cases (Figs. 17.1, 17.4). There is usually increased vascularity on color Doppler US when the mass is larger than 1.0 cm in diameter. On MRI these tumors present as isointense mass lesions on T1-weighted images and as sharply marginated, relatively homogeneous hypointense masses on T2-weighted images (Figs. 17.2b,c, 17.3b). Hemorrhage and necrosis, although rare in seminomatous tumors, cause areas of increased signal intensity on T2-weighted images (Fig. 17.5). Calcifications occasionally can be suspected because of the presence of decreased signal intensity.

### *17.2.1.2*
### *Nonseminomatous Germ Cell Tumors*

#### 17.2.1.2.1
EMBRYONAL CELL CARCINOMA

Embryonal cell carcinoma is the second most common germ cell neoplasm, accounting for almost 40% of nonseminomatous germ cell tumors (NSGCTs). It occurs most commonly during the third decade. With

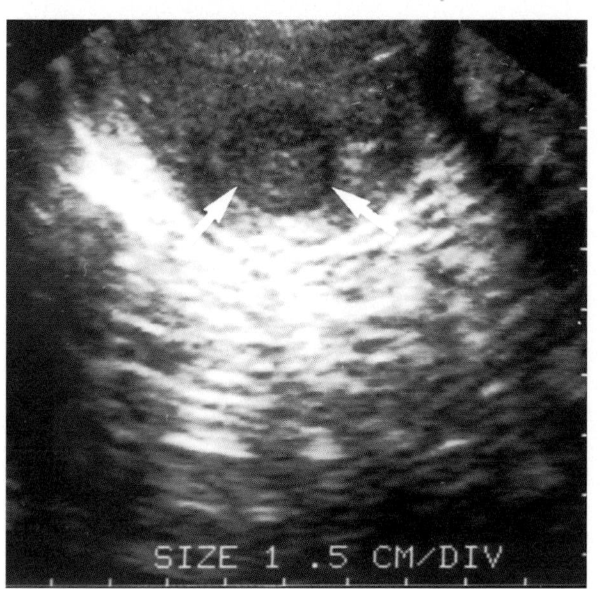

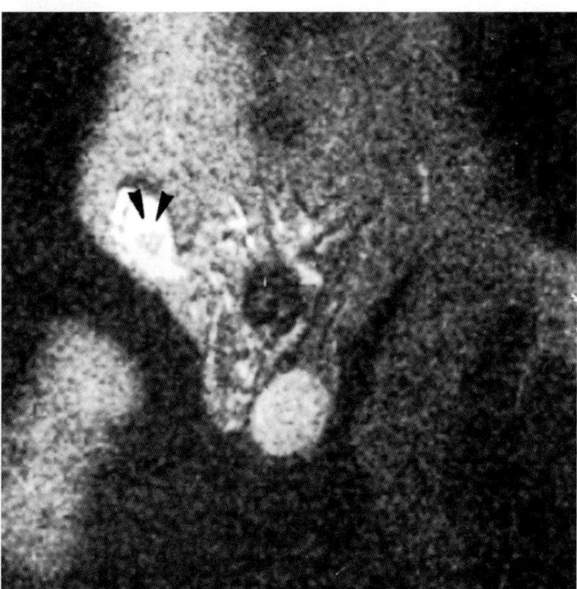

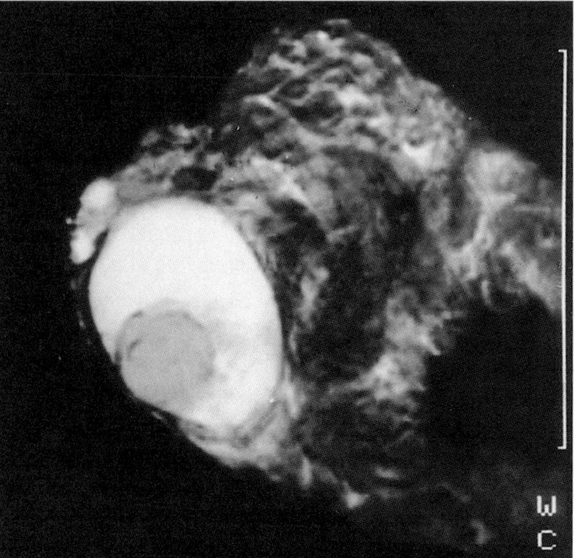

**Fig. 17.2 a–c.** Cryptorchidism and seminoma. US, MRI, and in vitro MRI of the resected specimen. Longitudinal US (**a**) shows a hypoechoic nodule (*arrow*) in the smaller right testis which was located in the inguinal canal. Coronal T2-weighted MR study (**b**) shows a hypointense nodule (*arrowhead*) in the cryptorchid right testis. In vitro T2-weighted MRI (**c**) confirms the hypointense appearance of the seminoma, surrounded by a hypointense halo

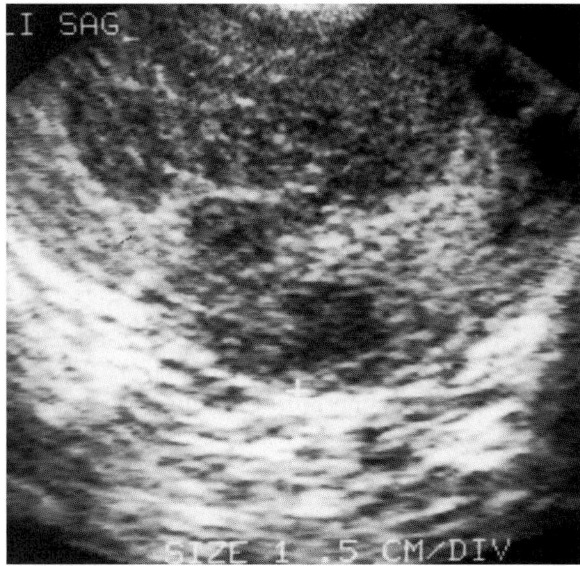

a

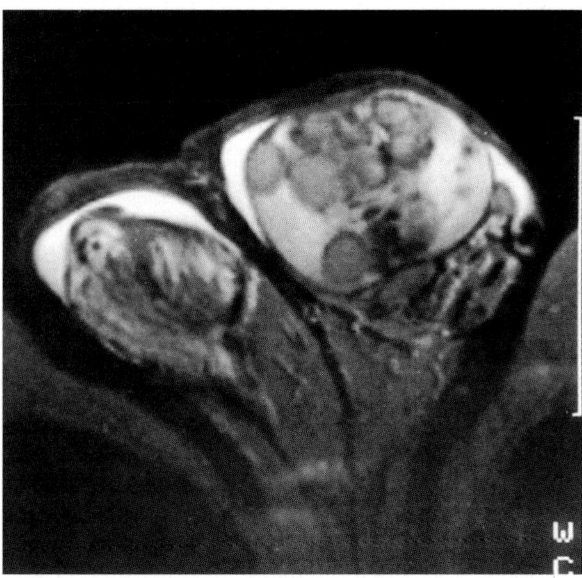

b

**Fig. 17.3 a,b.** Seminoma. US and MRI. Sagittal US (**a**) of the left testis shows a multinodular hypoechoic left testis, with focal bulging of the tunica albuginea. Axial T2-weighted MRI likewise illustrates the multinodular aspect and relatively lower signal intensity of this extensive testicular seminoma

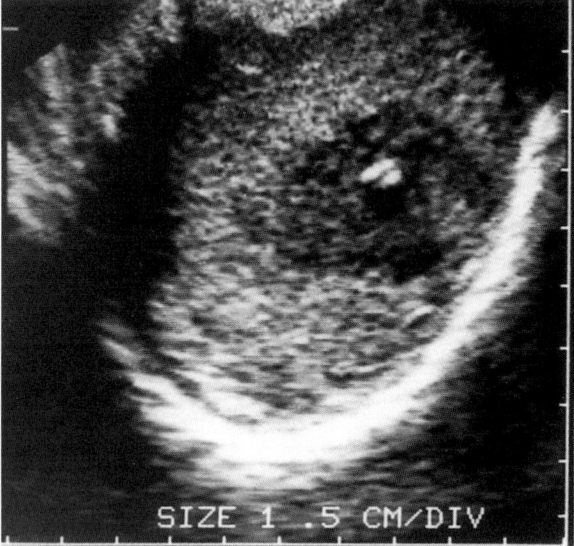

**Fig. 17.4.** Seminoma. US, transverse scan scan. Heterogeneous, predominantly hypoechoic lesion with central hyperechoic spot. Because of the heterogeneity, this was suggested to be a nonseminomatous germ cell tumor. This was a seminoma with areas of hemorrhage

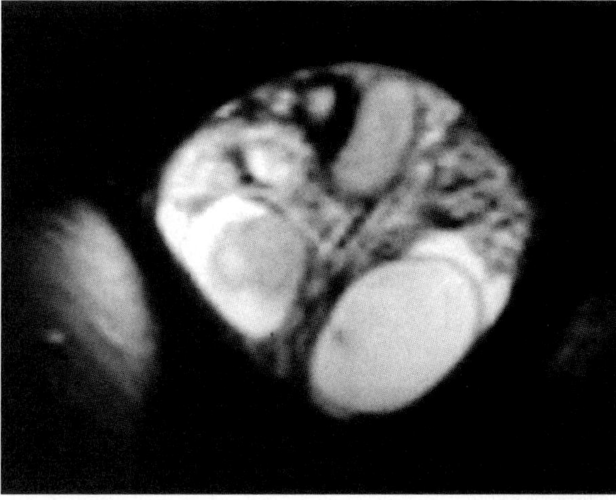

**Fig. 17.5.** Seminoma. MRI, T2-weighted image. Transverse scan shows a hypointense mass lesion in the right testis, indiscernible from the tunica albuginea. The lateral aspect of the lesion exhibits some hyperintense areas

the majority of embryonal cell carcinomas there are already metastases at the time of presentation. On US, these tumors may be hypoechoic but often are more heterogeneous than seminomas due to the presence of cystic changes and calcifications (Fig. 17.6a). Focal areas of hemorrhage may contribute to the increased echogenicity. Because of these characteristics, embryonal cell carcinomas tend also to be heterogeneous on MR images, with areas of high and low signal intensity (Figs. 17.6b, 17.7b). Heterogeneity of the mass has been found to be the most specific sign for a nonseminomatous tumor (compared to seminomas) followed by high signal intensity on T2-weighted images (JOHNSON et al. 1990).

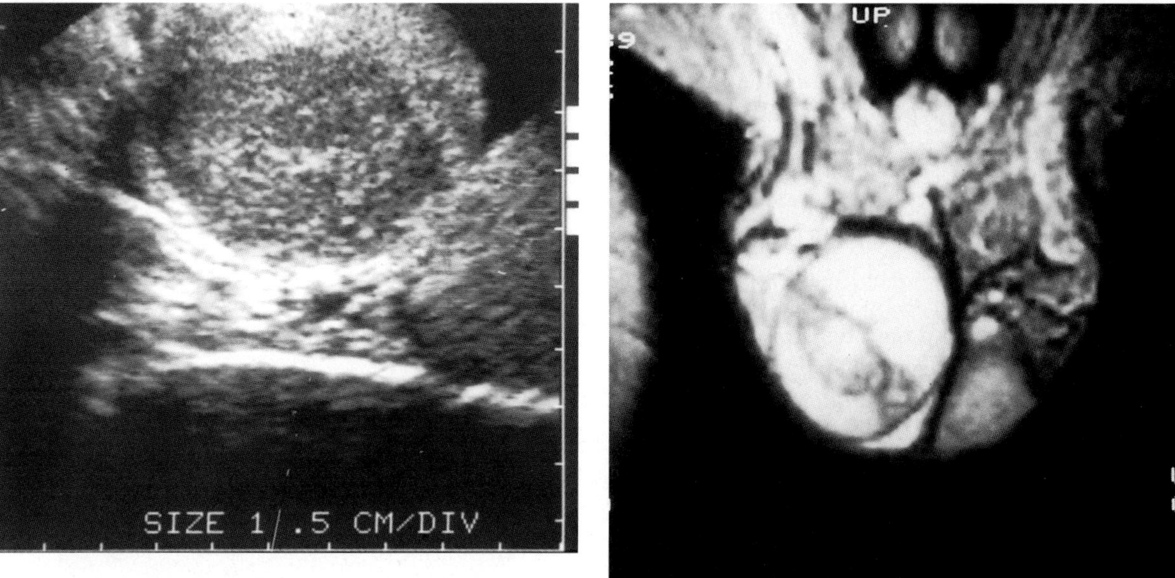

**Fig. 17.6 a,b.** Embryonal cell carcinoma. Transverse US (**a**) and coronal T2-weighted MRI (**b**). Hypoechoic, slightly heterogeneous mass in the right testis. The mass exhibits heterogeneous signal characteristics at MRI

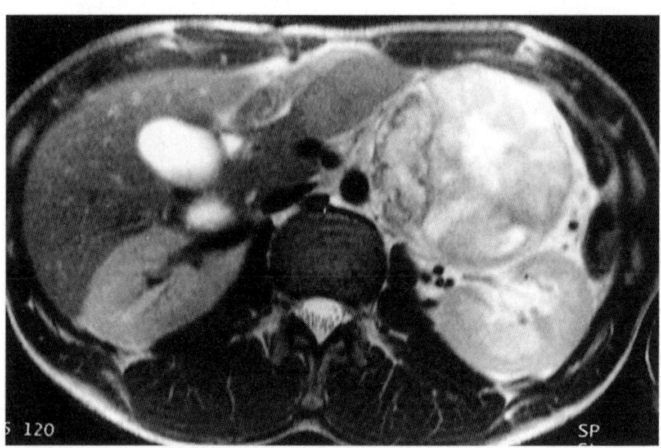

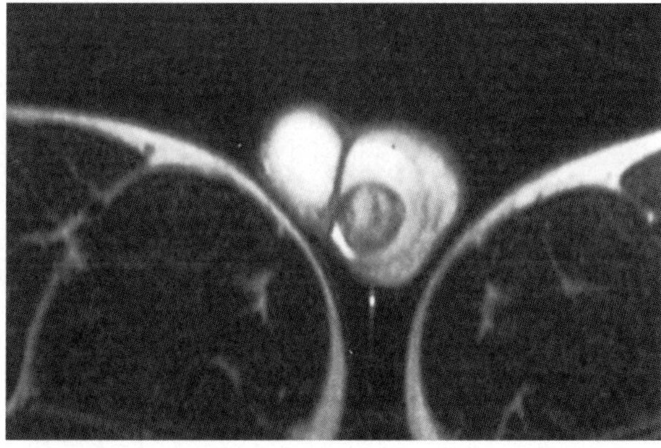

**Fig. 17.7 a,b.** Retroperitoneal metastases from a primary testicular nonseminomatous germ cell tumor (embryonal cell carcinoma) in a young male. MRI, transverse T2-weighted image of the abdomen (**a**) and of the scrotum (**b**). This patient was referred for MRI for a large retroperitoneal mass, which had heterogeneous signal intensities (**a**). Compression of the collecting system caused mild hydronephrosis. Because of the likelihood of retroperitoneal metastases from a testicular neoplasm, in addition MRI of the scrotum was performed. This showed a well-defined heterogeneous mass in the left testis

### 17.2.1.2.2
#### CHORIOCARCINOMA

Choriocarcinoma is the least common of all germ cell tumors and occurs most commonly during the second and third decades of life. US is nonspecific and may demonstrate heterogeneous solid masses with areas of hemorrhage, necrosis, and calcifications.

### 17.2.1.2.3
#### YOLK SAC TUMOR

The pure form is almost exclusively found in young children, where it is the most common malignant germ cell tumor; it is rare in postpubertal males. The tumor presents as a predominantly solid mass with heterogeneous echogenicity and anechoic spaces (THAVA et al. 1992; McENIFF et al. 1995).

### 17.2.1.2.4
#### TERATOMA

This germ cell neoplasm occurs most commonly in children. In this age group, their biologic behavior is that of a benign neoplasm. In adults, however, teratomas usually contain immature elements and behave as a malignant neoplasm. Indeed, despite its histologically benign appearance, primary pure teratoma of the testis is believed to have metastatic potential and to behave similarly to other NSGCTs. Metastatic disease may develop and the metastases may contain other subtypes of NSGCT in addition to teratoma (SIMMONDS et al. 1996). There is probably a reduced frequency of relapse, which should be considered when advising patients with stage I disease, but otherwise management should be the same as for other testicular NSGCTs and the prognosis is excellent (LEIBOVITCH et al. 1995; SIMMONDS et al. 1996). The US findings depend on the histologic tissue elements present in the lesion. Most are composed of areas of cystic and solid components. Bone or cartilage present as hyperechoic areas with acoustic shadow (LIU et al. 1991) (Fig. 17.8). Like other NSGCTs, teratomas are heterogeneous on MRI. Calcifications may account for areas of low signal intensity on both T1- and T2-weighted images. A band of low signal intensity surrounding the lesion is frequently appreciated (JOHNSON et al. 1990). This is likely to represent a fibrous pseudocapsule and is less commonly seen in seminomas (Fig. 17.2c).

#### 17.2.1.2.5
MIXED GERM CELL TUMORS

Any tumor that contains more than one histologic element is considered a mixed germ cell tumor. They actually account for 40% of primary testicular tumors and may present in a dozen possible combinations. Therefore, the US and MRI findings are

variable, with areas of cysts, hemorrhage, necrosis, and calcifications (Fig. 17.9). Heterogeneity of the mass has been found to be the most specific sign for a nonseminomatous tumor, followed by high signal intensity on T2-weighted images; a peritumoral pseudocapsule has only a rather low specificity (JOHNSON et al. 1990).

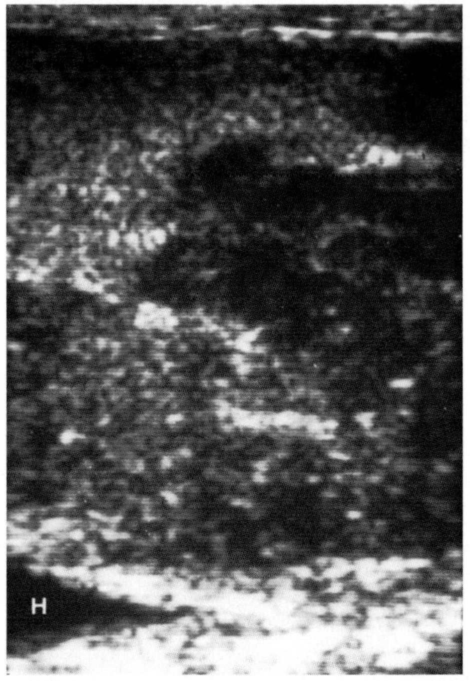

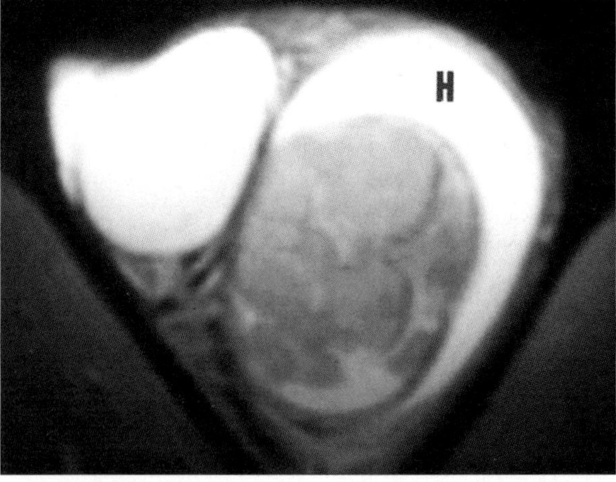

Fig. 17.9 a,b. Mixed germ cell tumor. US (a) and transverse T2-weighted image (b). Multinodular hypoechoic mass in the left testis (a), well marginated and hypointense on MRI. Note that the tumor is isointense to the tunica albuginea. Associated small hydrocele (*H*)

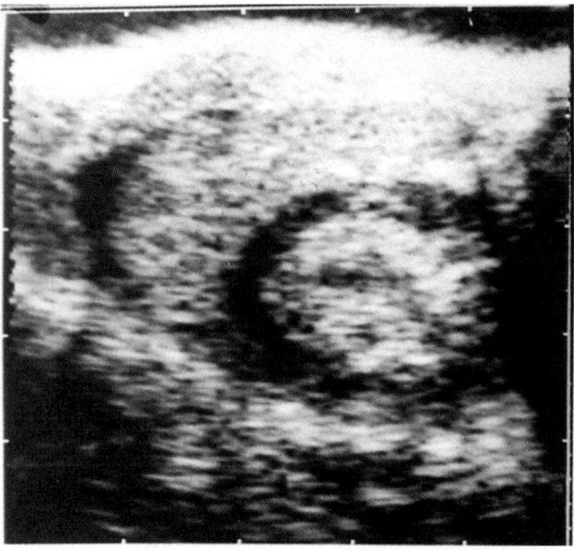

Fig. 17.8. Teratoma. US. Sagittal view of the right testis shows a heterogeneous mass, with hypoechoic and hyperechoic areas and focal calcifications

### 17.2.1.2.6
#### "BURNED-OUT" LESION

Rarely, a testicular scar is discovered in a patient with a presumed extragonadal germ cell tumor. Most patients are originally diagnosed with retroperitoneal germ cell tumors (COMITER et al. 1996). Scrotal US reveals an echogenic focus or foci in virtually all cases. Very rarely, a hypoechoic lesion is seen (Fig. 17.10). These lesions may correspond to intratubular hematoxyphilic bodies or to intratubular psammoma bodies close to a fibrous scar with hemosiderin deposition; they may contain foci of intratubular germ cell neoplasia (COMITER et al. 1996). These hematoxyphilic bodies and fibrosis with hemosiderin deposits are believed to represent remnants of testicular carcinoma. With a presumed retroperitoneal germ cell tumor and palpably normal testes, US demonstration of an echogenic lesion in the absence of a hypoechoic mass probably represents a burned-out primary neoplasm.

### 17.2.1.2.7
#### TESTICULAR MICROLITHIASIS

A high percentage of contralateral testes in men with unilateral testicular cancer have an abnormal echotexture (heterogeneous or with coarse echo-genic foci: "snowstorm" pattern) and carcinoma in situ is most likely to be found in these testes (LENZ et al. 1996) (Figs. 17.1, 17.11). In adults intratubular calcifications of the testes are rare and the pathogenesis is still poorly understood, although it is thought that it is a primary process of the testicles, rather than a sequel of an underlying process (SMITH et al. 1991). Testicular microlithiasis is seen at US as multiple echogenic spots in an otherwise normal testicular parenchyma (Fig. 17.11). Nevertheless, considerable variation is found in the number and distribution of occurrences of testicular microlithiasis (5–60 echogenic foci per transducer field; BACKUS et al. 1994). In some patients, peripheral clustering is seen. Most patients demonstrate side-to-side symmetry, but asymmetric distribution and unifocality may be seen, too, and are more frequent in our experience. In a large series of 1710 testicular sonograms, bilateral intratesticular microcalcifications were found in 11 cases (0.6%) (HOBARTH et al. 1992). In five cases, the microliths were associated with a testicular tumor. In Backus' series, 40% were associated with a testicular neoplasm, and therefore, testicular microlithiasis cannot continue to be considered a benign finding (BACKUS et al. 1994). On T2-weighted images, these small foci of calcifications may not be detected; on T1-weighted images, small scattered foci of low signal intensity have been described (HRICAK et al. 1995).

### 17.2.1.2.8
#### MALIGNANT TUMORS IN AN UNDESCENDED TESTIS

Carcinoma is far more common in an undescended testis than in a normally positioned testis. Seminoma and embryonal cell carcinoma are the two most

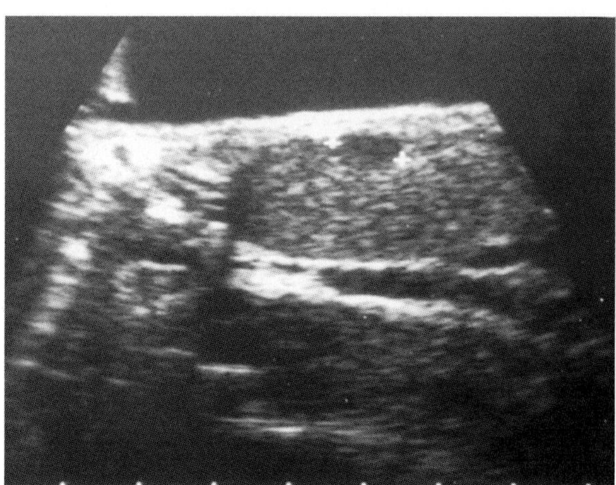

**Fig. 17.10.** "Burned-out" lesion. Longitudinal US. Small hypoechoic lesion at the anterior aspect of the testis (between +) in a patient with extensive retroperitoneal lymph nodes from an embryonal cell carcinoma. The testicular lesion turned out to be a scar, presumably from a prior primary neoplasm

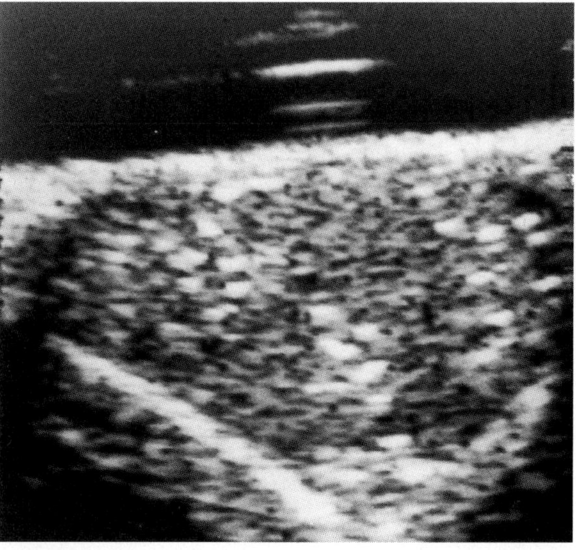

**Fig. 17.11.** Testicular microlithiasis. US. Transverse scan of a weak testis shows diffuse echogenic foci throughout the testis: microlithiasis

frequent neoplasms (ALTMAN and MALAMENT 1967; BATATA et al. 1980). The highest incidence is observed when the testis is located in an intra-abdominal position. The reported incidence of malignancy is variable, and it is generally believed that there is a 50 times higher frequency in an undescended testis (GARDNER 1990). Animal experiments have shown that orchiopexy does not necessarily protect against malignancy (ALTMAN and MALAMENT 1967). With bilateral cryptorchidism there is a 15% chance of developing a tumor in the opposite testis if one testis becomes involved with a tumor (GILBERT and HAMILTON 1940). In cases of bilateral intra-abdominal testes, if one testis becomes malignant there is a 30% chance of malignancy in the contralateral testis. Generally, the malignancy rate correlates with increasing distance of the testis from the scrotum; thus malignant change is six times more common in the abdominal testis than in the inguinal testis.

The ideal method for examining for malignant transformation of the undescended testis is MRI because of its ability to localize the testis (based on its capacity of multiplanar imaging) and, in addition, to characterize its internal structure (LORIGAN et al. 1989; OYEN et al. 1993; HRICAK et al. 1995) (Fig. 17.2).

## 17.2.2
### Adenocarcinoma of the Rete Testis

Adenocarcinoma of the rete testis is a rare but aggressive tumor. Nearly two-thirds of patients present with metastasis or develop metastasis within a year of presentation. US shows a solid mass consistent with a testicular tumor or multicystic septated lesions with intracystic solid echogenic nodules (STEIN et al. 1994; SANCHEZ-CHAPADO et al. 1995; GLAZIER et al. 1996). Metastases occur in the retroperitoneal lymph nodes, lung, liver, and elsewhere.

## 17.2.3
### Primary Carcinoid Tumor of the Testis

Primary carcinoid tumor of the testis is extremely rare and has been described more commonly in older patients. Again, the imaging findings are not specific. Hypoechoic lesions with well-defined borders and focal areas of necrosis have been described (ZAVALA-POMPA et al. 1993).

## 17.2.4
### Testicular Lymphoma/Leukemia

Malignant lymphoma (virtually limited to non-Hodgkin's lymphoma) of the testis is one of the most common neoplasms in men over age 50. Patients with testicular lymphoma or leukemia usually present with testicular enlargement. US usually shows either homogeneously hypoechoic testes in patients with diffuse infiltration or multifocal hypoechoic lesions of various sizes (mean lesion size 16 mm; range 8–26 mm) (MAZZU et al. 1995) (Fig. 17.12a). In some cases, parallel hyperechoic lines ra-

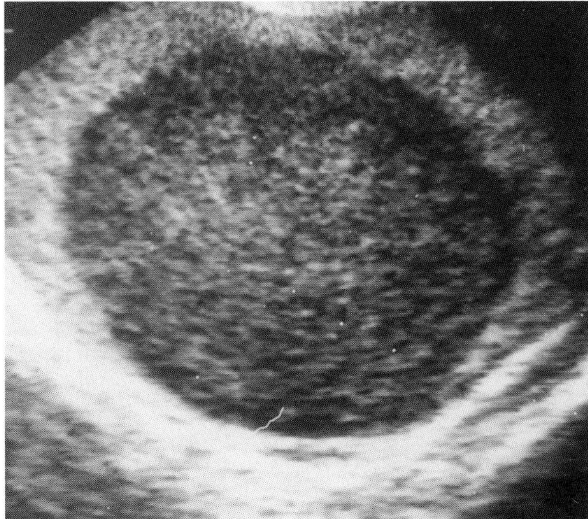

a

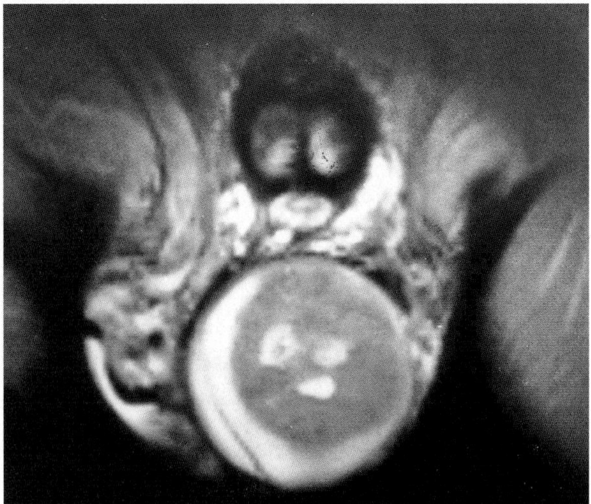

b

**Fig. 17.12.** Lymphoma. US and MRI. Sagittal US (**a**) shows a large hypoechoic nodule in the left testis, indiscernible from other histologic types of primary or metastatic testicular neoplasms. Likewise, the appearance on the T2-weighted MRI images is not specific for a testicular lymphoma (**b**)

diating peripherally from the mediastinum testis are seen, probably representing blood vessels crossing through the lesion (EMURA et al. 1996).

Color Doppler US reveals increased intralesional flow in all areas of lymphomatous or leukemic involvement irrespective of lesion size. Differentiation from inflammatory processes of the testis remains difficult; the clinical symptoms are often helpful. On T1-weighted images, the tumor is either hyperintense or homogeneously isointense. On T2-weighted images the tumor is homogeneously hypointense or homogeneously isointense with preservation of the basic morphology of the testis, epididymis, and spermatic cord (HRICAK et al. 1995; EMURA et al. 1996) (Fig. 17.12b). The tumor shows homogeneous or heterogeneous enhancement after Gd-DTPA administration.

## 17.2.5
### Testicular Metastases

The common primary sites include prostate, lung, gastrointestinal tract, skin (melanoma), and kidney but other primaries have been reported as well (including pancreas, urinary bladder, thyroid, neuroblastoma, schwannoma, and retinoblastoma).

As can be expected, imaging findings (US, MRI) are nonspecific and may indicate a focal mass.

## 17.2.6
### Miscellaneous Tumors

Primary testicular sarcoma is a rare indolent tumor with potential for distant metastases. Testicular sarcomas include rhabdomyosarcoma, spindle cell sarcoma, osteosarcoma, leiomyosarcoma, fibrosarcoma, granulocystic sarcoma, and chondrosarcoma (WASHECKA et al. 1996).

## 17.3
### Benign Testicular Tumors

### 17.3.1
### Gonadal Stromal Tumors

Gonadal stromal tumors generally are benign and hormonally silent. In adults, however, these tumors have a malignant potential and may produce metastases. They represent about 5% of all testicular neoplasms. When hormonally active, they may cause virilization or feminization. Klinefelter syndrome is associated with the development of breast and extragonadal germ cell tumors in some patients. Leydig cell tumor in association with Klinefelter syndrome is a rare entity (POSTER and KATZ et al. 1993).

There are two clear-cut types of large cell calcifying Sertoli cell tumor: those which are associated with complex dysplastic syndromes and which are bilateral and multifocal, and those which are not associated with such syndromes and are unilateral and focal. It is considered that conservative resection of the tumor is the treatment of choice in cases not associated with complex dysplastic syndromes, since the malignancy rate is low (DUDIAK et al. 1994; PLATA et al. 1995).

Granulosa cell tumor of the testis is rare, generally benign, and may occur in adults.

With gonadal stromal tumors, a palpable mass is not always present, and US may be required to identify such neoplasms. Single or multiple masses may be present; they may be either hypo- or hyperechoic, rarely with calcifications (Fig. 17.13). A diffusely heterogeneous pattern with increased echogenicity may be expected in large cell calcifying Sertoli cell tumor. On MRI, Leydig cell tumors are isointense on T1-weighted images and hypointense on T2-weighted images, and thus are indistinguishable from germ cell tumors (KAUFMAN et al. 1990; OYEN et al. 1993). Areas of necrosis and hemorrhage with high signal intensity on both T1- and T2-weighted images are rare (SCHNALL 1993). One case with MR images of a granulosa cell tumor has

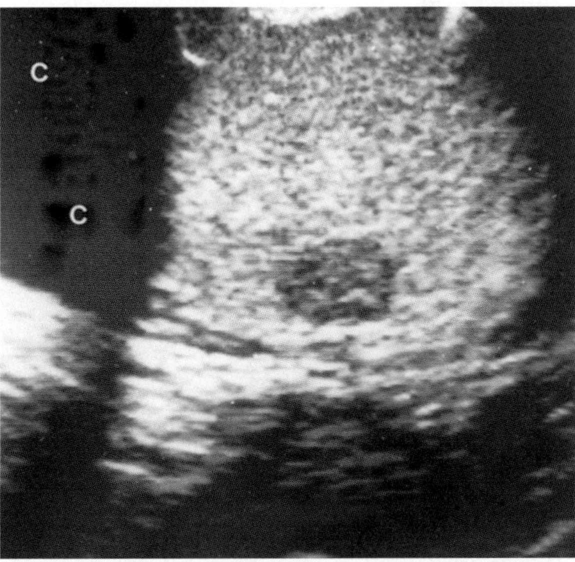

**Fig. 17.13.** Leydig cell tumor. US. This patient had an epididymal cyst (*C*), which was the reason for referral for US. A well-circumscribed hypoechoic solid lesion was seen in the testis. This occult, asymptomatic neoplasm was a Leydig cell tumor

been reported. The lesion demonstrated predominantly low signal intensity on both T1- and T2-weighted images, thought to correspond to its fibrous elements, and areas of higher signal intensity probably correlating with the granulosa cell components (NEMCEK et al. 1989).

## 17.3.2
## Adrenal Rests

Bilateral testicular adrenal rests may occur in untreated or poorly controlled congenital adrenal hyperplasia in children. These lesions are always hypoechoic multifocal nodules on US, and in most cases bilateral. Areas of fibrosis cause acoustic shadowing. The lesions have been described on MRI as bilateral, multiple, well-defined but irregularly bordered areas of decreased signal intensity on MRI (SEIDENWURM et al. 1987).

## 17.3.3
## Cystic Lesions

The differential diagnosis of intrascrotal cysts usually includes simple testicular cysts, intratesticular epidermoid and dermoid cysts, tunica albuginea cysts, epididymal cysts, and spermatoceles (KOENIGSBERG et al. 1995). Cysts originate in the testis parenchyma or in the tunica albuginea. The frequency increases with increasing age. The US appearance is similar to cysts elsewhere: an anechoic

and well-demarcated intratesticular lesion without a discernible wall (HAMM et al. 1988). It is postulated that tubular ectasia or cysts of the rete testis result from obstruction of the spermatic ductal system. They are bilateral in approximately 45% of cases and associated with an ipsilateral spermatocele in approximately 74% of cases. Ectasia of the seminiferous tubules at the level of the mediastinum is a recognized benign condition of the testes. Although it may have typical US features, the condition can at times be difficult to distinguish from tumors on the basis of US, especially by inexperienced sonographers. Rarely the cysts resemble dilated intratesticular veins (intratesticular varicocele). Color Doppler US then is essential to differentiate between cysts and dilated veins (Fig. 17.14). At presentation, most men are in their sixth decade. Most patients have a clinically palpable spermatocele (Fig. 17.15). On imaging, the intratesticular process is bilateral, involves the mediastinum testis, begins at the periphery adjacent to the spermatocele, and extends for a variable distance within the testis (TARTAR et al. 1993). The lesion is hypoechoic with coarse internal echoes. On MRI, lesions have a homogeneous signal similar to that of the coexisting spermatocele with all pulse sequences. They are hypointense relative to the testis on T1- and proton density-weighted images and, unlike tumors, are not visible on T2-weighted images (TARTAR et al. 1993).

Epidermoid cysts of the testis are very rare and account for approximately 1% of all testicular tumors (HEIDENREICH et al. 1995). Epidermoid cysts of the scrotum can become very large (500 ml). Testicular

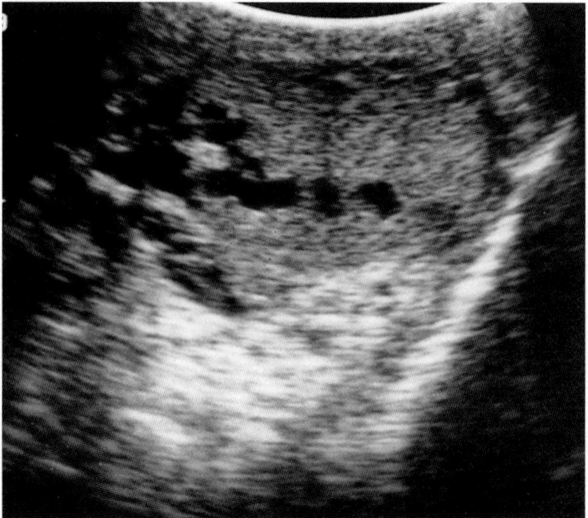
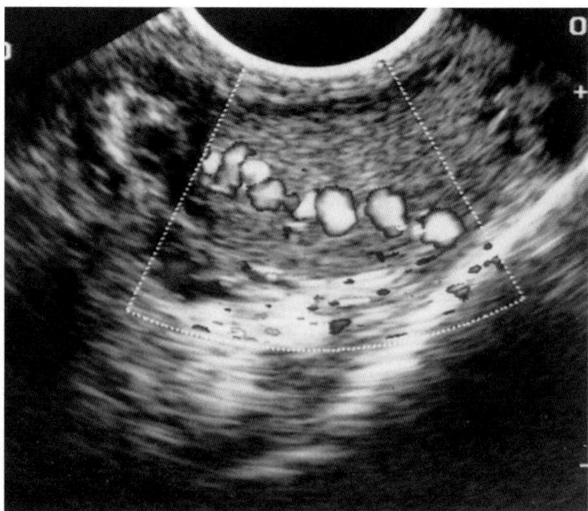

a

b

**Fig. 17.14 a,b.** Intratesticular varicocele. US. Longitudinal scan of the testis (**a**) and color Doppler sonography. Intratesticular anechoic cyst-like lesions (**a**), well vascularized at color Doppler US (**b**)

epidermoid cysts present as a single or as multiple intratesticular hypoechoic masses with a characteristic lamellar swirling configuration or concentric rings similar to the cross-section of an onion; alternatively, they have a target-like appearance (Fig. 17.16). Calcification of the wall or within the mass may also be present. A target or bull's-eye appearance has been reported on MRI as well, with a peripheral and central low signal intensity area, separated by an area of greater signal intensity, which likely corresponds to a high lipid content in degenerating exfoliated squamous cells (BRENNER et al. 1989).

## 17.4
## Benign Testicular Conditions Mimicking Malignancy

### 17.4.1
### Inflammatory Conditions

Granulomatous orchitis may present as focal or diffuse hypoechoic lesions in the testis, occasionally with calcifications. It can be indistinguishable from tumor (OKAJIMA et al. 1994; WEGNER et al. 1994). It predominantly affects men during the fifth and sixth decades. Approximately 150 cases have been reported in the literature.

Likewise, granulomatous epididymo-orchitis, indistinguishable from a testicular tumor, may develop as a (late) complication following use of Tice strain bacillus Calmette-Guerin for treatment of superficial bladder carcinoma (TRUELSON et al. 1992). Lesions are asymptomatic and on US demonstrate as a complex scrotal mass or a diffusely hypoechoic mass lesion (Fig. 17.17).

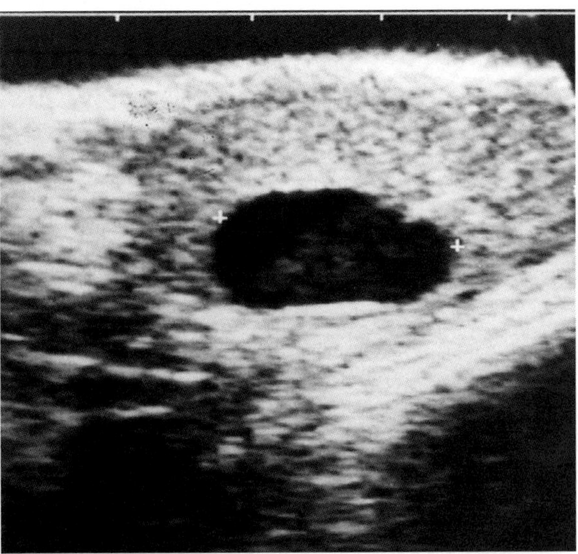

**Fig. 17.16.** Epidermoid cyst. Longitudinal US. Hypoechoic lesion with intraluminal fluid layer in the testis in a young male. Histologically proven epidermoid cyst containing keratinized material

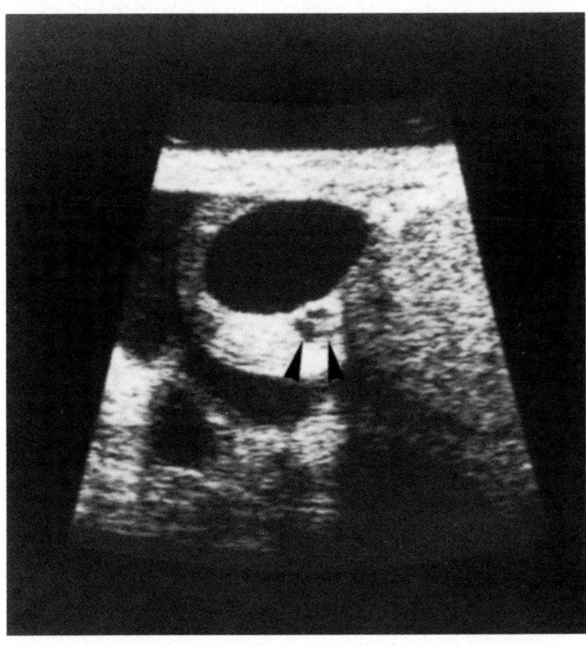

**Fig. 17.15.** Epididymal cyst (spermatocele). US. Longitudinal scan of the upper pole of the testis shows the typical anechoic aspect of a simple cyst in the epididymal head (spermatocele). Note the smaller cyst adjacent to it (*arrowheads*)

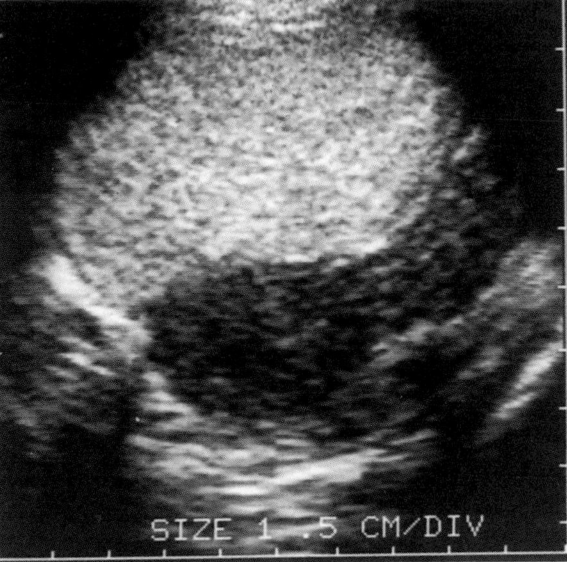


**Fig. 17.17.** Tuberculous epididymitis. US. Diffuse hypoechoic thickening of the entire epididymis in an asymptomatic male

Sarcoidosis with extrapulmonary manifestations in the testis, epididymis, and spermatic cord has been reported, but is rare, affecting fewer than 1% of patients with systemic sarcoidosis (GROSS et al. 1992). The patients usually present with an intrascrotal mass of unknown origin that suggests a testicular tumor both clinically and on imaging. US shows a hypoechoic mass in the epididymis or, more commonly, in the testis. Differentiation from a testicular neoplasm may not be possible.

## 17.4.2
### Testicular Infarction

Infarction of the testis or sequelae of partial infarction of the testis may atypically present as a testicular mass that may mimic a testicular neoplasm since the age of presentation is similar (FERNANDEZ-GOMEZ et al. 1996) (Fig. 17.18). On US, an ill-defined hypoechoic mass can be expected, which appears avascular on color Doppler US. On MRI the lesion is hypointense on T2-weighted sequences and avascular after injection of gadolinium.

## 17.4.3
### Fibrous Pseudotumor of the Tunica Albuginea

Focal fibrosis of the tunica albuginea may be seen following inflammatory conditions of the scrotum. On physical examination, the lesion may be difficult to distinguish from a testicular or an extratesticular neoplasm. On US, the tunica albuginea is focally

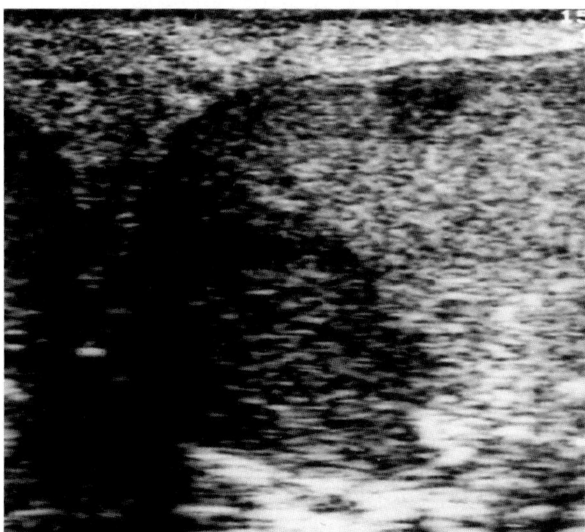

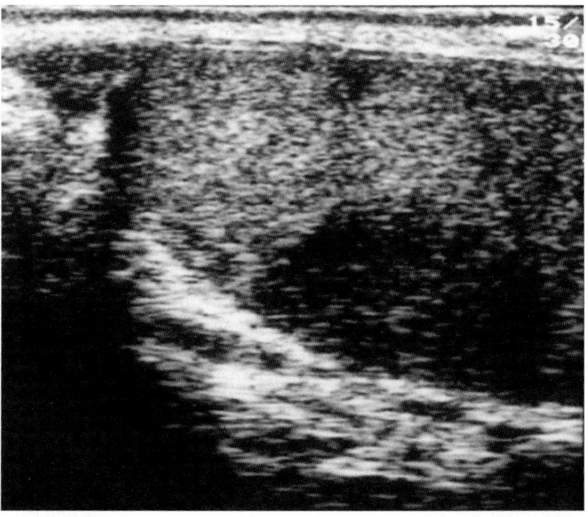

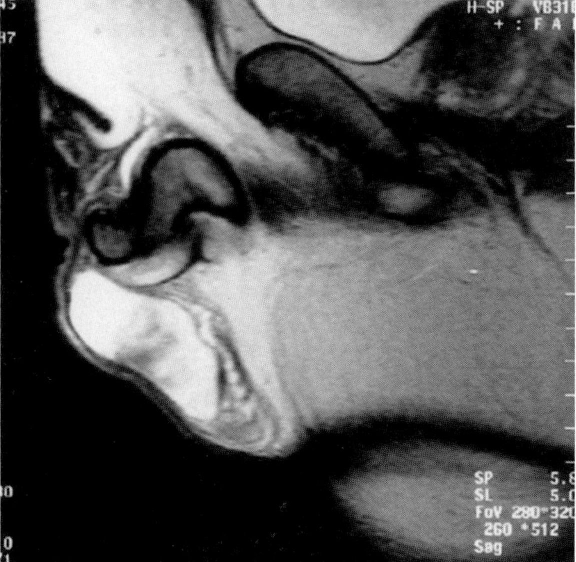

Fig. 17.18 a–c. Testicular infarction. US (a,b) and MRI (c). Transverse (a) and sagittal (b) US shows ill-defined hypoechoic areas in the left testis. These were avascular on color Doppler US. On the sagittal T2-weighted MR image, the lesion exhibits low signal intensities. The lesion is confined to the testis. Note the deformity of the testis. Histologically proved (orchiectomy) sequelae of testicular infarction

thickened and hypoechogenic. On MRI the thickening exhibits low signal intensity on both T1- and T2-weighted images.

## 17.4.4
## Miscellaneous

Testicular hematoma sometimes causes differential diagnostic problems, especially in those cases where there is no major trauma (Fig. 17.19). The aspect on imaging depends on the age of the hematoma. Differentiation from a neoplasm may be impossible. Occasionally calcifications may be found in the testis in an asymptomatic patient (Fig. 17.20). They are likely to be due to a previous intratesticular hemorrhage, although there is not always a clear history of relevant scrotal trauma. Sometimes, a single or several nonspecific hypoechoic lesions may be found on US (Fig. 17.21), but without evolution on follow-up scans. Perhaps they can be explained by fibrosis due to previous focal ischemia of inflammation.

## 17.5
## Extratesticular Masses

The frequency of malignant extratesticular masses seems to be higher than originally thought. In a recent report, FRATES et al. (1997) found a frequency of malignancy of 16%. This contrasts with prior reports suggesting a very low rate of malignancy among extratesticular masses. US and MRI are useful for identifying the extratesticular location of a mass but not for distinguishing the nature of the lesion.

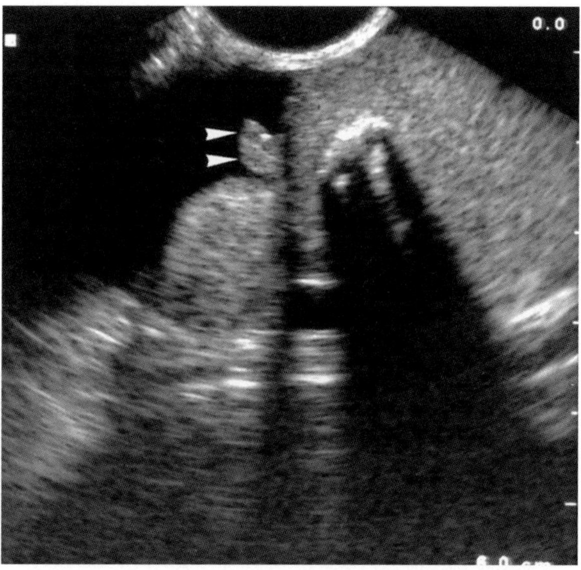

**Fig. 17.20.** Intratesticular calcified mass. US. Sagittal scan shows a calcified area in the upper pole of the testis. Note the epididymal head and a testicular appendage (*arrowheads*), well recognizable because of the small hydrocele

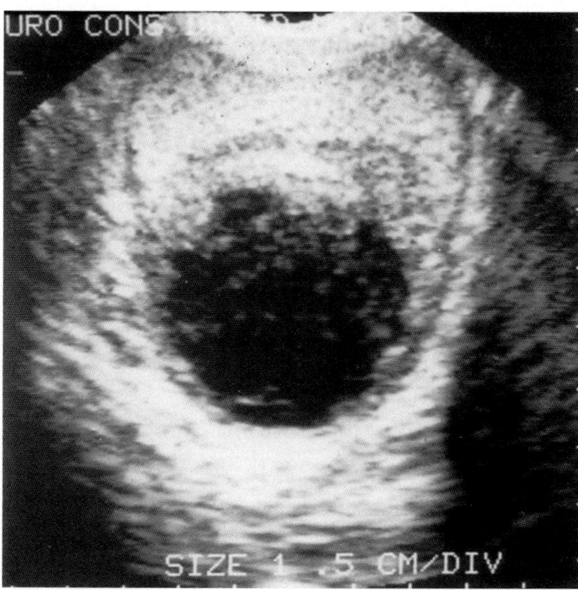

**Fig. 17.19.** Intratesticular hemorrhage. Transverse US. Heterogeneous mass with liquefied areas and a peripheral echogenic rim in the right testis. Because there had been no major trauma, and because of clinical suspicion of a testicular tumor, surgery had been performed. It proved to be an intratesticular hemorrhage without associated pathology

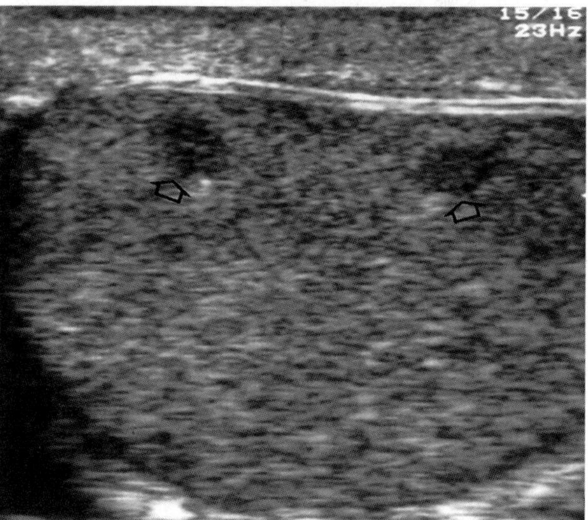

**Fig. 17.21.** Undefined lesions. US, longitudinal scan. Multiple (at least three) hypoechoic lesions (*arrows*) throughout the testicular parenchyma in a 48-year-old male. The lesions remain unchanged in shape and in size over a period of 1 year. The patient has refused therapy up to now

### 17.5.1
### Tumors of the Epididymis

Adenomatoid tumors are uncommon neoplasms of the paratesticular tissues, probably of mesothelial origin, and the majority of cases reported have involved the epididymis and the tunica albuginea. Currently it is well accepted that the origin of these tumors is in fact mesothelial cells, and it is better to term them as nonpapillary benign mesothelioma. They are the most common benign tumor arising from the epididymal tail, although they can also arise from the tunica albuginea, the spermatic cord, or even have an intratesticular origin. Most of them are almost isoechoic to the epididymis on US, oval to round, and have a rather coarse echopattern (VAN POPPEL et al. 1988). They can be hypoechoic to slightly hyperechoic nodules as well (MAKARAINEN et al. 1993) (Figs. 17.22). The clinical course of these tumors is benign, without local recurrence after local excision. The MRI appearance depends on the degree of fibrosis: the signal intensity varies from isointense to hypointense and is slightly higher than the signal intensity of the normal epididymis on T2-weighted images (HRICAK et al. 1995). On imaging, sperm granulomas exhibit similar appearances.

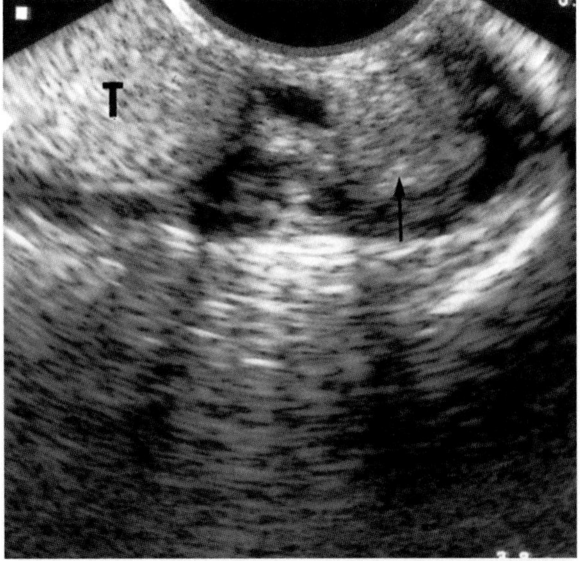


**Fig. 17.22.** Adenomatoid tumor of the epididymis. US. Sagittal scan of the lower pole of the left testis (*T*) and of the epididymal tail. Nodular, isoechoic lesion (*arrow*) at the inferior aspect of the epididymal tail. Histologically proven adenomatoid tumor. Sperm granuloma or mesothelioma may have a very similar appearance

### 17.5.2
### Tumors of the Tunica Vaginalis

Tumors of the tunica vaginalis testis (fibrous pseudotumor, mesothelioma) are usually incidentally discovered during hydrocelectomy or present as a painless mass of the hemiscrotum. Sometimes, US reveals a nodular mass on the epididymis and papillary projections on the surface of the tunica vaginalis (GREBENC et al. 1995; BERTI et al. 1997). The mass may be heterogeneous with acoustic shadowing. These tumors do not compromise the gonad and can be treated by a simple excision of the hydrocele (PELLICE-VILALTA et al. 1996).

There is a significant overlap in the US appearance of benign fibrotic lesions and testicular malignancies. When careful examination of a sonographically heterogeneous or focal hypoechoic lesion fails to reveal a mass and serum tumor markers are negative, an open biopsy with frozen section analysis should be considered rather than proceeding directly to orchiectomy. Homogeneously hyperechoic masses can be considered benign and do not require surgery (EINSTEIN et al. 1992) (Fig. 17.20).

### 17.5.3
### Lipoma/Liposarcoma

Most spermatic cord tumors are benign and are primarily lipomas. Liposarcomas of the spermatic cord and paratesticular liposarcomas are uncommon (SCHWARTZ et al. 1995). CT, MRI, and US reveal findings suggestive of either inguinal hernia (containing fat) or lipoma. Liposarcomas usually roll up the isolateral spermatic cord and testicular vessels (HRICAK et al. 1995; KITAMURA et al. 1996).

### 17.5.4
### Malignant Fibrous Histiocytoma

Malignant fibrous histiocytoma rarely affects the spermatic cord (GORE and AUBER 1993).

## 17.6
## Incidentally Found Testicular Tumors

The incidence of nonpalpable testicular masses on scrotal US examinations for other indications in the study of Horstman and co-workers was 9 on 1600 examinations (HORSTMAN et al. 1994). Of these nine lesions, seven were benign, including four Leydig cell tumors, two Sertoli cell tumors and one case of interstitial fibrosis. Two were malignant (teratocarcinoma and seminoma). Five lesions were less than 1 cm in diameter (four benign, one malignant), while four were 1–2 cm in diameter (three benign, one malignant). Seven lesions were hypoechoic, one was hyperechoic, and one was cystic. Incidentally discovered nonpalpable lesions are usually benign (Figs. 17.13, 17.20, 17.21). Management should include inguinal exploration with frozen section diagnosis. US follow-up should be used only if there is a strong clinical suspicion of a benign lesion, such as a recent trauma or infection. Nonpalpable tumors discovered in patients with metastatic germ cell tumor should be treated as malignant.

## 17.7
## Staging

### 17.7.1
### T-staging

The results for local staging of testicular tumors with US and MRI are disappointing (accuracy of 63% and 45% respectively) (THURNER et al. 1988). Whether this inaccuracy in staging is of clinical significance is controversial, as patients with suspected testicular malignancy require orchiectomy regardless of the local tumor stage and, in addition, pathologic stage remains the final prognosticator.

### 17.7.2
### N-staging

The primary route of dissemination of germ cell tumors is the lymphatic system. On the right the draining lymphatic channels from the testis most commonly terminate in lymph nodes at the level L1–L3 anterior, medial and lateral to the vena cava and anterior (but not lateral) to the aorta. Lymphatic drainage on the left is primarily to lymph nodes lateral and anterior (but not medial) to the aorta at the level of L1-L2, just caudal to the renal vessels (MACVICAR 1993). Suprahilar, retrocrural, and iliac nodal involvement is usually seen only with more advanced disease. Lymphatic drainage of the epididymis is to the external iliac chain.

Hematogenous metastases may occur via direct invasion of spermatic vessels or via venous commu-nications with lymphatics. Hence the thoracic duct with its direct venous drainage is a common route, and, as would be expected, the lung is the most common site of hematogenous dissemination, followed by the brain, kidney, gastrointestinal tract, bone, adrenal glands, peritoneum, and spleen (DIXON et al. 1986). Choriocarcinoma and embryonal cell carcinoma tend to produce early hematogenous metastases.

Computed tomography is the imaging procedure of choice for postorchiectomy staging of testicular cancers (HEIKEN et al. 1994), although similar results can be expected from MRI (Fig. 17.7a). Any number of nodes, regardless of size, in the expected primary retroperitoneal drainage area must be suspected of having a risk of harboring occult nodal disease (Fig. 17.23). The attenuation numbers of metastatic lymph nodes from testicular carcinoma are variable, and the occurrence of low attenuation (<30 HU) lymph nodes is well known (THOMAS et al. 1981). They may be seen before and after treatment. CT, however, is of limited utility for definitively characterizing residual masses (Fig. 17.24). NSGCTs demonstrate a significant incidence of malignancy in residual masses, whereas malignancy in residual masses of pure seminoma are less common (SCATARIGE et al. 1983). Neither residual mass size, nor attenuation, nor degree of shrinkage during chemotherapy can be used to reliably exclude residual malignancy or teratoma (STOMPER et al. 1985). For NSGCT, an enlarging mass generally represents residual malignancy but occasionally represents mature teratoma via tumor evolution or metastasis from a focus of mature teratoma in the primary tumor. These masses are unresponsive to chemotherapy but may be cured by surgical excision.

In a study of 201 testicular cancer patients [117 (58%) NSGCTs, 84 (42%) seminomas] who had both CT of the chest and radiographs of the chest in initial staging, chest radiography alone was found to be sufficient as initial chest staging in all seminoma patients and in NSGCT patients who had a negative abdominal CT (MOUL 1995). For low-stage patients without retroperitoneal adenopathy, chest CT had unacceptable false-positive rates, which precipitated additional invasive maneuvers. For higher stage NSGCT patients with retroperitoneal disease on initial abdominal CT, radiographs of the chest alone missed a significant number of occult thoracic metastases and chest CT remains indicated. In a study of 57 clinical stage I NSGCT all having negative staging abdominal CT followed by surgical staging, CT had an 67% accuracy in predicting retroperito-

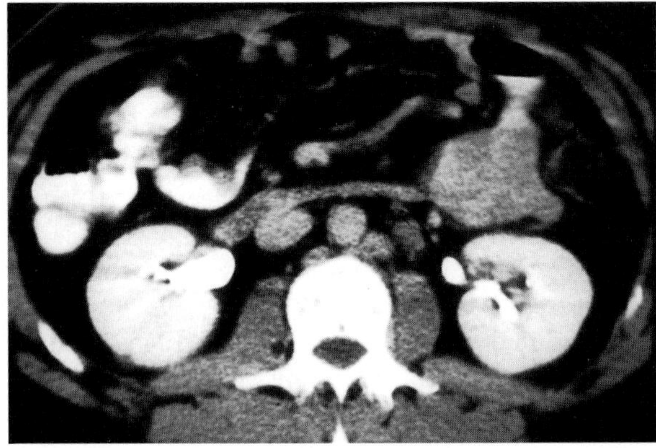

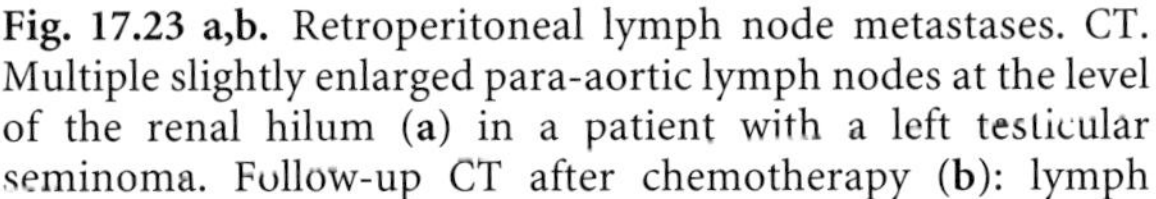

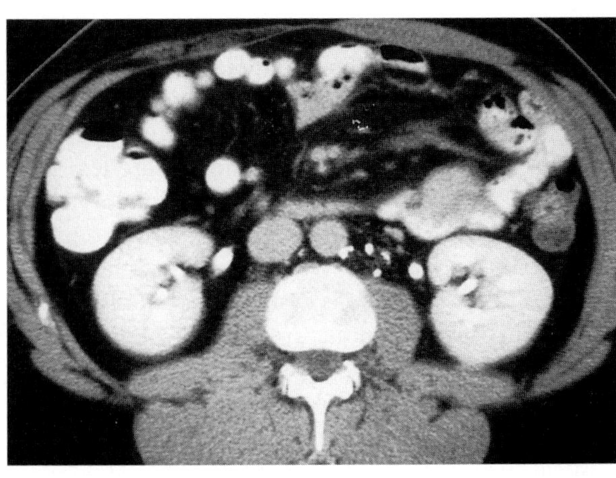

**Fig. 17.23 a,b.** Retroperitoneal lymph node metastases. CT. Multiple slightly enlarged para-aortic lymph nodes at the level of the renal hilum (**a**) in a patient with a left testicular seminoma. Follow-up CT after chemotherapy (**b**): lymph nodes have returned to normal size. The lymph nodes now appear hyperdense because of the lymphangiography which, at that time, was still being performed

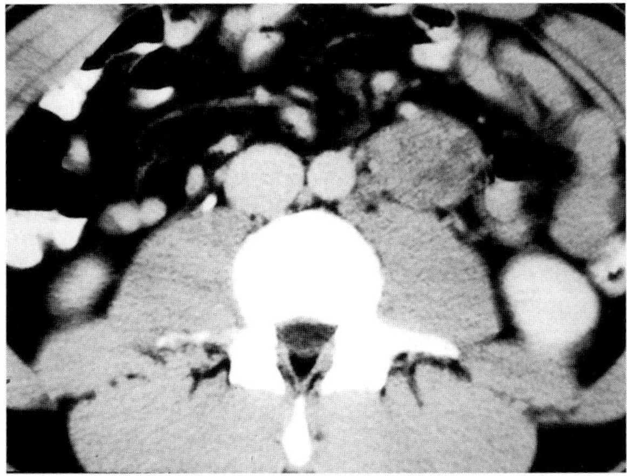

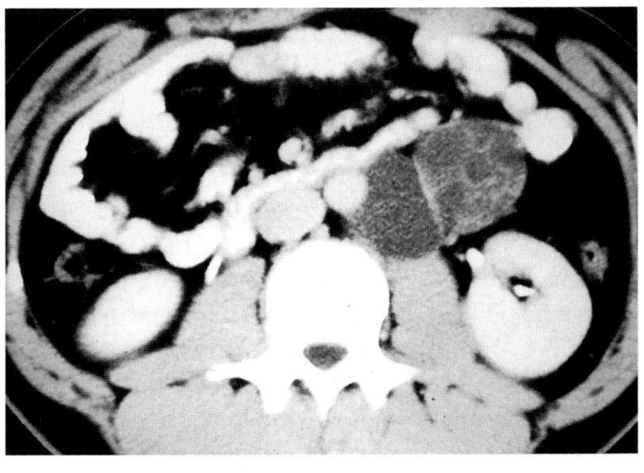

**Fig. 17.24 a,b.** Retroperitoneal lymph node metastases from a left testicular nonseminomatous germ cell tumor. At the time of the diagnosis, there were bulky para-aortic lymph node metastases with a predominantly solid consistency, except for some necrotic areas at the lateral aspect (**a**). Six months later, and after therapy, the lymph nodes have increased in size and now are predominantly cystic (medial aspect) or multicystic (lateral aspect) (**b**). Differential diagnosis between residual viable tumor and residual pseudocyst is not possible

neal metastases (MOUL 1995). This contemporary experience shows a 33% false-negative abdominal CT staging rate. Consideration of any lymph nodes, regardless of size, in the primary echelon retroperitoneal areas as indicative of retroperitoneal metastases may hold promise for improving accuracy of abdominal CT in low-stage NSGCT testicular cancer. In a study of 92 clinical stage I NSGCT patients, determination of primary tumor vascular invasion and percentage of tumor composed of embryonal carcinoma component was found to be a useful staging tool. A multivariate model using vascular invasion and percentage of embryonal carcinoma component was able to predict correct stage in 86% of the study cohort, and a probability table with these two variables was created (MOUL 1995). Using these histologic variables in a neural network artificial intelligence program, an expert correctly predicted stage in 92% of patients. Therefore, it can be recommended that chest staging should be tailored to tumor cell type and retroperitoneal disease status. Staging of the retroperitoneum utilizing abdominal CT remains problematic due to the inability to detect microscopic metastases. Primary tumor histologic factors, particularly vascular invasion and quantitation of embryonal carcinoma, are clinically useful tools.

## 17.8
## The Scrotum After Orchiectomy

A range of normal and abnormal US findings in patients after orchiectomy, including the appearances of the normal postorchiectomy space, acute and subacute hematomas, recurrent neoplasm, second primary tumor in the remaining testis, and testicular prostheses, has been described (EFTEKHARI and SMITH 1993).

The MRI appearance of a testicular prosthesis depends on the composition of the prosthesis. Somewhat older implants contain a viscous fluid with low signal intensity on T1- and T2-weighted images. Newer implants contain solid elastomers and exhibit low signal intensity on T1-weighted images, but exhibit high intensities on T2-weighted images, and cause no chemical shift artifact (SEMELKA et al. 1989).

## References


Altman BL, Malament M (1967) Carcinoma of the testis following orchiopexy. J Urol 97:498–504

Backus ML, Mack LA, Middelton WD, King BF, Winter TC, True LD (1994) Testicular microlithiasis: imaging appearances and pathologic correlation. Radiology 192:781–785

Batata MA, Whitmore WF Jr, Chu FCH (1980) Cryptorchidism and testicular cancer. J Urol 124:382

Berti E, Schiaffino E, Minervini MS, Longo G, Schmid C (1997) Primary malignant mesothelioma of the tunica vaginalis of the testis. Immunohistochemistry and electron microscopy. Pathology 29:96–99

Brenner JS, Cumming WA, Ros PR (1989) Testicular epidermoid cyst: sonographic and MR findings (letter). AJR 152:1344

Comiter CV, Renshaw AA, Benson CB, Loughlin KR (1996) Burned-out primary testicular cancer: sonographic and pathological characteristics. J Urol 156:85–88

Davis JW, Horstman WG, Schellhammer PF (1997) Segmental testicular ischemia mimicking testicular tumor. Br J Urol 80:187–188

Derouet H, Braedel HU, Brill G, Hinkeldey K, Steffens J, Ziegler M (1993) Nuclear magnetic resonance tomography for improving the differential diagnosis of pathologic changes in the scrotal contents. Urologe A 32:327–333

Dixon A, Ellis M, Sikora K (1986) Computed tomography of testicular tumors: distribution of abdominal lymphadenopathy. Clin Radiol 37:519–523

Dudiak CM, Vade A, Isaac RM (1994) Sonographic demonstration of bilateral large-cell calcifying Sertoli cell tumors of the testes. J Ultrasound Med 13:232–235

Eftekhari F, Smith JK (1993) Sonography of the scrotum after orchiectomy: normal and abnormal findings. AJR 160:543–547

Einstein DM, Paushter DM, Singer AA, Thomas AJ, Levin HS (1992) Fibrotic lesions of the testicle: sonographic patterns mimicking malignancy. Urol Radiol 14:205–210

Emura A, Kudo S, Mihara M, Masuo Y, Sato S, Ichigi Y (1996) Testicular malignant lymphoma: imaging and diagnosis. Radiat Med 14:121–126

Fernandez-Gomez JM, Martin-Huescar A, Rabade-Rey J, Sahagun JL, San-Martin A (1996) Testicular infarction as a cause of benign intrascrotal tumor. Arch Esp Urol 49:72–74

Frates MC, Benson CB, DiSalvo DN, Brown DL, Laing FC, Doubilet PM (1997) Solid extratesticular masses evaluated with sonography: pathologic correlation. Radiology 204:43–46

Gardner JN (1990) Urogenital system. In: Langman's medical embryology. Williams & Wilkins, Baltimore, p 272

Gilbert JB, Hamilton JB (1940) Incidence and nature of tumors in ectopic testes. Surg Gynecol Obstet 71:741–743

Glazier DB, Vates TS, Cummings KB, Antoun S (1996) Adenocarcinoma of the rete testis. World J Urol 14:397–400

Gore RL, Auber AE (1993) Ultrasonographic appearance of malignant fibrous histiocytoma of the spermatic cord: a case report. Mil Med 158:631–633

Grebenc ML, Gorman JD, Sumida FK (1995) Fibrous pseudotumor of the tunica vaginalis testis: imaging appearance. Abdom Imaging 20:379–380

Gross AJ, Heinzer H, Loy V, Dieckmann KP (1992) Unusual differential diagnosis of testis tumor: intrascrotal sarcoidosis. J Urol 147:1112–1114

Grunshaw ND, Gopichandran TD (1993) Case report: primary carcinoid tumor of the testis: ultrasound appearances. Clin Radiol 47:290–291

Hamm B (1997) Differential diagnosis of scrotal masses by ultrasound. Eur Radiol 7:668–679

Hamm B, Fobbe F, Loy V (1988) Testicular cysts: differentiation with US and clinical findings. Radiology 168:19–23

Heidenreich A, Engelmann UH, Vietsch HV, Derschum W (1995) Organ preserving surgery in testicular epidermoid cysts. J Urol 153:1147–1150

Heiken JP, Forman HP, Brown JJ (1994) Neoplasms of the bladder, prostate, and testis. Radiol Clin North Am 32:81–86

Hobarth K, Susani M, Szabo N, Kratzik C (1992) Incidence of testicular microlithiasis. Urology 40:464–467

Horstman WG, Haluszka MM, Burkhard TK (1994) Management of testicular masses incidentally discovered by ultrasound. J Urol 151:1263–1265

Hricak H, Hamm B, Kim B (eds) (1995) Imaging of the scrotum: textbook and atlas. Roven Press, New York

Johnson JO, Mattrey RF, Phillipson J (1990) Differentiation of seminomatous from nonseminomatous testicular tumors with MR imaging. AJR 154:539–543

Kaufman E, Akiya F, Foucar E, Grambort F, Cartwright KC (1990) Virilization due to Leydig cell tumor: diagnosis by magnetic resonance imaging. Clin Pediatr 29:414–417

Kitamura K, Kiyomatsu K, Noanka M, Sugimachi K, Saku M (1996) Liposarcoma developing in the paratesticular region: report of a case. Surg Today 26:842–845

Koenigsberg RA, Kelsey D, Friedman AC (1995) Ultrasound and MRI findings in a scrotal epidermoid cyst. Clin Radiol 50:576–578

Leibovitch O, Foster RS, Ulbright TM, Donohue JP (1995) Adult primary pure teratoma of the testis. The Indiana experience. Cancer 75:2244–2250

Lenz S, Shakkebaek NE, Hertel NT (1996) Abnormal ultrasonic pattern in contralateral testes in patients with unilateral testicular cancer. World J Urol 14 (Suppl 1):S55–58

Liu P, Phillips MJ , Edwards VDA, Ein S, Daneman A (1991) Sonographic findings of testicular teratoma with pathologic correlation. Pediatr Radiol 22:99–101

Lorigan JG, Shirkhoda A, Dexeus FH (1989) CT and MR imaging of malignant germ cell tumor of the undescended testis. Urol Radiol 11:113–117

MacVicar D (1993) Staging of testicular germ cell tumors. Clin Radiol 47:149–158

Makarainen HP, Tammela TL, Karttunen TJ, Mattila SI, Hellstrom PA, Kontturi MJ (1993) Intrascrotal adenomatoid tumors and their ultrasound findings. J Clin Ultrasound 21:33–37

Mazzu D, Jeffrey RB, Ralls PW (1995) Lymphoma and leukemia involving the testicles: findings on gray-scale and color-Doppler sonography. AJR 164:645–647

McEniff N, Doherty F, Katz J, Schrager CA, Klauber G (1995) Yolk sac tumor of the testis discovered on a routine annual sonogram in a boy with testicular microlithiasis. AJR 164:971–972

Moul JW (1995) Proper staging techniques in testicular cancer patients. Tech Urol 1:126–132

Nagler-Reus M, Guhl L, Volz C, Wuerstlin S, Arlart IP (1995) Magnetic resonance tomography of the scrotum. Experiences with 129 patients. Radiologe 35:494–503

Nemcek AA, Fischer MR, Leschorn E, Garnett J (1989) Mixed sexcord stromal tumor to the testis: evaluation by ulrasonography and magnetic resonance imaging. Uro l Radiol 11:186–189

Okajima E, Cho M, Maruyama Y (1994) Asymptomatic synchronous bilateral granulomatous orchitis: a case report. Hinyokika Kiyo 40:1123–1126

Oyen R, Verellen S, Drochmans A, Baert L, Marchal G, Moerman P, Baert AL (1993) Value of MRI in the diagnosis and staging of testicular tumors. J Belge Radiol 76:84–89

Pellice-Vilalta C, Cosme-Gimenez M, Casalots-Serramia J (1996) Neoplasm of the tunica of the testis. Report of 5 cases (3 mesothelial tumors and 2 fibrous pseudo-tumors). Arch Esp Urol 49:12–16

Plata C, Algaba F, Andujar M, Nistal M, Stocks P, Martinez JL, Nogales FF (1995) Large cell calcifying Sertoli cell tumor of the testis. Histopathology 26:255–259

Poster RB, Katz DS (1993) Leydig cell tumor of the testis in Klinefelter syndrome: MR detection. J Comput Assist Tomogr 17:480–481

Sanchez-Chapado M, Angulo JC, Haas GP (1995) Adenocarcinoma of the rete testis. Urology 46:468–475

Scatarige JC, Fishman EK, Kuhajda P (1983) Low attenuation nodal metastases in testicular carcinoma. J Comput Assist Tomogr 7:682–687

Schnall M (1993) Magnetic resonance imaging of the scrotum. Semin Roentgenol 28:19–30

Schwartz SL, Swierzewski SJ, Sondak VK, Grossman HB (1995) Liposarcoma of the spermatic cord: report of 6 cases and review of the literature. J Urol 153:154–157

Seidenwurm D, Smathers RL, Lo RK, Carroll CL, Bassett J, Hoffman AR (1987) Testis and scrotum: MR imaging at 1.5 T. Radiology 164:393–398

Semelka R, Anderson M, Hricak H (1989) Prosthetic testicle: appearance at MR imaging. Radiology 173:561–562

Simmonds PD, Lee AH, Theaker JM, Tung K, Smart CJ, Mead GM (1996) Primary pure teratoma of the testis. J Urol 155:939–942

Smith WS, Brammer HM, Henry M, Frazier H (1991) Testicular microlithiasis: sonographic features with pathologic correlation. AJR 159:1003–1004

Stein JP, Freeman JA, Esrig D, Chandrasoma PT, Skinner DG (1994) Papillary adenocarcinoma of the rete testis: a case report and review of the literature. Urology 44:588–594

Stomper PC, Jochelson MS, Garnick MB, Richie JP (1985) Residual abdominal masses after chemotherapy for nonseminomatous testicular cancer: correlation of CT and histology. AJR 145:743–746

Tartar VM, Trambert MA, Balsara ZN, Mattrey RF (1993) Tubular ectasia of the testicle: sonographic and MR imaging appearance. AJR 160:539–542

Thava V, Cooper N, Egginton JA (1992) Yolk sac tumor of the testis in childhood. Br J Radiol 63:1142–1144

Thomas JL, Bernardino ME, Bracken RB (1981) Staging of testicular carcinoma: comparison of CT and lymphangiography. AJR 137:991–996

Thurnher S, Hricak H, Carroll PR, Pobiel-RS, Filly RA (1988) Imaging of the testis: comparison between MR imaging and US. Radiology 167:631–636

Truelson T, Wishnow KI, Johnson DE (1992) Epididymoorchitis developing as a late manifestation of intravesical bacillus Calmette-Guerin therapy and masquerading as a primary testicular malignancy: a report of 2 cases. J Urol 148:1534–1535

Van Poppel H, Van Renterghem K, Claes H, Oyen R, Moerman P, Baert L (1988) Benign mesothelioma of the epididymis: case report. Urol Int 43:370–371

Washecka RM, Mariani AJ, Zuna RE, Honda SA, Chong CD (1996) Primary intratesticular sarcoma. Immuno histochemical ultrastructural and DNA flow cytometric study of three cases with a review of the literature. Cancer 77:1524–1528

Wegner HE, Loy V, Dieckmann KP (1994) Granulomatous orchitis – an analysis of clinical presentation, pathological anatomic features and possible etiologic factors. Eur Urol 26:56–60

Zavala-Pompa A, Ro JY, el-Naggar A, Ordonez NG, Amin MB, Pierce PD, Ayala AG (1993) Primary carcinoid tumor of testis. Cancer 72:1726–1732

# 18 Surgical Treatment for Early Germ Cell Tumors

E.C. SKINNER

CONTENTS



## 18.1
## Introduction

Germ cell cancer of the testis occurs in young men and is currently one of the most curable solid tumors in humans. The successful treatment of this disease requires a multidisciplinary approach, with close co-operation between the urologist, radiation oncologist, and medical oncologist.

## 18.2
## Diagnosis

Testis cancer occurs primarily between the ages of 17 and 40, with occasional cases appearing in older men and young children. It is rarely seen in African Americans. The etiology of this disease is unknown, with the only well-established risk factor being a history of cryptorchidism.

Most men present with a painless lump in the testicle which has been present for a few weeks to months. However, other presenting symptoms are common, including acute or chronic pain, a new hydrocele, or a history of recent scrotal trauma. Patients with these symptoms may be misdiagnosed, resulting in an unnecessary delay of appropriate treatment. Finally, some men present primarily with symptoms of metastatic disease, including back pain, neck mass, gynecomastia or hemoptysis.

Initial evaluation should include a scrotal ultrasound and serum levels of $\alpha$-fetoprotein (AFP), $\beta$-subunit human chorionic gonadotropin ($\beta$HCG), and lactic dehydrogenase (LDH). Once the diagnosis of testicular tumor is established, staging evaluation includes a chest x-ray and CT scan of the abdomen and pelvis. Patients with extensive disease should also have an MRI scan of the brain, and a bone scan if clinically indicated.

The clinical staging of the retroperitoneal lymph nodes continues to be relatively inaccurate in spite of modern imaging techniques. Most authors have identified approximately 20% false-positives and up to 40% false-negatives when comparing CT interpretation with pathologic staging in low-stage disease (DONOHUE et al. 1995). Other imaging techniques such as lymphangiography and magnetic resonance imaging have not proven any more accurate. Nodes greater than 2 cm are easily identified on CT, however. In general, CT tends to underestimate the extent of disease (RICHIE 1990).

## 18.3
## Staging

Several staging systems are currently in clinical use in the United States and elsewhere (Table 18.1). All divide patients into those with tumor confined to the testicle, those with tumor in retroperitoneal lymph nodes, and those with disease outside the retroperitoneum. The extent of the primary tumor within the scrotum (the T stage in the TNM system) adds additional prognostic information. Other variables have been identified which imply a poor prognosis in advanced disease, such as very high levels of $\beta$-HCG or involvement of liver, bone, or brain, and these are not currently included in the standard staging systems.

E.C. SKINNER, MD, Associate Professor of Clinical Urology, Department of Urology, University of Southern California, Norris Comprehensive Cancer Center, MS #74, 1441 Eastlake Ave., Suite 7414, Los Angeles, CA 90033, USA

**Table 18.1.** Staging systems for germ cell tumors of the testis

| | Royal Marsden[a] | Skinner[b] | Walter Reed[b] | TNM[b] |
|---|---|---|---|---|
| Confined to testis | I | A | I | T1 |
| Beyond tunica | | | | T2 |
| Into rete testis or epididymis | | | | T3 |
| Invades cord | | | | T4 |
| Regional nodes | | | | |
| Less than 2 cm[a] | IIA | | | |
| 2 cm, <5 cm[a] | IIB | | | |
| Less than 6 nodes, all <2 cm | | B1 | IIA | |
| More than 6 nodes, or >2 cm | | B2 | IIB | |
| Single unilateral node | | | | N1 |
| Multiple or bilateral nodes <5 cm | | | | N2 |
| Node >5 cm | IIC | B3 | IIC | N3 |
| Beyond retroperitoneum | III | C | III | M1 |

[a] Clinical staging.
[b] pathologic staging.

## 18.4
## Primary Orchiectomy

The first step in treatment of all germ cell tumors of the testis is inguinal (or "radical") orchiectomy. This accomplishes removal of the primary tumor and establishes the histologic type of the tumor. It should be performed through an inguinal incision and include early clamping or ligation of the spermatic cord at the level of the internal inguinal ring prior to manipulation of the testis itself. The cord should be ligated high with permanent suture so that the stump can be identified and removed at the time of retroperitoneal node dissection. There are few complications from this surgery, which is usually performed on an outpatient basis. The only real risk is retroperitoneal hemorrhage if the ligature on the cord should come off. A hematoma resulting from such a bleed might be mistaken for metastatic disease on a subsequent CT scan (BOCHNER et al. 1995).

Trans-scrotal biopsy of the testis is contraindicated because of potential tumor spill and contamination of the lymphatic drainage of the scrotum to the inguinal nodes. However, occasionally due to an error in diagnosis a testis tumor is inadvertently opened through a trans-scrotal approach. In the past this was thought to be a devastating occurrence with a very high incidence of local recurrence of the disease. However, current data suggest that most of these cases can be easily managed with little increased risk (CAPELOUTO et al. 1995). Gross tumor contamination is still worrisome and should be managed aggressively with either local radiotherapy or formal hemiscrotectomy (LEIBOVITCH et al. 1995).

## 18.5
## Retroperitoneal Lymph Node Dissection

### 18.5.1
### Indications

Retroperitoneal lymph node dissection is *not* indicated in cases of low-stage pure seminoma of the testicle. These patients should undergo prophylactic irradiation of the retroperitoneum and/or systemic chemotherapy. Surgical management of the patient with advanced seminoma is discussed in Chap. 19.

Considerable controversy now exists regarding the role of retroperitoneal lymph node dissection for men with clinical stage A (N0) nonseminomatous germ cell tumor. Other options for management of these patients include close surveillance or primary chemotherapy.

Multiple studies have been completed in the past 10 years using primary surveillance strategies for patients with stage A nonseminoma (GELDERMAN et al. 1987; DUNPHY et al. 1988; STURGEON et al. 1992; NICOLAI and PIZZOCARO 1995) On average 25%–35% of patients with clinical stage A will develop a recurrence and require further treatment on these protocols. Most recur in the retroperitoneum within the first 2–3 years; however, late recurrences are not uncommon, even beyond 5 years. Surveillance of the retroperitoneum requires frequent CT scans as well as monthly chest x-ray and serum markers. Survival on these protocols has generally been equivalent to primary surgical treatment, approaching 100%. Patients who are lost to follow-up, however, are at particularly high risk of failure.

Three pathologic variables have been identified as poor prognostic factors correlating with an increased risk of recurrence in surveillance protocols. These include higher T stage of the primary tumor (>pT1), presence of lymphovascular invasion, and a large proportion of embryonal cell histology. In addition, patients with mature teratoma in the primary tumor are at high risk of late recurrences with teratoma, which is unlikely to respond to chemotherapy. Most authors currently agree that patients with any of these risk factors should not be managed with surveillance alone. On the other hand, the absence of these factors has been associated with a risk of recurrence of less than 15% (WISHNOW et al. 1989; FREIHA and TORTI 1989).

Since survival is essentially equivalent, cost and quality of life are variables which should be taken into consideration when comparing these two approaches. Overall costs of surveillance may be somewhat less than primary surgical protocols (LOWE 1993; AASS et al. 1990). Quality of life for those who do not suffer recurrence is undoubtedly better, though the requirement of frequent studies and the risk of possible recurrence may take a psychological toll. Patients with recurrent disease in fact often require considerably more treatment than they may have needed with a primary surgical approach, usually including both full-course chemotherapy and surgical resection. Future fertility may be more compromised as well. Therefore these patients may have worse quality of life than if they had had primary surgery.

A short course of primary chemotherapy is currently being tested as an alternative approach for stage A nonseminomas in England and Europe (STUDER et al. 1993). Initial results are promising, but the risk of late recurrences is unknown. This approach may also require very long-term follow-up with at least annual CT scans of the abdomen.

There is also controversy about the best approach to the patient with minimal retroperitoneal disease evident on CT scan, or with elevated markers and negative CT scan (clinical stages IIA and IIB). The main advantage of initial node dissection is to avoid overtreatment in case of false-positive CT scan, or in cases with pure mature teratoma in the retroperitoneum (FOSTER et al. 1996). However, CT scan usually underestimates the extent of disease, and if there is any doubt about the ability to completely clear the retroperitoneum, then chemotherapy should be given first. In addition, patients with pure embryonal histology (no teratoma) treated with primary chemotherapy may not require node

dissection at all if they have a complete response to treatment (DONOHUE et al. 1995; LOGOTHETIS et al. 1982).

Our current approach favors nerve-sparing lymphadenectomy for most patients with stage A nonseminoma. However, treatment is individualized, taking into consideration the pathology of the primary tumor, the reliability of the patient for follow-up, and the patient's own concerns regarding surgery, chemotherapy, and surveillance. For stage IIA and IIB patients, those with questionable CT scans (nodes 1–3 cm in size) and normal markers or teratoma in the primary tumor generally are treated with primary node dissection followed by chemotherapy as indicated by the final pathology. Those with persistently elevated markers or a retroperitoneal mass >3 cm are generally treated with primary chemotherapy and delayed node dissection.

## 18.5.2
## Technique of Thoracoabdominal Retroperitoneal Lymph Node Dissection

### 18.5.2.1
### Choice of Surgical Approach

There are two main surgical approaches to the retroperitoneum, via either a thoracoabdominal or a standard midline incision. A laparoscopic approach has also been described (GERBER et al. 1994; STONE et al. 1993). We routinely use a thoracoabdominal incision, which provides the best exposure to the upper retroperitoneum with the renal hilum essentially in the middle of the operative field. This approach is especially helpful in a patient with a large retroperitoneal mass which requires an extensive suprahilar dissection. In patients with less disease this approach can be performed entirely extraperitoneally, reducing postoperative ileus and the risk of late small bowel obstruction.

The transabdominal approach offers a faster opening and closing time, and is more familiar to many surgeons. Exposure to the suprahilar area, however, requires mobilization of the pancreas and spleen. The chest is not entered, which decreases the potential pulmonary complications and decreases postoperative pain. However, mobilization of the bowel may result in a longer ileus, and puts the patient at risk for a late small bowel obstruction.

The laparoscopic approach is still new, but may offer the advantage of a more rapid postoperative recovery, perhaps at the cost of a longer operating time and a less thorough dissection. The learning curve has been steep for most laparoscopic procedures. No long-term data have yet been reported on effectiveness in terms of avoiding later retroperitoneal recurrence.

### 18.5.2.2
### Limits of Dissection

The limits of dissection have changed over time, primarily thanks to careful mapping studies by DONOHUE and colleagues in 1982. When grossly positive nodes are encountered in the retroperitoneum (stage IIB), a full bilateral dissection is necessary. This dissection extends to the opposite ureter, includes both suprahilar areas, and extends down over the presacral area to the level of the bifurcation of the common iliac artery. However, in stage I or IIA the dissection may be safely limited to reduce the risk of postoperative anejaculation. It is important to include the interaortocaval area in both right- and left-sided dissections. Our recommended limits of dissection are drawn in Fig. 18.1.

### 18.5.2.3
### Technique

A nerve-sparing thoracoabdominal node dissection begins by careful positioning of the patient (Fig. 18.2). He is placed near the edge of the table, with the

table flexed at the waist. The left arm is rotated over the head onto an adjustable arm rest. The lower leg is flexed 30° at the hips and 90° at the knee, and the upper leg is placed straight on a pillow. All pressure points are carefully padded. The table is flexed completely, and the patient is secured in place using wide adhesive tape.

An incision is made over the bed of the eighth or ninth rib from the midaxillary line to the midepigastrium, then carried inferiorly as a paramedian incision. The rib is resected subperiosteally and the anterior rectus fascia is divided. The rectus muscle is divided superiorly and retracted laterally, and the transversus abdominis is split in line with the incision. The pleural cavity is entered. Blunt Mayo scissors are passed behind the costochondral junction anterior to the peritoneum, and the cartilage divided. This allows the plane to be developed between the abdominal wall muscles and the peritoneal cavity. The posterior rectus fascia is freed from the peritoneum and is divided longitudinally.

With gentle downward traction on the spleen (or liver on the right), the attachments between the peritoneum and the underside of the diaphragm are divided back to the central tendon of the diaphragm. This allows complete mobilization of the peritoneal envelope medially. The diaphragm is then divided for a few centimeters. Palpation of the lung is carried out to detect any unexpected nodules.

The peritoneum and Gerota's fascia are then bluntly swept off the back muscles over to the side of the aorta. The fascia of the psoas muscle is incised longitudinally. The next step is to develop the plane

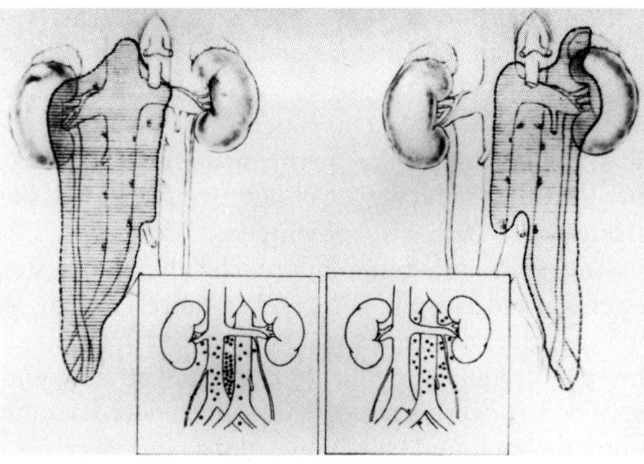

Fig. 18.1. Limits of dissection for a modified template or nerve-sparing retroperitoneal node dissection. Inset shows the areas of positive nodes in patients with negative preoperative CT scan (clinical stage I) in the study by DONOHUE et al. (1982). [Reprinted with permission from WALSH et al. (eds) (1998) Campbell's urology, 7th edn. Saunders, Philadelphia]

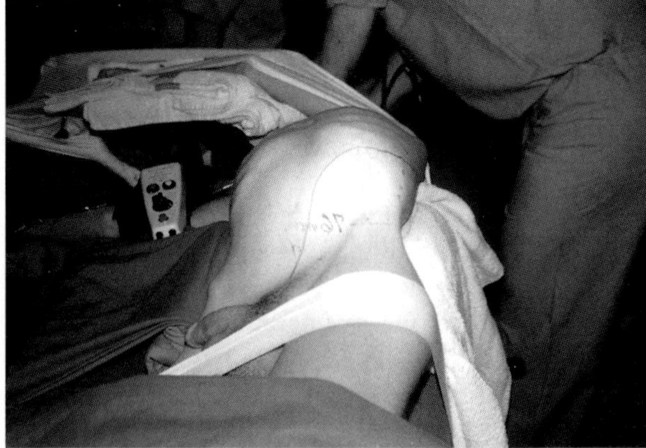

Fig. 18.2. Position for a left-sided thoracoabdominal node dissection. This incision places the high retroperitoneum in the center of the surgical field and allows the entire dissection to be performed in the retroperitoneal space

between the posterior peritoneum and the anterior surface of Gerota's fascia. A thin layer surrounds both the periotoneum and Gerota's fascia, and must be sharply incised. The avascular plane is then bluntly developed over to the aorta (Fig. 18.3). If a full bilateral dissection is planned for a left-sided tumor we routinely divide the inferior mesenteric artery (IMA), which allows access to the opposite common iliac vessels. This is safe except in elderly patients who may have compromised collateral blood supply to the left colon. In a limited or nerve-sparing dissection the IMA is usually left intact.

Once the peritoneum has been reflected medially, the next step is to identify the postganglionic nerve fibers coursing in the retroperitoneal fat overlying the anterior aorta from the each sympathetic chain. The fibers are variable, and coalesce with each other at various levels (Fig. 18.4). Identification of the fibers is relatively easy in a thin individual, but may be challenging in someone with significant retroperitoneal fat. Note that the right-sided fibers arise from behind the vena cava and pass anteriorly between the cava and the aorta. As each nerve is identified, it is carefully dissected free from the surrounding fat, and tagged with a fine vessel loop. The most important fibers to preserve are those arising from the third and fourth lumbar ganglia, which generally pass around the root of the IMA.

After identifying the nerve branches, the node dissection begins at the level of the root of the superior mesenteric artery (SMA). The left renal vein is mobilized, and the origin of the SMA is skeletonized, clipping the small lacteals which run alongside the vessel. The left crus of the diaphragm is identified and the tissue overlying it is clipped and divided. The left celiac plexus lies in this area, and may be mistaken for indurated nodes.

The dissection continues laterally, dividing the superior attachments of Gerota's fascia to the diaphragm. The adrenal gland may be left intact or may be removed with Gerota's fascia if there is disease in the hilum of the kidney. If the adrenal is to be preserved, the dissection should proceed across Gerota's fascia between the adrenal and the kidney.

The tissue over the top of the left renal vein is divided over to the anterior vena cava and inferiorly down the center of the vena cava. The adrenal, gonadal, and ascending lumbar veins draining into the left renal vein are ligated. The ipsilateral lumbar veins below the renal vein are carefully ligated with fine suture, taking care not to injure the sympathetic branches. In a bilateral dissection we continue the dissection over to the right ureter, and edn the lumbar veins are divided bilaterally. In either case, the right gonadal vein is generally ligated, and the dissection continues to the level of the IMA.

Attention is then turned to the anterior aorta. The tissue over the top of the aorta is split down to the origin of the IMA, carefully preserving the crossing sympathetic branches. The lumbar branches below the renal vessels are divided at their takeoff from the aorta. The left renal artery is identified and carefully dissected toward the hilum. The opposite renal artery is also dissected out, taking care to identify any accessory branches. The contralateral suprahilar area is generally not dissected in low-stage disease,

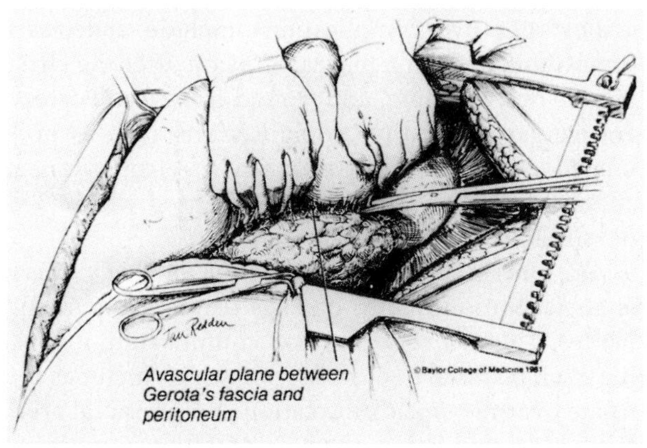


**Fig. 18.3.** The plane between Gerota's fascia and the posterior peritoneum is developed, incising the thin fascial covering which envelops the two. Once the fascia is incised the remainder of the dissection can be done bluntly. [Reprinted with permission from WALSH et al. (eds) (1998) Campbell's urology, 7th edn. Saunders, Philadelphia]

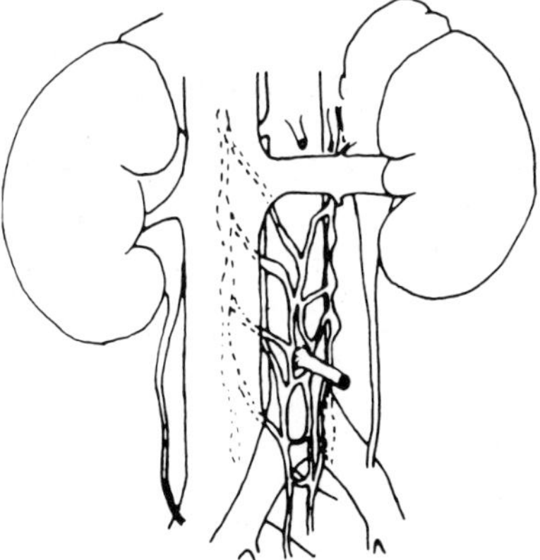

**Fig. 18.4.** Distribution of the postganglionic branches of the left and right lumbar sympathetic nerves as they course over the anterior aorta. [Reprinted with permission from WALSH et al. (eds) (1998) Campbell's urology, 7th edn. Saunders, Philadelphia]

so the opposite renal artery represents the upper limit of dissection. The tissue behind the right renal artery overlying the crus of the diaphragm should be carefully clipped, because it often contains the cysterna chyli.

At this point we divide Gerota's fascia over the lateral kidney, allowing half to pass posteriorly and half anteriorly. It is further taken off the hilum, allowing careful dissection of the branches of the renal artery and vein. The ureter is dissected out and mobilized away from the gonadal vessels. It is easily injured, and must be carefully protected during the dissection. The stump of the spermatic cord is then teased out of the internal iliac ring. Every effort should be made to identify and remove the suture which was placed on the end of the cord at the time of orchiectomy.

All of the tissue anterior to the great vessels has now been divided, and the limits of dissection clipped. The "split and roll" technique is then used to sweep the posterior lymphatic tissue to the ipsilateral side. We begin by elevating the vena cava slightly and clipping and dividing the tissue beneath the cava, carefully avoiding the sympathetic branches. This forms the medial posterior limit of dissection. The aorta can be completely elevated, and the tissue swept behind the aorta to the ipsilateral side, sharply dividing the attachments to the anterior vertebral ligaments. Each ligated lumbar artery and vein is encountered a second time as it enters the lumbar foramen and should carefully be clipped again at that level. The tissue is then swept off the psoas muscle and removed (Fig. 18.5).

A small chest tube is routinely placed, and generally removed the following morning. The diaphragm is closed with two layers of running No. 0 polyglycolic acid suture. The abdomen and chest are closed in a single layer of interrupted No. 1 nylon or other permanent suture. In the medial portion of the chest incision, the diaphragm should be included in this suture.

### 18.5.3
### Complications

Postoperative care is routine. Intravenous fluid requirements may be high for the first 24–48h because of third-spacing into the retroperitoneum. Overall complications occur in less than 3%–4% of patients (SKINNER et al. 1982; BANIEL et al. 1994). The most common operative complication is an inadvertent injury to one of the major vascular structures. The

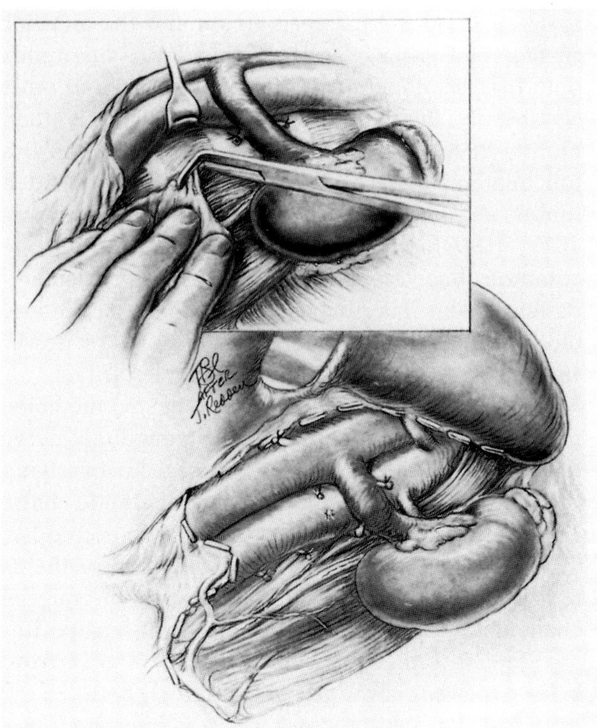

**Fig. 18.5.** Completing the posterior portion of the retroperitoneal node dissection, dividing the node packages off the anterior vertebral ligaments. Each lumbar branch is ligated as it enters the vertebral foramen. The sympathetic postganglionic nerves have not been preserved in this illustration. [Reprinted with permission from WALSH et al. (eds) (1998) Campbell's urology, 7th edn. Saunders, Philadelphia]

surgeon undertaking these operations must be prepared to perform some basic vascular techniques, such as repair of an injury to the aorta or vena cava.

Postoperative complications include atelectasis or accumulation of a pleural effusion after the chest tube is out, bleeding, and wound infection. Postoperative gastrointestinal complications such as prolonged ileus are very rare with a retroperitoneal approach. Most patients are discharged within 3–4 days following surgery.

The one long-term complication of this surgery is anejaculation due to damage to the sympathetic nerves. This is a very common complication following a full bilateral node dissection which includes the tissue over the aortic bifurcation and presacral area. It should occur in less than 5% of patients undergoing a nerve-sparing dissection (JEWETT et al. 1988; DONOHUE et al. 1993), and is seen in approximately 20% undergoing a modified template-type dissection which stops at the level of the IMA (DOERR et al. 1993).

# References


Aass N, Fossa SD, Ous S, Lien HH, Stenwig AE, Paus E, Kaalhus O (1990) Is routine primary retroperitoneal lymph node dissection still justified in patients with low stage non-seminomatous testicular cancer? Br J Urol 65:385–390

Baniel J, Foster RS, Rowland RG, Bihrle R, Donohue JP (1994) Complications of primary retroperitoneal lymph node dissection. J Urol 152:424–427

Bochner BH, Lerner SP, Kawachi M, Williams RD, Scardino PT, Skinner DG (1995) Post radical orchiectomy hemorrhage: should an alteration in staging strategy for testicular cancer be considered? Urology 46:408–411

Capelouto CC, Clark PE, Ransil BJ, Loughlin KR (1995) A review of scrotal violation in testicular cancer: is adjuvant local therapy necessary? J Urol 153:981–985

Colleselli K, Poisel S, Schachtner W, Bartch G (1990) Nerve-preserving bilateral retroperitoneal lymphadenectomy: anatomical study and operative approach. J Urol 144:293–298

Doerr A, Skinner EC, Skinner DG (1993) Preservation of ejaculation through a modified retroperitoneal lymph node dissection in low stage testis cancer. J Urol 149:1472–1474

Donohue JP, Zachary JM, Maynard BR (1982) Distribution of nodal metastases in nonseminomatous testis cancer. J Urol 128:315–320

Donohue JP, Thornhill JA, Foster RS, Rowland RG, Bihrle R (1993) Retroperitoneal lymphadenectomy for clinical stage A testis cancer (1965 to 1989): modifications of technique and impact on ejaculation. J Urol 149:237–243

Donohue JP, Thornhill JA, Foster RS, Bihrle R, Rowland RG, Einhorn LH (1995) The role of retroperitoneal lymphadenectomy in clinical stage B testis cancer: the Indiana University experience (1965–1989). J Urol 153:85–89

Dunphy CH, Ayala AG, Swanson DA, Ro JY, Logothetis C (1988) Clinical stage I nonseminomatous and mixed germ cell tumors of the testis: a clinicopathologic study of 93 patients on a surveillance protocol after orchiectomy alone. Cancer 62:1202–1206

Foster RS, Baniel J, Leibovitch I, Curran M, Bihrle R, Rowland R, Donohue JP (1996) Teratoma in the orchiectomy specimen and volume of metastasis are predictors of retroperitoneal teratoma in low stage nonseminomatous testis cancer. J Urol 155:1943–1945

Freiha F, Torti F (1989) Orchiectomy only for clinical stage I non-seminomatous germ cell testis tumors. Comparison with pathologic stage I disease. Urology 34:347–348

Gelderman WAH, Koops HS, Sleijfer DT, Oosterhuis JW, Marrink J, de Bruijn HWA, Oldhoff J (1987) Orchidectomy alone in stage I nonseminomatous testicular germ cell tumors. Cancer 578–580

Gerber GS, Bissada NK, Hulbert JC, Kavoussi LR, Moore RG, Kantoff PW, Rukstalis DB (1994) Laparoscopic retroperitoneal lymphadenectomy: multi-institutional analysis. J Urol 152:1188–1191

Jewett MAS, Kong Y-S, Goldberg SD, Sturgeon JFG, Thomas GM, Alison RE, Gospodarowicz MK (1988) Retroperitoneal lymphadenectomy for testis tumor with nerve sparing for ejaculation. J Urol 139:1220–1224

Leibovitch I, Baniel J, Foster RS, Donohue JP (1995) The clinical implications of procedural deviations during orchiectomy for nonseminomatous testis cancer. J Urol 154:935–939

Logothetis CJ, Samuels ML, Trindade A, Johnson DE (1982) The growing teratoma syndrome. Cancer 50:1629–1635

Lowe BA (1993) Surveillance versus nerve-sparing retroperitoneal lymph node dissection in stage I nonseminomatous germ-cell tumors. Urol Clin North Am 20:75–83

Nicolai N, Pizzocaro G (1995) A surveillance study of clinical stage I nonseminomatous germ cell tumors of the testis: 10 year followup. J Urol 154:1045–1049

Richie JP (1990) Clinical stage I testicular cancer: the role of modified retroperitoneal lymphadenectomy. J Urol 144:1160–1163

Skinner DG, Melamud A, Lieskovsky G (1982) Complications of thoracoabdominal retroperitoneal lymph node dissection. J Urol 127:1107–1110

Stone NN, Schlussel RN, Waterhouse RL, Unver P (1993) Laparoscopic retroperitoneal lymph node dissection in stage A nonseminomatous testis cancer. Urology 42:610–614

Studer UE, Fey MF, Calderoni A, Kraft R, Mazzucchelli L, Sonntag RW (1993) Adjuvant chemotherapy after orchiectomy in high-risk patients with clinical stage I nonseminomatous testicular cancer. Eur Urol 23:444–449

Sturgeon JF, Jewett MA, Alison RE, et al. (1992) Surveillance after orchidectomy for patients with clinical stage I nonseminomatous testis tumors. J Clin Oncol 10:564–568

Wishnow KI, Johnson DE, Tenney DM, et al. (1989) Identifying patients with low-risk clinical stage I nonseminomatous testicular tumors who should be treated by surveillance. Urology 34:339–343

# 19 Surgery for Advanced Stage Testis Cancer

E.C. SKINNER

CONTENTS



## 19.1
## Introduction

The survival of patients with advanced germ cell cancer of the testis was dismal before the advent of effective chemotherapy. Surgery still has a very important role in the cure of these patients today. The resection of large retroperitoneal metastases is one of the most challenging surgeries facing the urologist, and should probably be performed only in centers with considerable experience with this difficult operation.

## 19.2
## Staging

Advanced testis cancer is defined as bulky retroperitoneal adenopathy (stage B3 or IIC – usually defined as a mass greater than 5 cm) or metastases outside the retroperitoneum. Clinical staging usually includes computed tomography (CT) scan of the abdomen, pelvis, and chest. Magnetic resonance imaging of the brain should also be done in any patient with stage III disease to rule out brain metastases. Bone scan is reserved for patients with elevated alkaline phosphatase or bone pain.

E.C. SKINNER, MD, Associate Professor of Clinical Urology, Department of Urology, University of Southern California, Norris Comprehensive Cancer Center, MS #74, 1441 Eastlake Ave., Suite 7414, Los Angeles, CA 90033, USA

Several groups have identified risk factors which imply a poor prognosis in patients treated with conventional chemotherapy and surgery. The Indiana University suggested definition of "poor risk" is listed in Table 19.1. There is no consensus on the best approach to these patients, although most studies are focused on using higher dose chemotherapy, often with bone marrow transplantation (LAW et al. 1994).

## 19.3
## Surgery for Advanced Pure Seminoma

Patients with advanced pure seminoma are treated initially with platinum-based chemotherapy, with secondary radiation therapy in selected cases. Most cases will respond completely to these treatments (LOEHRER et al. 1987; PECKHAM et al. 1985). If the tumor bulk shrinks by >90% or minimal residual tissue is visible in the retroperitoneum or lung on follow-up scans, no surgery is recommended (SCHULTZ et al. 1989). However, occasionally a patient will be left with a considerable mass in the retroperitoneum after maximal chemotherapy. Some authors have recommended resection of the mass if it is >3 cm in diameter (MOTZER et al. 1991). A full node dissection is essentially impossible in this setting because of the intense scarring left after chemotherapy for seminoma. An alternative to resection would be close observation with frequent CT scans, with immediate resection if the mass enlarges.

## 19.4
## Surgery for Advanced Nonseminoma

Any patient with advanced nonseminoma (Fig. 19.1) must be treated initially with full-dose platinum-based chemotherapy. Response is monitored by the expected fall in serum markers according to their half-life, as well as radiologic response. Some authors have noted that failure of the markers to fall

**Table 19.1.** Indiana University Staging for advanced nonseminoma germ cell tumors

*Minimal extent*
1 Elevated markers only
2 Cervical nodes (+/− nonpalpable retroperitoneal disease)
3 Unresectable nonpalpable retroperitoneal disease
4 <5 pulmonary lesions per lung all <2 cm
   (+/− nonpalpable retroperitoneal disease)

*Moderate extent*
1 Palpable abdominal mass without
   supradiaphragmatic disease
2 5–10 lesions per lung field all <3 cm or solitary pulmonary
   lesion >2 cm (+/− nonpalpable retroperitoneal disease)

*Advanced extent*
1 >10 lesions per lung field or multiple lesions >2 cm or
   primary mediastinal tumor
2 Palpable abdominal mass plus supradiaphragmatic
   disease
3 Liver, bone, or central nervous system disease

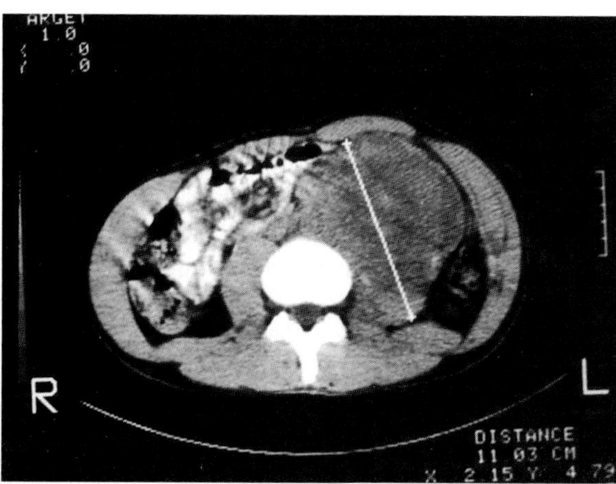


**Fig. 19.1.** CT scan following chemotherapy showing a large residual mass in the retroperitoneum, encasing the aorta

appropriately indicates high risk of incomplete response and should signal a change in chemotherapy strategy. A full discussion of this is beyond the scope of this chapter, but is detailed elsewhere (LAW et al. 1994).

In patients with retroperitoneal disease alone, a CT scan is done immediately after the last course of chemotherapy. If there has been a complete radiographic response (and markers have normalized), then node dissection can be omitted, especially in the case of pure embryonal cell tumors (DONOHUE et al. 1987). If there were teratomatous elements in the original testis, tumor node dissection should be performed regardless of the radiographic response because of the risk of late silent recurrence

(LOGOTHETIS et al. 1982). Any planned node dissection should follow within 4 weeks of completion of the chemotherapy to avoid potential regrowth of microscopic disease.

### 19.4.1
### Timing of Retroperitoneal Dissection in Stage III Nonseminoma

Timing of the node dissection is more problematic in patients with extensive disease outside of the retroperitoneum (TONER et al. 1990). These patients may require resection of extraperitoneal disease in addition to retroperitoneal node dissection. The order of these surgeries is decided on an individual basis. Neck dissection and thoracotomy for pulmonary disease are generally well tolerated with a short recovery time. These can be performed first with retroperitoneal dissection following soon after. Ipsilateral pulmonary disease can certainly be resected at the same time as the retroperitoneal dissection if a high thoracoabdominal incision is used. If the patient is found to have residual viable cancer in the neck or lungs, he may be referred for salvage chemotherapy prior to retroperitoneal dissection.

In some cases a large retroperitoneal mass needs to be resected first because of the risk of involvement of surrounding structures. Interestingly, in up to 40% of patients the histologic findings in different areas of resection may not be identical, and a smaller mass may harbor worse histology (GERL et al. 1994). Therefore it is important to proceed with retroperitoneal dissection even if initial pulmonary resection shows only fibrosis.

Patients with rising tumor markers are rarely cured with surgery alone. They should be treated with salvage chemotherapy prior to resection of any residual masses. Surgery is sometimes indicated as a heroic attempt to achieve a cure in a patient who has failed all chemotherapy, but the results are disappointing.

The histology of the residual mass in post-chemotherapy dissections is fibrosis or scar tissue in 27%–58%, mature teratoma in 22%–38%, and viable carcinoma in 12%–35% (CARTER et al. 1987; DONOHUE and ROWLAND 1984; LOEHRER et al. 1986; SAGALOWSKY et al. 1990). Patients with residual malignant elements should receive additional chemotherapy, with an expected long-term cure rate of 70% compared to <50% without it (SKINNER 1976). If such patients have already received salvage chemotherapy, however, continued chemotherapy does not appear to have any additional benefit (DONOHUE et al. 1994). Patients with pathologic findings of mature teratoma in the retroperitoneal dissection are generally followed without additional treatment.

## 19.4.2
## Technique of Retroperitoneal Node Dissection for Advanced Nonseminoma

### 19.4.2.1
### Preoperative Preparation

Patients who have been exposed to chemotherapy require special attention to prepare them for such extensive surgery. The white blood cell and platelet counts must be at normal levels prior to surgery. Patients who have received bleomycin should have pulmonary function assessed. The anesthesiologist must be advised about the need to maintain a low inspired oxygen level and low crystalloid replacement throughout the perioperative period (VILJOEN and THANGATHURAI 1989). In addition, patients may have other problems, such as renal insufficiency or anemia, which should be addressed.

A mechanical bowel preparation is employed, with full antibiotic preparation on those suspected to have small or large bowel involvement by tumor. In selected cases other consultants are involved, such as the vascular surgeon if replacement of the abdominal aorta or an external iliac vessel is anticipated.

### 19.4.2.2
### Surgical Technique

Patients with a significant retroperitoneal mass are best approached through a thoracoabdominal incision. Suprahilar dissections are necessary, often extending high into the retrocrural space, and the exposure to this area is clearly superior through a high (sixth to eighth rib) thoracoabdominal incision. In patients with minimal retroperitoneal disease, the dissection may be completed entirely retroperitoneally, as described above. With a significant mass, however, we routinely open the peritoneal cavity.

The patient positioning and initial steps of the exposure are identical to those described above for low-stage disease (see Chap. 18). The peritoneum is then opened, and the right colon and root of the small bowel mesentery are mobilized off of the retroperitoneum (Fig. 19.2). The bowel is placed in a plastic bag or wrap on the chest. It is not uncommon

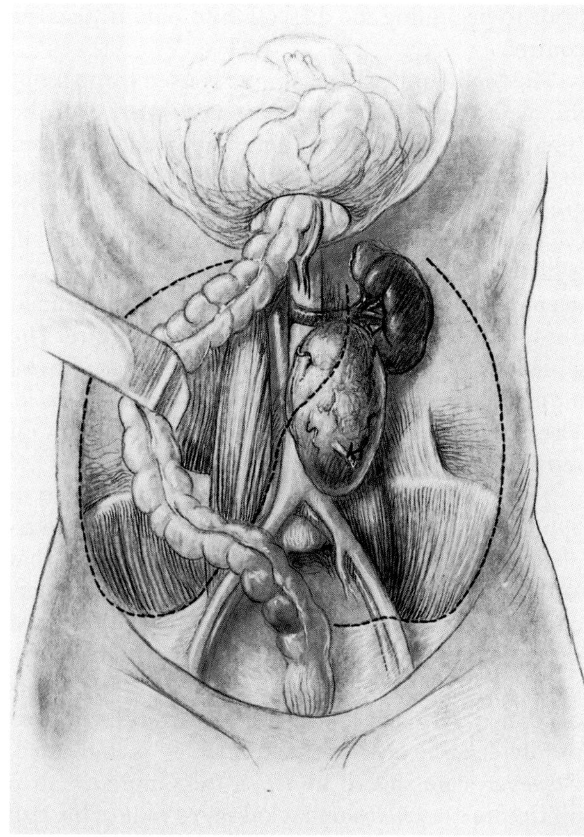

**Fig. 19.2.** Drawing showing the surgical exposure in a typical patient with a residual mass overlying the distal aorta. The right colon and small bowel mesenteries have been elevated off the retroperitoneum and the bowel is in a wrap on the chest. The sigmoid colon mesentery has been divided, and the inferior mesenteric artery ligated as it exits the tumor mass. [Reprinted with permission from Walsh, Retik, Vaughan, Wein, (eds) (1998) Campbell's Urology, 7th edn. Saunders, Philadelphia]

to find invasion of the duodenum by the mass, which may require partial duodenal resection. The posterior peritoneum is divided lateral to the left colon and the sigmoid mesentery is mobilized off of Gerota's fascia. The inferior mesenteric artery is divided if tumor extends to the inferior aorta. The sigmoid mesentery may also be invaded by tumor, and the mesenteric vessels may be divided providing the marginal artery and veins are left intact.

The superior mesenteric artery must be identified early, and its root dissected out, clipping the small lymphatic channels running along its surface. The renal vein is mobilized, and both the right and left renal arteries are dissected out. If this area is encased by tumor, normal areas of the vena cava and aorta should be mobilized above and below the tumor prior to beginning the dissection to obtain vascular control.

The "split and roll" technique is used throughout the dissection. The tumor mass is divided over the vena cava and aorta, finding the plane between the fibrous capsule of the tumor and the walls of the great vessels. If dissection proceeds too superficially (within the tumor capsule, for example), tumor spill is likely and an incomplete resection will result. Too deep dissection on the aorta will result in a thinned out wall which may result in a delayed rupture. The gonadal vessels are ligated bilaterally, as are all lumbar arteries and veins below the renal vessels. The latter may be difficult if a large amount of retroaortic disease is present.

The ureters should be dissected out early, prior to approaching the renal arteries. If one ureter is completely encased or directly invaded by tumor, that kidney may be sacrificed rather than risking an incomplete dissection. Once the ureters are free, the renal arteries bilaterally are dissected from the aorta to the renal hilum. Often multiple arteries make this dissection very difficult. If a polar artery is injured or divided, no attempt to repair it is indicated. However, care should be taken to completely strip off Gerota's fascia from that kidney to reduce the risk of late hypertension.

Superiorly, the tissue overlying the crus of the diaphragm is resected and swept inferiorly with the main nodal package. If there is any question of retrocrural disease, the crus should be divided alongside the vertebral body. The retrocrural tissue is dissected out as far superiorly as possible. The lumbar vessels should not be ligated bilaterally, since there is some risk of devascularization of the spine. On the right, the thoracic duct should be carefully clipped, and the hemiazygos vein may be ligated if necessary. The crus should be repaired after removing the nodal tissue.

When the great vessels have been fully mobilized, the tumor is dissected off the posterior body wall. The lumbar arteries and veins are again clipped as they dive into the foramina. Tongues of tumor may extend down into the foramina alongside the lumbar vessels, and should be teased out if possible. The anterior psoas fascia should be removed with the tumor, and if necessary some of the muscle itself may need to come with the tumor (Figs. 19.3, 19.4).

In the case of a large mass, no attempt is generally made to preserve the sympathetic trunks. If the prechemotherapy mass was centered around the inferior mesenteric artery (as shown in Fig. 19.2), then anejaculation is inevitable. One should remember

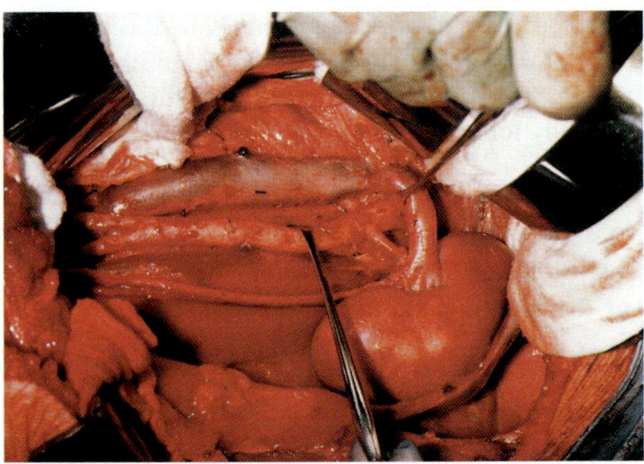

**Fig. 19.3.** The retroperitoneum is seen following a completed left-sided node dissection. All lumbar arteries and veins have been divided, and the entire nodal package removed, leaving the back muscles and anterior vertebral ligament exposed

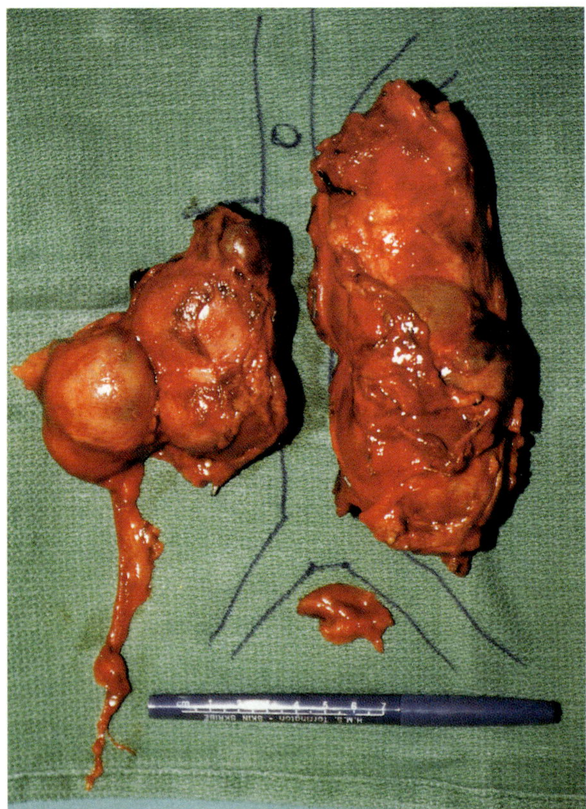

**Fig. 19.4.** Typical right-sided lymph node package which has been dissected using the "split and roll" technique. The outline of the aorta is drawn in relation to the tumor. Of note is the large amount of contralateral tumor in this patient. The right spermatic vessels are visible attached to the specimen. Histology showed mature teratoma

that fertility is already compromised in many of these patients because of effects of the chemotherapy. However, in selected patients the dissection may be more limited or one or more postganglionic nerve trunks may be salvaged (WOOD et al. 1992). The key is patient selection.

### 19.4.2.3
### Complications

Major intraoperative and postoperative complications are more common in patients with large volume retroperitoneal disease (BANIEL et al. 1995; SKINNER et al. 1982). Specialized vascular techniques may be required during the dissection, including suture repair, vascular patch graft, or complete replacement of the aorta, renal, or iliac vessels (Fig. 19.5) (KELLY et al. 1995). The vena cava may require repair or formal resection (AHLERING and SKINNER 1989). The latter can be safely ligated below the renal veins if tumor extends into it in the form of a tumor thrombus, or directly invades the wall. The patient may develop significant edema of the lower extremities, but this will gradually resolve.

Major postoperative complications occur in approximately 20% of patients (SKINNER et al. 1982; BANIEL et al. 1995). The perioperative mortality should be under 1%. The most devastating complication is fatal adult respiratory distress syndrome associated with bleomycin toxicity. GOLDFINGER and SCHWEIZER (1979) associated this risk with increased inspired oxygen and overhydration. This risk must be kept in mind constantly and requires the cooperation of the anesthesiologist, surgeon, and intensivists to avoid problems. Many other major complications have been reported, including other pulmonary complications, hemorrhage, thrombophlebitis, small bowel obstruction, wound infection or dehiscence, and pancreatitis. Pneumonia and wound infections accounted for nearly half of all of the complications seen (BANIEL et al. 1995).

In spite of the magnitude of this surgery, patients tolerate the procedure remarkably well, and there have been few long-term complications other than anejaculation. The efficacy of the procedure is attested to by the fact that retroperitoneal recurrences are exceedingly rare following a complete node dissection, even with advanced disease.

## References


Ahlering TA, Skinner DG (1989) Vena caval resection in bulky metastatic germ cell tumors. J Urol 142:1497–1499

Baniel J, Foster RS, Rowland RG, Bihrle R, Donohue JP (1995) Complications of post-chemotherapy retroperitoneal lymph node dissection. J Urol 153:976–980

Carter GE, Lieskovsky G, Skinner DG, Daniels JR (1987) Reassessment of the role of adjunctive surgical therapy in the treatment of advanced germ cell tumors. J Urol 138:1397–1401

Donohue JP, Rowland RG (1984) The role of surgery in advanced testicular cancer. Cancer 54:2716–2721

Donohue JP, Rowland RG, Kopechky K, et al. (1987) Correlation of computerized tomographic changes and histologic findings in 80 patients having radical retroperitoneal lymph node dissection after chemotherapy for testis cancer. J Urol 137:1170–1175

Donohue JP, Fox EP, Williams SD, Loehrer PJ, Ulbright TM, Einhorn LH, Weathers TD (1994) Persistent cancer in postchemotherapy retroperitoneal lymph-node dissection: outcome analysis. World J Urol 12:190–195

Gerl A, Clemm C, Schmeller N, et al. (1994) Sequential resection of residual abdominal and thoracic masses after chemotherapy for metastatic non-seminomatous germ cell tumours. Br J Cancer 70:960–965

Goldfinger PL, Schweizer O (1979) The hazards of anesthesia and surgery in bleomycin treated patients. Semin Oncol 6:121–124

Herr HW, Toner GC, Geller NL, Bosl GJ (1991) Patient selection for retroperitoneal lymph node dissection after chemotherapy for nonseminomatous germ cell tumors. Eur Urol 19:1–5

Kelly R, Skinner DG, Yellin AE, Weaver FA (1995) En bloc aortic resection for bulky metastatic germ cell tumors. J Urol 153:1849–1851

Law TM, Motzer RJ, Bajorin DF, Bosl GJ (1994) The management of patients with advanced germ cell tumors. Seminoma and nonseminoma. Urol Clin North Am 1994; 21:773–783

Loehrer PJ Sr, Hui S, Clark S, et al. (1986) Teratoma following cisplatin-based combination chemotherapy for nonseminomatous germ cell tumors: a clinico-pathological correlation. J Urol 135:1183–1189


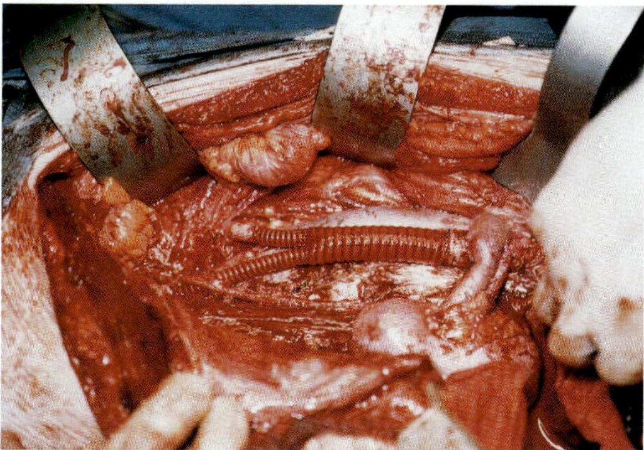

**Fig. 19.5.** Aortic replacement with a synthetic graft in the patient whose CT scan is shown in Fig. 19.1 above. Removal of the encased aorta allowed a complete dissection which would otherwise have been impossible

Loehrer PJ Sr, Birch R, Williams SD, Greco A, Einhorn LH (1987) Chemotherapy of metastatic seminoma: the Southeastern Cancer Study Group experience. J Clin Oncol 5:1212–1220

Logothetis CJ, Samuels ML, Trindade A, Johnson DE (1982) The growing teratoma syndrome. Cancer 50:1629–1635

Motzer RJ, Geller NL, Tan CC, et al. (1991) Salvage chemotherapy for patients with germ cell tumors. The Memorial Sloan Kettering Cancer Center experience (1979–1989). Cancer 67:1305–1310

Peckham MJ, Horwich A, Hendry WF (1985) Advanced seminoma: treatment with cis-platinum-based combination chemotherapy or carboplatin (JM8). Br J Cancer 52:7–13

Sagalowsky AI, Ewalt DH, Molberg K, Peters PC (1990) Predictors of residual mass histology after chemotherapy for advanced testis cancer. Urology 35:537–542

Schultz SM, Einhorn LH, Conces DJ Jr, Williams SD, Loehrer PJ (1989) Management of postchemotherapy residual mass in patients with advanced seminoma: Indiana University experience. J Clin Oncol 7:1497–1503

Skinner DG, Melamud A, Lieskovsky G (1982) Complications of thoracoabdominal retroperitoneal lymph node dissection. J Urol 127:1107–1110

Toner GC, Panicek DM, Heeland RT, et al. (1990) Adjunctive surgery after chemotherapy for nonseminomatous germ cell tumors: recommendations for patient selection. J Clin Oncol 8:1683–1694

Viljoen JF, Thangathurai D (1988) Anesthetic management in radical surgery for urologic malignancies. In: Skinner DG, Lieskovsky G (eds) Diagnosis and management of genitourinary cancer. Saunders, Philadelphia, pp 595–600

Wood DP Jr, Herr HW, Heller G, et al. (1992) Distribution of retroperitoneal metastases after chemotherapy in patients with nonseminomatous germ cell tumors. J Urol 148:1812–1816

# 20 Radiotherapy in Early Seminoma

L. VANUYTSEL

CONTENTS



## 20.1
## Introduction

Radiotherapy has a long track record as adjuvant treatment in stage I seminoma and as curative treatment in early stage II tumors. Although treatment results are excellent, concern has been raised in recent years about possible over-treatment, long-term toxicity, and induction of secondary tumours.

## 20.2
## Stage I Seminoma

### 20.2.1
### Adjuvant Radiation Treatment

#### 20.2.1.1
#### *Treatment Results*

It is well recognized that testicular seminoma follows an orderly pattern of progression. The predominant route of spread is through the lymphatics into the para-aortic, paracaval, and renal hilar lymph nodes.

Results of direct testicular lymphangiography show that the primary draining lymph nodes extend from the level of T11 down to L4, with the highest concentration existing around the renal hilar region

(BUSH et al. 1965). Subsequent drainage is into the iliac and inguinal lymph nodes.

Adjuvant radiotherapy to the para-aortic and ipsilateral pelvic ($\pm$ inguinal) lymph nodes has resulted in excellent relapse-free and cause-specific survival. Data of 12 reports, on a total of 1802 patients, published between 1991 and 1996, have been compiled in Table 20.1. The 5-year relapse-free survival ranges between 93% and 100%, and the 5-year cause-specific survival between 97% and 100%, indicating that most relapsing patients can be recovered with further treatment. These treatment outcomes confirm the results of a previous review on 2376 patients (ZAGARS 1991).

In contrast to previous reports on small series, it is now obvious from larger series (MIRIMANOFF et al. 1993; WEISSBACH and BUSSAR-MAATZ 1993) that human chorionic gonadotropin (HCG)-producing seminoma, when considered stage by stage, has the same natural history and prognosis as non-HCG-producing seminoma, even with HCG levels more than 100 times the upper normal limit.

In-field recurrences are nearly nonexistent, with four in-field recurrences reported in the aforementioned 1802 patients (0.2%). Recurrences outside of the radiation treatment field, mainly left supraclavicular and mediastinal lymph nodes and lung metastases, occurred in 47 patients, i.e., 2.6%. The median time to any relapse was 16–20 months, with a range of 3–121 months; 95% of all recurrences occurred within 5 years after treatment. The time pattern of recurrence after adjuvant radiotherapy and after watchful waiting is similar; the topographic pattern of recurrences, on the other hand, is completely different, with nearly no recurrences outside of the para-aortic and ipsilateral pelvic nodes in the surveillance series (see Sect. 20.2.2). Explanations for the observed difference are speculative, but it is tempting to suggest that it could at least partly be due to understaging in the radiation series. Most of the single-institution retrospective reports on adjuvant radiotherapy cover a long period of patient accrual, with a large number of patients treated before

L. VANUYTSEL, MD, PhD, Department of Oncology, Section of Radiotherapy, University Hospitals Gasthuisberg, Catholic University of Leuven, Herestraat 49, B-3000 Leuven, Belgium

274  L. Vanuytsel

**Table 20.3.** Seminoma stage I: secondary cancer

| Investigators | No. of patients | Period | Follow-up (in years) median | No. of second cancers | All | Skin MM | Skin Other | Skin All | L | S | P | C | R | K | P | B | Leu |
|---|---|---|---|---|---|---|---|---|---|---|---|---|---|---|---|---|---|
| Fossa et al. (1989) | 365 | 1970–82 | 9 | 15 | 1.44 | 0.63 | | | 1.60 | | | | | | | | 0.26 |
| Fossa et al. (1990) | 579[a] | 1956–77 | >10 | 46 | 1.32 | 1.32 | | | 1.40 | 1.75 | | 1.10 | | | | 2.00 | 0.85 |
| | 87[b] | 1956–77 | >10 | 14 | 4.13* | 7.69* | | | 7.69* | 8.33* | | 7.69 | | | | – | – |
| Glanzmann et al. (1991) | 289 | 1950–88 | >10 | 16 | 1.1 | | | | | | | | | | | | |
| Hamilton et al. (1986) | 232 | 1963–83 | 7 | 5 | 0.96 | | | | | | | | | | | | |
| Hanks et al. (1992) | 387 | 1973–74 | 15 | 14 | 3.4* | | | | | | | | | | | | |
| Hay et al. (1984) | 547 | 1950–69 | 15.4 | 57 | 1.87* | | | | | | | | | | | | |
| | | | | | 1.94*[c] | | | | | 0.94 | | 1.57 | 1.47 | | | | |
| | | | | | 1.99*[d] | | | 2.58* | 1.53 | | | | | 3.1[e] | 0.75 | 2.92[e] | |
| Horwich and Bell (1994) | 859 | 1961–85 | >10 | 37 | 1.27 | | | | | | | 1.5 | | 1.4 | 1.6 | 1.7 | 6.2* |
| Møller et al. (1993) | 3256 | 1943–87 | 11.6 | 337 | 1.5* | 1.3 | 1.8* | | 1 | 1.9* | 2.1* | 1.7* | 1.3 | 2.2* | 1.1 | 2.1* | 2.3* |
| van Leeuwen et al. (1993a)[f] | 907 | 1971–85 | 8.6 | NS | 1.8* | | | | | 4.4* | | | | | | | 5.2 |

NS, Not stated; L, lung; S, stomach; P, pancreas; C, colon; R, rectum; K, kidney; P, prostate; B, bladder; Leu, leukemia; MM, malignant melanomas.
*Significant at P < 0.05.
[a] Infradiaphragmatic RT only.
[b] Infradiaphragmatic + mediastinal RT.
[c] Within high-dose volume.
[d] Outside high-dose volume.
[e] All transitional cell carcinomas $P < 0.05$.
[f] Seminoma and nonseminoma.

In Table 20.3 the relative risk (RR) for secondary cancer after radiotherapy, both the overall risk and the risk for specific organ sites, has been listed. Most authors found a small but significant increase in RR overall. While it is difficult to come to hard conclusions concerning different organ sites owing to the small absolute numbers, there are some general conclusions to be drawn. Firstly, there is a clear time lag, with the highest increase in RR between 15 and 20 years (Hay et al. 1984; Møller et al. 1993; van Leeuwen et al. 1993a). Secondly, there is a tendency for an increased incidence of secondary tumours with larger treatment volumes (Fossa et al. 1990), although others (Hay et al. 1984) did find a similar increase in- and outside of the high-dose treatment volume. Thirdly, although there is probably no safe threshold dose, there are indications of an increasing risk with increasing radiation dose, e.g., van Leeuwen et al. (1993b) found a RR for stomach cancer of 26.3 (O/E 5/0.19) after 40–50 Gy and a RR of 3.2 (O/E 4/1.27) after 30 Gy (P < 0.001).

The available data indicate that there is a small risk of secondary tumors after radiation treatment for testicular cancer. The absolute numbers are small, and the risk for the individual patient is very low. This risk should be balanced against the advantages of treatment or against the possible hazards or disadvantages of withholding treatment.

## 20.2.2
## Surveillance

Several considerations have led a number of investigators to adopt a policy of postorchiectomy watchful waiting with treatment delayed until recurrence. The rationale for this approach is based on (a) the low incidence, about 10%, of microscopic nodal involvement in a report on retroperitoneal lymph node dissection in stage I seminoma (Maier et al. 1968), (b) the availability of CT scans from the early 1980s onward, which are believed to be able to detect low-volume retroperitoneal disease during follow-up, and (c) the availability and curative potential of cisplatin-based chemotherapy in the event of recurrence.

Data on the largest published series are listed in Table 20.4. Relapse-free survival and disease-specific survival at 5 years are 80%–82% and 99%–100% respectively.

Analysis of the relapse pattern yields information relevant for decision making on future treatment

**Table 20.4.** Seminoma stage I: surveillance

| Investigators | No. of patients | Period | Follow-up (in months) | | Time to relapse (in months) | | 5-year survival (%) | |
|---|---|---|---|---|---|---|---|---|
| | | | Range | Median | Range | Median | Relapse-free | Disease-specific |
| HORWICH et al. (1992) | 103 | 1983–1988 | 14–141 | 62 | 3–48 | NS | 82 | 100 |
| VON DER MAASE et al. (1993) | 261 | 1985–1988 | 6–67 | 48 | 2–37 | 14 | 80 | 98.9 |
| WARDE et al. (1995) | 172 | 1984–1991 | 7–121 | 50 | 3–108 | 16 | 81.9 | 99 |

[a] 4-year results.

**Table 20.5.** Seminoma stage I: surveillance – relapse

| Investigators | No. of patients | No. of recurrences | | | 2nd relapse |
|---|---|---|---|---|---|
| | | Total | Limited | Advanced | |
| HORWICH et al. (1992) | 103 | 17 | 12 | 5 | 4 |
| VON DER MAASE et al. (1993) | 261 | 49 | 37 | 12 | 4 |
| WARDE et al. (1995) | 172 | 27 | 22 | 5 | 3 |
| Total | 536 | 93 | 71 | 22 | 11 |

**Table 20.6.** Seminoma stage I: surveillance – pattern of relapse

| Investigators | Total | Para-aortic LN | Pelvic LN | Inguinal LN | Lung |
|---|---|---|---|---|---|
| HORWICH et al. (1992) | 17/103 | 17 | 0 | 1[a] | 1[a] |
| VON DER MAASE et al. (1993) | 49/261 | 41 | 5 | 2 | 1 |
| WARDE et al. (1995) | 27/172 | 23 | 1 + 1[a] | 1 + 1[b] | |

LN, Lymph nodes.
[a] Para-aortic LN at same time.
[b] Mediastinal LN at same time.

policy. About 17% of patients (93/536) suffered a recurrence, with an average time to recurrence of 14–16 months (Tables 20.4, 20.5). The range of time to relapse, however, was quite large, i.e., from 2 to 108 months. In the Toronto series (WARDE et al. 1995) 18% of relapses occurred more than 4 years from diagnosis, indicating the need for prolonged intensive follow-up.

Although all study protocols used intensive follow-up schedules, 4% of all cases (22/536, i.e., 23% of all relapses) were in an advanced stage, i.e., either large-volume (more than 5 cm) abdominal relapses or disseminated disease (Table 20.5). This surprising finding underscores the difficulty of detecting relapses in seminoma at an early stage, the main problem being the lack of a sensitive serum marker and the lack of sensitivity of CT scan in detecting small-volume disease. Patients with advanced relapse were treated with chemotherapy. Patients with limited relapse, i.e., small-volume (less than 5 cm) retroperitoneal disease, were treated with radiotherapy and in the event of a second relapse, with chemotherapy. In total, 6% of all patients (33/536) were treated with cisplatin-based chemotherapy.

The majority of relapses, 87% (81/93), occurred in the para-aortic lymph nodes. It is important to note that 10% (9/93) of relapses, i.e., 1.7% of all cases, occurred in the pelvic or inguinal lymph nodes as the only location (Table 20.6).

Unfortunately, the surveillance studies did not agree on patient- and disease-related parameters that could predict for relapse. In a multivariate analysis, VON DER MAASE et al. (1993) identified tumor size as the only factor with independent

**Table 20.7.** Seminoma stage II – radiotherapy: treatment results

| Investigators | Period | No. of pts. | Max. LN size | Follow-up (in years), median | Dose (Gy) | | Relapse-free survival (%) | | Cause-specific survival (%) | |
|---|---|---|---|---|---|---|---|---|---|---|
| | | | | | Infradiaphragmatic | Supradiaphragmatic | 5 yr | 10 yr | 5 yr | 10 yr |
| Speer et al. (1995) | 1964–1988 | 15 | <10 | 7 | 27.6 | 24.5 | 93 | 93 | NA | NA |
| Dosmann and | 1960–1983 | 39 | <10 | 12 | 35 | 25 | 92 | NA | NA | NA |
| Zagars (1993) | 1984–1991 | 16 | <10 | 2.5 | 35 | 0 | 73 | NA | NA | NA |
| Lai et al. (1993) | 1964–1988 | 33 | <5 | 6.7 | 34 | 27 | 93 | 93 | 97 | 97 |
| Whipple | 1966–1989 | 31 | <5 | 9.5 | 30 | 30 | 93 | NA | NA | NA |
| et al. (1997) | | 14 | >5 | 9.5 | 30 | 30 | 79 | NA | NA | NA |
| Hültenschmidt | 1978–1992 | 24 | <2 | 6 | 36 | 30 | 91.7 | 91.7 | 100 | 100 |
| et al. (1996) | | 13 | 2–5 | 6 | 36 | 30 | 76.9 | 76.9 | 100 | 100 |
| Schmidberger | 1991–1994 | 39 | <2 | 3 | 30 | 0 | 100[a] | 100[b] | 100 | 100 |
| et al. (1997) | | 19 | 2–5 | 3 | 36 | 0 | 94.1[a] | 87.4[b] | 100 | 100 |
| | | 58 | ≤5 | 3 | | | 98.1[a] | 96[b] | 100 | 100 |

[a] Relapse-free survival at 1 year.
[b] Relapse-free survival at 2 years.

prognostic significance. The 4-year relapse-free survival rates were 94%, 82%, and 64% for tumors smaller than 3 cm, 3–6 cm, and 6 or more cm, respectively. For the last-mentioned group of patients surveillance was not advocated. Tumor size was not a prognostic factor in the patient group followed by WARDE and colleagues (1995) when the same cut-off value of 6 cm was used. The latter group only identified age as a prognostic factor in a univariate analysis. Finally, the group of HORWICH et al. (1992) identified lymphatic and vascular invasion as a prognostic factor in univariate analysis. WARDE et al. (1995) did not retain this histologic factor as a prognostic factor.

In general it is believed that surveillance should not be used outside of a well-conducted prospective study. The main reason is the intensive prolonged follow-up necessary, given the wide time range of relapse and the lack of a serum marker, making regular abdominopelvic CT scans necessary. A second reason, of at least equal importance, is the difficulty in confirming a relapse when radiologic findings are suspicious, leading to a substantial number of large-volume relapses. These recurrences have to be treated with polychemotherapy, with its own associated toxicity.

## 20.3
## Stage II Seminoma

### 20.3.1
### Treatment Results

The treatment results of recently published series are listed in Table 20.7. The reported 5-year relapse-free survival ranges between 73% and 93%. There is a lack of uniformity in reporting owing to differences in patient grouping according to lymph node size and the varying percentage in each series of patients treated with mediastinal and supraclavicular irradiation. Interpretation of the data is therefore very difficult.

### 20.3.2
### Treatment Technique

#### 20.3.2.1
#### Treatment Fields

Although treatment results with infradiaphragmatic and supradiaphragmatic radiation treatment are excellent, elective mediastinal irradiation was gradually abandoned by most centers during the mid 1980s. The reasons were the excess morbidity and mortality due to cardiovascular and pulmonary complications, especially in patients aged 40 years or more (DOSMANN and ZAGARS 1993; HANKS et al. 1992), the availability and effectiveness of cisplatin-based chemotherapy as salvage therapy, and the impairment of bone marrow reserve for subsequent chemotherapy after extended radiotherapy (KELLOKUMPU-LEHTINEN and HALME 1990).

Only DOSMANN and ZAGARS (1993) separately reported patients according to the extent of treatment. They noticed a decrease in 5-year relapse-free survival from 92% to 73% when the supradiaphragmatic irradiation was omitted, mainly due to left supraclavicular nodal relapse. In an extensive literature review, SPEER et al. (1995) tried to define the incidence of mediastinal and supraclavicular relapses in relation to the size of the para-aortic lymph nodes when elective supradiaphragmatic radiation was not given. Estimates were as follows: 9% supradiaphragmatic relapses for abdominal lymph nodes smaller than 2 cm, 16% for lymph nodes between 2 and 5 cm, and 23% for lymph nodes larger than 5 cm. Further information comes from the data of SCHMIDBERGER et al. (1997) and the treatment results of relapsing patients in the seminoma stage I surveillance studies (see Sect. 20.2.2). SCHMIDBERGER et al. (1997) reported the results of a prospective study of seminoma stage II patients treated only to the para-aortic and ipsilateral pelvic nodes. The 1- and 2-year relapse-free survival rates for patients with lymph nodes smaller than 2 cm are 100% and 100%, respectively, while for patients with lymph nodes between 2 and 5 cm they are 94% and 87.5%, respectively. The surveillance studies (Table 20.5) identified 71 patients with a low-volume, i.e., less than 5 cm, infradiaphragmatic relapse. These patients were treated with para-aortic and ipsilateral pelvic radiation, and 11 of them, or 15.4%, experienced a second relapse, in all cases outside the treatment field.

It thus seems reasonable to estimate the probability of relapse after infradiaphragmatic radiation to be between 5% and 10% when lymph nodes are smaller or equal to 2 cm and between 10% and 15% when lymph nodes are between 2 and 5 cm.

### 20.3.2.2
### Radiation Dose

A radiation dose of 30 Gy in 2 Gy/fraction seems adequate for tumor control in lymph nodes up to 2 cm, while for lymph nodes between 2 and 5 cm a dose of 35 Gy appears required.

## 20.4
## General Conclusions

Radiotherapy is still a cornerstone modality in the treatment of early-stage seminoma. The use of radiotherapy as adjuvant treatment in stage I seminoma has yielded excellent disease-free and cause-specific survival results, with a low risk of long-term toxicity and secondary tumors. Surveillance has not established itself as a valid alternative outside the setting of prospective studies. Other adjuvant treatment, i.e., chemotherapy (OLIVER et al. 1994), will have to be validated in randomized trials allowing sufficient time for assessment of long-term side-effects.

In early stage II disease radiotherapy will cure the majority of patients when applied rigorously with limited doses and volumes, keeping chemotherapy in reserve for salvage.

## References

Bayens YC, Helle PA, Van Putten WLJ, et al. (1992) Orchidectomy followed by radiotherapy in 176 stage I and II testicular seminoma patients: benefits of a 10-year follow-up study. Radiother Oncol 25:97–102

Bush FM, Sayegh ES, Chenault O (1965) Some uses of lymphangiography in the management of testicular tumors. J Urol 93:490–495

Coia LR, Hanks GE (1988) Complications from large field intermediate dose infradiaphragmatic radiation and analysis of the patterns of care outcome studies for Hodgkin's disease and seminoma. Int J Radiat Oncol Biol Phys 15:29–35

Dosmann MA, Zagars GK (1993) Postorchiectomy radiotherapy for stages I and II testicular seminoma. Int J Radiat Oncol Biol Phys 26:381–390

Fossa SD, Aass N, Kaalhus O (1989) Radiotherapy for testicular seminoma stage I: treatment results and long-term post-irradiation morbidity in 365 patients. Int J Radiat Oncol Biol Phys 16:383–388

Fossa SD, Langmark F, Aass N, et al. (1990) Second non-germ cell malignancies after radiotherapy of testicular cancer with or without chemotherapy. Br J Cancer 61:639–643

Fossa SD, Horwich A, Russell JM, et al. (1996) Optimal field size in adjuvant radiotherapy of stage I seminoma – a randomized trial. Proc Am Soc Clin Oncol 15:239

Friedman LF (1982) Tables of the number of patients required in clinical trials using the log-rank test. Stat Med 1:121–129

Giacchetti S, Raoul Y, Wibault P, et al. (1993) Treatment of stage I testis seminoma by radiotherapy: long-term results – a 30-year experience. Int J Radiat Oncol Biol Phys 27:3–9

Glanzmann C, Schultz G, Lütolf UM (1991) Long-term morbidity of adjuvant infradiaphragmatic irradiation in patients with testicular caner and implications for the treatment of stage I seminoma. Radiother Oncol 22:12–18

Hamilton C, Horwich A, Easton D, et al. (1986) Radiotherapy for stage I seminoma testis: results of treatment and complications. Radiother Oncol 6:115–120

Hanks GE, Peters T, Owen J (1992) Seminoma of the testis: long term beneficial and deleterious results of radiation. Int J Radiat Oncol Biol Phys 24:913–919

Hay JH, Duncan W, Kerr GR (1984) Subsequent malignancies in patients irradiated for testicular tumours. Br J Radiol 57:597–602

Horwich A, Bell J (1994) Mortality and cancer incidence following radiotherapy for seminoma of the testis. Radiother Oncol 30:193–198

Horwich A, Alsanjari N, Nicholls J, et al. (1992) Surveillance following orchidectomy for stage I testicular seminoma. Br J Cancer 65:775–778

Hültenschmidt B, Budach V, Genters K, et al. (1996) Results of radiotherapy for 230 patients with stage I and II seminomas. Strahlenther Onkol 172:186–192

Joos H, Sedlmayer F, Gomahr A, et al. (1997) Endocrine profiles after radiotherapy in stage I seminoma: impact of two different radiation treatment modalities. Radiother Oncol 43:159–162

Kellokumpu-Lehtinen P, Halme A (1990) Results of treatment in irradiated testicular seminoma. Radiother Oncol 18:1–7

Kiricuta IC, Sauer J, Bohndorf W (1996) Omission of the pelvic irradiation in stage I testicular seminoma: a study of postorchiectomy paraaortic radiotherapy. Int J Radiat Oncol Biol Phys 35:293–298

Lai PP, Bernstein MJ, Kim J, et al. (1993) Radiation therapy for stage I and IIa testicular seminoma. Int J Radiat Oncol Biol Phys 28:373–379

Maier JG, Sulak MH, Mittemeyer BT (1968) Seminoma of the testis: analysis of treatment success and failure. Am J Roentgenol 102:596–602

Mirimanoff RO, Sinzig M, Krüger M, et al. (1993) Prognosis of human chorionic gonadotropin-producing seminoma treated by postoperative radiotherapy. Int J Radiat Oncol Biol Phys 27:17–23

Møller H, Mellemgaard A, Jacobsen GK, et al. (1993) Incidence of second primary cancer following testicular cancer. Eur J Cancer 29A:672–676

Niewald M, Waziri A, Walter K, et al. (1995) Short communication. Low-dose radiotherapy for stage I seminoma: early results. Radiat Oncol 37:164–166

Oliver RTD, Edmonds PM, Ong JYH, et al. (1994) Pilot studies of 2 and 1 course carboplatin as adjuvant for stage I seminoma: should it be tested in a randomized trial against radiotherapy? Int J Radiat Oncol Biol Phys 29:3–8

Schmidberger H, Bamberg M, Meisner C, et al. (1997) Radiotherapy in stage IIa and IIb testicular seminoma with reduced portals: a prospective multicenter study. Int J Radiat Oncol Biol Phys 39:321–326

Speer TW, Sombeck MD, Parsons JT, et al. (1995) Testicular seminoma: a failure analysis and literature review. Int J Radiat Oncol Biol Phys 33:89–97

Vallis KA, Howard GCW, Duncan W, et al. (1995) Radiotherapy for stages I and II testicular seminoma: results and morbidity in 238 patients. Br J Radiol 68:400–405

van Leeuwen FE, Stiggelbout AM, van den Belt-Dusebout AW, et al. (1993a) Second cancer risk following testicular cancer: a follow-up study of 1.909 patients. J Clin Oncol 11:415–424

van Leeuwen FE, Stiggelbout AM, van den Belt-Dusebout AW, et al. (1993b) Second tumors after radiation treatment of testicular germ cell tumors. Letter to the editor. J Clin Oncol 11:2286–2287

van Rooy EM, Sagerman RH (1994) Long-term evaluation of postorchiectomy irradiation for stage I seminoma. Radiology 191:857–861

von der Maase H, Specht L, Jacobsen GK, et al. (1993) Surveillance following orchidectomy for stage I seminoma of the testis. Eur J Cancer 29A:1931–1934

Warde P, Gaspodarowicz MK, Panzarella T, et al. (1995) Stage I testicular seminoma: results of adjuvant irradiation and surveillance. J Clin Oncol 13:2255–2262

Weissbach L, Bussar-Maatz R (1993) HCG-positive seminoma. Eur Urol 23:29–32

Whipple GL, Sagerman RH, van Rooy EM (1997) Long-term evaluation of postorchiectomy radiotherapy for stage II seminoma. Am J Clin Oncol 20:196–201

Zagars GK (1991) Management of stage I seminoma: radiotherapy. In: Horwich A (ed) Testicular cancer investigation and management. Chapman and Hall Medical, London, pp 83–107

# 21 Radiotherapy for Bulky Seminoma

C. Catton

CONTENTS



## 21.1 Introduction

Testicular germ cell neoplasms are rare, but are still the most common malignant tumors arising in young men. About half of these men will present with pure seminoma. Only 5% of these patients will present with distant metastases, but 20% will have radiologic evidence of retroperitoneal lymph node involvement. Half of these nodal masses will be greater than 2 cm in diameter (WARDE et al. 1998). This chapter will focus on the historical and current use of radiotherapy (RT) in the management of this group of patients.

The presence of bulky retroperitoneal metastases has long been recognized as an adverse prognostic factor for cure with RT but improvements in retroperitoneal imaging techniques have gradually changed the definition of what constitutes bulky disease, and reported outcomes that relate to the degree of tumor bulk must be interpreted with this in mind. Early reports that used lymphangiography to identify nodal disease classified tumor bulk into either palpable or nonpalpable disease (LAUKKANEN et al.

C. CATTON, MD, FRCPC, Department of Radiation Oncology, The Princess Margaret Hospital, 610 University Avenue, Room 4-728, Toronto, ON, M5G 2M9, Canada

1987; THOMAS et al. 1981; WILLAN and McGOWAN 1985). Attempts to conform to this policy during the transition to computerized tomographic (CT) staging prompted some investigators to classify patients into having bulky or nonbulky disease depending on whether the maximum cross-sectional diameter of the nodal mass seen on CT was larger or smaller than 10 cm (DOSMANN and ZAGARS 1993; MASON and KEARSLEY 1988; SMALLEY et al. 1985; SPEER et al. 1995). BALL et al. (1982) and PECKHAM (1981b) identified the prognostic significance of smaller volumes of nodal disease and incorporated this into the Royal Marsden Hospital staging classification. Modifications of this system, which includes the 1997 UICC classification, are now commonly used to define retroperitoneal tumor bulk, which is defined as the transverse diameter of the largest retroperitoneal lymph node mass. This chapter will use the Consensus Conference modification that THOMAS et al. (1990) adopted in 1989 to describe retroperitoneal tumor bulk (Table 21.1). There is no classification in general use that makes any provision for tumor bulk based upon the total number of involved nodes, and this may have prognostic significance following RT.

Until the advent of effective platinum-based chemotherapy regimens for germ cell tumors the standard therapy for any stage II seminoma was RT to the retroperitoneum, and often included prophylactic RT to the mediastinum and the supraclavicular lymph nodes. This treatment produced excellent local control of nodal disease and was usually curative for patients with all but the most bulky retroperitoneal disease. Even so, the routine use of RT for patients with more than minimal nodal bulk has declined, and the use of primary chemotherapy has increased. The optimal point for deciding who is best managed with primary chemotherapy or RT is not firmly established, but patients with nodal masses greater than 5 cm are usually recommended for primary chemotherapy, and those with retroperitoneal nodal bulk between 2 and 5 cm usually receive RT (HORWICH 1990). This chapter will review the results of RT for patients with retroperitoneal nodal bulk greater than 2 cm and attempt to define the role of RT for these patients in the chemotherapy era. There have been no randomized studies of treatment for these patients and the available data were retrospectively collected from small patient numbers. This, along with the changing definitions of tumor bulk and changing patterns of treatment, requires that the derived conclusions be interpreted with caution.

## 21.2
## Predictors of Outcome After Radiotherapy for Stage II Disease

Survival is the principal measure of treatment efficacy, and in the prechemotherapy era the presence of

a palpable retroperitoneal mass and stage III disease were associated with poorer survival than for impalpable stage II disease (Thomas et al. 1981). Since the advent of effective chemotherapy these differences in survival have been much less apparent (Fossa et al. 1995; Fossa and Horwich 1997; Horwich 1993; Mencel et al. 1994; Warde et al. 1998), and consequently relapse-free survival (RFS) is a better indicator of outcome after RT than survival. Table 21.2 presents a summary of RFS rates published for patients treated with RT for tumor bulk of greater than 2 cm in diameter since 1981. These studies were all retrospective and comprised relatively few patients due to the rarity of the presentation. The classification and determination of tumor bulk varied widely, but an attempt has been made to group the results by the degree of precision used to define the retroperitoneal tumor volume. Additionally, patients are identified who were treated with or without prophylactic mediastinal and supraclavicular irradiation.

**Table 21.1.** Consensus Conference seminoma staging classification (Thomas et al. 1990)

| | |
|---|---|
| Stage I: | No clinical evidence of metastases beyond testicle |
| Stage II: | Infradiaphragmatic lymph node metastases |
| | A) Maximum diameter $\leq 2$ cm |
| | B) Maximum diameter $> 2 \leq 5$ cm |
| | C) Maximum diameter $> 5 \leq 10$ cm |
| | D) Maximum diameter $>10$ cm |
| Stage III: | Supradiaphragmatic nodal involvement (Infradiaphragmatic nodes recorded as A, B, C, D, as for stage II) |
| Stage IV: | Parenchymal metastatic disease |

### 21.2.1
### Nodal Tumor Bulk

Almost all series using RT have demonstrated a relationship between retroperitoneal tumor bulk and outcome. The results presented in Table 21.2 showed that the RFS of patients treated with RT for tumor bulk described as being either less than 5 cm or stage

**Table 21.2.** Published RFS rates at 5 years or longer for stage II seminoma with nodes larger than 2 cm in diameter. Reports that combined stage IIA and B (described as 5 cm or less) have been grouped with those that described IIB separately. Reports that combined stage IIC and D (described as more than 5 cm) have been grouped with those that described stage IIC separately

| Authors | No. of patients | Relapse-free survival at 5 years or more | | | | |
|---|---|---|---|---|---|---|
| | | $\leq 5$ cm (or IIB) | $>5$ cm (or IIC) | Impalpable (or <10 cm) | Palpable (or >10 cm) | Mediastinal XRT |
| Thomas et al. (1981) | 86 | | | 92% | 52% | No |
| Willan and McGowan (1985) | 34 | | | 82% | 54% | Some yes |
| Mason and Kearsley (1988) | 49 | | | 89% | 64% | Most yes |
| Laukkanen et al. (1987) | 23 | | | – | 74% | Some yes |
| Smalley et al. (1990) | 20 | | | 100% | 75% | Most yes |
| Dosmann and Zagars (1993) | 68 | | | 87% | 69% | Most yes |
| Speer et al. (1995) | 21 | | | 83% | 75% | Yes |
| Evensen et al. (1985) | 77 | 94% | 78%[a] | | | Most yes |
| Gregory and Peckham (1986) | 34 | 82% | 72% | | | Some yes |
| Lederman et al. (1989) | 23 | 100% | 75% | | | Yes |
| Kellokumpu-Lehtinen and Halme (1990) | 82 | 74% | 60% | | | Some yes |
| Bayens et al. (1992) | 28 | 66% | 72% | | | No |
| Vallis et al. (1995) | 27 | 91% | 60% | | | Some yes |
| Warde et al. (1998) | 50 | 88% | 50% | | 0/2 patients | No |

[a] Some of these patients received chemotherapy with RT.

IIB, or for impalpable disease was excellent, and usually in the range of 82%–92% at 5 years. Bayens et al. (1992) and Kellokumpu-Lehtinen and Halme (1990) reported less favorable outcomes of 66% and 74% 5-year RFS respectively for patients with stage IIB disease, whereas Smalley et al. (1990) reported 100% 5-year RFS for patients with impalpable disease treated with para-aortic and mediastinal RT. Small patient numbers, variations in treatment techniques introduced over the years, and patient selection factors can partly explain these differences.

Patients with bulkier retroperitoneal disease, defined and grouped variously as masses greater than 5 cm or greater than 10 cm, or as stage IIC, or as palpable masses, did less well, with reported RFS in the 50%–75% range. For these patients, the highest relapse rates were in the patients who did not routinely receive prophylactic mediastinal or supraclavicular irradiation.

As will be discussed below, prophylactic therapy has influenced patterns of relapse without changing overall survival for patients with bulky stage II disease. When prophylactic therapy is not employed, the risk of a supradiaphragmatic nodal relapse increases from about 16% to 26% as retroperitoneal nodal bulk increases from between 2 and 5 cm to more than 10 cm in diameter (Speer et al. 1995). Extranodal metastases have been reported as an initial site of failure after RT in 10% of patients with palpable abdominal masses and much less frequently in patients with impalpable disease (Thomas et al. 1981).

## 21.2.2
## Treatment Volume

The indications for and value of prophylactic mediastinal and supraclavicular irradiation for patients with retroperitoneal metastases from seminoma are controversial. The mediastinum, and especially the supraclavicular fossa, are well-recognized sites of second echelon spread for patients with retroperitoneal nodal disease (Dosmann and Zagars 1993; Speer et al. 1995; Thomas et al. 1981; Warde et al. 1998), and prophylactic irradiation to these areas should improve RFS rates provided the patients are not also harboring micrometastatic disease elsewhere. The actual benefit of prophylaxis will depend on the risk of failure in these sites without prophylactic treatment, the effectiveness of the therapy in eradicating disease in the treated volume, the risk of the patient harboring micrometastatic disease in

other sites as well, and the toxicity of the additional therapy.

The available data show that the risk of supradiaphragmatic failure increases with the bulk of the retroperitoneal nodal disease, and a comprehensive review of the literature by Speer et al. (1995) demonstrated that the risk of mediastinal or supraclavicular failure was 16% for stage IIB, 23% for stage IIC, and 26% for stage IID.

Warde et al. (1998) identified a relapse in the supraclavicular fossa in 7/80 (9%) patients staged IIA–D who were treated without mediastinal irradiation, and an isolated supraclavicular fossa relapse represented 44% of all relapses seen in these patients. Dosmann and Zagars (1993) reported no supraclavicular fossa relapses in 39 patients with stage IIA–C disease treated with prophylactic mediastinal and supraclavicular fossa radiation, compared to 3/16 supraclavicular fossa relapses in similarly staged patients who did not receive prophylactic irradiation. On the other hand Vallis et al. (1995) reported that of five relapses (9% of all treated) in all their stage II patients, two were in the mediastinum of patients who had received prophylactic mediastinal irradiation.

The results taken together suggest that the risk of isolated mediastinal or supraclavicular failure is small for patients with stage IIA or IIB disease, and prophylactic therapy is not indicated. For patients with more advanced disease (stage IIC and D), prophylactic irradiation may improve RFS by as much as 25% over results obtained by abdominal nodal irradiation alone. This impression is supported by the generally better RFS rates reported for patients treated with prophylactic irradiation listed in Table 21.2, such as Speer et al. (1995), who reported an 83% 10-year RFS for patients with retroperitoneal masses of greater than 10 cm, and Lederman et al. (1989), who reported a 75% 10-year RFS for patients with stage IIC disease.

The possibility of improving RFS by up to 25% in this group (stage IIC and D) with prophylactic irradiation must be weighed against the fact that the majority of patients will not benefit from it, either because they do not need prophylaxis or because it is inadequate treatment for them. Additionally, it is very unlikely to improve overall survival, since salvage chemotherapy is now very effective. The addition of mediastinal fields may increase the overall toxicity of treatment, either in its own right or by increasing the toxicity of salvage chemotherapy (Lederman et al. 1989; Smalley et al. 1985; Whipple et al. 1997).

The routine use of primary chemotherapy for nodal disease greater than 5 cm has made this controversy largely a historical one. However, DOSMANN and ZAGARS (1993) recently suggested that in patients at risk of supradiaphragmatic relapse after abdominal RT the toxicity of primary chemotherapy or prophylactic mediastinal irradiation might be avoided by limiting prophylactic fields to the supraclavicular nodes. This hypothesis has not yet been tested.

### 21.2.3
### Radiation Dose

Seminoma is a very radiosensitive tumor (Figs. 21.1, 21.2). The radiation doses commonly employed for bulky disease are modest compared to the doses used in the radical therapy of other histologies, and failures within the radiation field are now rarely seen. Historically, local failure was an issue, and THOMAS et al. (1981) reported an abdominal in-field relapse rate of 5/17 (30%) for radiation doses between 28 and 39 Gy, and 11/27 (40%) for doses between 22 and 26 Gy for patients with palpable retroperitoneal disease. None of these patients had their treatment planned with cross-sectional imaging, and most of these failures were likely due to inadequate coverage of gross disease by the RT fields. In a more recent series from the same institution, WARDE et al. (1998) reported in-field failures in only 2/58 (3%) patients with stage IIB–D disease using radiation doses ranging from 25 to 40 Gy in 20–28 fractions over 4–6 weeks, and both cases relapsed as nonseminomatous germ cell tumors (NSGCT) despite histologically proven pure seminoma primaries. Most patients with disease stage IIB or greater received at least 30 Gy. Similarly, BABAIAN and ZAGARS (1988) reported that only 3/48 patients with stage II disease suffered relapse in para-aortic nodes using doses of 20–48 Gy. One case was choriocarcinoma on biopsy.

### 21.3
### Other Prognostic Factors

### 21.3.1
### Histology

VALLIS et al. (1995) reported that anaplastic seminoma was associated with a 43% failure rate after RT. A statistically significant difference in

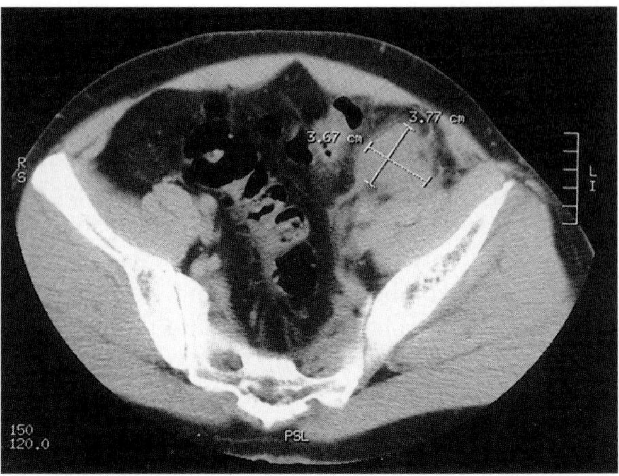

**Fig. 21.1.** An unusual presentation of stage IIB seminoma. This patient presented with a primary tumor in the left testis, and the staging CT scan demonstrated a 4 cm nodal mass at the junction of the left external and common iliac chains, without any other adenopathy present. This pattern of nodal spread is seen in about 5% of cases (PECKHAM 1981a)

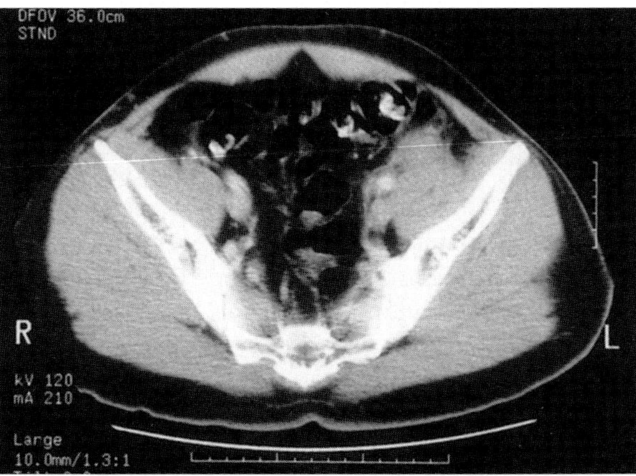

**Fig. 21.2.** An interim scan taken 2 weeks into the course of radiation therapy in the same patient as shown in Fig. 21.1. There has already been marked regression of the nodal mass after 12.5 Gy, demonstrating the extreme radiosensitivity of seminoma

relapse rates between the seminoma histologies has not been described by others, but anaplastic seminoma is an uncommon tumor and a somewhat higher risk of relapse compared to classical and spermatocytic histologies may be difficult to document (EVENSEN et al. 1985; WARDE et al. 1998).

### 21.3.2
### Tumor Markers

MENCEL et al. (1994), in a series of 142 patients with advanced seminoma treated with chemotherapy, observed that an elevated pretreatment βHCG level predicted for a higher relapse rate, and that the risk of dying of seminoma increased with the pretreatment level of βHCG or lactate dehydrogenase. This finding has not been identified in smaller series of patients treated with primary RT or chemotherapy (EVENSEN et al. 1987; MIRIMANOFF et al. 1993; VALLIS et al. 1995; WARDE et al. 1998).

### 21.3.3
### Relapse After Radiotherapy

MENCEL et al. (1994) reported that a history of radiation failure was associated with inferior survival in patients treated with chemotherapy. It is not clear whether this was because prior RT affected survival by limiting the effectiveness of salvage chemotherapy, or whether relapse after RT simply became a selection factor for poor prognosis disease. However, a similar finding was reported by LEDERMAN et al. (1989), who attributed the reduced chemotherapy salvage rate for their patients with stage IIC disease to loss of tolerance to chemotherapy following abdominal and thoracic radiotherapy.

## 21.4
## Management of the Residual Mass

The assessment of a complete response to treatment for metastatic seminoma can be complicated by a persistent residual mass. This is seen in 25%–30% of cases (PUC et al. 1996; SCHULTZ et al. 1989; WARDE et al. 1998) regardless of treatment modality. The surgical approach to a residual mass is less suitable for seminoma than for NSGCT since seminomas frequently contain only necrotic and fibrous tissue, and their infiltrative adherence to major vessels may make resection technically difficult (HERR et al. 1997). The most extensive experience in the management of residual masses has been by the MSKCC group following chemotherapy (PUC et al. 1996). They identified active residual disease after chemotherapy in 44% of their patients with residual masses 3 cm or larger, compared to only 3% of patients with smaller residual masses. They recommend that retroperitoneal lymph node dissection be limited to patients with residual masses of 3 cm or larger. Others have recommended a policy of observation as a reasonable strategy if a mass is stable or shrinking after therapy (CULINE and DROZ 1996; HORWICH et al. 1997; SCHULTZ et al. 1989; WARDE et al. 1998). In

The Princess Margaret Hospital experience using this approach, only 4% of patients required surgery (WARDE et al. 1998). Periodic CT examinations are mandatory when this approach is taken, and treatment with chemotherapy is indicated for residual masses that increase in size after RT. Pathologic confirmation is also required to direct the type of salvage chemotherapy, since a proportion of these patients will relapse with NSGCT (BABAIAN and ZAGARS 1988; WARDE et al. 1998).

The use of RT in patients with a post-chemotherapy residual mass has been shown to be of little benefit (DUCHESNE et al. 1997).

## 21.5
## Discussion and Conclusions

The majority of patients who present with metastatic seminoma will have retroperitoneal nodal masses no more than 5 cm in diameter (stage IIA or IIB) and a very high proportion of them will be cured with abdominal nodal RT and not suffer any significant long-term morbidity. The risk to these patients of an isolated supradiaphragmatic nodal relapse is small, and the salvage rate with chemotherapy is excellent, so the routine use of mediastinal and/or supraclavicular fossa prophylaxis is not warranted. Radiation fields for patients with stage IIB disease (Fig. 21.3) should include treating the para-aortic lymph nodes, both renal hila, and the ipsilateral pelvic nodes to 25 Gy. Many centers will also include the contralateral pelvic nodes in the volume. The dose to gross disease is then commonly brought up to 35–40 Gy.

The optimal use of RT for bulkier disease is controversial. The experiences of the Princess Margaret Hospital and others have shown that patients with nodal masses larger than 5 cm (IIC and D) are at increased risk of relapse after abdominal irradiation in both supradiaphragmatic nodal and extranodal sites, and that the overall risk of relapse can be as high as 50% for patients with palpable (greater than 10 cm) disease. There is no indication for treating these patients with abdominal irradiation alone, and 15%–25% will relapse even after prophylactic supradiaphragmatic nodal irradiation. Given the demonstrated efficacy of chemotherapy in inducing durable complete responses in advanced seminoma, a routine policy of primary radiotherapy with salvage chemotherapy is not justified for these patients. However, for the rare patient not suitable for curative chemotherapy, prophylactic supraclavicular

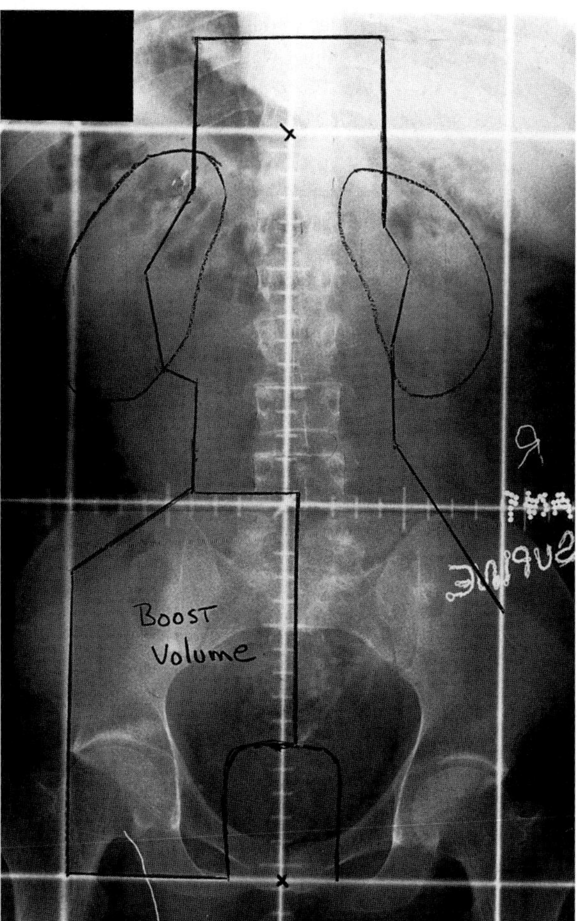



**Fig. 21.3.** The radiation portal used to treat the patient depicted in Figs. 21.1 and 21.2, and one which is typical of the radiation fields used to treat stage IIB seminoma at The Princess Margaret Hospital. The kidneys and the renal hilar nodes were localized onto the simulator film from a planning CT scan. This patient declined scrotal shielding, which would normally be used. The entire volume received 25 Gy in 20 fractions over 4 weeks, and the boost volume, which encompassed the original mass and adjacent lymph nodes, received an additional 10 Gy in five fractions over 1 week

irradiation adds little extra morbidity to treatment, and could be considered in addition to retroperitoneal nodal irradiation to improve the RFS.

An alternative approach to improving the results of radiotherapy while reducing the overall toxicity of the treatment regimen is to combine a single course of single-agent carboplatin with conventional abdominal radiotherapy. MacVicar and Horwich (1992) and Yao et al. (1994) have presented data suggesting that single-agent carboplatin is effective in eradicating micrometastatic disease, but less so for bulky disease. A phase II trial of combined single-course carboplatin with para-aortic and ipsilateral

pelvic radiotherapy for patients with stage IIA and B disease has produced 100% disease-free survival at a mean of 36 months' follow-up, with modest toxicity. This approach has not been tested on bulkier disease, but warrants investigation as a potentially less toxic alternative to standard combination chemotherapy protocols.

*Acknowledgements.* The author wishes to thank Drs. Carol Swallow, Pamela Catton, Mary Gospodarowicz, and Padraig Warde for their assistance in the preparation of this manuscript.

# References


Babaian R, Zagars G (1988) Testicular seminoma: the M.D. Anderson experience. An analysis of pathological and patient characteristics, and treatment recommendations. J Urol 139:311–314

Ball D, Barrett A, Peckham M (1982) The management of metastatic seminoma testis. Cancer 50:2289–2294

Bayens Y, Helle P, Van Putten W, Mali S (1992) Orchidectomy followed by radiotherapy in 176 stage I and II testicular seminoma patients: benefits of a 10-year follow-up study. Radiother Oncol 25:97–102

Culine S, Droz JP (1996) Optimal management of residual mass after chemotherapy in advanced seminoma: there is time for everything. J Clin Oncol 14:2884–2885

Dosmann M, Zagars G (1993) Postorchiectomy radiotherapy for stages I and II testicular seminoma. Int J Radiat Oncol Biol Phys 26:381–390

Duchesne G, Stenning S, Aass N, et al. (1997) Radiotherapy after chemotherapy for metastatic seminoma – a diminishing role. MRC Testicular Tumour Working Party. Eur J Cancer 33:829–835

Evensen J, Fossa S, Kjellevold K, Lien H (1985) Testicular seminoma: analysis of treatment and failure for stage II disease. Radiother Oncol 4:55–61

Evensen J, Fossa S, Kjellevold K, Lein H (1987) Testicular seminoma: histological findings and their prognostic significance for stage II disease. J Surg Oncol 36:166–169

Fossa S, Horwich A (1997) Current status of chemotherapy in advanced seminoma. Eur J Cancer 33:181–183

Fossa S, Droz J, Stoter G, Kaye S, Vermeylen K, Sylvester R, the members of the EORTC GU Group (1995) Cisplatin, vincristine and ifosphamide combination chemotherapy of metastatic seminoma: results of EORTC trial 30874. Br J Cancer 71:619–624

Gregory C, Peckham M (1986): Results of radiotherapy for stage II testicular seminoma. Radiother Oncol 6:285–292

Herr H, Sheinfeld J, Puc H, et al. (1997) Surgery for a post-chemotherapy residual mass in seminoma. J Urol 157:860–862

Horwich A (1990) Questions in the management of seminoma. Clin Oncol (R Coll Radiol) Sept 249–253

Horwich A (1993) Chemotherapy of seminoma. Eur Urol 2:26–28

Horwich A, Paluchowska B, Norman A, et al. (1997) Residual mass following chemotherapy of seminoma. Ann Oncol 8:37–40

Kellokumpu-Lehtinen P, Halme A (1990) Results of treatment in irradiated testicular seminoma patients. Radiother Oncol 18:1–8

Laukkanen E, Olivotto I, Jackson S (1987) Management of seminoma with bulky abdominal disease. Int J Radiat Oncol Biol Phys 4:227–233

Lederman G, Herman T, Jochelson M, et al. (1989) Radiation therapy of seminoma: 17-year experience at the joint center for radiation therapy. Radiother Oncol 14:203–208

MacVicar D, Horwich A (1992) Sites of relapse in seminoma treated with single agent carboplatin chemotherapy: implications for further management. Clin Oncol 4:209–213

Mason B, Kearsley J (1988) Radiotherapy for stage II testicular seminoma: the prognostic influence of tumor bulk. J Clin Oncol 6:1856–1862

Mencel P, Motzer J, Mazumdar M, Vlamis V, Bajorin D, Bosl J (1994) Advanced seminoma: treatment results, survival and prognostic factors in 142 patients. J Clin Oncol 12:120–126

Mirimanoff R, Sinzig M, Krueger M, et al. (1993) Prognosis of human chorionic gonadotropin-producing seminoma treated by postoperative radiotherapy. Int J Radiat Oncol Biol Phys 27:17–23

Peckham MJ (1981a) Investigation and staging: general aspects and staging classification. In: Peckham MJ (ed) The management of testicular tumors. Edward Arnold, London, p 89

Peckham MJ (1981b) Seminoma testis. In: Peckham MJ (ed) The management of testicular tumors. Edward Arnold, London, p 134

Puc H, Heelan R, Mazumdar M, et al. (1996) Management of residual mass in advanced seminoma: results and recommendations from the Memorial Sloan-Kettering Cancer Center. J Clin Oncol 14:454–460

Schultz S, Einhorn L, Conces D Jr, Williams S, Loehrer P (1989) Management of postchemotherapy residual mass in patients with advanced seminoma: Indiana University experience. J Clin Oncol 7:1497–1503

Smalley S, Evans R, Richardson R, Farrow G, Earle J (1985) Radiotherapy as initial treatment for bulky stage II testicular seminomas. J Clin Oncol 3:1333–1338

Smalley S, Earle J, Evans G, Richadson R (1990) Modern radiotherapy results with bulky stages II and III seminoma. J Urol 144:685–689

Speer T, Sombeck M, Parsons J, Million R (1995) Testicular seminoma: a failure analysis and literature review. Int J Radiat Oncol Biol Phys 33:89–97

Thomas G, Rider W, Dembo A, et al. (1981) Seminoma of the testis: results of treatment and patterns of failure after radiation therapy. Int J Radiat Oncol Biol Phys 8:165–174

Thomas G, Jones W, VanOosterom A (1990) Consensus statement on the investigation and management of testicular seminoma 1989. Prog Clin Biol Res 357:285–294

Vallis K, Howard G, Duncan W, Cornbleet M, Kerr G (1995) Radiotherapy for stages I and II testicular seminoma: results and morbidity in 238 patients. Radiology 68:400–405

Warde P, Gospodarowicz M, Panzarella T, Catton C, Sturgeon J, Moore M, Jewett M (1998) Management of stage II seminoma. J Clin Oncol 16:290–294

Willan B, McGowan D (1985) Seminoma of the testis: a 22-year experience with radiation therapy. Int J Radiat Oncol Biol Phys 11:1769–1775

Whipple G, Sagerman R, van Rooy E (1997) Long-term evaluation of postorchiectomy radiotherapy for stage II seminoma. Am J Clin Oncol (CCT) 20:196–201

Yao W, Fossa S, Dearnaley D, Horwich A (1994) Combined single course carboplatin with radiotherapy in treatment of stage IIA,B seminoma – a preliminary report. Radiother Oncol 33:88–90

# 22 Radiotherapy of Testicular Germ Cell Tumors: The German Experience

M. Bamberg and J. Classen

CONTENTS



## 22.1 Introduction

Testicular germ cell tumors are the most frequent malignancies of young men of 20–40 years of age. Seminoma represents approximately 40% of these tumors. Due to improvements in the field of diagnostic imaging, the development of new chemotherapy regimens, and the application of modern radiotherapeutic and surgical techniques, overall survival and disease-specific survival of patients with germ cell tumors have improved substantially over the past 20 years. Additionally, it has become evident that an interdisciplinary therapeutic approach by a team of urologists and radiation and medical oncologists is crucial for the excellent prognosis of these patients. Therefore, in Germany an interdisciplinary working group was set up in 1988 with the aim of defining standards for staging and treatment of patients with testicular germ cell tumors. The consensus which has been agreed upon by the working group has recently been published, thus providing guidelines for the management of testicular germ cell tumors in Germany (Bamberg et al. 1997).

This review will present the current opinion on the treatment of testicular germ cell tumors as expressed by the German Testicular Study Group. The chapter will focus on those topics particularly relevant to radiation management by concentrating on early stage testicular seminoma and the precursor lesion of testicular tumors, testicular carcinoma in situ (CIS), also known as testicular intraepithelial neoplasia (TIN). The latest results of clinical studies initiated by the study group will be discussed.

## 22.2 Staging and Classification

### 22.2.1 Tumor Markers

Patients presenting with clinical suspicion of testicular germ cell tumor should be referred for studies of tumor markers prior to surgery. As a routine procedure serum chorionic gonadotropin (HCG) and α-fetoprotein (AFP) are analyzed. In addition, analysis of placental alkaline serum phosphatase (PLAP) as a possibly more specific tumor marker for seminoma has been recommended (Bamberg et al. 1997). However, analysis of this marker is not yet commonly available outside of major medical centers. Additionally, the validity of PLAP for the detection of seminomatous tumors needs to be demonstrated in clinical trials.

Elevated levels of AFP exclude classification of the tumor as seminoma and should lead to thorough histologic reexamination of the tumor specimen (Warde et al. 1993). Elevated levels of HCG, however, are frequently observed in seminomas (Javadpour 1992). In previous years the topic of raised HCG values in patients with testicular semi-


M. Bamberg, MD, Professor, Department of Radiotherapy, Eberhard-Karls-Universität, Hoppe-Seyler-Strasse 3, D-72076 Tübingen, Germany

J. Classen, MD, Department of Radiotherapy, Eberhard-Karls-Universität, Hoppe-Seyler-Strasse 3, D-72076 Tübingen, Germany

noma was the subject of extensive discussions, and there was much concern whether these patients may be expected to have a worse prognosis than those without HCG elevation. However, it has now become evident that elevated values of HCG prior to surgery do not adversely affect the prognosis of seminoma patients, nor do they require specific treatment strategies (WEISSBACH and BUSSAR-MAATZ 1993; MIRIMANOFF et al. 1993).

## 22.2.2
## Staging

After high inguinal orchiectomy and histologic confirmation of pure testicular seminoma the patient undergoes a staging procedure comprising computed tomography of the chest, abdomen, and pelvis, conventional radiographs of the chest, and an abdominal ultrasound study. In the event of elevated tumor markers prior to surgery a repeated study of these markers should be performed 5–6 days after ablation. Clinical stage I disease may be diagnosed only in cases where tumor markers have returned to within normal limits (BAMBERG et al. 1997).

For clinical staging of seminoma patients the Royal Marsden Classification (RMC) is commonly used in Germany. According to the RMC stage I seminoma is characterized by a tumor restricted to the testis without lymph node or distant metastases. Metastatic involvement of regional lymph nodes less than 2 cm in diameter leads to classification as stage IIA seminoma whereas patients with metastatic lymph nodes 2–5 cm in diameter are classified as having stage IIB disease (PECKHAM et al. 1979).

## 22.3
## Testicular Seminoma

### 22.3.1
### Rationale for Treatment and Treatment Strategies

#### 22.3.1.1
#### Stage I

More than 70% of all patients presenting with seminoma at primary diagnosis are classified as clinical stage I. Without adjuvant therapy approximately 20% of these patients will relapse in the retroperitoneal lymph nodes due to microscopic metastases which cannot be visualized with the use of modern imaging techniques at the time of primary diagnosis. Furthermore, there are no established prognostic parameters predictive for lymph node relapse (WARDE et al. 1993; HORWICH et al. 1992). Radiotherapy to the draining lymph nodes in the retroperitoneum has therefore been well established for many decades and is considered as the standard treatment for stage I seminoma. With orchiectomy and subsequent radiotherapy, 95%–98% long-term disease-free survival can be achieved. Given the excellent rates of cure in relapsing patients, overall survival approaches 100% (BAMBERG and SCHMIDBERGER 1996; SCHMIDBERGER and BAMBERG 1995; BRUNT and SCOBLE 1992; THOMAS et al. 1982; FOSSA et al. 1989).

While the role of radiotherapy in stage I seminoma has been clearly defined, the parameters of treatment, i.e., treatment portals and total dose of radiation, have been the subject of controversy. Until recently, patients were treated with parallel opposed fields to the para-aortic and paracaval as well as ipsilateral iliac lymph nodes. While the inguinal region was usually not treated with radiotherapy, in the case of local T3 tumor ipsilateral inguinal and contralateral iliac lymph nodes were frequently integrated into the radiation field (ZAGARS 1991). Extension of treatment portals to include bilateral inguinal and contralateral iliac lymph nodes was recommended by several investigators for those patients with possible additional routes of lymphatic drainage, i.e., in cases of tumor infiltrating beyond the tunica albuginea (T2), or for those patients with a positive history of surgical manipulation at the scrotum or in the inguinal region (ZAGARS 1991, ZAGARS and BABAIAN 1987). For those rare cases of tumor infiltration of the scrotum (T4) or for patients with previous transscrotal biopsy, some authors recommend extending treatment portals to the affected hemiscrotum (ZAGARS 1991). However, this treatment strategy remains controversial, and no superiority of scrotal irradiation could be demonstrated (THOMAS et al. 1982). Furthermore, extension of the treatment fields to the inguinal region or the ipsilateral hemiscrotum substantially increases the dose of scattered radiation to the unaffected contralateral testis, thus increasing the risk of permanent infertility. On the other hand, some authors report that a small para-aortic/paracaval treatment field is sufficient for disease control (BRUNT and SCOBLE, 1992; FOSSA et al. 1996). This approach is promising insofar as reduced portals will minimize the risk of acute and possible late side-effects of the treatment.

### 22.3.1.2
### Stage IIA/B

Patients presenting with stage IIA/IIB seminoma have metastatic involvement of retroperitoneal lymph nodes. Due to the high radiosensitivity of seminoma, a high proportion of these patients can be cured with radiotherapy. Treatment results are stage dependent, with relapse rates of approximately 10% in stage IIA and up to 20% in stage IIB disease (SCHMIDBERGER and BAMBERG 1995; SCHMIDBERGER et al. 1997; ZAGARS and BABAIAN 1987). The radiation target volume includes metastatic lymph nodes and adjacent lymphatics. As for stage I patients, there is a wide variety of recommendations for optimal treatment portals and the total dose of radiation. In addition to the para-aortic/paracaval and ipsilateral iliac lymph nodes, some authors have in the past recommended irradiation of the mediastinum and the supraclavicular regions. However, extension of the target volume above the diaphragm has been shown to increase morbidity and mortality of treatment with only a marginal reduction in relapse rates (LEDERMAN et al. 1987). In addition, the bone marrow function may be substantially reduced for those patients who require chemotherapy as salvage therapy in the event of recurrent disease. Nowadays mediastinal radiation has to be considered obsolete, just as does retroperitoneal lymphadenectomy.

### 22.3.2

### Multicenter Clinical Trial for Radiotherapy of Stage I–IIA/B Testicular Seminoma

Due to the great variability of treatment parameters in the management of early stage seminoma, the German Testicular Study Group launched a multicenter clinical trial for radiotherapy of clinical stage I, IIA, and IIB seminoma. Patients were prospectively treated with small portals and low total radiation doses with the aim of reducing early and possible late side-effects of treatment. The trial was designed to sustain the high cure rates achieved with far more extensive treatment schedules. Treatment-related acute and late side-effects were systematically documented according to the recommendations of the European Organization for Research and Treatment of Cancer (EORTC) and Radiation Therapy Oncology Group (RTOG).

### 22.3.2.1
### Treatment Techniques

Patients with stage I disease were treated with parallel opposed para-aortic/paracaval fields extending from the upper border of T11 to the lower border of L4. Lateral margins were defined by the lateral edge of the lumbar tranverse processes (Fig. 22.1a). Patients with stage IIA/B disease were treated with a "hockey-stick" field extending from the upper border of T11 to the upper margin of the ipsilateral acetabulum, thus including the ipsilateral iliac lymph nodes (Fig. 22.1b). The total prescribed dose was 26 Gy for stage I disease, 30 Gy for stage IIA, and 36 Gy for stage IIB at 2-Gy daily fractions.

### 22.3.2.2
### Results

Between April 1991 and March 1994, 550 eligible patients who were staged and treated in accordance with the protocol were entered into the study. There were 43 participating clinical centers. Of the 550 patients treated, 493 (90%) were classified as having stage I disease, 39 (7%) as having stage IIA, and 18 (3%) as having stage IIA/B. Median follow-up was 36 months for stage I and 42 months for stage IIA/B disease.

To date there have been 18 cases of relapse in stage I, with a median time to relapse of 13 months. Fourteen patients (78%) failed in locoregional lymph nodes below the diaphragm but there were no "infield" recurrences (Table 22.1). Furthermore, there were two (11.1%) patients failing in the bone, one (5.5%) patient suffering from a recurrence in the mediastinum, and one (5.5%) patient relapsing in liver and lung. Sixteen patients could be successfully salvaged, mostly by the use of platinum-based polychemotherapy. One patient was lost to follow-up after the diagnosis of relapse, and one patient was referred for lymphadenectomy with lymphatic re-

**Table 22.1.** Sites of infradiaphragmatic relapse in lymph nodes

| Lymph nodes | Ipsilateral | | Contralateral | |
|---|---|---|---|---|
| | No. | % | No. | % |
| Iliac | 4 | 0.81 | 2 | 0.41 |
| Para-aortic | 3 | 0.61 | 0 | 0 |
| Inguinal | 2 | 0.41 | 0 | 0 |
| Iliac + para-aortic | 3 | 0.61 | 0 | 0 |

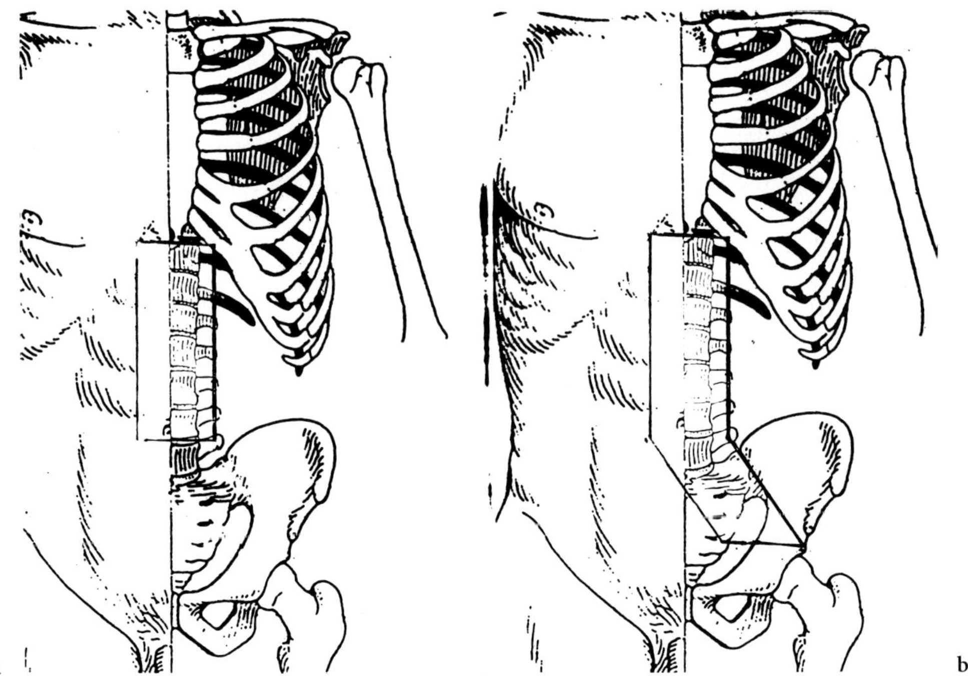

**Fig. 22.1. a** Para-aortic treatment field for stage I seminoma as used by the German Testicular Study Group. **b** Hockey-stick field as used in the German Testicular Study Group for the treatment of patients with stage IIA/B seminoma

currence below the diaphragm. This patient suffered from cerebral embolism after surgery and subsequently died.

There was one patient with relapse in locoregional lymphatics in stage IIA and two patients in stage IIB with distant metastases. All three patients could be salvaged with chemotherapy and are currently alive. Median time to relapse for stage IIA/B patients was 17 months.

The 3-year survival estimate for stage I calculated according to Kaplan and Meier was 95.7% (93.7%–97.7% confidence interval). The corresponding estimate at 4 years for stage IIA/B was 93% (85.3%–100% confidence interval). Overall disease-specific survival was 99.6% for stage I and 100% for stage IIA/B.

### 22.3.2.3
### *Treatment Complications*

Acute side-effects of the treatment were moderate (Table 22.2, Fig. 22.2). There were no cases of grade IV toxicity in this study. Statistical analysis of toxicity data showed a significant reduction of nausea and bowel dysfunction for stage I patients as compared to those with stage IIA/B disease.

Gastrointestinal side-effects were the predominant side-effects for all stages. Of stage I patients,

**Table 22.2.** Acute maximal side-effects (EORTC/RTOG) according to the clinical stage of disease

|  |  | Score Definition | Incidence (%) | |
|---|---|---|---|---|
|  |  |  | CS I | CS IIA/B |
| Nausea | 0 | No complaints | 42.9 | 18.6 |
|  | 1 | Nausea | 45.3 | 55.9 |
|  | 2 | Transient vomiting | 6.7 | 15.3 |
|  | 3 | Vomiting, treatment required | 4.5 | 10.2 |
|  | 4 | Intractable vomiting | 0 | 0 |
|  |  | Not obtained |  | 0.6 |
| Diarrhea | 0 | No complaints | 87.4 | 64.9 |
|  | 1 | Transient diarrhea <2 days | 9.3 | 14 |
|  | 2 | Tolerable diarrhea >2 days | 1.4 | 15.8 |
|  | 3 | Intolerable diarrhea, treatment required | 1.4 | 5.3 |
|  | 4 | Hemorrhagic diarrhea | 0 | 0 |
|  |  | Not obtained |  | 0.4 |
| Skin | 0 | No changes | 94.1 | 84.8 |
|  | 1 | Erythema | 4.9 | 15.3 |
|  | 2 | Dry desquamation | 0.4 | 0 |
|  | 3 | Moist desquamation | 0 | 0 |
|  | 4 | Necrosis | 0 | 0 |
|  |  | Not obtained | 0.6 |  |

CS, Clinical stage.

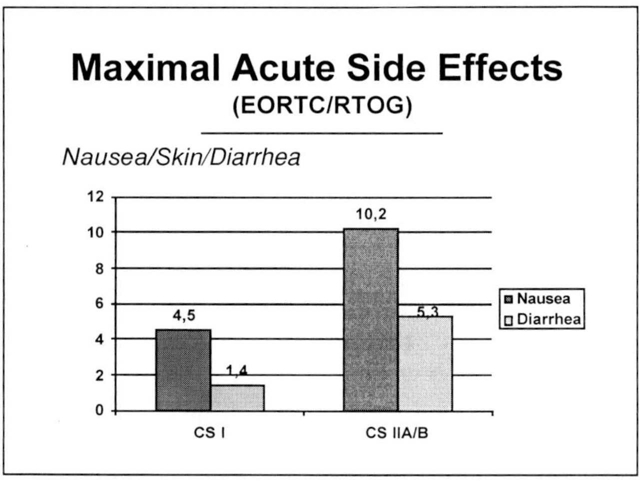


**Fig. 22.2.** Graphic representation of acute toxicity according to the recommendations of EORTC/RTOG. CS, Clinical stage

45.3% suffered from nausea (EORTC grade I), as did 55.9% of stage IIA/B patients. Vomiting requiring treatment (EORTC grade III) was observed in 4.5% for stage I and in 10.2% for stage IIA/B.

In 9.6% of stage I patients there were minor changes in bowel function (EORTC grade I) as compared to 15.3% in stage IIA/B. However, diarrhea requiring treatment (EORTC grade III) was a rare event, with a 1.2% incidence in stage I and a 5% incidence in stage IIA/B disease.

Acute skin reactions with mild erythema in the treatment field (EORTC grade I) were observed in 4.9% of stage I patients and in 15.3% of those with stage IIA/B disease. Dry desquamation (EORTC grade II) was documented for two (0.4%) patients in stage I but for no patients in stage IIA/B. The incidence of skin toxicity was not statistically different between the two treatment groups.

Sperm counts were performed in 133 patients after ablation of the testis before initiation of locoregional radiotherapy. Only 49 (37%) of these patients showed an unimpaired sperm count of $\geq 20 \times 10^6$ spermatocytes/ml (lower normal range according to WHO criteria). These data clearly demonstrated that preexisting factors influence the sperm quality prior to adjuvant treatment. There were, unfortunately, only nine patients with follow-up sperm counts so that no conclusions of statistical relevance can be drawn from these data. However, none of these nine patients showed a decrease in sperm count after completion of radiotherapy. One patient presented with persistent azoospermia while in three patients the sperm count improved from oligozoospermia to normozoospermia. These data show that impaired fertility is an inherent problem of testicular cancer patients independent of radiotherapy. Furthermore, Jacobsen et al. (1997) and Joos et al. (1997) could clearly demonstrate that scattered radiation to the testis is largely dependent on the field arrangement, with the least impairment of fertility occurring in those patients receiving a pure paraaortic treatment field; this finding provides support for our concept of reduced portals.

To date no major late adverse effects have been reported. One patient died 12 months after completion of radiotherapy for stage I seminoma as a consequence of a carcinoma of the esophagus. A second patient suffered from acute FAM M4 leukemia 16 months after radiotherapy and died 11 months later. Due to the short follow-up period between the course of radiotherapy and the two cases of second malignancy it seems rather unlikely that the second tumors could be ascribed to the preceding radiotherapy. However, the question of possible induction of second tumors can only be answered in more detail with a longer period of follow-up for the entire study population.

These data, although still of a preliminary nature, are in accordance with treatment results reported in the literature for considerably more intensive treatment regimens. Our preliminary conclusion is that reduction of total dose and treatment portals offers excellent cure rates for early stage testicular seminoma with few acute side-effects and, to date, virtually no late side-effects. This conclusion is supported by the data from Brunt and Scoble (1992) and a British Medical Research Council (MRC) randomized trial (Fossa et al. 1996). The latter study for stage I disease compared treatment of the paraaortic and ipsilateral iliac lymph nodes with irradiation of the para-aortic lymphatics only. The trial showed, just as did our study, that omission of pelvic irradiation does not decrease the high cure rates for stage I disease. The German Testicular Study Group therefore recommends as standard treatment para-aortic/paracaval irradiation with 26 Gy for stage I disease and a hockey-stick irradiation field as described above for stage IIA/B (Bamberg et al. 1997).

## 22.4
## Perspectives

Encouraged by treatment results in advanced testicular seminoma, systemic therapy with carboplatin was suggested for stage I seminoma by several authors. Data from nonrandomized trials provide evidence that single-agent carboplatin chemotherapy yields cure rates comparable to the standard adjuvant radiotherapy. However, to date no randomized data which enable a direct comparison between standard radiotherapy and carboplatin chemotherapy have been published.

Hence, the German Testicular Study Group initiated a multicenter randomized clinical trial for adjuvant treatment of stage I testicular seminoma. Standard para-aortic/paracaval radiotherapy with 26 Gy in 2-y daily fractions is compared with single-agent carboplatin given twice on day 1 and day 29. The study was opened for patient accrual in January 1996 and recruitment is still proceeding so that no data are available as yet. However, we expect the two treatment strategies to yield equivalent cure rates. Secondary criteria of the study, such as the patients' quality of life and socioeconomic aspects of both treatment modalities (e.g., treatment costs or working days missed due to therapy) may therefore finally gain particular importance.

## 22.5
## Testicular Intraepithelial Neoplasia

Testicular intraepithelial neoplasia (TIN) is a rare premalignant lesion which is located in the germinal epithelium of the testis. In 1972 Skakkebaek for the first time characterized the lesion as the precursor of invasive testicular tumor. Subsequently the challenging theory of TIN being the common precursor lesion of both seminoma and nonseminoma germ cell tumors with the exception of spermatocytic seminoma was put forward. This theory has found

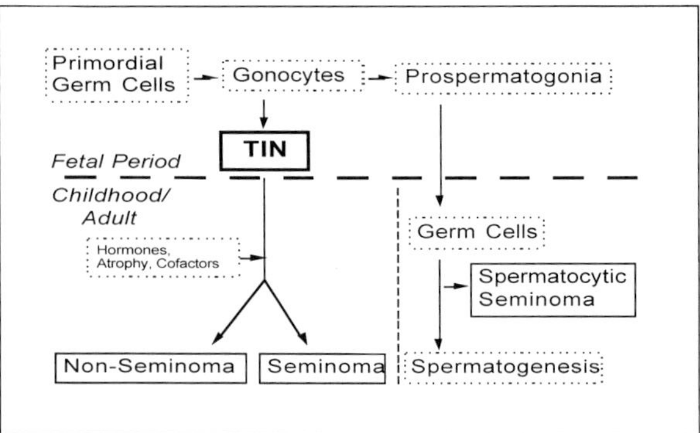


**Fig. 22.3.** Schematic representation of the concept of pathogenesis for TIN. (From Dieckmann and Loy 1993)

much support from epidemiologic data and is nowadays widely accepted (Giwercman et al. 1994; Skakkebaek et al. 1987) (Fig. 22.3).

## 22.5.1
## Natural History

The prevalence of TIN, as evaluated in Danish adult males, is approximately 0.8%. However, there are numerous factors associated with an increased incidence of TIN and a subsequently elevated risk for testicular tumor. Those men already harboring a testicular germ cell tumor are most prominently at risk for contralateral TIN. Dieckmann and Loy (1996) conducted a large prevalence study taking biopsy specimens from the contralateral testis in 1954 men with unilateral testicular cancer. The frequency of contralateral TIN was found to be 4.9%. This incidence has been confirmed in other series (Schmoll 1993; Mumperow et al. 1992). The natural course of TIN is unfavorable, with a high tendency towards the development of an invasive tumor. The rate of progression has been found to be 70% within 7 years (Skakkebaek et al. 1982; Giwercman et al. 1992).

## 22.5.2
## Management

Since spontaneous regression of TIN has never been described in the literature, treatment of the lesion is definitely required. While surgery is the treatment of choice for those men with unilateral TIN and an unaffected contralateral testis, the situation is different for those patients with TIN in a single testis after prior orchiectomy for testicular cancer or in bilateral

TIN. In these cases, which will constitute the majority of TIN patients seen in daily practice, the treatment of choice is local radiotherapy.

Radiotherapy for TIN was first introduced by von der Maase et al. in 1986. Treatment was given as local external beam irradiation to the whole scrotum with a total dose of 20 Gy in 2-Gy daily fractions. This fractionation schedule has been proven to provide safe eradication of TIN with virtually no acute side-effects. Thus definite cure of TIN patients can be achieved with low-dose radiotherapy. Histologic sections after local treatment show a Sertoli cell-only pattern with complete eradication of both TIN cells and cells of spermatogenesis (Fig. 22.4). Infertility is hence an unavoidable consequence of treatment. However, the majority of TIN patients showed

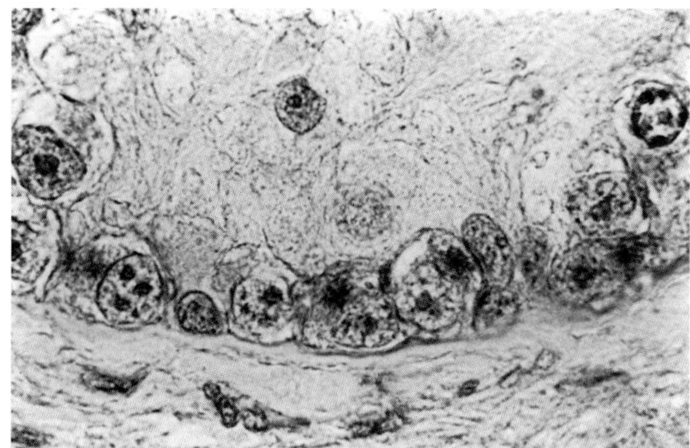

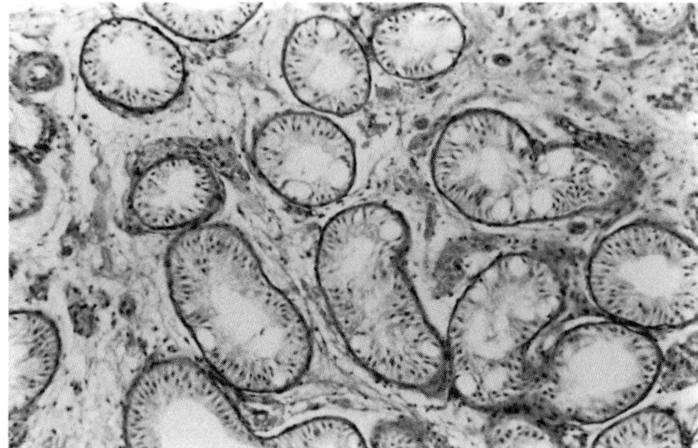

**Fig. 22.4. a** Contralateral testicular biopsy demonstrating typical features of TIN. TIN cells are located at the basal membrane of the tubules. The cytoplasm stains for PLAP. Magnification ×300. **b** Testicular biopsy obtained 3 months following the administration of local radiotherapy consisting of 20 Gy given in 2-Gy daily fractions. The biopsy shows typical Sertoli cell syndrome. There are only Sertoli cells left in the tubules (i.e., no germ cells) and there is no evidence of TIN. Foci of Leydig cells are present in the interstitium. Magnification ×33. (**a** and **b** were kindly provided by Prof. K.P. Dieckmann)

impaired fertility before radiotherapy. In a small study by Giwercman et al. (1993) sperm analysis of 16 patients presenting with TIN in a single testis showed an average of $0.3 \times 10^6$ spermatocytes/ml and only 1/16 patients had a normal sperm count. These data on the one hand underline that men harboring TIN in a single testis are destined to be infertile. On the other hand it should be pointed out that the presence of TIN does not necessarily exclude natural paternity. It is therefore crucial to discuss the problem of fertility individually with patients presenting with TIN.

The synthesis of testicular androgens may also be affected by the local treatment. Measurements of luteinizing hormone show a temporary elevation after irradiation while testosterone levels remain unchanged (Dieckmann et al. 1993; Giwercman et al. 1989, 1994). However, the more sensitive β-HCG stimulation test shows permanently lowered levels of testosterone as an indication of a significant decline in testicular androgen synthesis as a late sequela of treatment.

The current recommendation of the German Testicular Study Group concerning the total dose of local irradiation is 20 Gy as proposed by von der Maase (Bamberg et al. 1997). There are, however, sporadic reports that doses of 18 and 16 Gy might be equally efficient, while showing a lower rate of late effects. In the series of Dieckmann and Loy (1996), no relapse was observed after a total dose of 18 Gy, and Giwercman et al. (1994) reported two cases of successful eradication of TIN with only 16 Gy. To date, however, there have been no clinical studies systematically evaluating reduction of total doses with sufficient numbers of patients per dose level.

### 22.5.3
### Multicenter Clinical Trial

In light of the above, the German Testicular Study Group is currently conducting a multicenter clinical trial to evaluate the lowest total radiation dose necessary for the safe eradication of TIN. The first patients entered into the trial will be treated to the scrotum with 18 Gy. If this dose proves to ensure safe eradication of TIN as shown by control biopsy, the total dose will then be reduced to 16 Gy for the next patients. Likewise the total dose of radiation will subsequently be reduced in 2-Gy steps until a minimum of 10 Gy is reached or persisting TIN is shown in a control biopsy. The aim of the study is to offer the patients, who are usually young, a highly efficient yet well-tolerated treatment with the least possible side-effects. The study was opened in 1997; recruitment of patients is still ongoing so that no data are available as yet.

# References

Bamberg M, Schmidberger H (1996) Hoden. In: Scherer E, Sack H (eds) Strahlentherapie – Radiologische Onkologie, 4th edn. Springer, Berlin Heidelberg New York, pp 569–587

Bamberg M, Schmoll H-J, Weißbach L (1997) Interdisziplinäre Konsensus-Konferenz zur "Diagnostik und Therapie von Hodentumoren". Strahlenther Onkol 173:397–406

Brunt AM, Scoble JE (1992) Paraaortic nodal irradiation for early stage testicular seminoma. Clin Oncol 4:165–170

Dieckmann K-P, Loy V (1993) Testicular intraepithelial neoplasia: the precursor of testicular germ cell tumors. Onkologie 16:61–68

Dieckmann K-P, Loy V (1996) Relevance of contralateral testicular intraepithelial neoplasia in patients with testicular germ cell neoplasia. J Clin Oncol 14:3126–3132

Dieckmann K-P, Besserer A, Loy V (1993) Low-dose radiation therapy for testicular intraepithelial neoplasia. J Cancer Res Clin Oncol 119:355–359

Fossa SD, Aass N, Kaalhus O (1989) Radiotherapy for testicular seminoma stage I: treatment results and long-term post-irradiation morbidity in 365 patients. Int J Radiat Oncol Biol Phys 16:383–388

Fossa SD, Horwich A, Russell JM, Roberts JP, Jakes R, Stenning S (1996) Optimal field size in adjuvant radiotherapy (XRT) of stage I seminoma – a randomised trial. Proc Am Soc Clin Oncol, 15, 239

Giwercman A, Bruun E, Frimodt-Möller C, Skakkebaek NE (1989) Prevalence of carcinoma in situ and other histopathological abnormalities in testes of men with a history of cryptorchism. J Urol 142:998–1002

Giwercman A (1992) Carcinoma-in-situ of the testis: screening and management. Scand J Urol Nephrol Suppl 148:32

Giwercman A, von der Maase H, Rohrt M, Skakkebaek NE (1993) Semen quality in testicular tumour and CIS in the contralateral testis. Lancet I:384–385

Giwercman A , Maase von der H, Rorth M, Skakkebaek NE (1994) Current concepts of radiation treatment of carcinoma in situ of the testis. World J Urol 12:125–130

Horwich A, Alsanjari N, A'Hern R, et al. (1992) Surveillance following orchiectomy for stage I testicular seminoma. Br J Cancer 65:775–778

Jacobsen KD, Olsen DR, Fossa K, Fossa SD (1997) External beam abdominal radiotherapy in patients with seminoma stage I: field type, testicular dose, and spermatogenesis. Int J Radiat Oncol Biol Phys 38:95–102

Javadpour N (1992) Current status of tumor markers in testicular cancer. Eur Urol 21, Suppl:34–36

Joos H, Sedlmayer F, Gomahr A, et al. (1997) Endocrine profiles after radiotherapy in stage I seminoma: impact of two different radiation treatment modalities. Radiother Oncol 43:159–162

Lederman GS, Sheldon TA, Chaffey JT, et al. (1987) Cardiac disease after mediastinal irradiation for seminoma. Cancer 60:772–776

Mirimanoff RO, Sinzig M, Krüger M, et al. (1993) Prognosis of human chorionic gonadotropin-producing seminoma treated by postoperative radiotherapy. Int J Radiat Oncol Biol Phys 27:17–23

Mumperow E, Lauke H, Holstein AF, Hartmann M (1992) Further practical experiences in the recognition and management of carcinoma in situ of the testis. Urol Int 48:162–166

Peckham MJ, Barrett A, McElwain TJ, et al. (1979) Combined management of malignant teratoma of the testis. Lancet II:257

Schmidberger H, Bamberg M (1995) Therapieoptionen bei testikulären Seminomen in den frühen Stadien. Strahlenther Onkol 171:125–139

Schmidberger H, Bamberg M, Meisner C, Classen J, Winkler C, Hartmann M, Templin R, Wiegel T, Dornhoff W, Ross D, Thiel HJ, Martini C, Haase W (1997) Radiotherapy in stage IIA and IIB testicular seminoma with reduced portals: a prospective multicenter study. Int J Radiat Oncol Biol Phys 39:321–326

Schmoll H-J (1993) Management of early stages of testicular carcinoma: the current status. Recent Results Cancer Res 126:237–255

Skakkebaek NE (1978) Carcinoma in situ of the testis: frequency and relationship to invasive germ cell tumours in infertile men. Histopathology 2:157–170

Skakkebaek NE, Berthelsen JG, Müller J (1982) Carcinoma in situ of the undescended testis. Urol Clin North Am 9:377

Skakkebaek NE, Berthelsen JG, Giwercman A, Müller J (1987) Carcinom-in-situ of the testis: possible origin from gonocytes and precursor of all types of germ cell tumours except spermatocytoma. Int J Androl 10:19–28

Thomas GM, Rider WD, Dembo AL, et al. (1982) Seminoma of the testis: results of treatment and patterns of failure after radiation therapy. Int J Radiat Oncol Biol Phys 8:165–174

von der Maase H, Giwercman A, Skakkebaek NE (1986a) Radiation treatment of carcinoma-in-situ of testis. Lancet I: 624–625

von der Maase H, Rohrt M, Walbom-Jorgensen S, et al. (1986b) Carcinoma in situ of contralateral testis in patients with testicular germ cell cancer: study of 27 cases in 500 patients. Br Med J 293:1398–1401

Warde PR, Gospodarowicy MK, Goodman et al. (1993) Results of a policy of surveillance in stage I testicular seminoma. Int J Radiat Oncol Biol Phys 27:11–15

Warszawski N, Schmücking M, Samtleben M, et al. (1996) Die Strahlentherapie der regionären Lymphknoten stationen bei der Behandlung des Seminoms im Vergleich zur retroperitonealen Lymphadenektomie. Strahlenther Onkol 172:250–254

Weissbach L, Bussar-Maatz (1993) HCG-positiveseminoma. Eur Urol 23, Suppl 2:29–32

Zagars GK (1991) Management of stage I seminoma: radiotherapy. In: Horwich A (ed) Testicular cancer – investigation and management. Chapman and Hall Medical, London, pp 83–107

Zagars GK, Babaian RJ (1987) Stage I testicular seminoma: rationale for postorchiectomy radiation therapy. Int J Radiat Oncol Biol Phys 13:155–162

# 23 Chemotherapy for Seminoma

H. Dumez and A. Van Oosterom

CONTENTS



## 23.1
## Introduction

Testicular germ cell tumors represent only about 1%–2% of all human malignant tumors; however, they are the most common malignancies in young adult men. The vast majority of patients with disseminated germ cell tumors are curable with the currently available combination chemotherapy regimens. These results are in contrast to those obtained with chemotherapy for other disseminated malignancies.

About 40%–50% of testicular germ cell tumors are classified as seminomas. These cancers preferentially spread by lymphatic channels: from the retroperitoneal lymph nodes to the mediastinum, the supraclavicular lymph nodes, and the lungs. Therefore staging workup should include both chest radiography and computed tomography (CT) of the thorax and the abdomen. In pure seminomas elevated levels of lactate dehydrogenase (LDH) are common, although other tumor markers common in nonseminomatous germ cell tumors [$\alpha$-fetoprotein and $\beta$-human chorionic gonadotropin ($\beta$-HCG)] are not present in seminomas. An elevated $\alpha$-fetoprotein


H. Dumez, MD, Resident, Department of Oncology, University Hospitals Gasthuisberg, Catholic University of Leuven, Herestraat 49, B-3000 Leuven, Belgium
A. Van Oosterom, MD, PhD, Professor and Chairman, Department of Oncology, University Hospitals Gasthuisberg, Catholic University of Leuven, Herestraat 49, B-3000 Leuven, Belgium


level excludes the diagnosis of a pure seminoma, though some seminomas can present with a slight ($\leq$200 IU/l) elevation of $\beta$-HCG.

In 1979 Peckham et al. presented the Royal Marsden Hospital Classification System, according to which malignant teratomas of the testis were classified into four stages: stage I, no evidence of metastases; stage II, metastases confined to abdominal nodes (A <2 cm, B 2–5 cm, C >5 cm); stage III, involvement of supradiaphragmatic and infradiaphragmatic lymph nodes; stage IV, extralymphatic metastases. The International Germ Cell Cancer Collaborative Group (Mead et al. 1997) presented a prognostic classification for germ cell tumors. Approximately 90% of seminomas meet the criteria for good prognosis, i.e., any primary site, no nonpulmonary visceral metastases, and normal $\alpha$-fetoprotein level (any $\beta$-HCG level, any LDH level). The presence of nonpulmonary visceral metastases was the only factor used to identify an intermediate prognostic group for seminoma. No patients with a pure seminoma were classified as having a poor prognosis.

The treatment of patients with stage I testicular seminoma (70%–80%) or nonbulky stage II disease (i.e., less than 2 cm, stage IIa) consists in radiotherapy to the para-aortic and pelvic lymph nodes. Patients with large retroperitoneal masses ($\geq$5 cm, stage IIC) and patients with supradiaphagmatic or visceral metastases will nowadays receive chemotherapy as the treatment of first choice. It is not clear whether a patient with a retroperitoneal mass between 2 and 5 cm (stage IIb) should have radiotherapy or chemotherapy (see Chap. 21).

Patients with advanced seminoma in the good prognostic group have a 5-year survival rate of 86%. Patients with intermediate prognostic factors, including bone, liver, and brain metastases, have a 5-year survival rate of 73%. The overexpression of wild-type p53 in germ cell tumors possibly provides the basis for its chemosensitivity (Guillou et al. 1996). This p53 gene plays a key role in the DNA damage-related apoptosis, and mutations in this gene are considered to be related to chemo-resistance. Such mutations have not been detected in germ cell tumors. However, some other human cancer types also lack p53 mutations, while germ cell cancer stands alone in its curability. Therefore, other factors must also contribute to this chemosensitivity.

## 23.2
## History of Use of Chemotherapy for Seminoma

Primary radiation therapy showed unacceptably high failure rates of 40%–64% in patients with bulky abdominal disease and 70%–80% in stage III disease (see Chap. 21). In view of these results, chemotherapy should be considered the primary treatment of advanced seminoma.

Alkylating agents were the first drugs to be selected for the treatment of metastatic disease as a result of their radiomimetic properties. By the 1970s, several drugs, including actinomycin D, methotrexate, vinblastine, and bleomycin, produced objective responses with occasional long-term remissions. A major advance occurred with the introduction of cisplatin in combination chemotherapy. The initial cisplatin-, vinblastine-, and bleomycin-containing regimens, i.e., cisplatin, vinblastine, bleomycin, dactinomycin, and cyclophosphamide (VAB-6) or cisplatin, vinblastine, and bleomycin (PVB), resulted in a 70%–80% complete response rate. Treatment-related toxicity included hematologic toxicity, pulmonary fibrosis, neuropathy, Raynaud's phenomenon, and intestinal ileus (BOSL et al. 1988).

In a prospective, randomized clinical trial conducted by WILLIAMS et al. (1987), PVB was compared with cisplatin, etoposide, and bleomycin (BEP). The latter regimen was shown to be superior on the basis of the less severe toxicity (reduced rates of myalgia, constipation, and neurotoxicity) and an equally good if not improved therapeutic outcome for patients with advanced disease.

## 23.3
## First-line Chemotherapy for Advanced Seminoma

A prospective, randomized trial conducted by BOSL et al. (1988) in patients with "good-risk" germ cell tumors (which included all patients with seminoma)

showed equivalent efficacy and less toxicity for the two-drug regimen of cisplatin and etoposide, compared with the regimen based on cisplatin, vinblastine, and bleomycin (VAB-6). Hence, etoposide and cisplatin was the preferred regimen. The success of this combination in the treatment of advanced seminoma is confirmed by the findings of MENCEL et al. (1994), who reported that 130 of 140 patients (93%) thus treated achieved a favorable or a partial response with negative markers (HCG and LDH) and that 86% remained progression-free at a median follow-up duration of 43+ months. An extragonadal primary tumor site was not associated with an adverse prognosis. XIAO et al. (1997) indicated in a large retrospective study that four cycles of etoposide and cisplatin constitute effective therapy and can be offered to patients with good-risk germ cell tumors (including patients with pure seminoma histology, regardless of the primary site or sites of metastases).

Carboplatin seems to have similar activity to cisplatin in the treatment of ovarian carcinoma and can be administered on an outpatient basis. Compared to cisplatin, it does not cause renal damage, ototoxicity, or neuropathy, and has less gastrointestinal toxicity when used at standard doses. These advantages in practical handling and lower toxicity have prompted a phase II trial of single-agent carboplatin in patients with advanced seminoma (SCHMOLL et al. 1993). Myelosuppression, particularly thrombocytopenia, is the dose-limiting toxicity of carboplatin. The use of up-front carboplatin therapy appears not to compromise the ultimate curability of patients with advanced seminoma. At least 25% of patients, however, appear to fail carboplatin single-agent therapy and require cisplatin-based combinations for salvage. This high number of relapsed patients requiring exposure to a prolonged toxic treatment might finally outweigh the benefit of reduced toxicity with single-agent carboplatin treatment for the entire group. HORWICH et al. (1992) reported a study on 70 patients with metastatic seminoma treated with four to six courses of single-agent carboplatin (400 mg/m$^2$ every 3–4 weeks). Although the treatment was of low toxicity, approximately one in four patients relapsed and required combination chemotherapy. Because of this 25% failure rate with single-agent carboplatin therapy, and because more late relapses might still occur, at present carboplatin cannot be recommended as standard therapy outside of clinical studies, except in patients who are insufficiently fit for standard cisplatin-based therapy.

Bajorin et al. (1993) reported a study of 270 patients with good-risk germ cell tumors (including all patients with seminomas), randomized to receive four cycles of either etoposide and cisplatin or etoposide and carboplatin. This trial showed that combination therapy with carboplatin and etoposide had inferior relapse-free and event-free survival times and more hematologic toxicity than cisplatin and etoposide.

A phase II study of the HOP regimen (ifosfamide, vincristine, and cisplatin) conducted by Fossa et al. (1995) included 42 seminoma patients with abdominal masses $\geq 10\,cm$ or with relapses after previous radiotherapy. Response rates were as follows: complete remission, 65%; partial remission, 28%; 3-year survival, 90%. This regimen is highly effective in patients with advanced metastatic seminoma or those relapsing after previous radiotherapy, but is associated with a high risk of toxicity, in particular myelotoxicity.

Amato et al. (1995) described another phase II study, assessing the clinical efficacy and complications of a regimen containing carboplatin and ifosfamide, plus consolidation radiotherapy, in patients with a residual stable mass of 3 cm or more. Of the treated patients, 71% achieved a complete remission after chemotherapy alone, and 24% achieved a complete remission after chemotherapy plus consolidation; 91% of these patients remained free of disease after a median follow-up period of 35 months.

Several phase III studies to quantify the contribution of ifosfamide in poor-risk patients are now complete (Nichols 1996; Roth 1996). As first-line therapy in previously untreated patients, ifosfamide-based chemotherapy (VeIP/VIP) is therapeutically equivalent to standard therapy with etoposide and cisplatin but is associated with increased toxicity, especially myelosuppression.

## 23.4
## Salvage Therapy

In the salvage setting, it was not until ifosfamide was incorporated into cisplatin-based regimens that the percentage of durable complete responses increased, along with the number of long-term disease-free survivors (Nichols 1996; Roth 1996). Such clinical observations confirmed the observed preclinical synergy of cisplatin and ifosfamide. McCaffrey et al. (1997) reported on a study of 56 patients with advanced germ cell tumors (including 11 seminomas) resistant to one prior cisplatin-containing regimen. They were treated with a salvage chemotherapy regimen of ifosfamide, cisplatin, and either vinblastine or etoposide (VeIP/VIP). Of the 56 patients studied, 36% achieved a complete response and 23% were alive and continuously free of disease at a median follow-up of 52 months. Other authors confirm that while approximately half of the cisplatin-sensitive testicular cancer patients treated with ifosfamide-based salvage chemotherapy may achieve a disease-free status, only 25% will have durable complete remissions. This 50% relapse rate from complete remission in the salvage setting suggests the need for some additional therapy, such as oral etoposide or high-dose consolidation chemotherapy with carboplatin and etoposide. Nevertheless, this high-dose approach remains investigational.

Beyer et al. (1996) pointed out that progressive disease before high-dose chemotherapy, disease refractory to conventional-dose cisplatin, and HCG levels greater than $1000\,U/l$ are independent adverse prognostic variables for failure-free survival after high-dose chemotherapy. In third-line therapy, treatment with high-dose carboplatin-containing programs plus hematopoietic progenitor cell support results in long-term survival in 15%–21% of patients with resistant, progressive germ cell tumors (Motzer et al. 1996).

The backbone of most high-dose programs for germ cell tumors is carboplatin and etoposide, although there is a trend toward improved survival with the three-drug combination of carboplatin, etoposide, and either ifosfamide or cyclophosphamide.

High-dose chemotherapy can also be considered for patients with an incomplete response to first-line therapy, because these patients rarely achieve long-term survival on cisplatin and ifosfamide salvage therapy: the long-term no evidence of disease rate in this group was 15% according to Farhat et al. (1996).

Motzer et al. (1996) treated 58 patients with refractory germ cell tumors with high-dose carboplatin, etoposide, and cyclophosphamide plus autologous bone marrow transplantation. Cyclophosphamide was selected in this trial because of the lack of renal toxicity compared with ifosfamide. Nevertheless, myelosuppression was severe, and there were seven treatment-related deaths. This high-dose regimen results in a complete response rate of 40% and a 2-year survival rate of 31%.

BEYER et al. (1997) reported on 74 patients with recurrent and/or refractory germ cell tumors treated with 1500–2000 mg/m$^2$ carboplatin, 1200–2400 mg/m$^2$ etoposide, and 0–10 g/m$^2$ ifosfamide. The results were an overall survival rate of 38% and a failure-free survival rate of 31% at 5 years.

Some centers have extended the indications for high-dose chemotherapy, using it to intensity first salvage regimens, to treat patients with a slow response to conventional-dose chemotherapy, or even as a part of the first-line treatment of patients who present with advanced disease at the time of initial diagnosis. The role of dose intensification in these settings awaits clarification in future research.

As a single agent, paclitaxel is the first drug capable of inducing response rates greater than 20% in previously treated germ cell tumors. MOTZER et al. (1996) are studying paclitaxel as a component of conventional-dose and dose-intensive salvage therapy. In vitro cisplatin and the oxazaphosphorines have been found to be synergistic with paclitaxel (CHOU et al. 1994).

## 23.5
## Management of Residual Masses

PUC et al. (1996) reviewed 104 patients with advanced seminoma after cisplatin-based induction chemotherapy. Site failure correlated only with the size of the residual mass. Patients who have normal radiographs or residual masses of less than 3 cm after chemotherapy can be observed without further intervention. The following options exist for patients with a residual mass ≥3 cm, for which there is a 27% likelihood of persistent tumor: observation, radiotherapy, or surgical intervention. This author prefers surgery for several reasons. First, an immediate assessment of tumor response is accomplished; second, resistant tumor can in some instances be resected; third, it allows salvage chemotherapy to be administered in a timely fashion.

CULINE (1996) points to the difficulties and complications of surgery because of the severe fibrotic reaction in these tumors following chemotherapy, and the uselessness of surgery in the majority of the cases, where only fibrosis/necrosis is found. Fine-needle biopsies are not convenient because tiny tumor residues in large fibrotic masses could be missed. Whatever the drawbacks of surgery, radiotherapy also seems to be unsuitable because it fails in 80%–90% of cases. Therefore, surgery remains the postchemotherapy treatment that should be considered in patients in whom large masses persist; nevertheless, it is not necessary to operate immediately, allowing further shrinkage of residual mass. Surgical removal of residual masses is required only in those patients in whom shrinkage appears not to be satisfactory for up to 1 year after chemotherapy. Gallium scans are of minimal value in determining whether residual masses consist of viable tumor or necrotic fibrous tissue (WARREN and EINHORN 1995). Positron emission tomography can be useful for the detection of residual viable carcinoma in nonseminomas, but its role in seminomas has still to be established (STEPHENS et al. 1996).

## 23.6
## Conclusion

The combination of etoposide and cisplatin is considered to be the standard treatment for patients with advanced seminoma. This is in contrast with the standard treatment for patients with disseminated nonseminomatous germ cell tumors, which comprises the combination of bleomycin, etoposide, and cisplatin.

Single-agent carboplatin cannot be recommended as the first-line treatment because of a high incidence of late failure. Even the combination of etoposide and carboplatin is inferior compared to etoposide and cisplatin.

Postchemotherapy residual disease of less than 3 cm can be safely observed. Residual masses larger than 3 cm show persistent tumor in up to 30% of cases, and surgical evaluation of these residuals should be considered if shrinkage is not satisfactory after several months of follow-up.

While approximately half of the cisplatin-sensitive seminoma patients treated with ifosfamide-based salvage chemotherapy (cisplatin, ifosfamide, and etoposide or vinblastine) can achieve a disease-free status, only approximately 25% will have durable complete remissions. Consolidation therapy with high-dose regimens remains investigational.

A dose-intensive regimen containing carboplatin and etoposide ± ifosfamide or cyclophosphamide (plus hematopoietic stem cell support) can be considered for patients with advanced seminoma refractory to, or with an incomplete response to first-line therapy or for patients with recurrent disease after salvage therapy (third line).

Ongoing research efforts include randomized trials of high-dose chemotherapy in several settings, inclusion of paclitaxel in combination programs, and investigations of alternative means of achieving dose intensification.

## References

Amato RJ, Ellerhorst J, Banks M, Logothetis CJ (1995) Carboplatin and ifosfamide and selective consolidation in advanced seminoma. Eur J Cancer 31A:2223–2228

Bajorin DF, Sarosdy MF, Pfister DG, et al. (1993) Randomized trial of etoposide and cisplatin versus etoposide and carboplatin in patients with good-risk germ cell tumors: a multiinstitutional study. J Clin Oncol 11:598–606

Beyer J, Kramar A, Mandanas R (1996) High-dose chemotherapy as salvage treatment in germ cell tumors: a multivariate analysis of prognostic variables. J Clin Oncol 14:2638–2645

Beyer J, Kingreen D, Krause M, et al. (1997) Long term survival of patients with recurrent or refractory germ cell tumors after high dose chemotherapy. Cancer 79:161–168

Bosl GJ, Geller NL, Bajorin D, et al. (1988) A randomized trial of etoposide + cisplatin versus vinblastine + bleomycin + cisplatin + cyclophosphamide + dactinomycin in patients with good-prognosis germ cell tumors. J Clin Oncol 6:1231–1238

Chou T-C, Motzer RJ, Tong Y, et al. (1994) Computerized quantification of synergism and antagonism of Taxol, topotecan, and cisplatin against human teratocarcinoma cell growth: a rational approach to clinical protocol design. J Natl Cancer Inst 86:1517–1524

Culine S (1996) Optimal management of residual mass after chemotherapy in advanced seminoma: there is a time for everything. J Clin Oncol 14:2884–2885

Farhat F, Culine S, Théodore C, et al. (1996) Cisplatin and ifosfamide with either vinblastine or etoposide as salvage therapy for refractory or relapsing germ cell tumor patients. Cancer 77:1193–1197

Fossa SD, Droz JP, Stoter G, et al. (1995) Cisplatin, vincristine and ifosfamide combination chemotherapy of metastatic seminoma: results of EORTC trial 30874. Br J Cancer 71:619–624

Guillou L, Estreicher A, Chaubert P, et al. (1996) Germ cell tumors of the testis overexpress wild-type p53. Am J Pathol 149:1221–1228

Horwich A, Dearnaley DP, A'Hern R, et al. (1992) The activity of single-agent carboplatin in advanced seminoma. Eur J Cancer 28A:1307–1310

McCaffrey JA, Mazumdar M, Bajorin DF, et al. (1997) Ifosfamide- and cisplatin-containing chemotherapy as first-line salvage therapy in germ cell tumors: response and survival. J Clin Oncol 15:2559–2563

Mead et al., International Germ Cell Cancer Collaborative Group (1997) International Germ Cell Consensus Classification: a prognostic factor-based staging system for metastatic germ cell cancers. J Clin Oncol 15:594–603

Mencel PJ, Motzer R, Mazumdar M, et al. (1994) Advanced seminoma: treatment results, survival, and prognostic factors in 142 patients. J Clin Oncol 12:120–126

Motzer RJ (1996) Selecting patients with cisplatin-resistant germ cell tumors for high-dose chemotherapy. J Clin Oncol 14:2625–2626

Motzer RJ, Mazumdar M, Bosl GJ (1996) High-dose carboplatin, etoposide, and cyclophosphamide for patients with refractory germ cell tumors: treatment results and prognostic factors for survival and toxicity. J Clin Oncol 14:1098–1105

Nichols CR (1996) Ifosfamide in the treatment of germ cell tumors. Semin Oncol 23:65–73

Peckham MJ, Barret A, McElwain TJ, Hendry WF (1979) Combined management of malignant teratoma of the testis. Lancet II:267–270

Puc HS, Heelan R, Mazumdar M, et al. (1996) Management of residual mass in advanced seminoma: results and recommendations from the Memorial Sloan-Kettering Cancer Center. J Clin Oncol 14:454–460

Roth BJ (1996) The role of ifosfamide in the treatment of testicular and urothelial malignancies. Semin Oncol 23:19–27

Schmoll HJ, Harstrick A, Bokemeyer C, et al. (1993) Single-agent carboplatin for advanced seminoma. Cancer 72:237–243

Sleijfer DT, Mulder NH (1997) Treatment of advanced seminoma: an update. Anticancer Drugs 8:107–112

Stephens AW, Gonin R, Hutchins GD, Einhorn LH (1996) Positron emission tomography evaluation of residual radiographic abnormalities in postchemotherapy germ cell tumor patients. J Clin Oncol 14:1637–1641

Warren GP, Einhorn LH (1995) Gallium scans in the evaluation of residual masses after chemotherapy for seminoma. J Clin Oncol 13:2784–2788

Williams SD, Birch R, Einhorn LH, et al. (1987) Treatment of disseminated germ-cell tumors with cisplatin, bleomycin, and either vinblastine or etoposide. N Engl J Med 316:1435–1440

Xian H, Mazumdar M, Bajorin DF, et al. (1997) Long-term follow-up of patients with good-risk germ cell tumors treated with etoposide and cisplatin. J Clin Oncol 15:2553–2558

# 24 Nonseminomatous Germ Cell Tumors

H. Ozer

## CONTENTS



## 24.1
## Introduction

Germ cell tumors are derived from the malignant transformation of preanaphase I germ cells. These tumors most commonly originate in the gonads (testis or ovary) but similar neoplasms occasionally originate in midline structures (retroperitoneum, mediastinum, or pineal gland). Rarely, a germ cell tumor may originate in other sites. Many retroperitoneal germ cell tumors probably originate in occult testis primary sites whereas mediastinal germ cell tumors are likely distinct entities that arise in the mediastinum.

Germ cell tumors are classified as either seminoma, the cell type most closely resembling the primordial germ cell, or nonseminoma. Embryonal carcinoma is totipotential and can differentiate into extraembryonic malignant cell types (yolk sac tumor and choriocarcinoma) and more mature cell types (teratoma). Many germ cell tumors are mixtures of more than one cell type. A pure seminoma must be composed exclusively of seminoma; otherwise the tumor will have the clinical behavior of a nonseminomatous tumor (Williams 1998).

Nonseminomatous histology accounts for about 50% of all germ cell tumors and such tumors frequently present in the third decade of life. Most tumors are mixed, consisting of two or more cell types. Seminoma may be a component, but the definition of a pure seminoma *excludes* the presence of any nonseminomatous cell type. The presence of any nonseminomatous cell type (other than syncytiotrophoblasts) imparts the prognosis and management principles of a nonseminomatous tumor (Williams 1998).

Male relatives of testis cancer patients have a slightly increased risk of developing the disease. The other well-described predisposing factor is cryptorchidism. Males with a late descending testis should undergo orchiopexy before 5 years of age. Patients with testes not descending prior to puberty probably should undergo orchiectomy rather than orchiopexy. Patients with abdominal testes have a higher risk of malignancy and, as they cannot be examined, should undergo orchiectomy. It must be remembered that in about 25% of patients with a history of an undescended testis who develop testis cancer, the tumor will develop in the contralateral testis (Batata et al. 1982).

Testicular carcinoma in situ (CIS) has become increasingly well recognized. It is noted in the testis of most patients with adjacent invasive germ cell tumors. CIS is found occasionally in the workup of patients with infertility and is associated with a substantial risk of subsequent invasive carcinoma. Some patients with an invasive germ cell tumor will have CIS in the contralateral testis if a routine biopsy is done. The importance of this finding is not clear as a metachronous second primary testis cancer develops in only about 1%–2% patients not undergoing routine biopsy of the contralateral testis. Thus, most authorities do not recommend routine biopsy (Williams 1998; Daugaard et al. 1987).

H. Ozer, MD, Chief, Hematology/Oncology, Department of Medicine, Cancer Center Director, Allegheny University Hospitals, Hahnemann, Broad & Vine Streets, MS 487, Philadelphia, PA 19102-1192, USA

## 24.2
## Genetics

Cytogenetic studies show that male germ cell tumors are nearly always hyperdiploid, are frequently triploid or tetraploid, and have at least one X and one Y chromosome. This had been interpreted as implying that malignant transformation occurs in a premeiotic cell, and that endoreduplication of genetic material is an early event in germ cell transformation. However, separation of chromosomal complements does not occur until meiotic anaphase. Therefore, the timing of malignant transformation is more properly ascribed to a cell that is preanaphase I of the meiotic cycle (CHAGANTI et al. 1993). In 1983, ATKIN and BAKER (1983) described a small marker chromosome. Subsequent studies showed that this marker chromosome is an isochromosome of the short arm of chromosome 12 [i(12p)].

The isochromosome 12 [i(12p)] is present in more than 80% of germ cell tumors and is not seen in other malignancies. It is present in all histologic types, primary sites, and in primary and metastatic tumors as well as CIS (BOSL et al. 1994; VOS et al. 1990). Therefore, the i(12p) is probably the result of a very early event in germ cell tumorigenesis. This isochromosome can be identified by a variety of techniques including Southern analysis with FISH and the finding of this abnormality may provide diagnostic information in poorly differentiated tumors of uncertain origin. If i(12p) is present or if a high 12p copy number is demonstrated, then the patient has a germ cell tumor. Deletions on 12q are common and also diagnostic. These consistent findings suggest the presence of a tumor suppresser gene (RODRIQUEZ et al. 1992).

## 24.3
## Staging

Embryologically, the testes originate in the genital ridge and migrate into the scrotum. Thus, the lymphatic drainage of the testis is generally to the retroperitoneal lymph nodes. The inguinal lymphatics are rarely involved unless the scrotum has been contaminated or there has been prior inguinal or scrotal surgery. After the retroperitoneal nodes, retrocrural, mediastinal, and supraclavicular lymph nodes may be involved. Hematogenous spread ordinarily occurs to the lungs. Occasionally, liver involvement may be observed and rarely the newly diagnosed patient may have brain metastases.

Multiple staging systems are currently used to classify and manage patients with germ cell tumors. They differ in the number of stages (three versus four), clinical versus pathologic, the inclusion of tumor marker values, and the use of size and sites of the primary tumor and metastatic disease. Revision of the stage groupings of the American Joint Committee on cancer (AJCC) were recommended in January 1996, and the Union Internationale Contre le Cancrum (UICC) has approved the same classification. Broadly, stage I disease is confined to the testis; stage II disease is restricted to the retroperitoneum; and stage III disease represents involvement of supradiaphragmatic or other nodal sites, or visceral disease. Secondary classifications used for clinical trials of chemotherapy in patients with advanced disease, encompassing bulky retroperitoneal or supradiaphragmatic nodal disease and visceral metastases, vary considerably.

Studies that should be done for staging include an abdominal computed tomography (CT) scan, a chest radiograph, and, if this is normal, a chest CT scan. Completion of these studies will allow the assignment of a clinical stage. A simple and reproducible staging system is as follows (WILLIAMS 1998):

- Stage I: Tumor confined to the testis
- Stage II: Testis plus retroperitoneal nodes
    IIA: Abnormal nodes <2 cm
    IIB: Nodes 2–5 cm
    IIC: Nodes >5 cm
- Stage III: Supradiaphragmatic or visceral metastases

Patients with nonseminomatous tumors sometimes undergo retroperitoneal lymphadenectomy (RPLND) and can also be assigned a pathologic stage of the retroperitoneal nodes. The above system also proves useful in this situation. Alternatively, the TNM system is sometimes used. It is:

- Stage IIN1: Microscopic disease in five or fewer lymph nodes
- Stage IIN2a: Macroscopic disease in five or fewer lymph nodes, none greater than 2 cm
- Stage IIN3: Extranodal extension
- Stage IIN4: Bulky "unresectable" disease

## 24.4
## Tumor Markers

Measurement of serum $\alpha$-fetoprotein (AFP), human chorionic gonadotropin (HCG), and lactate dehydrogenase (LDH) is required for the management of all stages of disease. Persistently elevated or rising concentrations of AFP and/or HCG almost always imply active disease. AFP may, however, be elevated during hepatic regeneration or, rarely, for inexplicable reasons. HCG may be elevated due to relative or absolute hypogonadism, which may be seen in patients after chemotherapy or in those who have had bilateral orchiectomies and are not receiving adequate hormonal replacement. The half-lives of AFP and HCG are approximately 5 days and 30 h, respectively. An elevated AFP in a patient with otherwise pure seminoma denotes the presence of undetected elements of nonseminoma and alters treatment accordingly. HCG may also be elevated in patients with seminoma, but this does not alter management. LDH is less specific, but can be used to follow the progress of treatment, particularly in patients with seminoma.

## 24.5
## Therapy

Nonseminomatous germ cell tumor is relatively radioresistant. Therefore, radiation therapy plays no role in its initial management. If a patient has clinical stage I disease at the conclusion of initial staging, three management options remain, the choice of which depends on specific histologic features and status of serum tumor marker concentrations (BOSL et al. 1997).

After an inguinal orchiectomy has been performed, a CT scan of the abdomen, a chest x-ray, and tumor marker determinations should be done, as should a chest CT scan if the plain film is normal. If the radiographic studies are unequivocally normal and the markers return to normal, the patient has clinical stage I disease. Management decisions are complex in such patients, with alternatives being RPLND or surveillance. Both have cure rates that approach 100%. Chemotherapy for high-risk patients has been recommended by some, but at this time there are not adequate data to recommend this approach and a significant number of patients would receive unnecessary chemotherapy. If an RPLND is to be done, it should be performed by someone who has significant expertise with this surgical procedure and who can do a nerve-sparing procedure. Factors that must be considered are surgical expertise available, patient preference and compliance, estimated risk of relapse if surveillance is the choice, and concomitant illness.

Favorable prognostic factors for recurrence are the absence of vascular invasion, teratoma elements in the primary tumor, absence of embryonal carcinoma, and an elevated AFP concentration that returns to normal. The influence of T stage is less clear. Risk of relapse ranges from 15% to about 50% based upon these factors (WILLIAMS 1998). Vascular invasion is perhaps the most important feature but is not always reproducible among pathologists. Patients who elect surveillance should have monthly marker determinations, physical examinations, and chest x-rays for 1 year, with an abdominal CT scan every 2 months. During the second year, the marker determinations, physical examinations, and chest x-rays should be done every 2 months with the chest CT every 4 months. Appropriate follow-up during years 3 and 4 is less clear, but only a few patients will develop evidence of recurrent disease this long after orchiectomy. Management of patients undergoing RPLND is dependent upon pathologic stage. Patients with negative nodes are followed with physical examination, marker determinations, and chest x-ray monthly for 1 year and every other month during the second year. CT scans are unnecessary. Follow-up in years 3 and 4 can be infrequent as relapse is very rare. Management of patients with pathologic stage II disease is discussed subsequently.

The merits of RPLND versus observation can be summarized as follows (WILLIAMS 1998):

1. Provides pathologic staging and more certain natural history.
2. Brief adjuvant chemotherapy can be given to node-positive patients if desired (see Sect. 24.5.3).
3. Less reliance on patient and physician compliance during follow-up.
4. Risk of recurrence limited to 2 years.
5. Fewer tests required.
6. Fewer patients will require chemotherapy (those who have positive nodes do not receive adjuvant chemotherapy).

## 24.5.1
## Observation

The driving forces for early observation studies in clinical stage I patients were the infertility resulting from RPLND (due to retrograde ejaculation) and the apparent absence of therapeutic benefit (i.e., orchiectomy was a curative procedure or systemic disease occurred in the absence of retroperitoneal disease). The ability of cisplatin-based chemotherapy to cure systemic disease directly permitted observation studies because the rate of cure of low-burden disease exceeded 95% and treatment of relapse would not compromise survival. Relapse occurs in 25%–30% of patients who are observed (DUNPHY et al. 1988; GELS et al. 1995; READ et al. 1992; NICOLAI and PIZZOCARO 1995). A higher likelihood of retroperitoneal or systemic relapse was associated with T2–4 tumors and with lymphatic or vascular invasion in T1 tumors. Some studies suggested that a high percentage of embryonal carcinoma and other histologic features also predicted a higher likelihood of relapse. However, the correlation between lymphatic-vascular invasion and the presence of embryonal carcinoma is high, and general agreement on histologic criteria for relapse *independent* of vascular or lymphatic invasion does not exist. Therefore, vascular-lymphatic invasion is the critical pathologic predictor for relapse in tumors confined to the testis. The retroperitoneum is the site of relapse in approximately two-thirds of patients, the lungs in approximately one-third, and other visceral sites, much less frequently.

Patients with clinical stage I nonseminomatous germ cell tumor with a T1 tumor without vascular-lymphatic invasion and serum tumor markers that are normal or declining at half-life should be offered both surgical and observation options. If RPLND is chosen, it should be of the nerve-sparing type, thereby preserving ejaculatory capacity in the majority of patients. Frequent CT scans of the abdomen are unnecessary once an RPLND has been performed. If surveillance is chosen, then a possibly unnecessary RPLND is avoided, limiting therapy to orchiectomy alone in at least 70% of the patients (i.e., those who never relapse). The importance of patient compliance cannot be overemphasized. A physical examination, chest x-ray, and determinations of AFP and hCG levels are required at monthly intervals in the first year, every other month in the second year, quarterly in the third year, and less frequently thereafter. An abdominal CT scan is required quarterly in the first year, every 4 months in the second year, and every 6 months beginning in the third year. Visits and evaluations should be made annually in the fifth year and thereafter. In both situations, relapses are extremely uncommon after 2 years and have only very rarely been observed after 5 years, in contrast to the situation with seminoma (WILLIAMS 1998).

## 24.5.2
## Chemotherapy

There are few data regarding chemotherapy as initial treatment of clinical stage I disease when the risk of retroperitoneal disease is high. In three reports of patients receiving two cycles of cisplatin-based chemotherapy, fewer than 5% relapsed and about 1% died of germ cell tumor (PONT et al. 1996; NICOLAI and PIZZOCARO 1995; OLIVER et al. 1992; CULLEN et al. 1995). Although this approach avoids RPLND and the duration of therapy is brief, a majority of these patients would be exposed to the transient (e.g., myelosuppression), permanent (e.g., neuropathy), and delayed (e.g., Raynaud's phenomenon, acute leukemia) toxicities of chemotherapy. The data are not yet mature and follow-up is short; this approach should be considered investigational. Rarely, patients with clinical stage I disease are found to have persistently elevated serum concentrations of AFP or hCG after orchiectomy. If these markers increase or plateau at an elevated level after a period of observation (4 weeks or less), metastatic disease is present (DAVIS et al. 1994). This group of patients should receive initial systemic chemotherapy because the disease is often not limited to the retroperitoneum. An RPLND should be done only if clinical studies at the conclusion of therapy demonstrate new disease.

## 24.5.3
## Stage II Disease

Low-tumor-burden clinical stage II nonseminomatous germ cell tumor encompasses disease ipsilateral to the primary tumor, at or below the renal hilum, not associated with tumor-related back pain, and limited to the primary lymph nodes. The presence of suprahilar or retrocrural lymphadenopathy, bilateral retroperitoneal nodal metastases, back pain, or contralateral lymph node involvement (even if the ipsilateral lymph nodes do not appear to be involved) generally implies unresectable disease (e.g., tumor-associated back pain) or a higher likelihood of metastatic disease (suprahilar and retrocrural adenopathy), and initial chemotherapy is preferred. Ipsilateral solitary lymph nodes smaller than 3 cm are best handled by RPLND. Lymph nodes between 3 and 5 cm, even if solitary, may be associated with more extensive disease than can be detected on abdominal CT scan (WILLIAMS 1998).

Patients with clinical stage IIA disease should undergo an RPLND. Some patients will be candidates for a nerve-sparing procedure and some will not, depending upon intraoperative findings. One important reason for the procedure is that 20%–25% of patients with clinical stage II disease will have pathologic stage I tumors. The role of newer radiographic staging procedures (e.g., positron emission tomography) in this situation is not clear.

Many patients in clinical stage IIB and all stage IIC patients should be treated with chemotherapy with or without postchemotherapy surgery, as will be described subsequently. An occasional patient with small-volume IIB disease can undergo tumor resection, but most patients in these groups will have tumor that is difficult to resect completely and have a high likelihood of ultimately needing chemotherapy anyway.

A special situation is that in which the patient has normal radiographic studies but persistently elevated AFP or HCG after orchiectomy. Recent studies suggest that most patients with persistent AFP elevation in this situation have a high risk of relapse after RPLND and thus should be treated with chemotherapy rather than surgery (PIZZOCARO et al. 1984a; SKINNER and SCARDINO 1980). The optimum management of patients with persistent HCG elevation is not clear and either chemotherapy or RPLND may be considered. In one series, 24 patients underwent RPLND, seven had positive nodes, and six ultimately required chemotherapy (HARTLAPP et al. 1987; PIZZOCARO et al. 1984b).

Patients with positive nodes that have been completely resected and whose markers are normal after surgery may be observed or treated with adjuvant chemotherapy. Several clinical trials have shown that two courses of chemotherapy will nearly always prevent relapse. However, patients can also be observed after chemotherapy and those destined to be cured by surgery with "unnecessary" chemotherapy; those destined to suffer recurrence can be treated with three to four courses of chemotherapy when they have small volume tumor and a very high chemotherapy cure rate. Risk of recurrence ranges from 30% to 60% depending upon the size and number of involved nodes and extranodal extension. In compliant patients, these two approaches are equivalent and cure 98%–99% of patients. Patients receiving adjuvant chemotherapy have a very low risk of recurrence and need to be followed relatively infrequently. Observed patients should undergo physical examination, marker determinations, and chest x-ray monthly for 1 year and every other month in the second year.

Adjuvant chemotherapy remains a strong consideration in patients when six nodes or more are involved, any node is larger than 2 cm, or there is extranodal extension. In the late 1970s, treatment programs based on cisplatin, vinblastine, and bleomycin were given as adjuvant therapy following RPLND, and nearly 100% of patients survived relapse free. Considerable treatment-related morbidity was associated with these regimens, prompting efforts to reduce toxicity. Two cycles of cisplatin-based chemotherapy are nearly always effective in preventing relapse. A randomized trial showed that observation with standard treatment at relapse and two cycles of adjuvant chemotherapy yielded equivalent survival rates. Etoposide has replaced vinblastine in adjuvant regimens. A recent study suggests that etoposide plus cisplatin alone is adequate, and that bleomycin is unnecessary as part of adjuvant therapy (MOTZER et al. 1995).

## 24.5.4
## Stage III Disease

Approximately 70%–80% of patients with metastatic disease should be cured with chemotherapy with or without postchemotherapy surgery. More recent germ cell tumor clinical trials have divided patients into those most likely to achieve complete response (good risk) and those not likely to achieve a complete response (poor risk) (MOTZER et al. 1992c). In good-risk patients, the trial design attempted to reduce toxicity but maintain efficacy; in poor-risk patients, efficacy was a priority over toxicity. Unfortunately, until recently there has not been a generally agreed upon system that assigned patients to one group or the other. However, a consensus group recently reviewed data on more that 3500 patients and developed a prognostic factor system that is relatively simple and accurately assesses prognosis (Table 24.1). This system requires easily obtainable clinical data. It was highly reliable when validated in a test series (KAYE et al. 1995) and is being used in the ongoing international trial of high-dose chemotherapy with stem cell rescue in poor-prognosis patients.

Good-risk patients account for 70%–80% of the patient population and about 90% of them will survive. Patients with very small volume disease fare even better. Recent trials have attempted to reduce cost and toxicity of treatment. Results can be sum-

**Table 24.1.** Prognostic factor system for assessment of prognosis in patients with germ cell tumors

*Good prognosis:*
Nonseminoma    Testis/retroperitoneal primary *and*
               Good markers*
               No nonpulmonary visceral metastases
Seminoma       Any primary *and*
               Any markers *and*
               No nonpulmonary visceral metastases

*Intermediate prognosis:*
Nonseminoma    Testis/retroperitoneal primary *and*
               Intermediate markers* *and*
               No nonpulmonary visceral metastases
Seminoma       Any primary *and*
               Any markers *and*
               Nonpulmonary visceral metastases
                   present

*Poor prognosis:*
Nonseminoma    Mediastinal primary site or
               Testis/retroperitoneal primary with
                   either:
                   Nonpulmonary visceral metastases
                   or
                   Poor markers*
  *Good markers:   AFP < 1000 and
                   HCG < 5000 IU/l and
                   LDH < 1.5 × normal
  *Intermediate    AFP 1000–10 000 or
   markers:        HCG 5000–50 000 IU/l or
                   LDH 1.5–10 × normal
  *Poor markers:   AFP > 10 000 or
                   HCG > 50 000 IU/l or
                   LDH > 10 × normal

**Table 24.2.** Commonly used chemotherapy regimens for metastatic germ cell tumors

*Previously untreated – good risk*
Etoposide     100 mg/m$^2$ intravenously (IV) daily × 5 d
Cisplatin     20 mg/m$^2$ IV daily × 5 d
              Four cycles administered at 21-d intervals
Etoposide     100 mg/m$^2$ IV daily × 5 d
              Cisplatin 20 mg/m$^2$ IV daily × 5 d
Bleomycin     30 units IV weekly on d 2, 9, 16
              Three cycles administered at 21-d intervals

*Previously untreated – poor risk*
Etoposide     100 mg/m$^2$ IV daily × 5 d
Cisplatin     20 mg/m$^2$ IV daily × 5 d
Bleomycin     30 units IV weekly on d 2, 9, 16
              Four cycles administered at 21-d intervals

*Previously treated – first-line salvage therapy*
Ifosfamide    1.2 g/m$^2$ IV daily × 5 d
Mesna         400 mg/m$^2$ IV every 8 h × 5 d
Cisplatin     20 mg/m$^2$ IV daily × 5 d
              *plus either*
Vinblastine   0.11 mg/kg IV 1 and 2
              *or*
Etoposide     75 mg/m$^2$ IV daily × 5 d

marized as follows for regimens shown in Table 24.2.

1. Three courses of cisplatin, etoposide, and bleomycin (BEP) or four courses of etoposide and cisplatin (EP) are the standard of care.
2. If only three courses of chemotherapy are to be given, deletion of bleomycin significantly worsens therapeutic results.
3. Two large randomized trials have shown that the substitution of carboplatin for cisplatin is associated a higher risk of relapse and a worsened outcome.

Poor-risk patients fortunately comprise a minority of patients with germ cell tumors that require chemotherapy. Only about 50% will survive. At this time, there is no regimen that has been found to be therapeutically superior to four courses of standard dose BEP. A recent intergroup study compared BEP with cisplatin, ifosfamide, and etoposide (VIP) (NICHOLS et al. 1992). There were no therapeutic differences and the VIP regimen had more toxicity. The current ongoing international randomized trial in poor-prognosis patients is comparing four courses of BEP with a regimen comprising two courses of BEP followed by two courses of very high dose therapy with hematopoietic progenitor support.

### 24.5.5
### Salvage Therapy and Autologous Transplantation

Patients who do not achieve a complete response or who relapse from complete response have a less favorable prognosis but some are still potentially curable. For patients treated with conventional dose therapy, the regimen of choice is ifosfamide, vinblastine, and cisplatin (VeIP), assuming first-line therapy was EP or BEP. Four courses should be given. As first-line salvage therapy, this regimen will induce complete remissions in 40%–50% of patients (HARSTRICK et al. 1991; EINHORN et al. 1996; MOTZER et al. 1992b). About one-third will relapse and only about 25% of patients will be long-term survivors. Patients with seminoma and those who have a complete response to initial therapy fare better. This regimen in the salvage setting is considerably more toxic than BEP; severe neutropenia and thrombocytopenia are common. A hematopoietic growth factor should be administered prophylactically. Nephrotoxicity will occur occasionally. Mesna will almost always abrogate urothelial toxicity.

Several studies have shown that as third-line therapy, high-dose chemotherapy will induce durable complete remissions in about 10%–20% of patients (LINKESCH et al. 1992; BEYER et al. 1995). The most common chemotherapy is two courses of high-dose carboplatin and etoposide with or without cyclophosphamide or ifosfamide, each course being followed with hematopoietic progenitor support. Because of this activity in heavily pretreated patients, high-dose chemotherapy is being used earlier in the course of the disease. Some centers will give one course of VeIP followed by two courses of high-dose therapy with rescue as the initial salvage chemotherapy regimen. In a nonrandom trial about 40% of patients were long survivors (MOTZER et al. 1992b). However, this patient population was more favorable and it is not clear whether, as second-line treatment, high-dose chemotherapy is superior to four courses of standard dose VeIP; either approach is reasonable for most patients.

Patients with extragonadal primaries rarely if ever have durable complete remissions in response to any form of salvage therapy (either VeIP or high-dose therapy) and are candidates for phase II clinical trials. Patients who are overtly cisplatin refractory (progressive disease within 4 weeks of the last dose of cisplatin) should not be treated with VeIP and have less than a 5% chance of attaining a durable complete remission with high-dose therapy.

## 24.5.6
## Postchemotherapy Surgery

After serum tumor markers have normalized, postchemotherapy surgery remains an integral part of management for patients in whom a residual mass is indicated to be present by radiographic staging or clinical examination (DONOHUE et al. 1987). Approximately 45% of resected residual masses will contain fibrosis-necrosis and a similar number will contain immature or mature teratoma. About 10% will harbor residual carcinoma. Two additional cycles of chemotherapy should be given if viable malignant tumor is detected. All other patients have a low risk of relapse and do not require postoperative therapy. However, unresected postchemotherapy teratoma may progress over time and interfere with

organ function. Also, there is presumptive evidence that later malignant degeneration may occur. All residual masses at all sites should be resected. Most investigators define a residual retroperitoneal mass as persistent lymph nodes larger than 1 cm. However, patients whose primary tumors do not contain teratoma and who have at least a 90% regression of metastases do not need surgery. The occasional patient who has not undergone orchiectomy prior to chemotherapy should undergo this procedure after treatment as the testis may be a drug sanctuary.

Residual masses should be considered for resection only in patients whose serum tumor markers have completely normalized, except for patients with a solitary resectable residual site of metastasis (usually in the retroperitoneum) (FOSSA et al. 1992). All postchemotherapy surgery should be done by physicians with substantial expertise in the management of germ cell tumors. Similar surgical selection factors should be used for patients who have received salvage therapy and those with extragonadal tumors.

An area of controversy concerns patients with seminoma who have been treated with chemotherapy and have a residual mass; such residual masses are a common finding, particularly in those with very bulky disease. The residual mass is ordinarily densely fibrotic and adherent to adjacent structures. These patients are very unlikely to have residual teratoma, a major indication for surgery. It is very clear that those patients with residual masses less than 3 cm in diameter have a very low likelihood of having persistent seminoma. Data for those with larger masses are controversial. Some investigators favor surgical resection, while others favor observation. Radiotherapy to residual masses does not appear to affect outcome.

## 24.5.7
## Late Effects

An important consideration in these patients with high potential for cure is late effects of treatment. There have been anecdotal reports suggesting that cisplatin-based chemotherapy may be associated with an increased risk of cardiovascular disease. A recent study investigated the likelihood of these events in patients entered several years previously on a study that investigated therapeutic alternatives and outcome in early-stage tumors other than seminoma (GIETEMA et al. 1992). This study registered and observed patients with pathologic stage I tumors; some ultimately relapsed and required chemotherapy. Patients with stage II tumors randomly received either two courses of adjuvant chemotherapy or were observed. Relapsing patients received four courses of therapy. Thus, a prospectively defined patient population received either no chemotherapy or two or four courses of treatment. No differences were seen in the incidence of the development of cardiovascular disease or hypertension. The differences noted were in the frequencies of distal extremity paresthesias and Raynaud's phenomenon, primarily due to cisplatin, which were more likely to be present in patients who received longer chemotherapy.

Another concern is the discovery that etoposide is associated with the late development of a distinctive type of leukemia or myelodysplastic syndrome (BAJORIN et al. 1993; NICHOLS et al. 1992; PEDERSEN-BJERGAARD et al. 1991). This event appears to be dose related and is very rare in patients who receive less than a total dose of etoposide of 2000 mg/m$^2$. Among testis cancer patients this total dose is exceeded only in those who fail to enter durable complete remission with initial therapy.

The impact of chemotherapy on fertility is less than originally thought, but it is likely that at least some patients will have long-standing chemotherapy-induced oligospermia or azoospermia (STEPHENSON et al. 1995). However, many, if not most, will resume normal or nearly normal spermatogenesis and a significant number have fathered children.

## References


Atkin N, Baker M (1983) i(12p): specific chromosomal marker in seminoma and malignant teratoma of the testis? Cancer Genet Cytogenet 10:199–204

Bajorin DF, Mortzer RJ, Rodriquez E, Murphy B, Bosl GJ (1993) Acute nonlymphocytic leukemia in germ cell tumor patients treated with etoposide-containing chemotherapy. J Natl Cancer Inst 85:60–62

Batata M, Chu F, Hilaris B, Whitmore W, Golbey R (1982) Testicular cancer in cryptorchids. Cancer 49:1023–1030

Beyer J, Schwella N, Zingsem J, et al. (1995) Hematopoietic rescue after high-dose chemotherapy using autologous peripheral-blood progenitor cells or bone marrow: a randomized comparison. J Clin Oncol 13:1328–1335

Bosl GJ, Ilson DH, Rodriguez E, Motzer RJ, Reuter V, Chaganti RSK (1994) Clinical relevance of the i(12p) marker chromosome in germ cell tumors. J Natl Cancer Inst 86:349–355

Bosl G, Sheinfeld J, Bojorin DF, Motzer R (1997) Cancer of the testis. In: DeVita VT, Hellman S, Rosenberg SA (eds) Cancer: principles and practice of oncology, 5th edn. Lippincott-Raven, Philadelphia

Chaganti RSK, Rodriguez F, Bosl GJ (1993) Cytogenetics of male germ cell tumors. Urol Clin North Am 20:55–66

Cullen M, Stenning S, Parkinson M, et al. (1995) Short course adjuvant chemotherapy in high risk stage I nonseminomatous germ cell tumours of the testis (NSGCTT): an MRC(UK) study report [abstract]. Proc ASCO 14:244

Daugaard G, von der Masse H, Olsen J, Rorth M, Skakkebaek NE (1987) Carcinoma-in-situ of the testis in patients with assumed extragonadal germ-cell tumors. Lancet II:528–530

Davis B, Herr H, Fair W, Bosl GJ (1994) The management of patients with nonseminomatous germ cell tumors of the testis with serologic disease only after orchiectomy. J Urol 152:111–113

Donohue J, Rowland R, Kopecky K, et al. (1987) Correlation of computerized tomographic changes and histological findings in 80 patients having radical retroperitoneal lymph node dissection after chemotherapy for testis tumor. J Urol 137:1176–1179

Dunphy C, Ayala A, Swanson D, Ro J, Logothetis C (1988) Clinical stage I nonseminomatous and mixed germ cell tumors of the testis. Cancer 62:1202–1206

Einhorn LH, Weathers T, Loehrer P, Nichols C (1996) Long-term follow up of second line chemotherapy with vinblastine, ifosfamide, and cisplatin in disseminated germ cell tumors [abstract]. Proc ASCO 15:240

Fossa SD, Qvist H, Stenwig AF, et al. (1992) Is post chemotherapy retroperitoneal surgery necessary in patients with nonseminomatous testicular cancer and minimal residual tumor masses? J Clin Oncol 10:569–573

Gels M, Hoekstra H, Sleijfer D, et al. (1995) Detection of recurrence in patients with clinical stage I nonseminomatous testicular germ cell tumors and consequences for further followup: a single center 10-year experience. J Clin Oncol 13:1188–1194

Gietema J, Sleijfer D, Willemse P, et al. (1992) Long term follow up of cardiovascular risk factors in patients given chemotherapy for disseminated nonseminomatous testicular cancer. Ann Intern Med 116:709–715

Harstrick A, Schmoll HJ, Wilke H, et al. (1991) Cisplatin, etoposide, and ifosfamide salvage therapy for refractory or relapsing germ cell carcinoma. J Clin Oncol 9:1549–1555

Hartlapp JH, Weissbach I, Bussar-Maatz R (1987) Adjuvant chemotherapy in nonseminomatous testicular tumor stage II. Int J Androl 10:277–284

Kaye SB, Mead GM, Fossa S, et al. (1995) An MCR/EORTC randomized trial in poor prognosis metastatic teratoma, comparing BEP with BOP-VIP [abstract]. Proc ASCO 14:246

Linkesch W, Krainer M, Wagner A (1992) Phase I/II trail of ultrahigh carboplatin, etoposide, cyclophosphamide with ABMT in refractory or relapsed nonseminomatous germ cell tumors. Bone Marrow Transplant 10 (Suppl 2);28

Motzer RJ, Bjorin DF, Valamis V, Weisen S, Bosl GJ (1992a) Ifosfamide-based chemotherapy for patients with resistant germ cell tumors: the Memorial Sloan-Kettering Cancer Center Experience. Semin Oncol 19:8–11

Motzer RJ, Gulati SC, Crown JP, et al. (1992b) High-dose chemotherapy and autologous bone marrow rescue for patients with refractory germ cell tumors: early intervention is better tolerated. Cancer 69:550–556

Motzer RJ, Bjorin DF, Bosl GJ (1992c) "Poor-risk" germ cell tumors: current progress and future directors. Semin Oncol 19:206–214

Motzer RJ, Gulati SC, Tong WP, et al. (1993) Phase I trial with pharmacokinetic analyses of high-dose carboplatin, etoposide, and cyclophosphamide with autologous bone marrow transplantation in patients with refractory germ cell tumors. Cancer Res 53:3730–3735

Motzer RJ, Sheinfeld J, Mazumdar M, et al. (1995) Etoposide and cisplatin adjuvant therapy for patients with pathologic stage II germ cell tumors. J Clin Oncol 13:2700–2704

Nichols CR, Breeden ES, Leohrer PJ (1992) Secondary leukemia associated with a conventional dose of etoposide: review of serial germ cell tumor protocols. J Natl Cancer Inst 85:36–40

Nicolai N, Pizzocaro G (1995) A surveillance study of clinical stage I nonseminomatous germ cell tumors of the testis: 10 year followup. J Urol 154:1045–1049

Oliver RTD, Raja M, Ong J, Gallagher C (1992) Pilot study to evaluate impact of a policy of adjuvant chemotherapy for high risk stage I malignant teratoma on overall relapse rate of stage I patients. J Urol 148:1453–1455

Pedersen-Bjergaard J, Hansen ST, Larsen SO, Daugaard G, Philip R, Rorth M (1991) Increased risk of myelodysplasia and leukaemia after etoposide, cisplatin, and bleomycin for germ-cell tumors. Lancet 338:359–363

Pizzocaro G, Piva L, Salvioni R, Pasi M, Pilotti S, Monfardinai S (1984a) Adjuvant chemotherapy in resected stage II nonseminomatous germ cell tumors of the testis. In which cases is it necessary? Eur Urol 10:151–158

Pizzocaro G, Zanoni F, Milani A, et al. (1984b) Retroperitoneal lymphadenectomy and aggressive chemotherapy in non-bulky clinical stage II nonseminomatous germinal testis tumors. Cancer 53:1363–1368

Pont J, Albrecht W, Postner G, et al. (1996) Adjuvant chemotherapy for high-risk clinical stage I nonseminomatous testicular germ cell cancer: long-term results of a prospective trial. J Clin Oncol 14:441–448

Read G, Stenning S, Cullen M, et al. (1992) Medical Research Council prospective study of surveillance for stage I testicular teratoma. J Clin Oncol 10:1762–1768

Rodriguez E, Mathew S, Reuter V, et al. (1992) Cytogenetic analysis of 124 prospectively ascertained male germ cell tumors. Cancer Res 52:2285–2291

Skinner DG, Scardino PT (1980) Relevance of biochemical tumor markers and lymphadenectomy in management of nonseminomatous testis tumors: current perspective. J Urol 123:378–382

Stephenson W, Poirier S, Rubin L, Einhorn I (1995) Evaluation of reproductive capacity in germ cell tumor patients following treatment with cisplatin, etoposide, and bleomycin. J Clin Oncol 13:2278–2280

Vos A, Oosterhuis W, de Jong B, Buist J, Koops H (1990) Cytogenetics of carcinoma in situ of the testis. Cancer Genet Cytogenet 46:75–81

Williams S (1998) Germ cell tumors. In: Cheson BD (ed) MKSAP IV. American College of Physicians

# 25 Is a Policy of Surveillance Warranted in Early Stage Testicular Cancer Following Orchiectomy?

A. Pawinski, W. Wynendaele, and A. Van Oosterom

CONTENTS



## 25.1 Introduction

The progress in imaging modalities and in the available treatment options in recent decades has rendered, stage I testicular cancer, the most frequent malignancy in the young male population, highly curable. Seventy percent of seminomas and 50% of nonseminoma testicular tumors are diagnosed as stage 1 disease (Bosl and Motzer 1997; Fossa and Horwich 1989). High inguinal orchiectomy has been the standard initial diagnostic and treatment approach for a patient with a suspected testicular tumor. In the past, even patients with no clinical signs of cancer dissemination were additionally subjected to adjuvant retroperitoneal lymph node dissection (RPLND) or locoregional radiotherapy. There were certainly reasons justifying this cautious approach. Patients with stage I testicular cancer, a highly aggressive disease, had a good prog-

nosis, but due to the insufficient accuracy of clinical staging and a low probability of curing patients with relapsed disease, survival rates were usually proportional to the incidence of relapse and ranged at that time from 70% to 90% (Carter 1983; Maier and Sulak 1973; Whitmore 1979; Peckham and McElwain 1974). Although not proven by randomized trials, some authors believed that a combined approach, which often included chemotherapy, gave a decrease in relapse rate and a higher overall survival.

## 25.2 Is Adjuvant Treatment Necessary?

The introduction of modern imaging modalities and cisplatin-based chemotherapy substantially improved the likelihood of cure of patients with a relapse, resulting in a further increase in overall survival. Elective treatment of the retroperitoneal area with radiotherapy or surgery, in combination with cisplatin-based chemotherapy offers a real prospect of cure for primary stage I and relapsed (20%–30%) testicular cancer patients. The technical progress in the surgical treatment of nonseminomas, orchiectomy, and RPLND resulted in a decrease in the incidence of surgical complications but did not significantly influence the prognosis (Richie 1990; Bosl et al. 1997; Small and Torti 1995; Foster and Donohue 1992; Williams et al. 1987; Nichols et al. 1992; McLeod et al. 1991). Despite this progress, in 11%–23% of these surgical procedures considerable morbidity has been reported (Donohue 1987). Fifteen percent of the operated patients have ejaculatory impotence (Donohue et al. 1993a, b). Ten to 25% will relapse and will have to receive additional salvage chemotherapy (McLeod et al. 1991; Klepp et al. 1990).

The technical progress in radiotherapeutic treatment of seminomas, with reduction of dose and fields, resulted in a significantly decreased incidence of relapse. This is expected to decrease the incidence

A. Pawinski, MD, Department of Oncology, University Hospitals Gasthuisberg, Catholic University of Leuven, Herestraat 49, B-3000 Leuven, Belgium
W. Wynendaele, MD, Department of Oncology, University Hospitals Gasthuisberg, Catholic University of Leuven, Herestraat 49, B-3000 Leuven, Belgium
A. van Oosterom, MD, PhD, Professor and Chairman, Department of Oncology, University Hospitals Gasthuisberg, Catholic University of Leuven, Herestraat 49, B-3000 Leuven, Belgium

of radiotherapy-related late side-effects (FOSSA et al. 1989; HAMILTON et al. 1986; DOSMANN et al. 1993; HANKS et al. 1992; VAN LEEUWEN et al. 1993).

As a third possible adjuvant method, cisplatin-based chemotherapy has been successfully used in the treatment of both seminomas and nonseminomas. The high response rate of this systemic treatment has been considered to justify its use despite the substantial toxicity (CULLEN et al. 1996; STUART et al. 1990; DIECKMANN et al. 1996). Myelosuppression, infertility, reduced lung function, and sporadic drug toxicity-related deaths are possible severe toxicities. Although the incidence of recurrence after cisplatin-based chemotherapy in stage I testicular cancer is low (3%–6%), relapse can be fatal because of the lack of an equally effective second-line treatment (CULLEN et al. 1996; PONT et al. 1996; MADEJ and PAWINSKI 1991a, b). In the opinion of some authors, the latter makes adjuvant chemotherapy unsuitable in this population of patients with a small risk of recurrence (RORTH 1992; PONT et al. 1990; CULLEN and JAMES 1996).

To summarize, patients undergoing orchiectomy for stage I testicular cancer have a very high probability of long-lasting disease-free survival, irrespective of the adjuvant treatment applied. This raises the question of whether the application of an additional harmful and costly approach after orchiectomy is justifiable.

## 25.3
## Surveillance

Most important is the fact that 70% of stage I patients treated with any form of adjuvant therapy undergo an unnecessary additional, harmful, and costly treatment (McLEOD et al. 1991). Based on these data, Peckham proposed a new strategy of surveillance with screening by means of computed tomography (CT) scanning and tumor marker tests [human chorionic gonadotropin (HCG) and $\alpha$-feto-protein (AFP) during close follow-up and treatment with chemotherapy in the event of a relapse (PECKHAM et al. 1982). Due to the introduction of this procedure, most patients do not need adjuvant treatment, while a minority, in whom a relapse will be detected at an early stage, can be adequately treated with chemotherapy.

Nonseminoma appeared to be the best model for the implementation of this surveillance policy. The availability of reliable tumor markers facilitates the detection of an early relapse. Most recurrences are diagnosed in the first year, thus limiting the period during which intensive surveillance is required. The extreme chemosensitivity of this cancer guarantees a high probability of cure even after a relapse. Only a minority of patients will have a second relapse after chemotherapy and less than 10% need additional surgery (BOKEMEYER et al. 1996). The results of several nonrandomized studies confirm the efficacy of this approach (Table 25.1).

Thirty percent of patients who have no detectable metastatic disease after orchiectomy still harbor micrometastases. This 30% could be an underestimate, according to KLEPP et al. (1990). In their study, 279 patients with clinical stage I disease underwent postorchiectomy retroperitoneal lymphadenectomy. Seventy-five patients (27%) had pathological stage 2 disease and 30 (11%) additional patients with no apparent metastases at operation relapsed within the median follow-up time of 50 months. These authors concluded that at least 37.6% of the clinical stage I population have subclinical metastatic disease at the

**Table 25.1.** Relapse rate in various surveillance trials in stage I testicular nonseminomas

| Reference | Number of patients | Median follow-up (months) | Relapse rate (%) | Survival (%) |
|---|---|---|---|---|
| HOSKIN et al. (1986) | 126 | 42 | 28 | 99 |
| GELDERMAN et al. (1987) | 54 | 29 | 20 | 98 |
| SWANSON et al. (1987) | 82 | Unknown | 29 | 99 |
| PIZZOCARO et al. (1987) | 85 | 42 | 27 | 99 |
| FREEDMAN et al. (1987) | 259 | 30 | 32 | 98 |
| SOGANI and FAIR (1988) | 102 | 40 | 25 | 97 |
| RAGHAVAN et al. (1988) | 46 | 40 | 28 | 96 |
| RORTH et al. (1991) | 79 | 64 | 30 | 98 |
| READ et al. (1992) | 396 | 60 | 27 | 98 |
| STURGEON et al. (1992) | 105 | 60 | 35 | 99 |
| VAN OOSTEROM et al. (1998) | 139 | 87 | 27 | 99 |
| Total | 1473 | 4–10 years | 29 | 98 |

time of orchiectomy (KLEPP et al. 1990). Although similar data were reported by DONOHUE et al. (1993b), Klepp's results have not been confirmed by the clinical practice of other investigators. In the combined analysis of 11 studies including almost 1500 patients with nonseminoma clinical stage I disease and at least 4 years' follow-up, the median incidence of relapse was 29%. Tumor-related mortality was 2% (Table 25.1). The discrepancy between pathological staging (DONOHUE et al. 1993b; KLEPP et al. 1990) and the observed relapse rate in the published surveillance studies (Table 25.1) (CULLEN and JAMES 1996; PIZZOCARO et al. 1995) could be explained either by inadequate staging in Klepp's patients or by a too short follow-up in several of the clinical reports or simply by a statistical chance.

Despite earlier suggestions to the contrary, surveillance in nonseminomas did not prove to be more expensive than traditional adjuvant treatment (BANIEL et al. 1996). However, some authors stress that surveillance can be troublesome for both the patient and the medical staff. According to early reports, some patients find the process of surveillance stressful. Frequent examinations remind patients of their cancer history and of their continuing risk of relapse (MOYNIHAN 1987). Although recent psychometric investigations have shown that doctors tend to overestimate the degree of psychological distress in patients on the surveillance program (FOSSA et al. 1996b), insufficient patient compliance can become the reason for advanced recurrent disease at the time of detection. This lack of compliance can become a reason for bulky relapse with possible development of drug-resistant clones and subsequent fatal outcome (FOSSA et al. 1996b; HOWARD et al. 1995). A patient should therefore only be admitted into a surveillance program if he agrees to the regular follow-up visits.

## 25.4
## Prognostic Factors

One of the most important advantages of a surveillance program is the "ex juvantibus" identification of the 70% of patients who do not need any other treatment after orchiectomy. Since this is only a theoretical estimation, the most important challenge for this policy is to discover early screening tests for patients with a high risk of relapse. Research has recently been focused on two endpoints: (1) to identify early prognostic factors predictive for present disease dissemination; and (2) to increase the sensitivity and

specificity of the imaging methods that can allow early noninvasive detection of low-volume metastatic disease.

Several retrospective studies have identified histological evidence of vascular or lymphatic invasion in the primary tumor as a predictor of either relapse or occult nodal involvement in patients with clinical stage I disease (CS1) (KLEPP et al. 1990; HOSKIN et al. 1986; MEAD et al. 1992; JACOBSEN et al. 1990). The Testicular Intergroup Study observed venous or lymphatic invasion in 24% and 9% of CS1 specimens, respectively. Relapse was seen in 6% of patients who demonstrated no vascular invasion and in 19% of those with vascular invasion (SESTERHENN et al. 1992). The presence of embryonal carcinoma elements was reported to be the second most important prognostic factor in early stage nonseminoma disease (SESTERHENN et al. 1992; WISHNOW et al. 1989). One of the largest Medical Research Council (MRC) trials of surveillance in 259 patients resulted in a prognostic model based on the following parameters: (1) tumor vascular invasion, (2) presence of embryonal cell carcinoma, and (3) absence of yolk sac tumor. The presence of these parameters identifies a high-risk group of stage I patients with approximately 50% chance of recurrence (FREEDMAN et al. 1987). The following prospective study validated this prognostic index and allowed the identification of patients for whom adjuvant chemotherapy had been offered (READ et al. 1992). In a recently updated prospective European Organization for Research and Treatment of Cancer (EORTC) trial, tumor specimens of 137 patients at surveillance were reassessed by one review pathologist. Out of 16 variables analyzed, invasion of tunica albuginea and the presence of hemorrhage within the tumor were the only important risk factors reported (VAN OOSTEROM 1998). Other proposed prognostic factors were: (1) absence of AFP before orchiectomy (KLEPP et al. 1990; WISHNOW et al. 1989), (2) high T stage (HOSKIN et al. 1986), and (3) recently discovered tumor proliferative activity measured by a high level of MIB-1 antibody (ALBERS et al. 1997).

Computed tomography and magnetic resonance imaging (MRI) are not able to differentiate between malignant and nonmalignant tissue. Positron emission tomography (PET), a new imaging technique based on quantification of glucose uptake in tumors and normal tissue, can help to identify tumor and differentiate it from the normal tissue (STRAUSS and CONTI 1991). Early results of studies confirmed a superior positive predictive value and accuracy of PET as compared to CT in the diagnosis of testicular cancer. However, PET scan was not able to detect micrometastases and thus at this preliminary level of investigation does not represent an alternative to a surgical diagnostic approach, if one believes that such an approach is indeed necessary (BENDER et al. 1997; NUUTINEN et al. 1997).

## 25.5
## Risk-Related Surveillance Policy

Risk-related surveillance policy (RRSP) is a multimodal treatment strategy based on inclusion of all stage I testicular cancer patients in the surveillance program, except those with a high risk of relapse. The latter patients should be treated with adjuvant chemotherapy. The experience of several centers has validated this new treatment approach. In the MRC adjuvant chemotherapy study two cycles of BEP chemotherapy were given to high-risk stage I nonseminoma testicular cancer patients. High-risk patients were identified by the use of the study's own prognostic model (FREEDMAN et al. 1987). Two of 114 patients relapsed and one died with chemotherapy-resistant tumor. The median follow-up time was 4 years (CULLEN et al. 1996). In a similar series of the Warsaw Group, 70 patients with vascular invasion or advanced local T stage were treated with two or three cycles of adjuvant BEP or PVB chemotherapy. Seventy-two other, low-risk patients were only kept under surveillance. In the treatment and the surveillance arm, similar relapse rates were noted, at 7% and 5%, respectively . After a median follow-up time of 5 years, an overall survival of 99% was reported (PALUCHOWSKA et al. 1995). PONT et al. (1996) selected 29 patients for adjuvant chemotherapy on the basis of presence of venous invasion. The median follow-up was 79 months. Two of the 29 patients relapsed and one tumor-related death was reported. OLIVER et al. (1992) entered 22 patients into their pilot study of adjuvant chemotherapy. In patients in whom a maximum of only two MRC risk factors (recurrence risk <25%) were present, the authors observed only a single relapse (OLIVER et al. 1992). STUDER et al. (1993) selected 43 patients for adjuvant treatment based on the presence of vascular invasion, stage pT > 1, and the presence of embryonal cancer in the primary tumor specimen. One relapse occurred in this study and the patient was cured by second-line chemotherapy treatment.

The value of RRSP needs further confirmation in randomized trials; however, the results of the mentioned studies suggest that with RRSP or adjuvant chemotherapy, similarly high rates of cure in stage I nonseminoma can be obtained. The overall recurrence rate of <10% in RRSP is comparable with the best results of adjuvant chemotherapy or RPLND alone, while the risk of treatment side-effects is restricted only to the small group of patients at high risk of relapse or with a subsequent relapse. In RRSP, cisplatin-based therapy remains the adjuvant therapy of choice because of its high response rate in relapsed disease.

## 25.6
## Surveillance as a Management Option for Seminoma

Radiotherapy has been considered the standard adjuvant treatment of early stage seminomas for the last 30 years. The exceptional radiosensitivity of the tumor results in universally high cure rate, relatively low costs, and acceptable acute treatment toxicity (DOSMANN et al. 1993; HANKS et al. 1992). The relapses observed in 2%–9% of patients, however, are almost always systemic, and a 1%–2% disease-related death rate has been noted (FOSSA et al. 1989, 1996a; HANKS et al. 1992; CULLEN and JAMES 1996). The list of reported side-effects include: (1) common nausea, (2) peptic ulcers, and (3) oligospermia; long-term sequelae in this relatively young population included the increased risk of carcinogenesis (HANKS et al. 1992; VAN LEEUWEN et al. 1993; SCHOVER et al. 1986). After several preliminary reports, this was confirmed in a large epidemiological study, where this type of radiotherapy was found to be associated with an excess incidence of cancers of the stomach, bladder, and pancreas (CHOW et al. 1997).

Since the 1970s seminomas have also been proved to be sensitive to chemotherapy (HORWICH and DEARNALEY 1992; MOTZER et al. 1988; PAWINSKI et al. 1992). However, in the treatment of patients with no parent tumor, only a low toxic regimen can be accepted as a good alternative for radiotherapy. Carboplatin, introduced by OLIVER et al. in 1990, seems a new option for adjuvant treatment for stage I seminoma. In 300 patients treated in several pilot studies with one or two courses of adjuvant carboplatin only four relapses were seen (DIECKMANN et al. 1996; OLIVER et al. 1996; KRATZIK et al. 1993). A single outpatient visit for a short infusion of the drug, with low immediate and apparently no late toxicity, makes carboplatin a very attractive alternative to radiotherapy. The results of a phase III study (radiotherapy vs single cycle carboplatin) will be available soon (CULLEN and JAMES 1996).

The relapse rate of early stage seminomas is lower than in nonseminoma (NS) patients, in whom the surveillance programs have already proved to be effective. Review of the literature shows that as many as 83% stage I seminoma patients do not need additional treatment after orchiectomy (Table 25.2). Moreover, the predominant pattern of relapse after surveillance is within para-aortic lymph nodes. Subsequent salvage local or systemic therapy results in cause-specific survival rates identical to those obtained with conventional radiotherapy (WARDE et al. 1995; HORWICH et al. 1992; VON DER MAASE et al. 1993). In a Canadian study based on 364 patients treated with adjuvant radiotherapy or managed by surveillance, 6% and 16% of patients relapsed, respectively. Overall cause-specific survival rate for all patients was 99.7% (WARDE et al. 1995). In 103 patients of the Royal Marsden Hospital study, no patient died within a median follow-up of 62 months (HORWICH et al. 1992). Similar results were reported by other authors (MADEJ and PAWINSKI 1991a; VON DER MAASE et al. 1993; ALLHOFF et al. 1991).

Surveillance in seminoma is, however, a less convenient treatment policy than in nonseminoma. In spite of a higher relapse rate in nonseminoma, 80% of the recurrences appear in the first 12 months after orchiectomy, while the same relapse rate in seminomas can be detected only after 3–4 years (READ et al. 1992; WARDE et al. 1995; VON DER MAASE et al. 1993; RORTH et al. 1991). This, together with the lack of a sensitive and specific serum marker to facilitate early relapse detection, necessitate a longer and close follow-up program, which generates more medical and patient attention than after adjuvant treatment. In a recent study by SHARDA et al.(1996), surveillance was also reported to be significantly more expensive than adjuvant radiotherapy. This calculation was largely dependent on the design of the follow-up program. The maximum cost difference between the two treatment arms occurs at 5 years with the cost equivalence point at 2.5 years following orchiectomy. The main criticism of this study is that the risk of radiation-induced carcinogenesis or inhibition of spermatogenesis was not included in the model (SHARDA et al. 1996).

Since identification of a risk group within an almost nonrelapsing population of irradiated patients is very difficult, the lack of reliable prognostic factors becomes an important weakness of the surveillance policy in seminomas. Among the few proposed, and not yet validated factors are tumor type (anaplastic), tumor size (>6 cm) (VON DER MAASE et al. 1993), vascular invasion (HORWICH et al. 1992), and patient age (WARDE et al. 1995). The only known data on risk-related treatment policy in seminomas were reported by the Warsaw group. Vascular invasion, tumor type (anaplastic vs typical), and >T1 stage were considered as risk factors. Eighty-six patients at risk for recurrence received two adjuvant cycles of BEP/PVB, while 74 other patients were kept under surveillance. In this study only ten relapses were observed (6%): one (1%) after chemotherapy and nine (12%) under surveillance. The median follow-up was 44 months with a range of 1–120 months. In nine patients the relapse was locoregional and in one patient concomitant lung metastases were observed. The only disease-related death in the surveillance group was reported for a patient with a concomitant hepatic cirrhosis, for whom the administration of the full-dose salvage systemic treatment was contraindicated (MADEJ et al., unpublished work).

The above results suggest that RRSP may become the third management option in the treatment of seminoma. Moreover, further decrease in the relapse rate should be possible, provided by a successful application of more efficient prognostic models. Again, however, the possible advantage of this new management policy over any other method discussed above needs confirmation in randomized trials.

**Table 25.2.** Relapse rate in various surveillance trials in stage I testicular seminomas

| Reference | Number of patients | Median follow-up (months) | Relapse rate (%) | Survival (%) |
|---|---|---|---|---|
| ALLHOFF et al. (1991) | 33 | 48 | 11 | 100 |
| HORWICH et al. (1992) | 103 | 62 | 16 | 100 |
| VON DER MAASE (1993) | 261 | 48 | 19 | 98 |
| WARDE et al. (1995) | 172 | 60 | 16 | 98 |
| Total | 569 | 4–10 years | 17 | 99 |

## 25.7
## Ethical Issues in Surveillance

The decision to give adjuvant therapy in the treatment programs was usually based on the risk of recurrence, since tumor relapse was inevitably associated with a worsening of prognosis. Due to the important progress in treatment options, the relapse itself is no longer a real threat to survival for patients with early stage testicular cancer. Regarding both seminomas and nonseminomas, only a few patients died in the entire group of 2000 investigated patients. The most often reported cause of death was resistance of the tumor to chemotherapy. This definitively changes the future scope on treatment strategy. The surveillance policy is focused on two main objectives: (1) to identify relapsing patients at the earliest possible level of tumor development; and (2) to save all active treatment modalities until they become necessary. However, these endpoints need professional organization of a follow-up program in which patient compliance and close cooperation with the general practitioner are mandatory. None of the discussed treatment methods can guarantee 100% curability, since patients can suffer or die because of either treatment toxicity or refractory relapsed disease. Thus the option of adjuvant treatment for all stage I testicular cancer patients may not be accepted by everyone. Given that it is impossible to weigh any individual, cancer- or treatment-related death against the quality of life of others, and since patient compliance is a crucial determinant for successful outcome, the final decision as to the most acceptable price for the patient's cure should in large part be made by the patient himself. An important role of the physician in this optional treatment program is to provide the patient with complete and understandable information on the treatment methods and possible threats, stressing at the same time the necessity of his close compliance.

## 25.8
## Conclusions

Surveillance policy in the management of stage I germ cell tumors is becoming an important alternative to the standard local and systemic adjuvant programs. In the treatment of nonseminomas, surveillance policy is attractive for patients with a low risk of relapse, saving unnecessary harmful medication for the majority of these patients. For stage I seminomas, risk-related surveillance policy may become (together with the classical radiotherapy and low toxicity chemotherapy) the third treatment option, however, definitive confirmation of its role needs final validation in randomized trials.

Since 100% curability is the main objective of surveillance policy, a professionally designed, optimal follow-up program that is able to assure full patient compliance is mandatory. Investigations with respect to this optimal program are being defined in current trials and their results are awaited.

## References

Albers P, Bierhoff E, Neu D, Fimmers R, Wernert N, Muller SC (1997) MIB-1 immunochemistry in clinical stage I nonseminomatous testicular germ cell tumors predicts patients at low risk for metastasis. Cancer 79:1710–1716

Allhoff EP, Liedke S, de Riese W, Stief C, Schneider B (1991) Stage I seminoma of the testis. Adjuvant radiotherapy or surveillance. Br J Urol 68:190–194

Baniel J, Roth BJ, Foster RS, Donohue JP (1996) Cost- and risk-benefit considerations in the management of clinical stage I nonseminomatous testicular tumors. Ann Surg Oncol 3:86–93

Bender H, Schomburg A, Albers P, Ruhlmann J, Biersack H-J (1997) Possible role of FDG-PET in the evaluation of urologic malignancies. Anticancer Res 17:1655–1660

Bokemeyer C, Kuczyk MA, Serth J, Hartmann JT, Schmoll HJ, Jonas U, Kanz L (1996) Treatment of clinical stage I testicular cancer and a possible role for new biological prognostic parameters. J Cancer Res Clin Oncol 122:575–584

Bosl GJ, Motzer RJ (1997) Testicular germ-cell cancer. N Engl J Med 337:242–253

Bosl GJ, Bajorin D, Sheinfeld J, Motzer R (1997) Cancer of the testis. In: De Vita VT, Hellman S, Rosenberg SA (eds) Cancer: principles and practice of oncology. 5th edn. Lippincott-Raven, Philadelphia, pp 1397–1425

Carter SK (1983) The management of testicular cancer. Recent Results Cancer Res 85:70–97

Chow WH, Lindblad P, Gridley G, et al. (1997) Risk of second malignant neoplasms among long-term survivors of testicular cancer. J Natl Cancer Inst 89:1429–1439

Cullen MH (1996) Management of stage I non-seminoma: surveillance and chemotherapy. In: Horwich A (ed) Testicular cancer: investigation and management. Chapman and Hall Medical, London, pp 149–166

Cullen M, James N (1996) Adjuvant therapy for stage I testicular cancer. Cancer Treat Rev 22:253–264

Cullen MH, Stenning SP, Parkinson MC, et al. (1996) Short-course adjuvant chemotherapy in high-risk stage I nonseminomatous germ cell tumors of the testis: a MRC report. J Clin Oncol 14:1106–1113

Dieckmann KP, Krain J, Kuster J, Bruggeboes B (1996) Adjuvant carboplatin treatment for seminoma clinical stage I. J Cancer Res Clin Oncol 122:63–66

Donohue JP (1987) Controversies in testis cancer management. In: Kernion J, Paulson D. Genitourinary cancer management. Lea & Febiger, Philadelphia, pp 161–186

Donohue JP, Thornhill JA, Foster RS, Rowland RG, Bihrle R (1993a) Primary retroperitoneal lymph node dissection in clinical stage A non-seminomatous germ cell testis cancer: review of the Indiana University experience. Br J Urol 71:326–335

Donohue JP, Thornhill JA, Foster RS, Rowland RG, Bihrle R (1993b) Retroperitoneal lymphadenectomy for clinical stage A testis cancer: modifications of technique and impact on ejaculation. J Urol 149:237–243

Dosmann MA, Gunar K, Zagars MD (1993) Postorchiectomy radiotherapy for stage I and II testicular seminoma. Int J Radiat Oncol Biol Phys. 26:381–390

Fossa SD, Horwich AH (1989) The staging and treatment of testicular cancer: management of stage I disease. In: Smith PH (ed) Combination therapy in urological malignancy. Springer, London Berlin Heidelberg New York, pp 173–189

Fossa SD, Aass N, Kaalhus O (1989) Radiotherapy for testicular seminoma stage I: Treatment results and long term post-irradiation morbidity in 365 patients. Int J Radiat Oncol Biol Phys 16:383–388

Fossa S, Horwich A, Russell J, Roberts JP, Jakes R, Stenning S (1996a) Optimal field size in adjuvant radiotherapy of stage I seminoma – a randomized trial. Proc Am Soc Clin Oncol 15:239

Fossa SD, Moynihan C, Serbuti S (1996b) Patients' and doctors' perception of long-term morbidity in patients with testicular cancer clinical stage I. Support Care Cancer 4:118–128

Foster RS, Donohue JP (1992) Surgical treatment of clinical stage I nonseminomatous testis cancer. Semin Oncol 19:166–170

Freedman LS, Parkinson MC, Jones WG, et al. (1987) Histopathology in the prediction of relapse of patients with stage I testicular teratoma treated by orchiectomy alone. Lancet II:294–298

Gelderman WAH, Schraffordt Koops H, Sleijfer DT (1987) Orchiectomy alone in stage I nonseminomatous testicular germ cell tumours. Cancer 59:578–580

Hamilton C, Horwich A, Easton D, Peckham MJ (1986) Radiotherapy for stage I seminoma testis: results of treatment and complications. Radiother Oncol 6:115–120

Hanks GE, Peters T, Owen J (1992) Seminoma of the testis: long term beneficial and deleterious results of radiation. Int J Radiat Oncol Biol Phys 24:913–919

Horwich A, Dearnaley DP (1992) Treatment of seminoma. Semin. Oncol. 19:171–183

Horwich A, Alsanjari N, Hern RA, Nicholls J, Dearnaley DP, Fisher C (1992) Surveillance following orchiectomy for stage I testicular seminoma. Br J Cancer 65:775–778

Hoskin P, Dilly S, Easton D, Horwich A, Hendry W, Peckham MJ (1986) Prognostic factors in stage I non-seminomatous germ-cell testicular tumors managed by orchiectomy and surveillance: implications for adjuvant chemotherapy. J Clin Oncol 4:1031–1036

Howard GCW, Clarke K, Elia MH (1995) A Scottish National Audit of current patterns of management for patients with testicular non-semiomatous germ cell tumors. Br J Cancer 72:1303–1306

Jacobsen GK, Rorth M, Osterlind K (1990) Histopathological features in stage I non-seminomatous testicular germ cell tumors correlated to relapse. APMIS 98:377

Klepp O, Olsson AM, Henrikson H, et al. (1990) Prognostic factors in clinical stage I nonseminomatous germ cell tumors of the testis: multivariate analysis of a prospective multicenter study. J Clin Oncol 8:509–518

Kratzik C, Kuhrer I, Wiltsche C, Amman G (1993) Carboplatin-monotherapie bei Seminomen in Stadium I. Acta Chir Aust 25:27–28

Madej G, Pawinski A (1991a) Risk-related adjuvant chemotherapy for stage I non-seminoma of the testis. Clin Oncol R Coll Radiol 3:270–272

Madej G, Pawinski A (1991b) Preliminary evaluation of prognostic factors in selecting the methods of treatment of patients with stage I testicular seminoma. Nowotwory 40:181–185

Maier JG, Sulak MH (1973) Radiation therapy in malignant testis tumors. Part II Carcinoma. Cancer 32:1217–1226

McLeod DG, Weiss RB, Stablein DM, et al. (1991) Staging relationships and outcome in early stage testicular cancer: a report from the TCIG. J Urol 145:1178–1183

Mead GM, Stenning SP, Parkinson MC (1992) The second MRC study of prognostic factors in nonseminomatous germ cell tumors. J Clin Oncol 10:85–88

Motzer RJ, Bosl GJ, Geller NL (1988) Advanced seminoma. The role of chemotherapy. and adjunctive surgery. Ann Intern Med 108:513–521

Moynihan C (1987) Testicular cancer: the psychosocial problems of patients and their relatives. Cancer Surv 6:478–510

Nichols CR, Roth BJ, Einhorn LH (1992) Managing testicular cancer. Contemp. Oncol May/June: 13

Nuutinen JM, Leskinen S, Elomaa I, et al. (1997) Detection of residual tumors in postchemotherapy testicular cancer by FDG-PET. Eur J Cancer 33: 1234–1241

Oliver RTD, Love S, Ong J (1990) Alternatives to radiotherapy in the management of seminoma. Br J Urol 65:61–67

Oliver RTD, Ong J, Blandy JP, Altman DG (1996) Testis conservation studies in germ cell cancer justified by improved primary chemotherapy response and reduced delay, 1978–1994. Br J Urol 78:119–124

Oliver RTD, Raja MA, Ong J, Gallagher CJ (1992) Pilot study to evaluate impact of a policy of adjuvant chemotherapy for high risk stage I malignant teratoma on overall relapse rate of stage 1 cancer patients. J Urol 148:1453–1456

Paluchowska B, Madej G, Wiechno P, et al. (1995) Adjuvant chemotherapy dependent on the presence of risk factors in a non-seminomatous testicular tumors of a clinical stage I. Urologia Pol. 3A Suppl: 117

Pawinski A, Madej G, Gajl D (1992) Evaluation of the results of combined treatment of patients with testicular seminoma in the II stage of clinical advancement. Pol Tyg Lek 47:540–541

Peckham MJ, McElwain TJ (1974) Radiotherapy of testicular tumors. Proc R Soc Med 67:400–404

Peckham MJ, Barret A, Husband JE, Hendry WF (1982) Orchiectomy alone in testicular stage I non-seminomatous germ cell tumors. Lancet II:678–680

Pizzocaro G, Zanoni F, Salvioni R, Milani A, Piva L, Pilotti S (1987) Difficulties of a surveillance study omitting retroperitoneal lymphadenectomy in clinical stage I nonseminomatous germ cell tumors of the testis. J Urol 138: 1393–1395

Pizzocaro G, Salvioni R, Nicolai N (1995) The role of adjuvant treatment in low-stage germ cell testicular tumors. Eur Urol 28:267–272

Pont J, Holtl W, Kosak D, Machacek E, Kienzer H, Julcher H, Honetz N (1990) Risk adapted treatment choice in stage I nonseminomatous testicular germ cell cancer by regarding vascular invasion in the primary tumor. J Clin Oncol 8:16–19

Pont J, Albrecht W, Postner G, Sellner F, Angel K, Holtl W (1996) Adjuvant chemotherapy for high risk clinical stage I nonseminomatous testicular germ cell cancer: long term results of a prospective trial. J Clin Oncol 14:441–448

Raghavan D, Colls B, Levi J (1988) Surveillance for stage I nonseminomatous germ cell tumors of the testis: the optimal protocol has not yet been difined. Br J Urol 61:522–526

Read G, Stenning SP, Cullen MH, Parkinson MC, Horwich A, Kaye SB, Cook PA (1992) MRC prospective study of surveillance for stage I testicular teratoma. J Clin Oncol 10:1762–1768

Richie JP (1990) Clinical stage 1 testicular cancer: the role of modified retroperitoneal lymphadenectomy. J Urol 144: 1160–1163

Rorth M (1992) Therapeutic alternatives in clinical stage I nonseminomatous disease. Semin Oncol 19:190–198

Rorth M, Krag Jacobsen G, von der Maase H, Madsen EL, Nielsen OS, Pedersen M, Schultz H (1991) Surveillance alone versus radiotherapy after orchiectomy for clinical stage I nonseminomatous testicular cancer. J Clin Oncol 9:1543–1548

Schover LR, Gonzales M, von Eschenbach A (1986) Sexual and marital relationships after radiotherapy for seminoma. Urology 27:117–123

Sesterhenn IA, Weiss RB, Mostofi FK, et al. (1992) Prognosis and other clinical correlates of pathologic review in stage I and II testicular carcinoma: a report from the TCIS. J Clin Oncol 10:69–78

Sharda NN, Kinsella TJ, Ritter MA (1996) Adjuvant radiation versus observation: a cost analysis of alternate management schemes in early-stage testicular seminoma. J Clin Oncol 14:2933–2939

Small E, Torti FM (1995) Testes. Management of low stage disease. In: Abeloff MD, Armitage JO, Lichter AS, Niederhuber JE (eds) Clinical oncology. Churchill Livingstone, New York, pp 1504–1511

Sogani PC, Fair WR (1988) Surveillance alone in the treatment of clinical stage I nonseminomatous germ cell tumor of the testis. Semin Urol 6:53–56

Strauss LG, Conti PS (1991) The applications of PET in clinical oncology. J Nucl Med 32:623–648

Stuart NSA, Woodroffe CM, Grundy R, Cullen MH (1990) Long term toxicity of chemotherapy for testicular cancer – the cost of cure. Br J Cancer 61:479–484

Studer UE, Fey MF, Calderoni A, Kraft R, Mazzucchelli L, Sontag RW (1993) Adjuvant chemotherapy after orchiectomy in high risk patients with clinical stage I nonseminomatous testicular cancer. Eur Urol 23:444–449

Sturgeon JFG, Jewett MAS, Alison RE, et al. (1992) Surveillance after orchiectomy for patients with clinical stage I nonseminomatous testis tumors. J Clin Oncol 10:564–568

Swanson D, Johnson D, von Eschenbach A (1987) Five years experience with orchiectomy of clinical stage I nonseminomatous germ cell testicular tumors. J Urol 137:211A

van Leeuwen FE, Stiggelbout AM, van den Belt-Dusebout AW, et al. (1993) Second cancer risk following testicular cancer: a follow-up study of 1909 patients. J Clin Oncol 11:415–424

Van Oosterom A, Neijt JP, Theodore C, Keizer HJ, Ten Bokkel Huinink W, Collette L (1998) Management of stage I nonseminomatous testicular cancer with unilateral orchidectomy alone. Eur J Cancer (to be published)

Von der Maase H, Specht L, Jacobsen GK, et al. (1993) Surveillance following orchiectomy for stage I seminoma of the testis. Eur J Cancer 29A:1931–1934

Warde P, Gospodarowicz MK, Panzarella T, et al. (1995) Stage I testicular seminoma: results of adjuvant irradiation and surveillance. J Clin Oncol 13:2255–2262

Whitmore WF (1979) Surgical treatment of adult germ cell tumors. Semin Oncol 6: 55–69

Williams SD, Stablein DM, Einhorn LH, et al. (1987) Immediate adjuvant chemotherapy vs. observation with treatment at relapse in pathologic stage II testicular cancer. N Engl J Med 317:1433–1436

Wishnow KI, Johnson DE, Dunphy CH, et al. (1989) Identifying patients with low-risk clinical stage I nonseminomatous testicular tumors who should be treated by surveillance. Urology XXXIV:339–343

# 26 Fertility Following Treatment of Testicular Carcinoma

D.J.M.K. DE RIDDER and L. BAERT

CONTENTS



## 26.1
## Introduction

Testicular cancer usually occurs in young men, many of whom have not yet established a family at the time at which the diagnosis of cancer is made. Most of the tumors are germ cell tumors, which are highly curable with surgery, radiotherapy, chemotherapy, or multimodality treatment. The primary goal for urologists, radiotherapists, and medical oncologists is, of course, to cure the patient. Despite the obvious stress to the patient caused by the news of a diagnosis of testicular cancer, one must take time to discuss the fertility issues with the patient. Unlike Hodgkin's disease, which also affects young men of reproductive age and is highly curable, testicular cancer involves an organ intrinsically linked with fertility, sexuality, and self-image (see Chap. 36). RIEKER et

al. (1990) showed that there were different fertility-related behaviors in these patients. Young childless patients without a stable relationship were more interested in sperm banking, while men who also lost their ejaculatory function after treatment had the greatest risk of continued distress regarding infertility. RIEKER et al. showed that adjustment to infertility is a complex process that begins at diagnosis and extends long after treatment has been completed.

## 26.2
## Pretreatment Fertility

Most authors agree that the fertility potential of patients with testicular cancer is already diminished at the time of diagnosis. Although there are some methodological problems in assessing the fertility potential at the time of diagnosis, 15%–50% of all patients will have oligoasthenospermia (FOSTER et al. 1994; PRESTI et al. 1993). Stress related to the diagnosis of carcinoma may be one influencing factor, but other organic mechanisms are probably of greater importance.

### 26.2.1
### Sperm Abnormalities Before Treatment

The most obvious changes in sperm characteristics are a decreased concentration and impaired motility. The literature data are summarized in Table 26.1. These changes do not seem to be permanent in all patients since recovery of sperm parameters has been described (CARROLL et al. 1987; FOSSA et al. 1990; HANSEN P.V. et al. 1990). Methodologically there are some points that need to be addressed when interpreting these results. First of all there is the natural variance in the sperm concentration depending on a number of factors. Secondly, these sperm samples have been delivered in a very stressful situation, which in itself can already have an effect on sperm quality (BELL and ALDER 1994).

D.J.M.K. DE RIDDER, MD, Consultant Urologist, Department of Urology and Fertility Center Leuven, University Hospitals Gasthuisberg, Catholic University of Leuven Herestraat 49, B-3000 Leuven, Belgium
L.V. BAERT, MD, PhD, Chairman, Department of Urology, University Hospitals Gasthuisberg, Catholic University of Leuven Herestraat 49, B-3000 Leuven, Belgium

**Table 26.1.** Incidence of oligospermia (<20 million/ml) in patients with testicular cancer

| Authors | Year of publication | No. of patients | % oligo spermia |
|---|---|---|---|
| THACIL et al. | 1981 | 42 | 52% |
| DRASGA et al. | 1983 | 30 | 77% |
| JEWETT et al. | 1983 | 86 | 27% |
| WEISSBACH et al. | 1985 | 76 | 51% |
| FRITZ and WEISSBACH | 1985 | 36 | 17% |
| NIJMAN et al. | 1987 | 25 | 72% |
| CARROLL et al. | 1987 | 15 | 60% |
| HORWICH et al. | 1988 | 97 | 48% |
| HANSEN et al. | 1989 | 97 | 53% |
| FOSSA et al. | 1989b | 147 | 69% |
| FOSTER et al. | 1994 | 51 | 45% |

Thirdly, usually only one sample has been evaluated, whereas in modern spermiology study of multiple samples is preferred (MORTIMER 1994). Moreover there is well-documented and important variation in the laboratory skills of people examining these samples, which can lead to differences in the reported sperm concentrations and morphology. Data on more elaborate sperm studies are rarely reported. FOSTER et al. (1994) found that DNA histograms were normal in 33 out of 35 men with testicular cancer when compared to a control group. HANSEN S.W. et al. (1990) showed that the penetration capacity of spermatozoa was preserved even after chemotherapy. Data on other tests such as fructose contents and capacitation potential are not yet available for routine use but could give better insight into the sperm abnormalities encountered in these patients.

## 26.2.2
### The Role of Endocrine Dysfunction

Testicular tumors can be endocrinologically active. Alterations in the levels of the following are the most common changes found in the sera of these patients: (1) $\alpha$-fetoprotein (AFP), (2) $\beta$-human chorionic gonadotropin ($\beta$HCG), (3) luteinizing hormone (LH), (4) follicle-stimulating hormone (FSH), (5) estrogen, and (6) testosterone. Obviously these observations usually refer to nonseminoma tumors. The role of $\beta$HCG in altering the fertility potential was recognized during the 1980s by several investigators (BERTHELSEN and SKAKKEBAEK 1983; NIJMAN et al. 1987), although the exact mechanism of action was initially unclear. MORRISH et al. (1990) published a

well-designed study on this subject. These authors found elevated concentrations of total serum estradiol and serum estradiol not bound to sex hormone binding globulin, impaired spermatogenesis and sperm motility, and a blocking of multiple enzymes for steroidogenesis in tumor tissue but not in the normal remaining tissue. They concluded that this paracrine-endocrine mechanism in which tumor-produced $\beta$HCG stimulates the production of estradiol by the "normal" testicular tissue but not tumor tissue is responsible for the impaired spermatogenesis. A second source for estradiol is tumor aromatization of dehydroepiandrosterone sulfate to estradiol. Elevated serum levels of estrogens will inhibit the production of FSH and subsequently also result in decreased spermatogenesis (Joos et al. 1993). It is also known that in normal men after $\beta$HCG administration, FSH is decreased, resulting in increased production of inhibin. On the other hand, in patients with high FSH levels before the treatment, FSH seems to be a poor prognostic factor for sperm recovery after treatment (FOSSA et al. 1990).

Concerning the function of the pituitary gland in men with testicular cancer, there are conflicting reports in the literature. Both normal and abnormal concentrations of LH, FSH, and prolactin have been described (CARROL et al. 1987; THACHIL et al. 1981). Dynamic testing showed no impairment of pituitary function and indicated that basal LH elevations were artifacts of the cross-reactivity of the LH assay with HCG (MORRISH et al. 1990). HANSEN S.W. et al. (1989), however, found elevated LH concentrations in patients with normal $\beta$HCG values. In these patients the increased LH is considered a compensatory mechanism for the decreased Leydig cell function (WILLEMSE et al. 1983). The effect of an increased AFP level on spermatogenesis is unknown, although an association between high levels of AFP and decreased spermatogenesis has been described (PRESTI et al. 1993).

## 26.2.3
### Sperm Antibodies

Sperm antibodies are present in about 7% of fertile adult men and about 30% of subfertile men (HÖBARTH et al. 1994). In patients with testicular cancer incidences between 21% and 73% have been reported by PRESTI et al. (1993). Destruction of the testis-blood barrier by the tumor with secondary immune responses is the probable mechanism behind the appearance of these antibodies. In a study by Höbarth et al. (1994), four (18%) of 22 patients with testicular cancer had positive serum antibodies, compared with one (5%) out of 20 patients with normogonadotrophic oligoastheno-teratozoospermia. However, only two patients with testicular cancer had had an abnormal spermiogram.

The role of antisperm antibodies in male infertility remains unclear. With increasing availability of advanced in vitro fertilization techniques such as intracytoplasmic injection, the importance of these antibodies is progressively decreasing.

### 26.2.4
### The Role of the Contralateral Testis

Carcinoma in situ (CIS) of the testis is still the subject of ongoing debate. It is present in the contralateral testis in about 6% of all patients with unilateral testicular cancer (Von der Maase et al. 1986). Since these men have bilateral neoplasia, the local paracrine-endocrine effects can persist after orchiectomy. A persistently increased FSH level posttreatment may identify patients at risk of harboring CIS (Wanderas et al. 1990). It is noteworthy that in the infertile male without cancer, the incidence of CIS is also increased and that, when present, sperm counts are usually lower than in other infertile men (Jorgensen et al. 1990).

### 26.2.5
### Psychological Considerations

The diagnosis and treatment of testicular carcinoma obviously create a lot of stress for the patient and his partner. Not only the oncological aspect is of importance, but also the fertility and sexuality issues. Hemicastration can lead to an altered self-image and a less satisfactory sexuality or relationship subsequently (Presti et al. 1993). The option of a testicular prosthesis may be offered to the patient to alleviate at least partially the effect of hemicastration. The study of Rieker et al. (1990) showed that infertility distress correlates well with the level of education of the patient and with the existence of a relationship at the time of diagnosis. Patients undergoing retroperitoneal lymph node dissection or patients who had lost their ejaculatory function were at higher risk of long-term infertility distress. Some of these patients might benefit from professional counseling.

### 26.2.6
### The Female Factor

Almost all studies on subfertility in relation to testicular cancer lack information on the possible subfertility of the female partner. Paternity and not the spermiogram is still the gold standard for normal fertility. Generally speaking, only about 25% of all cases of infertility are due to male-only factors. In 50% of the cases there is a problem with both partners. To what extent taking into account the female factor would change the data on testicular cancer-related male infertility cannot be objectively evaluated at present. On the other hand, one must be careful in interpreting paternity results, and especially those from fathers with very poor sperm counts, since proof of paternity is usually lacking.

## 26.3
## Fertility After Surgical Treatment

### 26.3.1
### Unilateral Orchiectomy and Fertility

According to Ferreira et al. (1991), orchiectomy in itself leads to a considerable decrease in fertility potential regardless of the reason for which it is performed. In this study semen analysis was performed in 54 men after hemicastration for cryptorchidism, testicular torsion, trauma, or testicular cancer. Between 50% and 57% of these patients had oligospermia, without any significant difference between the individual groups. In testicular cancer, only selected patients with early-stage disease are candidates for a surveillance policy after inguinal orchiectomy. In these patients conflicting results have been published concerning the fertility potential. S.W. Hansen et al. (1990) reported, in nine patients, a mean sperm count of 17 million per ml with a range from 0 to 87 million. Four of the study patients attempted to have a child and two (50%) succeeded. P.V. Hansen et al. (1991) found that three out of nine patients (33%) became fathers after orchiectomy alone. These findings did not differ significantly from those in patients who underwent chemotherapy or radiotherapy. Bar-Chama et al. (1992) reported a very optimistic 84% paternity rate in 19 patients on a surveillance protocol.

### 26.3.2
### Retroperitoneal Lymph Node Dissection and Fertility

Retroperitoneal lymph node dissection (RPLND) is a treatment option for patients with nonseminoma tumors or for seminoma patients with residual mass after chemotherapy (see Chaps. 18 and 19). RPLND has no direct effect on spermatogenesis as far as we know, but can severely impair ejaculatory function. The techniques and boundaries for lymph node dissection have changed (LANGE et al. 1987). Spontaneous return of ejaculation was previously described in 19% (FOSSA et al. 1985) to 92% (GARNICK and RICHIE 1986) of treated patients. More recently nerve-sparing techniques have been introduced (DONOHUE et al. 1990). These nerve-sparing techniques have been successfully used in stage I disease (FOSTER et al. 1994) with preservation of ejaculatory function in 99% and a posttreatment paternity rate of 76%. Moreover, even in patients who underwent this procedure following chemotherapy, ejaculatory function could be preserved in 76.5% with a paternity rate of 16%. In the latter patient group, COOGAN et al. (1996) reported the rate of normal ejaculation to be 73.8% even following bilateral lymph node dissection.

If ejaculation fails to return, sympathomimetic drugs may be tried, although knowledge about use of these drugs in this patient population is merely anecdotal (LANGE et al. 1987). If this therapy fails, electroejaculation is the treatment of choice. In a study of 23 men who had undergone RPLND, seminal emission was successfully achieved in all 23 after electrical stimulation (OHL et al. 1991). Nineteen couples underwent artificial insemination with the electroejaculated sperm, resulting in a 36.8% pregnancy rate for a 9% cycle fecundity.

## 26.4
## Chemotherapy and Fertility

The issue of fertility changes after chemotherapy for germ cell tumors is difficult to assess. First of all there is the intrinsic subfertility related to the tumor itself, as described above. Secondly, improvement of the pretreatment fertility status has been observed after chemotherapy. AASS et al. (1991) reported the pretreatment fertility status to be a more important factor in recovery than the administration of chemotherapy itself.

Chemotherapeutic agents can have an effect on both endocrine and exocrine functions. Alkylating agents seem to have the most profound effect on the fertility potential. Most of the patients undergoing chemotherapy become azoospermic approximately 7–8 weeks after the beginning of treatment. This is in keeping with the kinetics of human spermatogenesis, because the anticancer drugs act mostly on the sperm cells during cell division and thus destroy mainly the rapidly proliferating type B spermatogonia. If all stem cell spermatogonia (type A spermatogonia) survive, spermatogenesis can be expected to recover 12 weeks after treatment (PONT and ALBRECHT 1997).

Cisplatin, which is frequently used in chemotherapy programs for testicular cancer, has proven to be toxic for type A spermatogonia in animal studies (RUSSEL and RUSSEL 1991). Cisplatin itself is not an alkylating agent, but has a similar mechanism of action. If the cumulative dose of cisplatin does not exceed 400 mg (equivalent to four courses of state-of-the-art treatment), chemotherapy is unlikely to cause irreversible damage to fertility. When administered at conventional doses, vinblastine, etoposide, bleomycin, and ifosfamide do not appear to affect long-term fertility. Data for taxanes are not yet available (PONT and ALBRECHT 1997).

Besides a direct effect on spermatogenesis, endocrine abnormalities have also been described. HANSEN S.W. et al. (1990) showed that in some patients there was a persistent elevation of LH and FSH, with a normal or slightly decreased testosterone level, indicative of a subclinical or compensated Leydig cell dysfunction. This observation was confirmed by PALMIERI et al. (1996). BRENNEMANN et al. (1997) looked at the testosterone to LH ratio as a more sensitive marker of the Leydig cell function. This ratio was still abnormal in 31.6% of 232 patients more than 60 months following chemotherapy. The investigators concluded that the partial impairment of testosterone secretion is based upon a primary testicular defect, since persistent higher LH secretion is necessary to allow testosterone secretion. The impact on spermatogenesis is more important with high-dose chemotherapy (PALMIERI et al. 1996). Testicular atrophy of the remaining testicle has been recognized as a poor prognostic factor for recovery (NIJMAN et al. 1987; HANSEN S.W. et al. 1990). FOSSA et al. (1990) showed that oligoasthenozoospermia was transient in at least 50% of patients, except in those with an elevated FSH. PALMIERI et al. (1996) confirmed these findings, but noted that patients with high βHCG levels were more prone to have high FSH levels and a poor sperm concentration. Additionally, these authors also proved the age of the patient to be an important factor. The poor prognostic factors for sperm recovery after chemotherapy and radiotherapy are listed in Table 26.2.

As to the fathering of children, HANSEN P.V. et al. (1991) found that there was no statistical difference between patients under surveillance and those who underwent either chemotherapy or radiotherapy. In addition they concluded that low sperm counts do not differentiate fertile from infertile men. But in their study population 53% of the patients remained infertile after 5 years of follow-up.

There is no evidence of an elevated relative risk of malformations in children fathered by patients with germ cell tumors after chemotherapy, just as there is no increased risk of malignancies in these children (SENTURIA and PECKHAM 1990; MULVIHILL et al. 1987). At one time some authors favored the use of LHRH analogs to temporarily suppress spermatogenesis in order to protect it from the damaging effects of chemotherapy. Despite the interesting theoretical advantages, this approach did not prove to be successful (KREUSER et al. 1993).

**Table 26.2.** Poor prognostic factors for sperm quality recovery during and after adjuvant treatment for testicular cancer

---

*Chemotherapy*
Atrophy of the remaining testicle
Pretreatment azoospermia with FSH >2× upper limit of
  normal
Patient age >25 years
High-dose chemotherapy (>400 mg cumulative dose of
  cisplatin)
High preoperative βHCG levels
Multimodality treatment (radiotherapy and chemotherapy)
Subfertility prior to testicular carcinoma
Contralateral carcinoma in situ

*Radiotherapy*
Inadequate shielding of remaining testis during
  radiotherapy
Radiotherapy on the remaining testis for carcinoma in situ
Multimodality treatment
Low pretreatment sperm count
Patient age >25 years

*Surgery*
Loss of ejaculatory function

---

## 26.5
## Radiotherapy and Fertility

Radiation has a direct effect on spermatogenesis. In healthy males a transient depression of spermatogenesis has been observed after a single dose of radiation (PRESTI et al. 1993). Scatter radiation affecting the remaining testis has been a point of major interest. HANSEN et al. (1990) calculated that about 1.7 Gy (range 1.2–4.1 Gy) reached the remaining unshielded testis. Of the 49 evaluable patients, 20 underwent additional chemotherapy as well. At 2 years after treatment all of the 45 evaluable patients had low sperm counts, and after 8 years of follow-up 82% still had low sperm counts. The investigators performed a regression analysis of sperm recovery and concluded that recovery was dependent on the radiation dose. Adjuvant chemotherapy prolonged the recovery period and it was less successful in patients with initial low sperm counts and in those older than 25 years. FOSSA et al. (1989b) reported that of 53 patients who had gonadal shielding during radiotherapy, only 23% remained infertile after infradiaphragmatic radiation therapy. Gonadal shielding is thus imperative during radiotherapy for testicular carcinoma.

In the presence of carcinoma in situ of the remaining testis, a Sertoli cell-only pattern was described invariably after curative radiotherapy of 20 Gy given in ten equal fractions (GIWERCMAN et al. 1991). Biopsies of the remaining testicle 2 years after the treatment failed to show any recovery (GIWERCMAN et al. 1991).

## 26.6
## Treatment Options

The treatment of ejaculatory dysfunction has already been described. The issue of importance here is whether one should offer sperm banking to patients with germ cell tumors. As mentioned earlier, nearly half of the patients with testicular tumors will have abnormal sperm counts at the time of diagnosis. It is expected that some of these patients will recover and could father children in a natural way (FOSSA et al. 1989a). Such recovery, however, is not always predictable and therefore sperm banking prior to therapy is indicated. Additionally, sperm banking has a strong beneficial psychological effect on the treated patient. Low sperm counts should not preclude patients from having sperm banking. The earlier eligibility criteria of a sperm count of 40 million per ml and 60% motility need to be reconsidered owing to the increasing availability of modern in vitro fertilization techniques such as intracytoplasmic injections (LANGE et al. 1987; SANGER et al. 1992). A recent study used a sperm count of 20 million per ml and 30% motility as the lowest values for cryopreservation, and reported a high incidence of successful insemination and pregnancy (KLIESCH et al. 1996). In patients treated with radiotherapy for Hodgkin's disease even lower sperm counts have resulted in successful in vitro fertilization (TOURNAYE et al. 1991). The management of the infertile noncancer patient is becoming more and more aggressive and at the present time intratesticular sperm or spermatids can be used for intracytoplasmic injections. Even frozen-thawed testicular sperm have been used successfully for in vitro fertilization. This includes sperm obtained from testes with very little spermatogenic activity. In such testes preserved zones of spermatogenesis can be found and sperm successfully obtained and used for in vitro fertilization. This evolution opens new possibilities for patients with severe oligospermia. So far, the use of these options has not been reported in patients with germ cell tumors.

## 26.7
## Conclusion

Fertility changes secondary to testicular cancer are complex and unpredictable. Many factors are involved. Pretreatment fertility seems to be the best, but certainly not a perfect prognostic factor of what the patient might expect after completion of his treatments. Chemotherapy and radiotherapy do allow sperm recovery if applied in a state-of-the-art fashion. Sperm banking should be offered to the patient and the possibility of utilization of modern in vitro fertilization techniques has to be discussed with the patient and his spouse in a realistic way. Investment of adequate time to explain these complex issues to the patient prior to the administration of definitive therapy will ultimately result in a better quality of life for the patient.

## References


Aass N, Fossa SD, Theodorsen L, Norman N (1991) Prediction of long term gonadal toxicity after standard treatment for testicular cancer. Eur J Cancer 27:1087–1091

Baniel J, Roth BJ, Foster RS, Donohue JP (1995) Cost and risk benefit in the management of clinical stage II non-seminomatous testicular tumors. Cancer 75:2897–2903

Bar-Chama N, Herr HW, Sogani PC, et al. (1992) The fertility of males with stage I NSGCT managed on surveillance alone. J Urol 147:337A

Bell JS, Alder EA (1994) Psychology of infertility and management. In: Hargreave TB (ed) Male infertility. Springer, London Berlin Heidelberg New York, pp 177–185

Berthelsen JG, Skakkebaek NE (1983) Gonadal function in men with testis cancer. Fertil Steril 39:68–71

Brennemann W, Stoffel-Wagner B, Helmers A, Mezger J, Jäger N, Klingmüller D (1997) Gonadal function of patients treated with cisplatin based chemotherapy for germ cell cancer. J Urol 158:844–850

Carroll PR, Morse MJ, Whitmore WF Jr, et al. (1987) Fertility status of patients with clinical stage I testis tumors on a surveillance protocol. J Urol 138:70–72

Coogan CL, Hejase MJ, Wahle GR, Foster RS, Rowland RG, Bihrle R, Donohue JP (1996) Nerve sparing post-chemotherapy retroperitoneal lymphnode dissection for advanced testicular cancer. J Urol 156:1656–1658

Donohue JP, Foster RS, Rowland RG, Bihrle R, Jones J, Geier G (1990) Nerve-sparing retroperitoneal lymphadenectomy with preservation of ejaculation. J Urol 144:287–290

Drasga RE, Einhorn LH, Williams SD, et al. (1983) Fertility after chemotherapy for testicular cancer. J Clin Oncol 1:179–183

Ferreira U, Netto NR Jr, Esteves SC, Rivero MA, Schirren C (1991) Comparative study of the fertility potential of men with only one testicle. Scan J Urol Nephrol 25:255–259

Fossa SD, Ous S, Abyholm T, et al. (1985) Post treatment fertility in patients with testicular cancer: influence of retroperitoneal lymph node dissection on ejaculatory potency. Br J Urol 57:204–209

Fossa SD, Aass N, Molne K (1989a) Is routine pretreatment cryopreservation of semen worthwhile in the management of patients with testicular cancer? Br J Urol 64:524–529

Fossa SD, Aass N, Kaalhus O (1989b) Long-term morbidity after infradiaphragmatic radiotherapy in young men with testicular cancer. Cancer 64:404

Fossa SD, Theodorsen L, Norman N, Aabyholm T (1990) Recovery of impaired pretreatment spermatogenesis in testicular cancer. Fertil Steril 54:493–496

Foster RS, Rubin LR, McNulty A, et al. (1991) Detection of antisperm antibodies in patients with primary testicular cancer. Int J Androl 14:179–182

Foster RS, McNulty A, Rubin LR, et al. (1994) The fertility of patients with clinical stage I testis cancer managed by nerve sparing retroperitoneal lymph node dissection. J Urol 152:1139–1143

Fritz K, Weissbach L (1985) Sperm parameters and ejaculation before and after operative treatment of patients with germ-cell testicular cancer. Fertil Steril 43:451–454

Garnick MB, Richie JP (1986) Toward more rational management for stage I testicular cancer. J Clin Oncol 4:1021–1023

Giwercman A, von der Maase H, Berthelsen JG, Rorth M, Bertelsen A, Skakkebaek NE (1991) Localized irradiation of testes with carcinoma in situ: effects on Leydig cell function and eradication of malignant germ cells in 20 patients. J Clin Endocrinol Metab 73:596–603

Hansen PV, Trykker H, Andersen J, Helkjaer PE (1989) Germ cell function and hormonal status in patients with testicular cancer. Cancer 64:956–961

Hansen PV, Trykker H, Svennekjaer IL, Hvolby J (1990) Long-term recovery of spermatogenesis after radiotherapy in patients with testicular cancer. Radiat Oncol 18:117–125

Hansen PV, Glavind K, Panduro J, Pedersen M (1991) Paternity in patients with testicular germ cell cancer: pretreatment and post-treatment findings. Eur J Cancer 27:1385–1389

Hansen SW, Berthelsen JG, von der Maase H (1990) Long-term fertility and Leydig cell function in patients treated for germ cell cancer with cisplatin, vinblastine and bleomycin versus surveillance. J Clin Oncol 8:1695–1698

Höbarth K, Klingler HC, Maier U, Kollaritsch H (1994) Incidence of antisperm antibodies in patients with carcinoma of the testis and in subfertile men with normogonadotropic oligoasthenoteratozoospermia. Urol Int 52:162–165

Horwich A, Nicholls EJ, Hendry WF (1988) Seminal analysis after orchiectomy in stage I teratoma. Br J Urol 62:79

Jarow JP (1994) Life-threatening consitions associated with male infertility. Urol Clin North Am 21:409–415

Jewett MAS, Thachill JV, Harris JF (1983) Exocrine function of testis with germinal testicular tumour. Br Med J 286:1849–1851

Joos H, Chandra I, Frick J (1993) Endokrinologie und Fertilität beim Hodentumor im Stadium I. Helv Chir Acta 60:367–370

Jorgensen N, Müller J, Giwercman A, Skakkebaek NE (1990) Clinical and biological significance of carcinoma in situ of the testis. Cancer Surv 9:287–302

Kliesch S, Behre HM, Jürgens H, Nieschlag E (1996) Cryopreservation of semen from adolescent patients with malignancies. Med Pediatr Oncol 26:20–27

Kreuser ED, Klingmüller D, Thiel E (1993) The role of LHRH analogues in protecting gonadal functions during chemotherapy and irradiation. Eur Urol 23:157–164

Lange PH, Chang WY, Fraley EE (1987) Fertility issues in the therapy in nonseminomatous testicular tumors. Urol Clin North Am 14:731–747

Morrish DW, Venner PM, Siy O, Barrron G, Bhardway D, Outhet D (1990) Mechanisms of endocrine dysfunction in patients with testicular cancer. J Natl Cancer Inst 82:412–418

Mortimer D (1994) Semen analysis and other standard laboratory tests. In: Hargreave TB (ed) Male infertility. Springer, London Berlin Heidelberg New York, pp 37–42

Mulvihill JJ, Meyers MH, Connelly R, et al. (1987) Cancer in offspring of long term survivors of childhood and adolescence cancer. Lancet II:813

Nijman JM, Schraffordt Koops H, Kremer J, et al. (1987) Gonadal function after surgery and chemotherapy in men with stage II and III nonseminomatous testicular tumors. J Clin Oncol 5:651

Ohl DA, Denil J, Bennet CJ, Randolph JF, Menge AC, McCabe M (1991) Electroejaculation following retroperitoneal lymphadenectomy. J Urol 145:980–983

Oliver RTD, Oliver JC (1996) Endocrine hypothesis for declining sperm count and incidence of cancer. Lancet 347:339–340

Palmieri G, Lotrecchiano G, Ricci G, Lombardi G, Bianco AR, Torino G (1996) Gonadal function after multimodality treatment in men with testicular germ cell cancer. Eur J Endocrinol 134:431–436

Pont J, Albrecht W (1997) Fertility after chemotherapy for testicular germ cell cancer. Fertil Steril 68:1–5

Presti JC, Herr HW, Carroll PR (1993) Fertility and testis cancer. Urol Clin North Am 20:173–179

Rieker PP, Fitzgerald EM, Kalish LA (1990) Adaptive behavioral responses to potential infertility among survivors of testis cancer. J Clin Oncol 8:347–355

Russel LD, Russel JA (1991) Short-term morphological response of the rat testis to administration of five chemotherapeutic agents. Am J Anat 192:142–168

Sanger WG, Olson JH, Sherman JK (1992) Semen cryobanking for men with cancer – criteria change. Fertil Steril 58:1024–1027

Senturia YD, Peckham CS (1990) Children fathered by men treated with chemotherapy for testicular cancer. Eur J Cancer 26:429–432

Thachil JW, Jewett MAS, Rider WD (1981) The effects of cancer and cancer therapy on male fertility. J Urol 126:141–145

Tournaye H, Camus M, Bollen N, Wisanto A, Van Steirteghem AC, Devroey P (1991) In vitro fertilization techniques with frozen-thawed sperm: a method for preserving the progenitive potential of Hodgkin patients. Fertil Steril 55:443–445

Von der Maase H, Rorth M, Walbom-Jorgensen S, et al. (1986) Carcinoma in situ of contralateral testis in patients with testicular germ cell cancer: study of 27 cases in 500 patients. BMJ 293:1398–1401

Wanderas EM, Fossa SD, Meilo A, et al. (1990) Serum follicle stimulating hormone: predictive of cancer in the remaining testes in patients with unilateral testicular cancer. Br J Urol 66:315

Weissbach L, Boedefield EA, Oberdorster W (1985) Modified RLND as a means to preserve ejaculation. In: Khoury S, Kuss R, Murphy GP, et al. (eds) Testicular cancer. Liss, New York

Willemse PHB, Sleijfer D, Sluiter WI, et al. (1983) Altered Leydig cell function in patients with testicular cancer: evidence for bilateral testicular defect. Acta Endocrinol 102:616–619

# 27 Testicular Tumors in Prepubertal Boys: Assessment and Treatment

J.A.L.L. BAERT and R.J.M. NIJMAN

CONTENTS



## 27.1 Introduction

As in many subjects of pediatric urology, distinct differences exist between the natural history of testicular tumors in children and adults. The attempt to extrapolate the experience in adults creates confusion in the classification, therapy, and prognosis of testis cancer in children.

Testicular tumors in children represent approximately 1% of all childhood malignancies and occur at an incidence of 0.5–2 per 1 000 000 children. They


J.A.L.L. BAERT, MD, Pediatric Urologist, Beatrix Children's Hospital, University Hospital Groningen, Postbus 3001, 9700 RB Groningen, The Netherlands
R.J.M. NIJMAN, MD, PhD, Head, Department of Pediatric Urology, Sophia Children's Hospital, University Hospital Rotterdam, Postbus 2060, 3000 CB Rotterdam, The Netherlands


are the seventh most common neoplasm in children. The cause of this rare cancer in children remains unclear. Because prepubertal testicular tumors are uncommon, only small series, with the exception of a few multicenter studies, have been reported. This makes valid conclusions difficult to reach and many questions remain unanswered. LI and FRAUMENI (cited in COPPES et al. 1994) have pointed out the extreme rarity of testicular tumors in black and Asiatic children. They suggested that the racial differences as well as the occasional occurrence of familial testis cancer and the rare gonadoblastoma in dysgenetic gonads lead to a genetic predisposition.

Others claim that the incidence of testicular tumors in children under 15 years of age is similar for white and black boys. The frequency of testicular cancer in whites in the United States starts to rise at 15–19 years of age to a peak at 25–29 years of age. There is no corresponding peak for blacks and Japanese. GILBERT and HAMILTON (1940) first pointed out the relationship between cryptorchidism and subsequent development of testicular cancer. He noted orchiopexy may not protect children against development of testicular cancer.

## 27.2 Classification

In morphological terms, testicular tumors are a varied and heterogeneous group of neoplasms. The classification is based on the histological appearance. Separation of testicular tumors into germ cell tumors and nongerm cell tumors, formalized in the classification of the World Health Organization, is now generally used. In children, however, Kaplan proposed a classification of prepubertal testicular tumors, sponsored by the Section of Urology of the American Academy of Pediatrics (COPPES et al. 1994; BROSMAN 1979). This proposed classification is presented in Table 27.1.

**Table 27.1.** Classification of prepubertal testicular tumors (COPPES et al. 1994)

Germ cell tumors
   a) Yolk sac tumor
   b) Teratoma
   c) Seminoma
   d) Mixed germ cell tumor
Gonadal stromal tumors (nongerminal tumors)
   a) Leydig cell
   b) Sertoli cell
   c) Granulosa cell
   d) Mixed gonadal stromal tumor
Gonadoblastoma
Tumors of the supporting tissues
   Fibroma, fibrosarcoma, leiomyoma, leiomyosarcoma,
     hemangioma
Lymphomas and leukemias
Tumor-like lesions
   a) Epidermoid cyst
   b) Hyperplastic nodule secondary to congenital adrenal
     hyperplasia
Secondary tumors
Tumors of the adnexa
   Rhabdomyosarcoma, fibroma, fibrosarcoma, leiomyoma,
     leiomyosarcoma, hemangioma, lipoma

## 27.3
## Diagnosis

Almost 85% of boys with a testicular tumor present with a scrotal painless mass, present for one to several months (Fig. 27.1). Less frequent presenting symptoms are trauma, swelling, and hydrocele formation. The differential diagnosis includes hydrocele, testicular infarction, torsion, mumps orchitis and epididymo-orchitis.

In the neonatal period, a healed stage of meconium peritonitis, which initially presents as a scrotal mass, often turns out to be a diagnostic problem and raises the question of a testicular tumor. There are reports in the literature of such cases leading to unnecessary removal of the testis (FOROUHAR 1982; DAGANY 1975).

In prepubertal children with hormonally active tumors, the diagnosis may be considered due to precocious puberty, even when scrotal examination is unremarkable. The available diagnostic procedures are of limited value. Successful transillumination of the scrotal mass may induce a false sense of security and cause an underlying tumor to be misdiagnosed.

The preoperative evaluation of a child suspected of having a testicular malignancy should include a complete blood count, serum studies of hepatic and renal function, a urinalysis with a microscopic examination of the urine sediment, and determina-

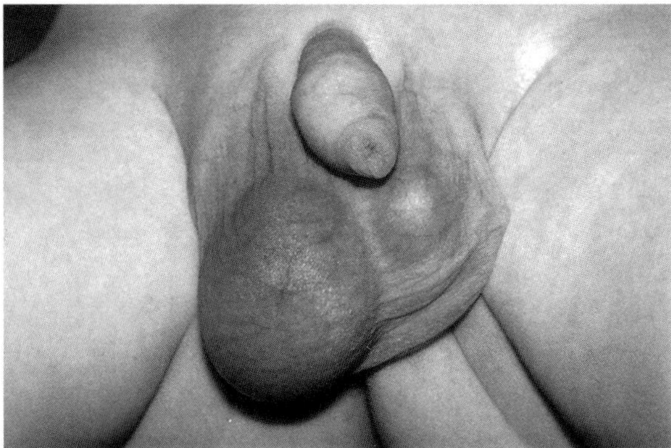

**Fig 27.1.** Typical presentation of a right testicular tumor

tions of α-fetoprotein (AFP) and the β subunit of human chorionic gonadotropin (β-HCG).

The diagnosis of a testicular tumor is established after examination and removal of the testis. Transscrotal ultrasonography can be performed in patients with a scrotal mass to determine the composition and tumor extent. If torsion is suspected, the blood flow should be evaluated. Transscrotal ultrasonography is a simple and noninvasive imaging technique. However, some investigators claim ultrasound studies to be less accurate in delineating a testicular neoplasm, especially in the neonate (LEVY et al. 1994).

The operative procedure is performed through an inguinal incision. At the internal inguinal ring the entire spermatic cord is isolated and cross-clamped by an atraumatic vascular clamp. The testis is mobilized into the inguinal canal and the tumor in the testicular or paratesticular tissue is confirmed. At this level the spermatic cord is divided and ligated at the proximal end (Fig. 27.2). Aspiration of a testicular tumor or a biopsy while the testis is still within the scrotal sac creates local tumor spill and increases the probability of recurrence.

Further studies should be performed once a diagnosis of a testicular tumor is confirmed histologically. Retroperitoneal lymph nodes, lungs, and liver should be evaluated for the presence of metastatic disease. Abdominal and supraclavicular palpation, ultrasonography, computed tomographic (CT) examination of the abdomen and pelvis, and radiographs of the chest are the most important staging procedures. Chest radiographs will detect most lung metastases, but CT of the chest is needed to detect pulmonary lesions smaller than 0.5 cm in diameter.

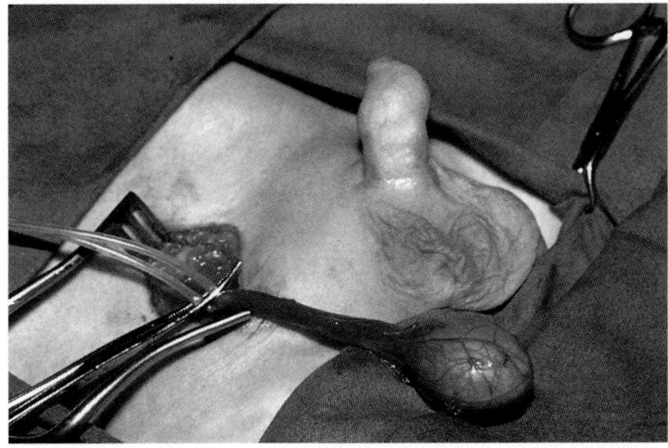

**Fig 27.2.** Inguinal orchiectomy with a clamp applied at the proximal end of the spermatic cord

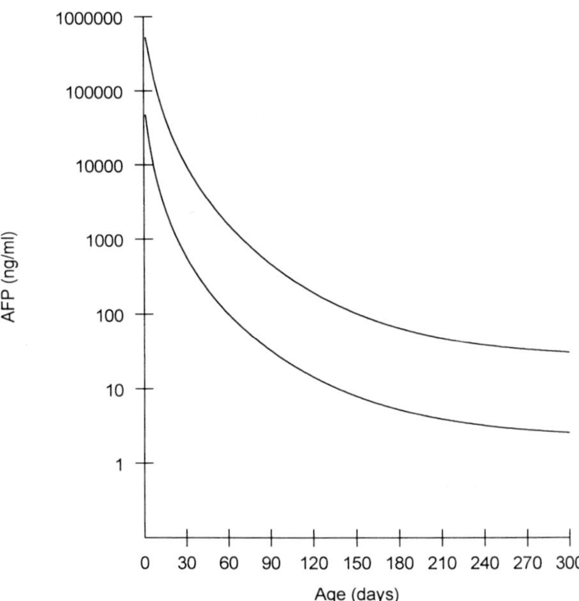



**Fig 27.3.** Normal levels of α-fetoprotein in the first 300 days of life (MASTERSON et al. 1985)

Biochemical parameters play an important role in the evaluation of children with testicular tumors. AFP is a major serum binding protein produced by the fetal yolk sac, the liver, and the gastrointestinal tract. Its half-life is 5 days. In neonates AFP levels are very high and will remain elevated until the age of 8–12 months (Fig. 27.3) (ABLIN 1982). The β subunit of HCG is elevated in all patients who have tumors with trophoblastic components.

## 27.4
## Germ Cell Tumors

Primordial germ cells originate in the yolk sac endoderm and find their way into the developing fetus by the 5th or 6th week of fetal life, through the dorsal artery of the hind gut and then to the urogenital ridge. When these cells or their progeny undergo malignant transformation, tumors occur in the gonadal site for those cells which have reached their target; alternatively, when neoplastic transformation occurs earlier, extragonadal tumors may be the result. Malignant germ cell tumors account for approximately 3% of neoplasms in children.

### 27.4.1
### Yolk Sac Tumors

Of the various types of germ cell tumors, the endodermal sinus tumor is the most common among the pediatric population, and it occurs almost exclusively in children. This tumor was first described by White in 1910. Many synonyms have been used to describe this tumor, including adenocarcinoma of the testis, orchioblastoma, embryonal cell carcinoma, juvenile embryonal cell carcinoma, and endodermal cell tumor of Teilum.

Microscopically, the yolk sac tumor is well recognized. The morphology of the yolk sac tumors is uniform and composed of epithelial, glandular, and mesenchymal elements. The presence of a perivascular Schiller-Duval bodies is the most distinguishing feature. It consists of a labyrinth of interconnecting cavities associated with endodermal sinus structures containing AFP.

#### 27.4.1.1
#### Clinical Course

The peak incidence of this tumor is between the ages of 12 and 24 months. Congenital anomalies including cryptorchidism, inguinal hernia, and hydrocele can occur in association with this tumor. Less than 1% of patients have bilateral involvement at the time of initial presentation.

The presenting level of AFP has not been shown to be a good prognostic sign. However, it is of great concern if the AFP level fails to decrease or normalize after radical orchiectomy. If this is not the case in children older than 1 year of age, the patient is suspected to have metastatic disease and careful workup is obligatory.

### 27.4.1.2
### Staging

Once the histological diagnosis has been established, the patient must be thoroughly staged to exclude the presence of metastatic disease. This staging includes a CT scan of the chest, abdomen, and pelvis. However, none of these studies are completely reliable in detecting metastatic disease. If tumor spread to the bone or brain is suspected, bone scan or CT scan of the brain is indicated. The initial levels of AFP are of major importance in the further follow-up of the disease.

### 27.4.1.3
### Treatment

The management of the yolk sac tumor has become clearer but is still not scientifically proven. Metastatic disease and death are rare in patients with yolk sac tumor.

A treatment protocol and management of patients were outlined by GEARHART and CONNOLLY (1993) (Fig 27.4). Following radical inguinal orchiectomy, adjuvant therapy in stage 1 disease remains controversial, and this is especially true of the role of retroperitoneal lymphadenectomy (RLND). At the time of diagnosis, the tumor is localized in the testis in 80% of the patients. Hematogenous tumor spread is more common than lymphatic involvement. Some authors still propose retroperitoneal lymphadenectomy as a diagnostic and therapeutic procedure, because a few studies have indicated an improved survival rate even when lymph nodes were free of tumor (CONNOLLY and GEARHART 1993).

Major complications of RLND (up to 19%) include: bowel obstruction, intussusception, and chylous ascites. Following bilateral RLND the retroperitoneal and sympathetic nerves that form the superior hypogastric plexus may result in dry or retrograde ejaculation and infertility. Exploration of the retroperitoneum should therefore be reserved to patients with stage 1 disease and persistently elevated or increasing AFP values, a normal CT scan of the chest, and a normal bone scan. Patients older than 2 years of age at diagnosis have a worse prognosis and should also be

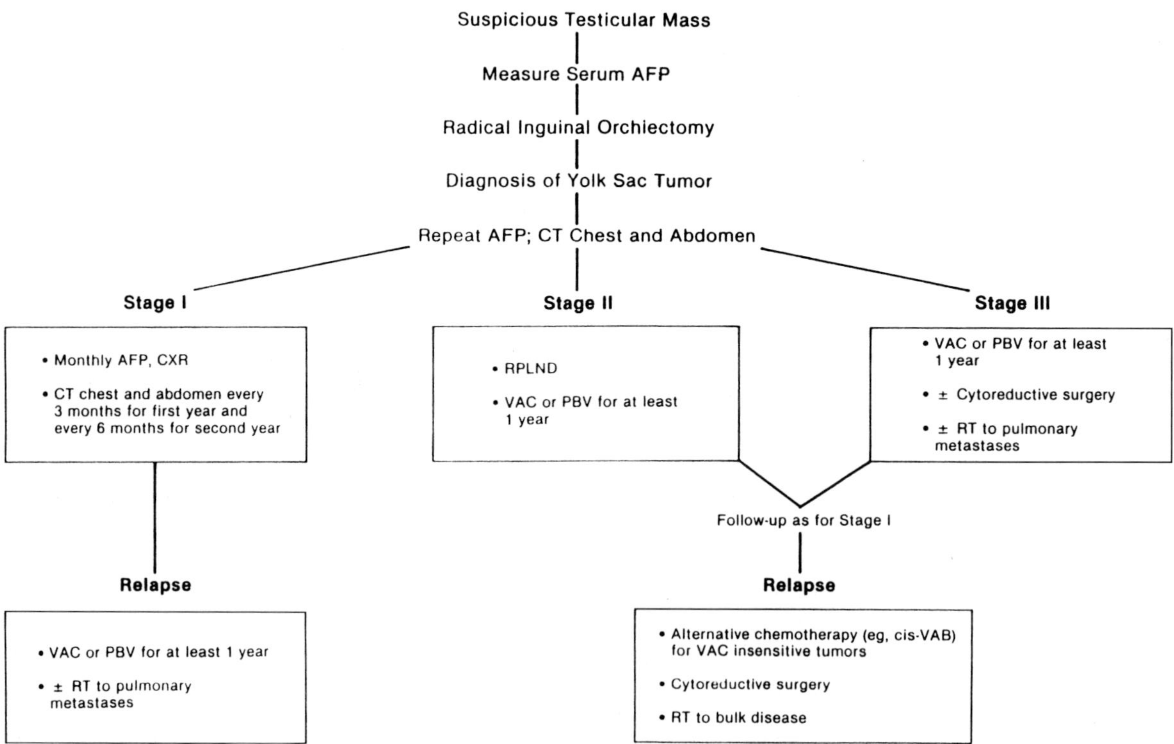



**Fig 27.4.** Schematic representation of the management pathway in pediatric patients with yolk sack tumors

considered for RLND with preservation of the sympathetic nerves.

Prophylactic chemotherapy is considered since metastatic spread is mostly hematogenous.

Chemotherapeutic agents, however, have severe side-effects, and evidence of improved prognosis is lacking in patients with organ-confined disease; accordingly, adjuvant chemotherapy should not be given in stage 1 patients under the age of 1 year. Stage I patients older than 2 years at diagnosis may benefit from the use of adjuvant chemotherapy because their prognosis is generally poor.

All children with stage II and III disease should be treated by combination chemotherapy, consisting of vincristine, dactinomycin, and cyclophosphamide or cisplatin, vinblastine, and bleomycin. At this time there are no clear therapeutic recommendations for the treatment of advanced yolk sac tumors. Patients with advanced yolk sac tumors should be treated in a national clinical protocol(s) to gain better understanding of this rare condition.

### 27.4.1.4
### Prognosis

The prognosis of children with a testicular yolk sac tumor is very good, with an overall reported survival rate of 87%. Testicular yolk sac tumors are mostly organ confined, and metastatic spread is less frequently seen than in adults. Some authors have explained this by the absence of intratubular germ cell neoplasia or carcinoma in situ commonly associated with the adult germ cell tumor of the testis (MANIVEL et al. 1988).

### 27.4.2
### Teratoma

Teratoma is the second most common germ cell tumor in children. It occurs both in children and adults, but in childhood teratoma accounts for approximately 14%–27% of germ cell tumors of the testis. The testis is the third most common site of origin following the sacrococcygeal region and the ovaries (HERR et al. 1993). Some investigators have suggested a familial occurrence of teratoma. Teratoma has a mean age of occurrence of 18 months but may also be seen at the neonatal period. Most patients present under the age of 4 years. In prepubertal children teratoma of the testis is a benign neoplasm because it invariably presents as a mature

teratoma and the tumor does not spread. Most patients have a painless swelling of the involved testis, with only 15% of patients suffering pain. The mass does not transilluminate, but a translucent mass does not exclude a testicular tumor. Often a hydrocele is present, causing confusion and leading to a misdiagnosis (LEVY et al. 1994).

Macroscopically the tumor appears lobulated and contains cysts of various size, filled with gelatinous and mucinous material. Ultrasound examination of a teratoma typically reveals multiple cystic areas (Fig. 27.5). Microscopically these tumors consist of elements resembling structures derived from the ectoderm, mesoderm, and endoderm. The ectoderm may be represented by squamous epithelium, the mesoderm by smooth muscles, cartilages, or bone, and the endoderm by intestinal, pancreatic, or respiratory tissue. On examination, the testis is diffusely enlarged but sometimes a nodule is felt in the lower or upper pole. Metastases in prepubertal children have not been reported. However, pubertal and postpubertal boys should be regarded as adults, in whom metastatic disease does occur. Serum tumor marker levels remain normal in prepubertal patients, unlike in patients with a yolk sac tumor of the testis. Preoperative ultrasound examination may delineate cystic and solid areas in which calcifications may be seen to be differentiated from neuroblastoma, meconium, or hemorrhage.

The standard therapy is inguinal orchiectomy without adjuvant treatment as teratomas in prepubertal children do not metastasize. As prepubertal teratomas are encapsulated, it is reasonable to consider enucleation of the lesion in selected cases with reconstruction of the tunica albuginea. In those patients in whom an epidermoid cyst of the testis is considered, careful follow-up of the lesion by

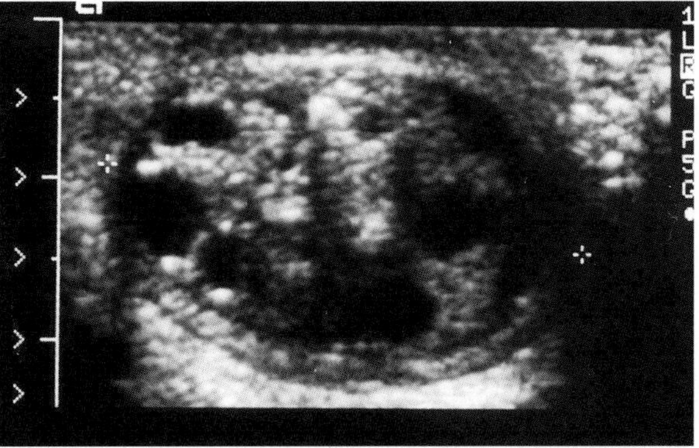

**Fig 27.5.** Ultrasound examination of the testis demonstrates the presence of multiple cystic areas characteristic of teratoma

ultrasound may be employed. When changes occur, inguinal orchiectomy should be performed. This measure is not appropriate in pubertal and postpubertal teratoma, where intratubular germ cell neoplasia exists in the adults.

### 27.4.3
### Seminoma

Seminomas are the most common testicular tumors in adults but they are very rare in children. The explanation for this phenomenon is that seminomas are related to spermatogenesis. However, they have been described in children. Therapy should be the same as in adults.

## 27.5
## Gonadal Stromal Tumors

Gonadal stromal tumors represent about 6% of testicular tumors in prepubertal boys according to the Prepubertal Testicular Tumor Registry.

### 27.5.1
### Leydig Cell Tumors

In the neonate Leydig cells in the testis are absent and they normally appear by the time puberty is reached. The age distribution in Leydig cell tumor is bimodal, with the first peak occurring between 5 and 10 years of age (in children with precocious puberty) and the second peak between 30 and 35 years of age. The mean time between onset of symptoms and diagnosis varies from 6 months to 4 years. In most children with unilateral testicular enlargement in combination with precocious puberty, a testicular Leydig cell tumor is found. However, congenital adrenal hyperplasia with ectopic adrenal tissue in the testis also causes precocious puberty and testicular enlargement. The differential diagnosis should be made prior to surgery. In most patients with congenital adrenal hyperplasia with ectopic adrenal tissue, testicular volume will decrease with glucocorticoid therapy [luteinizing hormone-releasing hormone (LH-RH) administration on two occasions] and surgery can be avoided. Urinary pregnanetriol and 17-ketosteroids, and plasma testosterone and androstenedione determinations are useful in differentiating between these two conditions (URBAN et al. 1978).

Physiologically patients with a Leydig cell tumor have elevated levels of plasma testosterone. However, a case of Leydig cell tumor without precocious puberty has been reported.

Microscopic examination of Leydig cell tumors shows typical Reinke's crystalloids in 40% of the cases.

Preoperatively, children should undergo endocrinological screening including serum levels of testosterone, follicle stimulating hormone (FSH), luteinizing hormone (LH), and determination of bone age. Ultrasound examination of the scrotum can provide additional information in many cases. No large series of Leydig cell tumors of the testis have been published in the literature. The generally accepted therapy, however, is inguinal orchiectomy. Tumor enucleation has only rarely been performed. It should be pointed out that no case of malignant Leydig cell tumor has been described so far in children. In adults late onset of metastases have been described and for that reason children probably also need long-term follow-up.

### 27.5.2
### Sertoli Cell Tumors

In general, gonadal stromal tumors are benign. Only some rare variants have been described by the Prepubertal Testicular Tumor Registry. The clinical course of Sertoli cell tumor is in general also benign, and orchiectomy alone should be a curative treatment. In one case metastatic disease was reported and even in this special case surgical extirpation of metastatic lesions was curative. However, due to an unpredictable tumor behavior, long-term follow-up is necessary.

### 27.5.3
### Granulosa Cell Tumors

Benign granulosa cell tumors account for 15% of all gonadal stromal tumors reported in the Prepubertal Testicular Tumor Registry by 1986. The usual age at presentation is in the first months of life, with the majority of patients presenting in the neonatal period.

Granulosa cell tumors have been reported in descended and cryptorchid testes. These tumors are hormonally inactive and patients with a cryptorchid granulosa cell tumor of the testis have structural abnormalities of the Y chromosome or mosaicism.

Some of these patients have mixed gonadal dysgenesis or ambiguous genitalia. Ultrastructural analysis of this tumor confirms the presence of granulosa and theca cell types and reveals a cellular structure similar to that of primitive Sertoli cell tumors and ovarian granulosa cell tumors. This tumor probably already develops in utero. CORTEZ and KAPLAN (1993) suggest hormonal factors during gestation affecting the immature gonadal blastema or Sertoli cells inducing growth of this tumor.

Scrotal ultrasound examination typically reveals a multicystic pattern. In differential diagnosis a cystic teratoma or cystic yolk sac tumor as well as cystic degeneration following testicular torsion and cystic dysplasia of the testis have to be ruled out. The classical therapy is inguinal orchiectomy. The clinical course of this tumor remains benign.

### 27.5.4
### Mixed Gonadal Stromal Tumors

This is a particular group of gonadal stromal tumors that cannot be further classified histologically. Despite the fact that a lot of mitotic activity can be identified in such tumors, in childhood they are considered to be benign.

## 27.6
## Gonadoblastoma

Gonadoblastoma is seen in intersex patients with dysgenetic gonads. The majority (80%) are phenotypic female patients who have various degrees of virilization. A minority (20%) are male patients with hypospadias and cryptorchidism. Most gonadoblastomas occur after puberty and in general under the age of 20 years. In prepubertal children, gonadoblastoma has rarely been described.

This tumor is benign but can potentially degenerate into a malignant neoplasm, usually into a dysgerminoma. It contains a mixture of germ cells and stromal cells. One-half of the reported cases have a predominant growth of the germ cell component. Germ cell tumors that have developed in this context metastasize in about 10% of patients.

Screening of patients with XY gonadal dysgenesis or mixed gonadal dysgenesis (XO\XY -mosaicism) is recommended, as they may have a risk of developing a germ cell tumor. The mechanism predisposing genotypically normal male siblings of phenotypic females with dysgenetic gonads to develop germ cell neoplasms is poorly understood.

Gonadoblastoma may be bilateral and more commonly appears after puberty. All patients with gonadal dysgenesis and a Y cell line are at risk for developing gonadoblastoma and should be closely followed. They should undergo laparoscopy and excision of the dysgenetic gonads. However, if the testis is localized in the scrotum, there is no consensus as to whether orchiectomy is required.

## 27.7
## Patients with Ambiguous Genitalia in Adolescence

The diagnosis and management of patients born with intersex characteristics should be worked out within the first few days of life. Except perhaps for the 46XY with complete androgen insensitivity this should usually not present a diagnostic problem. It is, however, surprising that these intersex characteristics in many patients are not recognized immediately after birth. Normally, by the time of puberty the sex of rearing should already have been long established. Problems may arise when the child fails to conform to that sex, cannot perform sexually, or has gonads with neoplastic potential. Because the accuracy of diagnosis is currently much higher than it was 15 years ago, we now face the problem of drawing conclusions from patients whose original diagnosis was uncertain.

The decision on gender assignment, assuming the diagnosis is made accurately, in male pseudohermaphrodites with ambiguous genitalia is relatively easy. Patients with largely female genitalia and little or no gonadal source of testosterone usually have a reconstructible vagina and are reared as females. This group includes patients with pure gonadal dysgenesis, mixed gonadal dysgenesis unless there is a descended testis, 17-ketosteroid reductase deficiency, and 5 α-reductase deficiency. Because the gonads are usually removed early in infancy there is no longer any potential for neoplastic transformation by the time of puberty. Patients with pure gonadal dysgenesis (46XY) appear to be normal females. They may even have a uterus and tubes but no ovaries, necessitating estrogen replacement therapy. Prolonged estrogen treatment may precipitate endometrial carcinoma in those who have a uterus and gonadal dysgenesis. At puberty some may even have sufficient testosterone production to show penile development. Surprisingly these patients may develop an estrogen-secreting gonadal neoplasm.

In other patients androgen production in utero is sufficient for the development of male characteristics. At birth patients have some penile development and may have a descended testis. They should be brought up as boys even though they may have some internal female structures. This group includes patients with mixed gonadal dysgenesis and dysgenetic male pseudohermaphrodites. The management of the gonads requires a particularly accurate diagnosis because of the risk of development of benign or malignant neoplasia.

A true hermaphrodite has both ovarian and testicular tissue with about half of the patients demonstrating 46XX, 20% 46XY, and 30% mosaics. Especially in this group there is a high rate of late diagnosis. The well-known high risk of neoplasia is one of the most influential factors in the management of patients with intersex. A biopsy may be necessary to define both the type of gonad present and the neoplastic risk. The majority of neoplasms are of germ cell origin and therefore some germ cells must be present in the gonads, although they may be primitive and small in number. The risk of neoplasia is higher with more dysplastic germ cells or with the coexistence of ovarian and testicular tissue in the same gonad.

In gonadal dysgenesis the gonads may contain testicular tissue, but sometimes the gonad is nothing more but a streak. A streak gonad containing testicular is at highest risk. Such a testicle has a 30% probability of developing gonadoblastoma, which may become invasive. A dysgerminoma/seminoma may arise in a streak gonad. The risk of neoplasia is highest in the patients with pure gonadal dysgenesis with 46XY chromosomes. These patients were reported to have a 20%–30% incidence of gonadoblastoma, of which about a third will progress to malignancy (SAVAGE and LOWE 1989). The majority of tumors develop during the period of puberty, but they may occur earlier in life.

Gonadoblastoma is composed of Sertoli cells and germ cells with only sporadic Leydig cells. Such tumors are typical of the streak and dysgenetic gonad. A gonadoblastoma never metastasizes as a gonadoblastoma and may undergo spontaneous regression. Metastases of a gonadoblastoma are composed only of germ cell elements. It is therefore believed that the germ cell portion of the gonadoblastoma develops malignant change and then metastasizes rather than the whole lesion being malignant from the beginning. The endocrine cells may produce active hormones, especially testosterone.

Dysgerminoma (classical seminoma arising in the ovary) is a malignant germ cell neoplasia from the outset, although this tumor tends to metastasize late.

True hermaphrodites with a Y chromosome have a high risk of gonadal malignancy, and those patients with a testis rather than ovotestis are at the highest risk of tumor development. Both gonadoblastoma and seminoma have been described. Also the ovarian gonads may be at risk of tumor development. A juvenile granulosa cell tumor has been described (ZALOUDEK and NORRIS 1982). These tumors may produce estrogen, and they have a low malignant potential. Patients with complete androgen insensitivity are at risk of developing malignant tumors in childhood or later in life. Gonadal biopsies in childhood have identified atypical cells which appear to precede the development of carcinoma in situ in adulthood (MULLER et al. 1984). These abnormal cells have similar features to seminoma cells. In male phenotypes that are 45XO/46XY these features are considered to be an indication for gonadectomy.

In male patients with congenital adrenal hyperplasia who are poorly controlled, adrenocortical rests in the testes may develop hyperplasia, usually in both testes but not always synchronously. These tumors will disappear when the adrenals are properly suppressed with dexamethasone (CUNNAH et al. 1989).

The indications for removal of the gonads are inappropriate gonadal type for the sex of rearing and the risk of malignancy, which is partly dependent on the diagnosis. The highest risk of neoplasia is in those patients with gonadal dysgenesis and a lower risk is present in true hermaphrodites and patients with testicular feminization. In congenital adrenal hyperplasia there is no increased risk of neoplasia. In true hermaphrodites the risk of neoplasia is higher in those with a Y chromosome. Also, the position of the gonads is of importance, with the risk of malignancy in abdominal gonads being very high, warranting their removal.

But what should one do with palpable gonads? Should they all be removed at puberty? Some investigators have suggested regular biopsies to diagnose carcinoma in situ or regular ultrasound studies. At the present time there does not seem be a clear consensus on the management of these patients. In patients with a significant risk of neoplasia the gonads are probably best removed with placement of a prosthesis and subsequent testosterone replacement therapy. When the risk is considered to be acceptable, a careful follow-up policy should be instituted.

## 27.8
## Tumors of the Supporting Tissue

Tumors of the supporting tissue are extremely rare and generally seen in adult patients. Testicular tumors of the supporting tissue may be benign, including fibroma, leiomyoma, and hemangioma. Following excision, the outcome of pathological examination will dictate further management. Most patients will be cured of these tumors, but in the occasional malignant tumor (leiomyosarcoma, fibrosarcoma), further assessment and therapy will resemble the treatment given to adult patients.

## 27.9
## Lymphomas and Leukemias

Testicular lymphoma and leukemia is often seen at a site of persistence of leukemic cells after chemotherapy for acute lymphoblastic leukemia (ALL). There are multiple explanations for this phenomenon. The incidence of these tumors ranges from 10% to 30% in boys with ALL during or following the treatment course. The first manifestation of lymphoma is often a painful enlargement of the testis in a leukemia patient. Transscrotal ultrasound examination and magnetic resonance imaging are not diagnostically helpful. In addition, testicular biopsies are difficult to interpret and interpretation can differ between several observers. Routine pretreatment biopsies of the testis and end of therapy for leukemia are of no clinical value. Testicular leukemia is extremely radiosensitive. The classical treatment consists of a radiation dose of 2400 and 3000 cGy with an additional dose of salvage systemic chemotherapy. Iatrogenic gonadal toxicity is a well-known phenomenon in patients receiving chemotherapy as well as in those treated with radiotherapy and it often results in future infertility.

## 27.10
## Tumor-Like Lesions

### 27.10.1
### Epidermoid Cysts

Epidermoid cysts are rarely seen in prepubertal boys and represent less than 2% of childhood testicular tumors. The epidermoid cyst of the testis is a benign intraparenchymal squamous epithelium-lined cyst with a fibrous wall and intraluminal keratinized debris. They are distinguished from teratomas because they do not have all layers of the germinal epithelium. Because of the intraparenchymal localization of these lesions, it may be difficult to make a correct preoperative diagnosis. Ultrasound examination may demonstrate the presence of a heterogeneous mass. This finding, however, is rather nonspecific for epidermoid cyst.

The recommended therapy for epidermoid cyst is radical inguinal orchiectomy, but if the diagnosis can be suspected preoperatively, enucleation of the lesion is possible. If enucleation is performed, biopsy of the normal testis should be performed to rule out carcinoma in situ in other locations.

### 27.10.2
### Hyperplastic Nodules Secondary
### to Congenital Adrenal Hyperplasia

Hypertrophic adrenal rests in the testis secondary to adrenal hyperplasia have to be considered in the differential diagnosis of a Leydig cell tumor. Both of these conditions are present with precocious puberty and testicular enlargement. The differential diagnosis can frequently be difficult. Both lesions can be unilateral. Some authors recommend the use of biochemical differentiation, which is, however, not totally reliable. Pathological differentiation between adrenal rests and interstitial cell tumors is equally difficult, if not impossible.

Clinically it is relevant to note that adrenal rest cells occur frequently but usually not in the substance of the testis and that interstitial cell tumors are rare. On histological examination, Reinke crystalloids are suggestive, but not diagnostic, of interstitial cell tumors.

Empirically regression of a testicular mass after glucocorticoid therapy suggests an adrenal origin but sometimes high and prolonged steroid administration is required. Failure to reduce the size of the testicular mass, however, does not prove the existence of an interstitial cell tumor.

## 27.11
## Testis Cancer and the Undescended Testis

Undescended testis occurs in 1 of 400–500 men. The risk of developing a testicular tumor is 20–40 times greater in this group of patients than in the normal descended testicle patient population. About 85% of the testes are descended normally at birth. Discovery of a nondescended testis at the present time results in earlier treatment administration than a decade ago. However, the protective effect of orchiopexy against the development of testicular tumors has not yet been confirmed. The peak incidence of tumor development in these patients, as in other forms of testicular cancer, is in the third and fourth decades of life whether the cancerous testis is located in the abdomen, groin, or scrotum and irrespective of modes of correction. The time between orchiopexy and development of a testicular tumor averages 20 years and some studies describe no prognostic difference whether there was a spontaneous testicular descent at a later age or as a result of hormonal or surgical treatment. Testicular cancer is associated with previous testicular atrophy. The incidence of cancer recurrence is similar whether the cryptorchidism has been corrected or not, and correction has no effect on the initial tumor stage. The relative incidence of pure seminoma and germinal carcinoma is similar in corrected and non-corrected cases. (Even the initial cancer stage is similar.)

Some authors postpone orchiectomy rather than orchiopexy in a unilateral postpubertal smaller cryptorchid testis to prevent ipsilateral carcinogenesis. Testicular biopsies during the orchiopexy to detect carcinoma in situ (CIS) give no relevant information since CIS occurs not earlier than 4 years before tumor development. To date no evidence has been found for the presence of histological premalignant changes. Flow cytometric analysis of testicular aspirates offers as important information as classical histology. It may permit prediction regarding the fertility and malignant potential of undescended testes in postpubertal children. Patients should be instructed to perform self-examinations of the scrotum for an indefinite period of time.

## 27.12
## Paratesticular Rhabdomyosarcoma

Rhabdomyosarcoma is the most common soft tissue sarcoma of childhood and accounts for about 10% of all malignant diseases in children (see Chap. 35). Of all rhabdomyosarcomas, from 13%–20% develop in the urogenital tract. Paratesticular rhabdomyosarcoma accounts for about 10% of all intrascrotal tumors.

The diagnostic assessment as well as the primary treatment are identical to those in the other testicular tumors. In patients undergoing incomplete excision some authors advocate the use of hemiscrotectomy in order to avoid the need for radiation to the groin and scrotum. After surgical and pathological confirmation, patients should undergo staging, consisting of radiographs of the chest, CT scan of the retroperitoneum, and a scintigraphic bone scan. Paratesticular rhabdomyosarcomas are divided into two pathological subtypes: those with an alveolar pattern and those without this pattern. Those without an alveolar pattern are prognostically the best and comprise almost 97% of the paratesticular rhabdomyosarcomas. At the time of diagnosis about 20% of patients have distant metastases and more than 50% have para-aortic and paracaval lymph node involvement.

The indication for extended retroperitoneal lymphadenectomy remains controversial since a high incidence of major complications has been reported and some investigators believe that chemotherapy can sterilize microscopic lymph node metastasis. However, a safer nerve-sparing lymphadenectomy sharply reduces the incidence of surgical complications. It has been reported that less than 20% of patients will be confronted with retrograde ejaculation and lymphedema. In modern series such complications are infrequently seen, and with the use of contemporary fertility-supporting techniques such as intracytoplasmatic sperm injection, fertility remains possible following RLND. Other treatments such as radiotherapy and chemotherapy also have serious side-effects.

Because of the rarity of this disease, multicenter studies such as the IRS-III (Intergroup Rhabdomyosarcoma Study III) clinical protocol and a rhabdomyosarcoma study of the Society of Paediatric Oncology (SIOP) were initiated (see Chap. 35). The IRS-III consists of a staging system classifying tumors into groups from 1 to 4 with appropriate treatment advised for each group (SHAPIRO and STROTHER 1992). Overall the prognosis of a paratesticular rhabdomyosarcoma especially in younger age patients is very good. The 3-year survival rate was reported to range from 65% to 90% depending on the stage at diagnosis. The good prognosis of this particular tumor means that care must be taken that the treatment should not be more dangerous than the tumor itself.

## References

Ablin A (1982) Malignant germ cell tumors in children. Front Radiat Ther Oncol 16:141–149

Batata MA, Chu FCH, Hilaris BS, Whitmore WF, Golbey RB (1982) Testicular cancer in cryptorchids. Cancer 49:1023–1030

Brosman SA (1979) Testicular tumors in prepubertal children. Urology 8:581–588

Brosman SA, Cohen A, Fay R (1974) Rhabdomyosarcoma of the testis and spermatic cord in children. Urology III-5:568–572

Coppes MJ, Rackley R, Kay R (1994) Primary testicular and paratesticular tumors in childhood. Med Pediatr Oncol 22:329–340

Cunnah D, Perry L, Dacie JA, et al. (1989) Bilateral testicular tumors in congenital adrenal hyperplasia. Clin Endocrinol 30:140–147

Dagany AM (1975) Obscure bilateral calcified swellings of paratesticular tissues. Urology 6:101–104

Exelby PR (1980) Testicular cancer in children. Cancer 45:1803–1809

Forouhar F (1982) Meconium peritonitis. Am J Clin Pathol 208–213

Gearhart JP, Connolly JA (1993) Management of yolk sac tumors in children. Urol Clin North Am 20:7–14

Gilbert JB, Hamilton JB (1940) Studies in malignant testis tumors. III. Incidence and nature of tumors in ectopic testis. Surg Gynecol Obstet 71:731–743

Green DM (1986) Testicular tumors in infants and children. Semin Surg Oncol 2:156–162

Herr HW, et al. (1993) Management of teratoma. Urol Clin North Am 20:145–152

Kaplan GW, Firlit CF (1980) Treatment of testicular yolk sac carcinoma in the young child. J Urol 126:663–664

Kaplan GW, Cromie WC, Kelalis PP, Silber I, Tank ES (1988) Prepubertal yolk sac testicular tumors – report of the Testicular Tumor Registry. J Urol 140:1109–1111

Levy DA, Kay R, Elders JS (1994) Neonatal testis tumors: a review of the Prepubertal Testis Tumor Registry. J Urol 151:715–717

Loughin KR, Retik AB, Weinstein HJ, et al. (1989) Genitourinary rhabdomyosarcoma in children. Cancer 6:1600–1606

Manivel SC, Simoulon S, Wold LE, et al. (1988) Absence of intralobular germ cell neoplasm in testicular yolk sac tumors in children: a histochemical and immunohistochemical study. Arch Pathol Lab Med 112:641–645

Muller J, Skakkebaek NE, Neilson OH, Graem N (1984) Cryptorchidism and testis cancer: atypical germ cells followed by carcinoma in situ in adult age. Cancer 54:629–634

Newell ME, Lippe BM, Ehrlich RM (1977) Testis tumors with congenital adrenal hyperplasia: a continuing diagnostic and therapeutic dillemma. J Urol 117:256–258

Parkinson MC, Swerdlow AJ, Pike MC (1994) Carcinoma in situ in boys with cryptorchidism: when can it be detected? Br J Urol 73:431–435

Ring KS, Burbige KA, Benson MC, Karp FK, Hensle TW (1990) The flow cytometric analysis of undescended testes in children. J Urol 144:494–513

Savage MO, Lowe DG (1989) Gonadoblastoma: a review of 74 cases. Cancer 25:1340–1356

Shapiro E, Strother D (1992) Pediatric genitourinary rhabdomyosarcoma. J Urol 148:1761–1768

Urban MD, Lee PA, Plotnick LP, Migeon CJ (1978) The diagnosis of Leydig cell tumors in childhood. Am J Dis Child 132:494–497

Vries de JDM (1995) Paratesticular rhabdomyosarcoma. World J Urol 13:219–225

Woodhouse CRJ (1997) Patients born with ambiguous genitalia in adolescence and adulthood. ESPU annual course on paediatric uro-endocrinology

Zaloudek C, Norris HJ (1982) Granulosa cell tumors of the ovary in children: a clinical and pathologic review of 32 cases. Am J Surg Pathol 6:503–512

# Carcinoma of the Penis and Scrotum

cations poses another drawback to recommending routine use of LND in all patients presenting with penile cancer (ORNELLAS et al. 1994; JOHNSON and LO 1984). Retrospective analyses of data on patients with penile carcinoma treated in our medical center and also treated by others have identified clinically lymph node-negative patient groups at high risk of having occult metastases (McDOUGAL 1995; AYYAPPAN et al. 1994; HORENBLAS et al. 1993; FRALEY et al. 1989).

Patients with carcinoma in situ or T1 or small T2 tumors (tumors smaller than 2 cm and tumors of 2–5 cm with minimal invasion respectively, HARMER 1978) have a fairly low risk of metastatic spread. Additionally the degree of tumor differentiation indicates the probability of dissemination to the regional lymph nodes (HORENBLAS et al. 1993; FRALEY et al. 1989). Nevertheless, even when LND is reserved for the high-risk group, we found in our clinical experience that in up to 40% of patients no tumor was present in the resected specimen (HORENBLAS et al. 1993). In order to decrease the number of unnecessary LNDs and to improve the detection of occult metastases, better staging procedures are mandatory. HORENBLAS et al. (1991) have shown that occult metastases cannot be detected by the currently available imaging modalities.

About 20 years ago, CABANAS (1977) investigated the existence of a so-called sentinel node, a specific lymph node location being the first site of metastasis. Identification of tumor cells in this lymph node would indicate the need for LND. The absence of tumor cells would obviate the need for subsequent LND, assuming a sequential pattern of metastatic spread. On the basis of lymphangiography performed via dorsal lymphatics of the penis, CABANAS (1977) labeled the lymph node close to the superficial epigastric vein as the sentinel node. The removal of this node was recommended based on static anatomical landmarks. More recently, MORTON and co-workers (1994) extended the concept of the sentinel lymph node to include patients with melanoma. They identified the sentinel node through individual visualization of lymphatic channels originating in the primary tumor using vital dyes. We prospectively investigated this new approach in patients with penile cancer. In addition to the blue dye technique, we explored the value of lymphoscintigraphy with technetium-99 m nanocolloid as a tracer for preoperative evaluation and the value of a gamma detection probe for intraoperative guidance.

## 28.3.2
## Innovations in Surgical Treatment of the Regional Lymph Nodes: Dynamic Sentinel Node Procedure

Since January 1994 all clinically lymph node-negative patients with squamous cell carcinoma of the penis have been submitted to the so-called dynamic sentinel node procedure. Patients with T1 tumors or carcinoma in situ have been excluded from this study because of the assumed low risk of occult metastases. To date the study population consists of 40 consecutive patients. Scintigraphy of lymphatic drainage is performed on the day before surgery. Sixty MBq of $^{99m}$Tc-nanocolloid in a volume of 0.3–0.4 ml is injected around the tumor. Immediately after this injection dynamic image acquisition is started for a period of 20 min using a gamma camera to study the lymphatic flow. Subsequently anterior and lateral static views are obtained for 5 min each (Fig. 28.7), and repeated 2 h after the injection. Sentinel lymph nodes are defined as nodes receiving direct drainage from the site of injection. The location of the sentinel node is subsequently marked on the skin with a dye. The following day, 1 ml of patent blue dye is injected around the tumor in a similar fashion (Fig. 28.8). A few minutes later, a small incision is made over the skin mark. The sentinel node is searched for by tracing blue lymphatic channels leading to blue lymph nodes and by using the gamma detection probe in the wound (Figs. 28.9–28.11). Once identified, the sentinel node is removed and the wound is scanned for remaining radioactivity. Regional LND is reserved for patients with a sentinel node positive for metastases.

After the surgery all patients are seen at 2-month intervals during the first 2 years following treatment. In the 40 patients studied we identified 88% of sentinel nodes. Of these, 70% were identified with both the probe and blue dye, while 30% were located with the probe only. The mean total duration of exploration was 12 min. In nine (22.5%) of the 40 study patients metastases were found, necessitating an inguinal LND. The LND specimens showed additional lymph node metastases in two patients only, underscoring the reliability of the procedure. There were no complications following the procedure. The average period of follow-up for all patients was 16 months (range: 0.6–45.6 months). To date we have been confronted with one (2.5%) false-negative dynamic sentinel lymph node procedure. In contrast to the procedure described by CABANAS (1977, 1992),

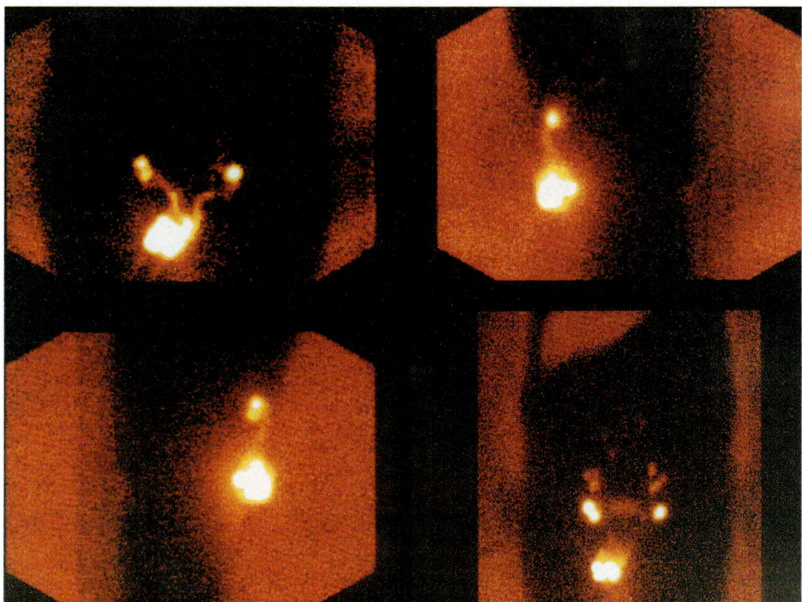

**Fig. 28.7.** Lymphoscintigram of a 67-year-old patient with a T2 tumor. The site of injection (tumor) drains onto two sentinel nodes in the left and right groin. A large number of nonsentinel nodes are clearly visible

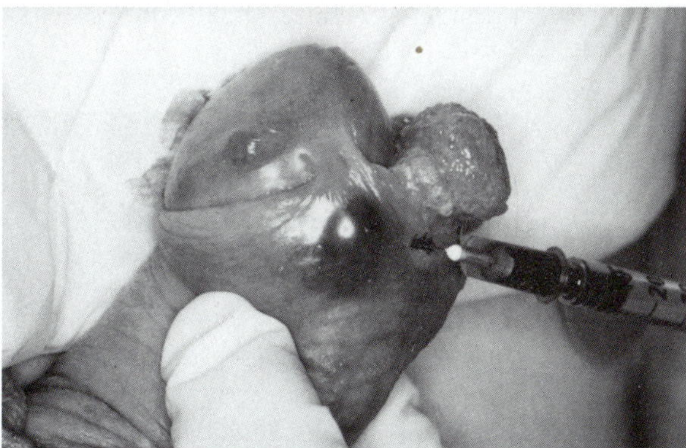

**Fig. 28.8.** Injection of patent blue dye around the tumor

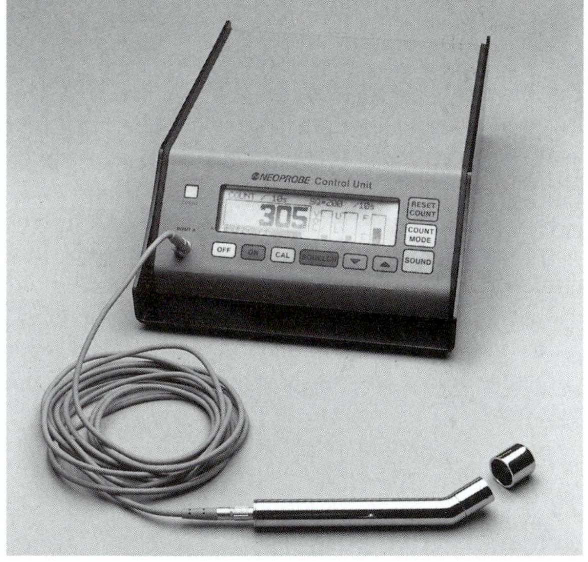

**Fig. 28.9.** A gamma detection probe and the control unit as used in this study

this procedure takes into account the individual drainage pattern of each tumor and the diversity of the anatomy of lymphatic drainage. Given the encouragement provided by the favorable results in melanoma, the sentinel node concept is now being explored in other malignancies such as breast cancer and carcinoma of the vulva (GIULIANO et al. 1994; LEVENBACK et al. 1995). The results in carcinoma of the vulva deserve mention because of the similarities in behavior when compared with carcinoma of the penis. LEVENBACK and co-workers identified the sentinel node in 19 (66%) of 29 groins using only the blue dye technique. No false-negative results were obtained with inguinal LND as the gold standard. The probability of a false-negative result underscores the need for a strict follow-up schedule.

During the first 2 years after a dynamic SN procedure, patients are seen every second month. Utilizing this close follow-up allows for an early diagnosis of tumor progression and administration of early therapy.

The occurrence of a false-negative sentinel node may be partially explained by the presence of metastases blocking the lymphatic flow, as shown in our experience with lymphoscintigraphy of prostatic

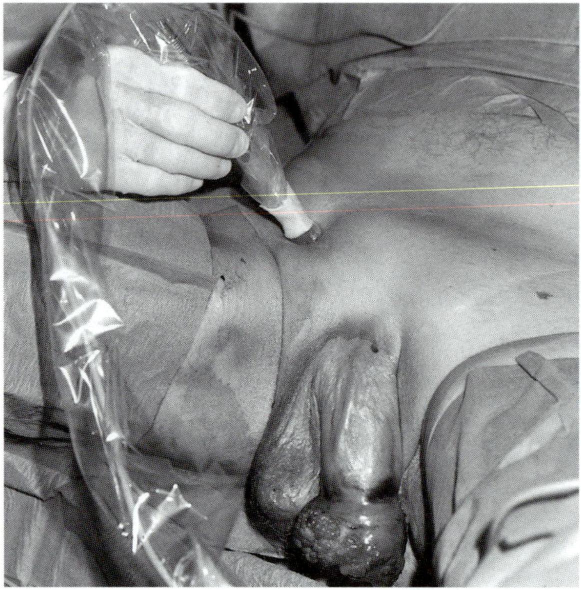

Fig. 28.10. The use of the gamma detection probe at the marked spots on the skin surface

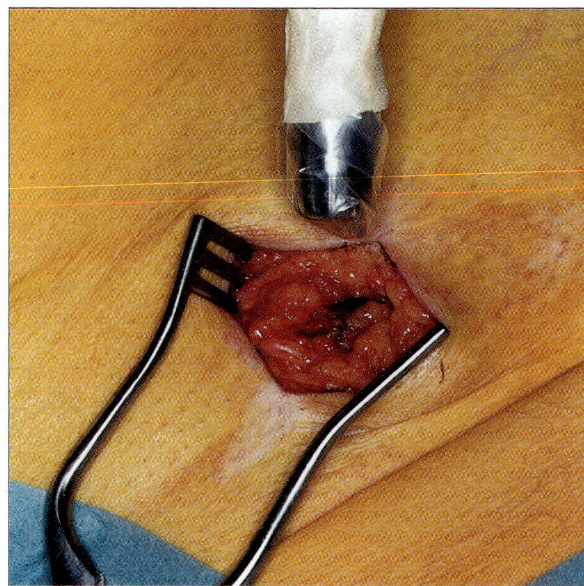

Fig. 28.11. The use of the gamma detection probe following incision of the skin to expose the lymph node-bearing area

cancer (HORENBLAS et al. 1992b). The tracer is then diverted to another lymph node that is falsely labeled as the sentinel node. It is not clear from our experience whether this occurs only in cases where gross metastatic invasion is present or whether microscopic invasion may produce the same effect. More clinical research is required to answer this important question. This technique is minimally invasive and holds great promise in identifying patients with clinically occult metastasis at an early stage of the disease.

## 28.4
## Reconstructive Surgery

Various innovations in reconstructive surgery have made possible mitigation of the ablative effects of primary surgery. Traditionally myocutaneous island flaps have been used to cover large skin defects or to reconstruct the penis (HAGE et al. 1993). Well-known flaps used to cover inguinal or perineal surgical defects include the following: (1) the tensor fascia lata island flap; (2) the rectus abdominis flap; and (3) the gracilis flap. Tubularized flaps were rotated to the penile amputation zone to reconstruct the penis. Free flaps revascularized by microvascular anastomosis and "skin stretching" (MELIS et al. 1998) have greatly increased the scope of reconstructive surgery.

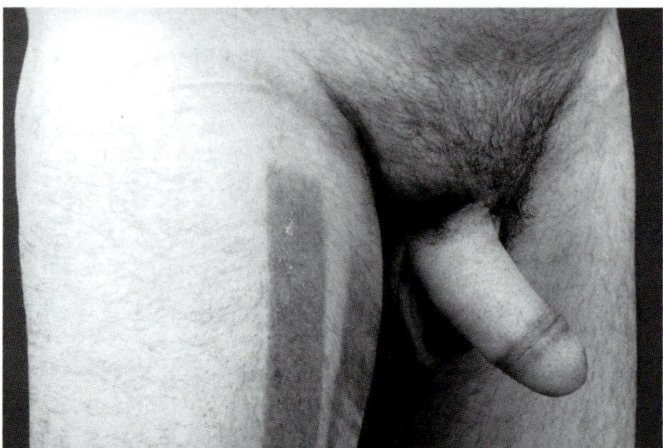

Fig. 28.12. Total penile reconstruction in a 44-year-old patient after penile amputation. The indication for this procedure was tumor recurrence following a course of radiation therapy. The reconstruction was performed using the radial forearm flap. (Courtesy of J.J. Hage, MD PhD, Department of Plastic and Reconstructive Surgery, Academisch Ziekenhuis Vrije Universiteit, Amsterdam, The Netherlands)

### 28.4.1
### Reconstructive Surgery of the Penis After Treatment of Carcinoma of the Penis

The use of free flaps revascularized by microvascular anastomosis has led to a major improvement in total penile reconstruction. The use of the radial forearm flap with microvascular anastomosis to the penile stump has given very satisfactory cosmetic results (Fig. 28.12). Micturition can be done standing after

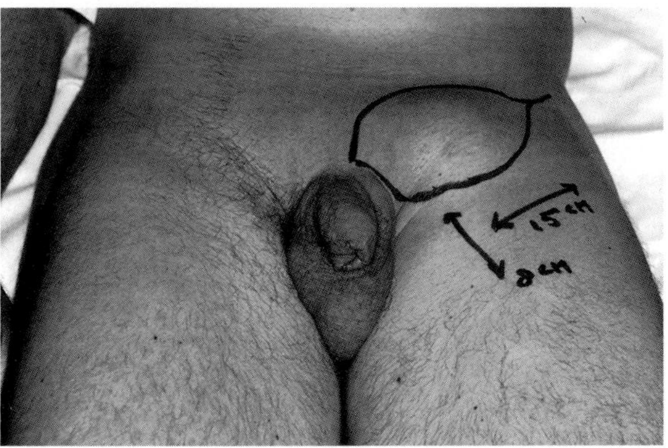

**Fig. 28.13.** Delineation of skin incision around a large left inguinal nodal mass

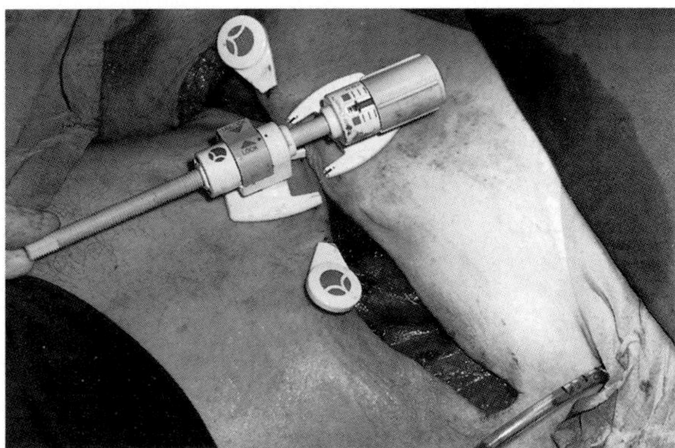

**Fig. 28.15.** After placing two needles in the dermis parallel to each other, the skin-stretching device is anchored in place behind the two needles. Approximation of the skin edges occurs by turning the tension screws of the device

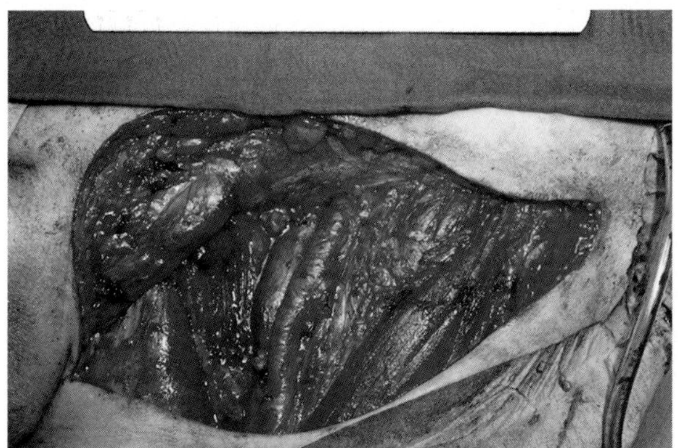

**Fig. 28.14.** A large skin defect following ilioinguinal LND

complete urethral reconstruction by way of tubularized skin. Disadvantages of this penile reconstruction include the following: (1) poor sexual function; (2) impaired cosmetic aspect of the donor site; and (3) hair growth on the reconstructed penis. Implantation of penile prostheses has not been successful as yet. A new technique was published recently, using a free tibial flap incorporating a part of the tibia in order to give some rigidity to the reconstructed penis (CAPELOUTO et al. 1997; HAGE et al. 1997; SADOVE et al. 1993a,b). Satisfactory intercourse has been reported following this penile reconstruction.

### 28.4.2
### Reconstructive Surgery After Lymph Node Dissection

Removal of large inguinal masses with fixation of the skin sometimes leads to a skin defect that cannot be closed primarily. Standard reconstructive procedures include various myocutaneous flaps or so-called free flaps. These techniques are time consuming, technically demanding, and often necessitate the closure of the donor site with a skin graft. Closing a large defect primarily with the use of a skin-stretching technique has been used with success in our medical center (MELIS et al. 1998). Stretching and relaxing the skin in a controlled fashion, so-called cycle loading, allows the skin to stretch beyond its inherent extensibility. Groin defects of approximately 10–12 cm can be closed primarily (Figs. 28.13–28.15). This procedure can be performed without the need for undermining, so vascular impairment is very likely avoided. The advantages of a skin-stretching technique include the elimination of a donor skin defect and its associated morbidity. The stretched skin is an ideal match in color, and hair-bearing properties and the cutaneous innervation are preserved. Despite the fact that previous radiation therapy is considered a contraindication to the use of this procedure, we have also used the skin-stretching device in a patient after radiotherapy to the inguinal region, without subsequent complications (Figs. 28.16–28.18).

### 28.5
### Combination Therapy

Adjuvant treatment with radiation therapy is a time-honored treatment after circumcision and/or local tumor excision, especially in cases with positive surgical margins. As mentioned earlier, we have been disappointed by the sexual function of the irradiated

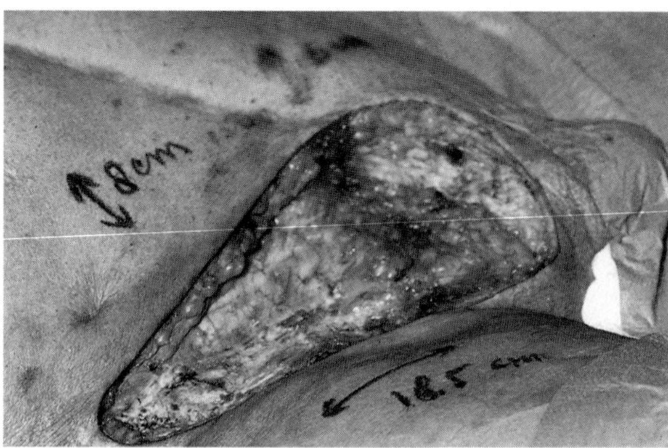

**Fig. 28.16.** Skin defect after removal of a local recurrence following inguinal LND, adjuvant radiation therapy, and neoadjuvant chemotherapy

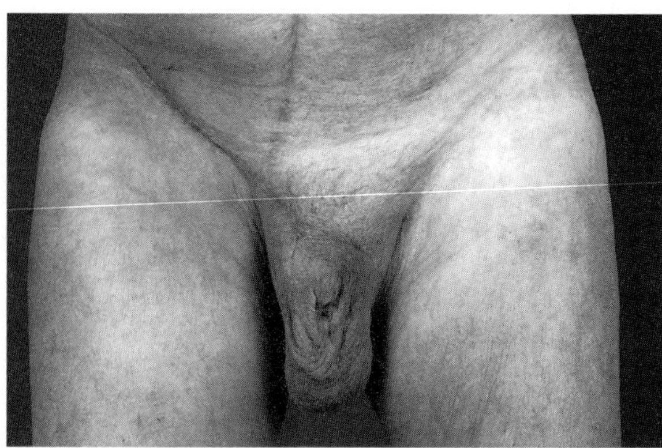

**Fig. 28.18.** Primary healing 6 months after surgery

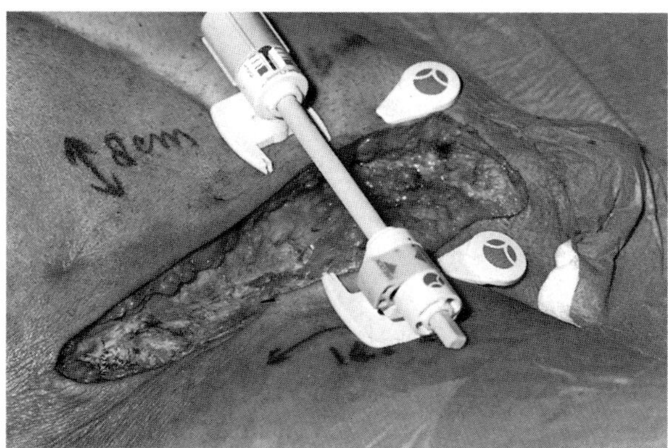

**Fig. 28.17.** Gradual approximation of the skin edges after placing the needles and the skin-stretching apparatus

penis. The vulnerable skin with its radiation-induced changes is prone to bleeding, laceration, and subsequent cellulitis following sexual activity. Admittedly these experiences are based on "old" radiotherapy series, and recently published series have shown excellent sexual function after penile irradiation (Fossa et al. 1987). At present the potential of adjuvant chemotherapy after surgery of the primary tumor remains to be assessed. Surgery plays the most important role in the cure of patients presenting with locoregional disease. The presence of unresectable metastases is a challenging issue. Favorable results of preoperative radiation therapy, permitting subsequent surgical removal, have been reported. In the absence of randomized studies it is unclear whether survival is improved in these cases. The use of combination chemotherapy in patients with locally unresectable disease appears to be able to achieve major responses in approximately two-thirds of patients. Resectability has been reported in about 50% and durable disease-free survival in 15%–

30% of patients (Pizzocaro et al. 1995). These treatment results are based on two combination chemotherapy regimens: (1) cisplatin and 5-fluorouracil and (2) vincristine, bleomycin, and methotrexate (Dexeus et al. 1991; Shammas et al. 1992). The curative potential of surgery is restricted by the presence of poor prognostic factors such as high tumor grade and extensive metastatic disease. Does adjuvant treatment improve survival in cases with poor prognostic factors? In the absence of prospective randomized trials a definitive answer cannot be given. The experience in other primary sites of squamous cell carcinoma can be of help. Based on experience with head and neck surgery we have given adjuvant radiation therapy in all patients with: (1) two or more lymph node metastases, (2) extracapsular tumor growth, and (3) pelvic lymph node metastases. The major goal of this treatment is increased local tumor control. From 1979 to 1990 adjuvant combination chemotherapy was used by Pizzocaro and co-workers in 25 patients with radically resected nodal metastases (Pizzocaro and Piva 1988; Pizzocaro et al. 1995). Chemotherapy consisted of vincristine, bleomycin and methotrexate. However, analysis of the data showed that most of those patients were in need of adjuvant treatment (bilateral metastases, pelvic lymph node involvement) and fared poorly, raising doubts as to the efficacy of this adjuvant regimen.

## 28.6
## Carcinoma of the Scrotum

While being interesting from a medical history point of view as an occupational cancer, scrotal cancer is extremely rare (Lowe 1992). A regionally variable incidence of scrotal carcinoma was reported by the World Health Organization (WHO). While the incidence in the United States was reported to be fewer than ten cases per year (Doll et al. 1976), the incidence in the United Kingdom was reported to be 10 times higher. Again, the most common scrotal tumor is squamous cell carcinoma. The biological behavior is not very much different from that of penile carcinoma, i.e. locoregional spread with inguinal metastasis and late onset of hematogenous metastasis.

The same principles apply to the surgical management of carcinoma of the scrotum as to that of carcinoma of the penis, the aim being to achieve total local tumor excision. With respect to the regional lymph nodes (inguinal), histopathological evidence of aggressive behavior of the primary tumor would justify an elective LND in the absence of a reliable wait-and-see program. To date no reports are available on treatment outcomes, but knowledge from squamous cell carcinoma at other sites in the human body is readily applicable. This also applies to the dynamic sentinel node procedure in cases with scrotal cancer: no reports have been published so far (Lowe 1992).

# References

Abi-Aad AS, deKernion JB (1992) Controversies in ilioinguinal lymphadenectomy for cancer of the penis. Urol Clin North Am 19:319–324

Ansink A (1992) Squamous cell carcinoma of the vulva, etiology, treatment and prognosis. Thesis, Rijksunversiteit Utrecht

Ayyappan K, Ananthakrishnan N, Sankaran V (1994) Can regional lymph node involvement be predicted in patients with carcinoma of the penis? Br J Urol 73:549–553

Boon TA (1988) Sapphire probe laser surgery for localized carcinoma of the penis. Eur J Surg Oncol 14:193–195

Cabanas RM (1977) An approach for the treatment of penile carcinoma. Cancer 39:456

Cabanas RM (1992) Anatomy and biopsy of sentinel lymph nodes. Urol Clin North Am 19:267–276

Capelouto CC, Orgill DP, Loughlin KR (1997) Complete phalloplasty with a prelaminated osteocutaneous fibula flap. J Urol 158:2238–2239

Dexeus FH, Logothetis CJ, Sella A, Amato R, Kilbourn R, Fitz K, Striegel A (1991) Combination chemotherapy with methotrexate, bleomycin and cisplatin for advanced squamous cell carcinoma of the male genital tract. J Urol 146:1284–1287

Doll R, Payne P, Waterhouse J (1976) Cancer incidence in five continents. International Agency for Research on Cancer, Lyon, France

Fossa SD, Hall KS, Johannessen NB, Urnes T, Kaalhus O (1987) Cancer of the penis, experience at the Norwegian Radium Hospital 1974–1985. Eur Urol 13:372–377

Fraley EE, Zhang G, Manivel C, Niehans GA (1989) The role of ilioinguinal lymphadenectomy and significance of histological differentiation in treatment of carcinoma of the penis. J Urol 142:1478–1482

Giuliano AE, Kirgan DM, Guenther JM, Morton DL (1994) Lymphatic mapping and sentinel lymphadenectomy for breast cancer. Ann Surg 220:391–398

Hage JJ, Bloem JJAM, Suliman HM (1993) Review of the literature for phalloplasty with emphasis on the applicability in female to male transsexuals. J Urol 150:1093–1098

Hage JJ, Winters HAH, van Lieshout J (1997) Fibula free flap phalloplasty: modifications and recommendations. Microsurgery 17:358–365

Harmer MH (1978) TNM classification of malignant tumours, 3rd edn. International Union Against Cancer, Geneva

Horenblas S (1994) Squamous cell carcinoma of the penis: update on diagnosis, staging and management. Eur Urol Update Series, vol 3/8

Horenblas S, van Tinteren H (1994) Squamous cell carcinoma of the penis. IV. Prognostic factors of survival: analysis of tumor, nodes and metastasis classification system. J Urol 151:1239–1243

Horenblas S, van Tinteren H, Delemarre JFM, Moonen LMF, Lustig V, Kröger R (1991) Squamous cell carcinoma of the penis: accuracy of tumor, nodes and metastasis classification system, and role of lymphangiography, computerized tomography scan and fine needle aspiration cytology. J Urol 146:1279–1283

Horenblas S, van Tinteren H, Delemarre JFM, Boon TA, Moonen LMF, Lustig V (1992a) Squamous cell carcinoma of the penis. II. Treatment of the primary tumor. J Urol 147:1533–1538

Horenblas S, Nuyten MJC, Hoefnagel CA, Moonen LMF, Delemarre JFM (1992b) Detection of lymph node invasion in prostatic carcinoma with iliopelvic lymphoscintigraphy. Br J Urol 69:180–182

Horenblas S, van Tinteren H, Delemarre JFM, Moonen LFM, Lustig V, Van Waardenburg EW (1993) Squamous cell carcinoma of the penis. III. Treatment of the regional nodes. J Urol 149:492–497

Johnson DE, Lo RK (1984) Complications of groin dissection in penile cancer. Experience with 101 lymphadenectomies. Urology 24:312–314

Kulkarni JN, Kamat MR (1994) Prophylactic bilateral groin node dissection versus prophylactic radiotherapy and surveillance in patients with N0 and N1–2a carcinoma of the penis. Eur Urol 26:123–128

Levenback C, Burke TW, Gershenson DM, Morris M, Malpica A, Lucas KR, Gershenson DM (1995) Potential applications of intraoperative lymphatic mapping in vulvar cancer. Gynecol Oncol 59:216–220

Lowe FC (1992) Squamous cell carcinoma of the scrotum. Urol Clin North Am 19:397–405

McDougal WS (1995) Carcinoma of the penis: improved survival by early regional lymphadenectomy based on the histological grade and depth of invasion of the primary lesion. J Urol 154:1364–1366

McDougal WS, Kirchner FK Jr, Edwards RH, Killion LT (1986) Treatment of carcinoma of the penis: the case for primary lymphadenectomy. J Urol 135:38–41

Melis P, Bos KE, Horenblas S (1998) Primary skin closure of a large skin defect after inguinal lymphadenectomy for penile cancer using a skin stretching device. J Urol 159:185–187

Morton DL, Wen D, Wong JH, Economou JS, Cagle LA, Storm FK, Foshag LJ, Cochran AJ (1994) Technical details of intraoperative lymphatic mapping for early stage melanoma. Arch Surg 127:392–399

Ornellas AA, Seixas ALC, Marota A, Wisnescky A, Campos F, de Moraes JR (1994) Surgical treatment of invasive squamous cell carcinoma of the penis: retrospective analysis of 350 cases. J Urol 151:1244–1249

Pizzocaro G, Piva L (1988) Adjuvant and neoadjuvant vincristine, bleomycin and methotrexate for inguinal metastases from squamous cell carcinoma of the penis. Acta Oncol 27:823–824

Pizzocaro G, Piva L, Nicolai N (1995) Lymphadenectomy for cancer of the penis. In: Donohue JP (ed) Lymph node surgery in urology. Isis Medical Media, Oxford, pp 118–130

Sadove RC, McRoberts JW, Wells MD (1993a) Total phallic reconstruction with the free fibula osteocutaneous flap [letter] [see comments]. Plast Reconstr Surg 89:1001

Sadove RC, Sengezer M, McRoberts JW, Wells MD (1993b) One stage total penile reconstruction with a free fibula osteocutaneous flap. Plast Reconstr Surg 92:1314–1323

Schellhammer FP, Jordan GH, Schlossberg SM (1992) Tumors of the penis. In: Walsh PC, Retik AB, Stamey TA, Vaughan ED (eds) Campbell's urology, 6th edn. Saunders, Philadelphia

Shammas FV, Ous S, Fossa SD (1992) Cisplatin and 5-fluorouracil and advanced cancer of the penis. J Urol 147:630–632

Theodorescu D, Russo P, Zhang ZF, Morah C, Fair W (1996) Outcomes of initial surveillance of invasive squamous cell carcinoma of the penis and negative nodes. J Urol 155:1626–1631

Windahl T, Hellsten S (1995) Laser treatment of localized squamous cell carcinoma of the penis. J Urol 154:1020–1023

# 29 Radiotherapy in Cancer of the Penis, Male Urethra, and Scrotum

B.K. Lee and L.W. Brady

CONTENTS



B.K. Lee, MD, Department of Radiation Oncology, Allegheny University of the Health Sciences, Allegheny University Hospitals, Hahnemann, 230 North Broad Street, Mail Stop 200, Philadelphia, PA 19102-1192, USA
L.W. Brady, MD, Hylda Cohn/American Cancer Society Professor of Clinical Oncology, and Professor, Department of Radiation Oncology, Allegheny University of the Health Sciences, Allegheny University Hospitals, Hahnemann, 230 North Broad Street, Mail Stop 200, Philadelphia, PA 19102-1192, USA

## 29.1 Carcinoma of the Penis

### 29.1.1 Anatomy

The penis is composed of two corpora cavernosa and the corpus spongiosum encased in the dense Buck's fascia (Chao and Perez 1997). A loose connective tissue separates this fascia from overlying skin. The corpus spongiosum expands into the glans penis distally and it is covered by the skin fold known as the prepuce.

### 29.1.2 Epidemiology

Penile cancer is an uncommon malignancy in developed countries, representing 2%–5% of all urogenital tumors (Herr et al. 1997). It is a significant clinical problem in populations in which circumcision is not a common practice and proper hygiene is lacking. It accounts for up to 20% of male concerns in certain areas of Africa, Asia, and South America. In the United States, it accounts for 0.3%–1% of all cancers in men (Chao and Perez 1997).

### 29.1.3 Etiology

The most consistent etiologic factor is the presence of an intact foreskin and the irritative effect of smegma combined with the products of poor hygiene within the preputial sac (Stadler et al. 1996). In the United States, the risk of penile carcinoma in uncircumcised males is threefold higher than the risk in circumcised men and approaches the rate seen in some Third World nations (Stadler et al. 1996). The protective effects of circumcision appear to be abrogated when it is performed during adolescence or later years (Stadler et al. 1996). Phimosis is found in a higher proportion of penile cancer patients and chronic infection developing beneath a phimotic foreskin may be of significance. There are also many epidemiologic studies attempting to link viral etiology with penile malignancy, namely, human papilloma virus types 16 and 18. But there are no compelling data to support the assertion that penile cancer is a sexually transmitted disease (HERR et al. 1997).

### 29.1.4
### Natural History

Nearly all cases of carcinoma of the penis originate within the preputial area, with the glans being the most common site followed by the prepuce (CHAO and PEREZ 1997). It is characterized by slow local and regional progression. The inguinal lymph nodes are the most common site of metastatic spread. Among the patients who present with clinically palpable inguinal lymph nodes, about 50% have pathologic evidence of metastasis (CHAO and PEREZ 1997). In patients with clinically nonpalpable inguinal lymph nodes, about 20% are found to have micrometastasis. Distant metastasis is uncommon, being present in about 10% of the cases (CHAO and PEREZ 1997). Most patients die from septic complications and/or erosion of large vessels in the groin.

### 29.1.5
### Pathology

Ninety-five percent of penile cancers are squamous cell carcinomas (STADLER et al. 1996). Other primary tumors include: basal cell carcinoma, melanoma, sarcoma, and Kaposi's sarcoma. Metastatic lesions to the penis have infrequently been reported.

The early premalignant lesions include Bowen's disease and Queyrat's erythroplasia, which is being considered as a penile carcinoma in situ. The descriptions of other premalignant lesions of the penis are summarized in Table 29.1 (HERR et al. 1997).

### 29.1.6
### Clinical Presentation

The most common presenting manifestation of penile cancer is a mass, persistent sore, or ulcer of the glans or prepuce (HERR et al. 1997). Most penile carcinomas are painless. The patient also experiences fear and embarrassment, which probably contribute to delayed diagnosis. It has been estimated that more than half of the patients delay more than 1 year before seeking treatment after the initial appearance of the lesion. Assessment of the primary lesion may be obscured by the presence of phimosis. Secondary infection and associated foul smell are also common. Urethral obstruction is rare.

In a collective series of 552 patients with penile carcinoma, the presenting symptoms were: mass lesion (78%), pain or itching (12%), bleeding (7%), groin mass (7%), and urinary symptoms (4%) (CHAO and PEREZ 1997). Inguinal lymph nodes are palpable on presentation in 30%–45% of the patients. Among these patients with palpable lymph nodes, in only half is a positive histologic diagnosis made following surgery. Diagnosis of penile cancer requires obtaining a detailed history with careful examination of the balanopreputial area, which may demonstrate small lesions. Regional lymph nodes,

**Table 29.1.** Premalignant lesions of the penis

| Lesions | Characteristics | Treatment |
| --- | --- | --- |
| Leukoplakia | White plaque | Local excision |
| Erythroplasia of Queyrat | Raised, red, velvet lesion; cellular disorientation with multiple mitosis; identical to carcinoma in situ of skin; 10%–20% may develop areas of squamous cell carcinoma. May be painful | Local excision; topical 5-fluorouracil; radiation therapy |
| Bowen's disease | Red plaque | Local excision |
| Balanitis xerotica obliterans | Scaly, atrophic with fissure or ulcerations; meatus often involved | Local excision; topical steroids |
| Buschke-Löwenstein tumor | Large verrucous lesion, histologically benign; may undergo malignant degeneration | Local excision with negative margins; topical therapy doubtful; radiation therapy has limited effectiveness |

especially inguinal lymph nodes, should be evaluated thoroughly. Chest radiographs and intravenous pyelogram are routinely obtained during patient workup. Urethroscopy and cystoscopy are considered to be essential diagnostic procedures.

The use of lymphangiography is of a questionable value due to the difficulty in interpretation of findings in the lymph nodes with extensive inflammatory changes as well as the pattern of lymphatic filling with contrast in a dorsopedal injection (CHAO and PEREZ 1997). Computed tomography (CT) scan is a useful study in the identification of enlarged pelvic and periaortic lymph nodes in patients with involved inguinal lymph nodes.

## 29.1.7
## Staging

The staging system proposed by Jackson is most commonly used for penile carcinoma. This staging system is summarized in Table 29.2. The American Joint Committee Staging System is shown in Table 29.3.

## 29.1.8
## Lymphatic Drainage

The penis is a midline structure with bilateral lymphatic drainage. Lymph flow from the prepuce, glans, and skin drains to the superficial inguinal lymph nodes. The glans and corpora cavernosa drain into the deep inguinal and external iliac lymph nodes. The 5-year survival rate for patients without lymph node involvement ranges from 85% to 90% (CHAO and PEREZ 1997). For those with positive inguinal lymph nodes, the 5-year survival rate decreases sharply to 40%–50%, and patients with pelvic lymph node involvement at diagnosis show a 5-year survival of less than 20% (CHAO and PEREZ 1997).

## 29.1.9
## General Management

Penile carcinoma metastasizes to regional lymph nodes by embolization rather than permeation of regional lymphatics (CHAO and PEREZ 1997). Therapeutic intervention has been performed in two phases. The first phase consists of initial management of the primary tumor followed by the management of the regional lymphatics.

**Table 29.2.** Staging system for carcinoma of the penis proposed by JACKSON

| Stage | Characteristics |
| --- | --- |
| I | Tumor confined to glans and/or prepuce |
| II | Tumor extending onto shaft of penis |
| III | Tumor with malignant, but operable, inguinal lymph nodes |
| IV | Inoperable primary tumor extending off the shaft of the penis, or inoperable groin nodes or distant metastases |

**Table 29.3.** American Joint Committee Staging System for carcinoma of the penis

*Primary tumor (T)*

| | |
| --- | --- |
| Tx | Primary tumor cannot be assessed |
| T0 | No evidence of primary tumor |
| Tis | Carcinoma in situ |
| Ta | Noninvasive verrucous carcinoma |
| T1 | Tumor invades subepithelial connective tissue |
| T2 | Tumor invades corpus spongiosum or cavernosum |
| T3 | Tumor invades urethra or prostate |
| T4 | Tumor invades other adjacent structures |

*Regional lymph nodes (N)*

| | |
| --- | --- |
| Nx | Regional lymph nodes cannot be assessed |
| N0 | No regional lymph node metastasis |
| N1 | Metastasis in a single superficial inguinal lymph node |
| N2 | Metastasis in multiple or bilateral superficial inguinal lymph nodes |
| N3 | Metastasis in deep inguinal or pelvic lymph node(s), unilateral or bilateral |

*Distant metastasis (M)*

| | |
| --- | --- |
| Mx | Presence of distant metastasis cannot be assessed |
| M0 | No distant metastasis |
| M1 | Distant metastasis |

Lesions of the glans penis have traditionally been treated by partial penectomy. However, newer microsurgical techniques have shown local excision to be an acceptable and desirable option with small superficial lesions, because sexual and urinary functions can be preserved (CHAO and PEREZ 1997). Larger or more invasive lesions (stage III) can be treated by partial or total penectomy. Partial penectomy is the procedure of choice if a surgical margin of 2 cm can be achieved (CHAO and PEREZ 1997). Total penectomy with a perineal urethrotomy is warranted if an adequate margin cannot be achieved or if local recurrence has occurred (see Chap. 28).

The sensitivity of clinical staging of the lymph nodes ranges from 40% to 60%, and the false-negative rate is 10%–20%. The relatively low incidence of metastatic disease (10%–20%) in patients with clinically normal lymph nodes has led to management by observation with delayed intervention when signs of lymph node involvement appear (CHAO and PEREZ 1997). For clinically positive lymph nodes, bilateral inguinal dissection is routinely performed. This is required because of the richly anastomotic network of lymphatic channels draining the penis. The frequency of contralateral metastasis approaches 50%. Approximately 20% of patients with palpable lymph node involvement can be salvaged by radical pelvic lymphadenectomy (CHAO and PEREZ 1997).

Patients with clinically negative lymph nodes who are at high risk for microscopic metastasis can be managed with elective radiation to the inguinal lymph nodes with a high probability of tumor control and low incidence of treatment complications (CHAO and PEREZ 1997).

## 29.1.10
### Radiation Oncology

The main advantage of radiation therapy is preservation of the penis. Modalities of radiation delivery include megavoltage external beam irradiation, iridium-192 mold plesiotherapy, and interstitial implant using iridium-192 wires. Using external beam irradiation, Grabstald and Kelley reported 90% local tumor control in ten patients with stage I lesions treated to 50 Gy over a 6-week period (CHAO and PEREZ 1997). Duncan and Jackson reported 90% local control for Stage I lesions delivering 50 to 57 Gy (CHAO and PEREZ 1997). Patients who experienced local failure after radiation therapy are salvaged by surgery. Of those patients who present with nonpalpable inguinal lymph nodes, 20% can be expected to develop positive lymph nodes at a later date (CHAO and PEREZ 1997). A control rate of 95% is achieved in patients who receive prophylactic radiation therapy to the inguinal lymph nodes. For those who present with palpable lymph nodes, bilateral groin dissection becomes necessary.

## 29.1.11
### Chemotherapy

The role of chemotherapy in the management of penile cancer has not been established. Chemotherapeutic agents including cisplatin, doxorubicin, bleomycin, and methotrexate have been mentioned for management of advanced stage lesions but the treatment results have been poor.

## 29.1.12
### Radiation Therapy Techniques

If the prepuce is intact, circumcision must be performed prior to initiation of radiation therapy to minimize radiotherapy-associated morbidity.

External beam radiation therapy with specially designed apparatus for the penis is employed to achieve a homogeneous dose distribution to the entire penis. Typically a plastic box with a central opening that can be fitted over the penis is used. The space between the skin and the box is then filled with a tissue-equivalent material. The penis then can be treated with parallel opposed radiation beams. It is of importance to note the need to angle the beams in such a way as to avoid delivery of high doses of radiation to deeper pelvis structures and to allow matching inguinal fields when this becomes necessary. Many of the series have reported 2.5- to 3.5-Gy daily fractions to a total dose of 50–55 Gy. However, a smaller daily fraction size of 1.8–2 Gy and a higher total dose are preferred to reduce the incidence of late fibrosis and tissue damage (CHAO and PEREZ 1997). For prophylactic lymph node irradiation, the field should include inguinal, external iliac, and hypogastric lymph nodes. The posterior pelvis may be partially spared by anterior loading of the radiation beams. Total dose may be limited to 50 Gy for clinically negative lymph nodes. In patients with palpable lymph nodes, approximately 70–75 Gy over a period of 7–8 weeks with field reduction after 50 Gy is advised (CHAO and PEREZ 1997).

## 29.1.13
### Brachytherapy

Brachytherapy can be employed by using the technique of plesiobrachytherapy or interstitial implantation. Plesiobrachytherapy involves building a customized box or a cylinder mold with a central opening and channels for placement of radioactive sources in the periphery of the device. Doses of 60–65 Gy at the surface and approximately 50 Gy to the urethra are delivered over 6–7 days (STADLER et al. 1996). Implementation of this technique requires the presence of nonbulky tumor (stage I and II) and a cooperative patient. The mold can be applied continuously, in which case an indwelling catheter should be in place or worn for 8–10 h a day. Local control rates of 50%–67% have been reported with the use of this treatment technique (STADLER et al. 1996). The reported incidence of urethral stricture is low, at 12%.

Interstitial implantation is performed under general anesthesia. A urinary catheter is inserted to ensure that the radioactive sources are not passed through the urethra. Usually a two-plane implant is necessary to surround the target volume by the 85% isodose line. A dose of 60–65 Gy is delivered to the 85% isodose line, usually over a period of 6–7 days (STADLER et al. 1996). The dose rate is 0.3–0.5 Gy per hour. Local control rates of up to 91% for T1 tumors, 78% for T2, 71% for T3, and 50% for T4 lesions have been reported (STADLER et al. 1996). Most authors recommend T3 tumors or lesions greater than 40 mm in diameter should not be treated with interstitial implantation.

## 29.1.14
### Side-effects

Acute effects of radiotherapy are mucosal and skin reactions leading to edema, moist desquamation, and dysuria. Delayed effects include telangiectasia, fibrosis, urethral stenosis, and focal necrosis. Patients are advised that sexual intercourse may be resumed 3 or 4 months after the completion of treatment. Following administration of radiotherapy a routine penile biopsy should be avoided and performed only in patients in whom local recurrence is suspected.

## 29.2
### Carcinoma of the Male Urethra

Carcinoma of the male urethra is extremely rare, only about 600 cases having been reported worldwide (HERR et al. 1997). No definitive etiologic factors have been identified. However, chronic inflammation appears to play a role in initiation of the disease process. The peak incidence occurs at 58 years of age and there is no evidence of racial predisposition.

## 29.2.1
### Symptoms

Urethral carcinoma has a rather insidious onset. The most common presentation is that of a palpable urethral mass or the presence of obstructive symptoms.

Elderly patients may present with pain associated with urethral fistula or periurethral abscess.

## 29.2.2
### Pathology

The male urethra can be divided into three segments: prostatic urethra, bulbomembranous urethra, and penile urethra. The bulbomembranous urethra is the most common site of urethral carcinoma, representing about 60% of cases; the penile urethra is involved in about 30%, and the prostate urethra in about 10% (STADLER et al. 1996). Histologically, 80% of male urethral tumors are squamous cell carcinoma, 15% are transitional cell carcinoma, and about 5% are adenocarcinoma or undifferentiated carcinoma (STADLER et al. 1996).

Male urethral carcinoma primarily spreads by direct extension with hematogenous spread being uncommon. Metastasis occurs by lymphatic embolization to regional lymph nodes. The lymphatics from the penile urethra drain into superficial and deep inguinal lymph nodes and occasionally also external iliac lymph nodes. The lymphatics from bulbomembranous and prostatic urethra drain into the external iliac, obturator, and hypogastric lymph nodes. Approximately 20% of patients at diagnosis have clinically positive lymph nodes and they almost always are positive for tumor (STADLER et al. 1996).

## 29.2.3
### Diagnostic Workup

Diagnosis of urethral carcinoma requires a detailed history and complete physical examination. Examination under anesthesia aids in evaluating the extent of local involvement by tumor. Cystourethroscopy and transurethral needle biopsy are also performed at this time. Complete blood count, serum chemistries, and urinalysis are also obtained. Radiologic studies including chest radiographs, intravenous urography, and CT scan of the abdomen and pelvis should be obtained to complete the process of staging.

## 29.2.4
### Staging

The most commonly used staging system is that pro-

**Table 29.4.** Staging system for male urethra carcinoma proposed by Ray and associates

| Stage | Characteristics |
| --- | --- |
| 0 | Tumor confined to mucosa only |
| A | Tumor extension into but not beyond lamina propria |
| B | Tumor extension into but not beyond substance of corpus spongiosum or into but not beyond prostate |
| C | Direct extension into tissues beyond corpus spongiosum or beyond prostatic capsule |
| D1 | Regional metastasis including inguinal and/or pelvic lymph nodes |
| D2 | Distant metastasis |

**Table 29.5.** American Joint Committee Staging System for carcinoma of the urethra

*Primary tumor (T)*

| | |
| --- | --- |
| Tx | Primary tumor cannot be assessed |
| T0 | No evidence of primary tumor |
| Ta | Noninvasive papillary, polypoid, or verrucous carcinoma |
| Tis | Carcinoma in situ |
| T1 | Tumor invades subepithelial connective tissue |
| T2 | Tumor invades corpus spongiosum or prostate or periurethral muscle |
| T3 | Tumor invades corpus cavernosum or beyond prostatic capsule, or the anterior vagina or bladder neck |
| T4 | Tumor invades other adjacent organs |

*Regional lymph nodes (N)*

| | |
| --- | --- |
| Nx | Regional lymph nodes cannot be assessed |
| N0 | No regional lymph node metastasis |
| N1 | Metastasis in a single lymph node, <2 cm in greatest dimension |
| N2 | Metastasis in a single lymph node, >2 cm but not >5 cm in greatest dimension, or multiple lymph nodes none >5 cm in greatest dimension |
| N3 | Metastasis in a lymph node >5 cm in greatest dimension |

*Distant metastasis (M)*

| | |
| --- | --- |
| Mx | Presence of distant metastasis cannot be assessed |
| M0 | No distant metastasis |
| M1 | Distant metastasis |

posed by Ray and associates, and this system is summarized in Table 29. 4. The American Joint Committee Staging System is shown in Table 29.5.

## 29.2.5
### General Management

Traditionally, surgical excision with or without combined radiation therapy has been the treatment of choice for carcinoma of the male urethra (Stadler et al. 1996). Although there are reports of tumor control by radiation therapy alone, because of the rarity of this disease, comparison of cure rates with radiation therapy or surgery is difficult. The principal advantage of radiation is preservation of the organ. Noninvasive carcinoma of the penile urethra can be treated with transurethral resection. For distal urethral carcinoma, 5-year survival rates following penectomy or radiation therapy are comparable, at 50% versus 60%, respectively (Chao and Perez 1997). Lymphadenectomy is indicated for patients with clinically involved regional lymph nodes.

Penile urethral carcinoma can be treated by transurethral resection, local excision, partial amputation, or radical amputation with or without orchiectomy. For tumors infiltrating the corpus and localized to the distal half of the penis, partial amputation with a 2-cm margin is an accepted and generally successful treatment. For infiltrative tumor involving the entire urethra or located in the proximal penile urethra, radical amputation should be considered.

Early lesions of bulbomembranous urethra have been treated successfully by transurethral resection or resection of the involved urethral segment with an end-to-end anatomosis. Unfortunately, most patients with bulbomembranous urethral carcinoma present with locally advanced disease and overall survival is poor despite a radical surgical approach. This has led to combined preoperative radiation (2000–6000 cGy in 2–6 weeks) followed by surgical resection of the inferior pubic rami. This approach offered small but distinct advantages in terms of better local control and improved overall survival. Carcinoma arising from the prostatic urethra is rare. The serum acid phosphatase and prostate-specific antigen concentrations generally are normal (Herr et al. 1997). Superficial lesions of the prostatic urethra in a majority of patients are successfully treated by transurethral resection. Unfortunately, most patients present with tumor involvement of the bulk of the prostate with variable extension to the bulbomembranous urethra, bladder neck, and trigone. For these patients, cystoprostatectomy and urethrectomy are the treatment of choice. Overall 5-year survival of these patients is poor, with rates of 10%–20% being reported (Herr et al. 1997).

Radiation therapy techniques for carcinoma of penile urethra are similar to those for carcinoma of the penis. Bulbomembranous urethral carcinoma can be treated with the setup of parallel opposed fields covering the groin and the pelvis followed by perineal and inguinal boost. The prostatic urethral carcinoma can be treated with techniques and radiation doses similar to those used for treatment of carcinoma of the prostate.

Concomitant chemoradiation combination employing 5-fluorouracil and mitomycin C has been reported to be effective for local and advanced urethral carcinomas in organ preservation protocols (CHAO and PEREZ 1997).

## 29.2.6
## Conclusion

Patients with early-stage lesions of the urethra may be treated successfully with surgery or radiation alone. Advanced disease may best be treated with a combination of surgery, irradiation, and chemotherapy.

## 29.3
## Carcinoma of the Scrotum

Carcinoma of scrotum became widely known as chimney sweeper's disease as a result of the work by Pott in 1775. This tumor was the first known environmentally related neoplasm (MCDONALD 1982). A carcinogen related to the soot that accumulated in the sweeper's clothing and contaminated the scrotum was responsible for induction of neoplasia. The cases of scrotal cancer in shale oil workers were presented by Joseph Bell in 1876 (WALDRON 1983). In the 1920s and 1930s, Kennaway discovered that those who handled tar and tar products at high temperatures had a higher incidence of scrotal carcinoma (WALDRON 1983). Cook and his colleagues isolated a highly carcinogenic 3,4-benzpyrene compound from distillate of pitch. Mineral oil used by cotton mule spinners was also found to be carcinogenic (WALDRON 1983).

Fortunately, with an increase in the awareness of etiologic factors responsible for scrotal carcinoma and consequent alterations in the work environment, considerably fewer cases of scrotal carcinoma are seen at this time.

## 29.3.1
## General Information

The term scrotum is derived from Latin, from the word meaning a bag. The organ is a pouch designed to house the testes and regulate the temperature of the testes. Tumor may originate from any structure in the wall of the scrotum. The most frequently encountered lesions are pigmented nevi and epidermal inclusion cysts (sebaceous cysts). The most common cancer is squamous cell carcinoma followed by basal cell carcinoma (MCDONALD 1982). Other malignancies are exceedingly rare.

## 29.3.2
## Epidemiology

Scrotal cancer is practically nonexistent in nonindustrialized rural areas. It is seen most frequently in those who pay the least attention to local hygiene. The disease is found most often during the fifth or sixth decade of life (GERBER 1985). The lesion usually involves the lower and anterior region of the scrotum. The most common complaint on presentation is pruritis which leads to an area of roughened dense scaly skin. Over the subsequent several months this leads to a small papule or a wart. The lesion then becomes larger and ulcerated. Carcinoma should be suspected in any patients with a warty, scaly, or ulcerated scrotal lesion that fails to heal, particularly if there has been prolonged exposure to irritants such as soot, mineral oils, or petroleum products. Multifocality of tumor is found in up to 25% of patients (GERBER 1985). Diagnosis can be established only by biopsy.

## 29.3.3
## Pathology

Histologically, the typical patterns of squamous cell carcinoma with moderate differentiation are present. The tumor spreads from overlying epidermis into the adjacent dermis with various degree of finger-like projections. The cells are large and polyhedral, and may show a distinct pearl formation (GERBER 1985). There is usually an abundant dense, sclerotic supporting stroma with infiltration by chronic inflammatory cells.

The disease spreads by slow but relentless local extension. The spread is facilitated by lack of protective substratum in the scrotal wall, and by repetitive trauma. Also, there is an extremely rich lymphatic network within the scrotal wall with a free bilateral lymphatic communication. The incidence of clinical involvement of inguinal lymph nodes at the time of diagnosis has been reported to range from 30% to 71% (GERBER 1985). Hematogenous spread with distant metastasis is rare. Death is usually due to inanition from excessive local disease and the presence of large, tender, ulcerated, and necrotic infected lymph node involvement. A sudden exsanguination may occur from eroded femoral vessels.

### 29.3.4
### Staging

The most commonly used clinical staging system for carcinoma of the scrotum was proposed by Ray and Whitmore, and it is summarized in Table 29.6.

### 29.3.5
### Treatment Recommendations

The treatment of choice for localized scrotal carcinoma is wide local excision with care taken to ensure generous margins of both skin and subcutaneous tissue around the tumor (McDonald 1982).

Inguinal lymph node dissection should be withheld until there is a clinical suspicion of lymph node metastasis. There is a high incidence of inflammatory nonmalignant adenopathy in these patients (McDonald 1982).

**Table 29.6.** Ray and Whitmore clinical staging system for scrotal carcinoma

| Stage | Characteristics |
| --- | --- |
| A1 | Disease localized to the scrotum |
| A2 | Local extension to adjacent structures by continuity but without evidence of metastasis |
| B | Regional (nodal) metastasis resectable |
| C | Regional (nodal) metastasis, nonresectable |
| D | Distant metastasis (beyond regional nodes) |

In general, treatment results with the use of radiation therapy have been disappointing, although successful in a few isolated cases. Radiation therapy has been successfully employed in combination with surgery in patients who have presented with advanced inguinal lymph node metastasis.

Bleomycin has been reported to be an effective agent against scrotal carcinoma and should be considered as the first-line chemotherapy in this disease. Cisplatin has also shown some effectiveness against scrotal carcinoma originating in the penis and deserves trial in patients with scrotal carcinoma. Chemotherapy should be given when the disease has progressed to the point of surgery, or if surgery in combination with radiation therapy cannot effect a cure.

## References


Chao KS, Perez CA (1997) Penis and male urethra. In: Perez CP, Brady LW (eds) Principles and practice of radiation oncology, 3rd end. Lippincott-Raven, Philadelphia, pp 1717–1731

Gerber WL (1985) Scrotum malignancies: the University of Iowa experience in review of the literature. Urology 26:337–342

Grigsby PW, Herr HW (1996) Urethral tumors. In: Vogelzang NJ, Scardino PT, Shipley WV, Coffey DS (eds) Comprehensive textbook of genitourinary oncology. Williams & Wilkins, Baltimore, pp 1117–1123

Herr HW, Fuks ZY, Scher HI (1997) Cancer of the urethra and penis. In: DeVita VT Jr, Hellman S, Rosenberg SA, Turin B (eds) Cancer: principle and practice of oncology, 4th edn. J.B. Lippincott, Philadelphia, pp 1386–1395

McDonald NW (1982) Carcinoma of the scrotum. Urology 19:269–274

Stadler WM, Elwell CM, Jones WG (1996) Penile cancer. In: Vogelzang NJ, Scardino PT, Shipley WV, Coffey DS (eds) Comprehensive textbook of genitourinary oncology. Williams & Wilkins, Baltimore, pp 1097–1116

Waldron HA (1983) A brief history of scrotal cancer. Br J Ind Med 40:390–401

# Carcinoma of
the Female Urethra

# 30 Urethral Carcinoma of the Female Urethra: Surgical Management

C.E. SALEM and E.C. SKINNER

CONTENTS



## 30.1 Introduction

Urethral cancer accounts for less than 1% of all cancers occurring in women, but represents the only genitourinary cancer that is more common in the female population, with a female to male ratio of 4:1 (JOYNER and McDOUGAL 1997). It is more prevalent in Caucasians (88%) than in African Americans (12%), except when associated with a urethral diverticulum (NARAYAN and KONETY 1992). Urethral cancer is primarily a disease that occurs in the sixth and seventh decades of life; however, extreme age ranges have been reported in the literature, from 25 to 90 years (NARAYAN and KONETY 1992; MAYER et al. 1987).

Urethral carcinoma usually has an insidious onset with a long interval between the first symptoms and the diagnosis. This cancer is usually associated with a poor prognosis unless it is confined to the anterior or distal third of the urethra.


C.E. SALEM, MD, Urologic Oncology Fellow, USC School of Medicine, Department of Urology, 1441 Eastlake Ave, Suite 7414, MS-74, Los Angeles, CA 90033, USA
E.C. SKINNER, MD, Assistant Professor of Medicine, USC School of Medicine, Department of Urology, 1441 Eastlake Ave, Suite 7414, MS-74, Los Angeles, CA 90033, USA


## 30.2 Urethral Anatomy

The female urethra is approximately 4 cm in length as it passes through the pelvic and urogenital diaphragms. It is commonly divided into the anterior urethra (the distal third) and the posterior urethra (the proximal two-thirds). While this anatomic differentiation has significant implications regarding types of treatment, it has no relation to the histology of the urethral mucosa. The proximal third of the urethra is lined by transitional cell epithelium and the distal two-thirds is lined by stratified squamous epithelium (MOORE 1985).

Periurethral glands are present along the length of the female urethra. These are primarily lined with pseudostratified columnar and stratified columnar epithelium. One pair of paraurethral glands, Skene's glands, are homologous to the prostate gland in the male and drain into the distal urethra (MOORE 1985).

The blood supply to the female urethra is rich with contributions from the inferior vesical, internal pudendal, and vaginal arteries. The lymphatics of the anterior urethra (distal third) drain preferentially into the superficial inguinal lymph nodes, primarily the medial and central groups. These then drain into the deep inguinal lymph nodes or to the external-iliac lymph nodes. The posterior urethral (proximal two-thirds) lymphatics drain into the external iliac, internal pudendal, or presacral lymph nodes (MOORE 1985).

## 30.3 Urethral Pathology

Urethral cancer can present with a wide variety of histologic types, including transitional cell carcinoma, squamous cell carcinoma, adenocarcinoma, melanoma, and undifferentiated carcinoma. A review of the literature from 1980 to 1997 is represented in Table 30.1, comprising the experience of 11

**Table 30.1.** Various histologic cell types of 251 female urethral carcinoma specimens found in the recent literature

| | |
|---|---|
| Transitional cell | 47 (18.7%) |
| Squamous cell | 130 (51.8%) |
| Adenocarcinoma | 53 (21.1%) |
| Melanoma | 7 (2.8%) |
| Undifferentiated | 14 (5.6%) |

institutions (JOHNSON and O'CONNELL 1983; ELKON et al. 1980; DESAI et al. 1973; HEDDEN et al. 1993; TURNER and HENDRY 1980; BENSON et al. 1982; MOINUDDIN et al. 1988; HAHN et al. 1991; WEGHAUPT et al. 1984; MAYER et al. 1987; BOLDUAN and FARAH 1981). The epithelial lining of the urethra results in the varied histopathology of urethral carcinoma. In the female, the proximal urethra usually develops transitional cell carcinoma and the distal urethra usually develops squamous cell carcinoma. The most common histologic type overall is squamous cell. While it is conceivable how the transitional and squamous cell varieties develop based on the normal histologic anatomy of the urethra, it is not known how the adenomatous variety develops. Furthermore, malignant melanoma is an uncommon neoplasm, representing only 2% of all malignant tumors (KATZ and GRABSTALD 1976). However, the urethra is the most common genitourinary site of melanoma. Primary melanoma of the urethra usually occurs anteriorly, but is associated with a worse prognosis than the other histologic tumor types at this location (KATZ and GRABSTALD 1976; POW-SANG et al. 1988).

Urethral diverticular cancer is a very uncommon disease (CLAYTON et al. 1992). Because these urethral tumors tend to present earlier, they are associated with a better prognosis. Adenocarcinoma is the most common cell type occurring in urethral diverticular cancers, accounting for 56% of cases. Transitional cell carcinoma, squamous cell carcinoma, and undifferentiated carcinoma have been reported, accounting for 29%, 15%, and <1%, respectively (CLAYTON et al. 1992; GONZALEZ et al. 1985; EVANS et al. 1981).

## 30.4
## Etiology of Urethral Carcinoma

There has been no definitive causal etiologic factor for urethral carcinoma. However, several etiologic factors have been implicated. Inflammatory diseases have long since been associated with urethral cancer, though because of the rarity of urethral cancer no definitive causal relationship has been established (JOYNER and McDOUGAL 1997). Chronic irritation, caruncles, fibrosis, and urethral diverticular disease have all been found to be associated with urethral cancer. A few cases documented in the literature suggest an association between human papillomavirus (HPV), especially genotype 16, and carcinoma of the male and female urethra (WIENER and WALTHER 1994; MEVORACH et al. 1990; WIENER et al. 1992).

## 30.5
## Diagnosis of Urethral Carcinoma

Female patients with urethral cancer present most commonly with urethral bleeding, though the presenting symptoms can vary depending on the location and extent of the lesion (Table 30.2) (JOHNSON and O'CONNELL 1983; ELKON et al. 1980; Desai et al. 1973; TURNER and HENDRY 1980; BENSON et al. 1982; MOINUDDIN et al. 1988; MAYER et al. 1987). The range of symptom duration prior to diagnosis is 3–9 months (MAYER et al. 1987; JOHNSON and O'CONNELL 1983; ELKON et al. 1980; BENSON et al. 1982; MAYER et al. 1987). Furthermore, all of the symptoms associated with urethral cancer can be attributed to benign diseases of the urethra and this is often the reason for the frequent delay in diagnosis. It is therefore important to have a high index of suspicion for any seemingly benign urethral lesion that does not resolve after standard therapy.

Following a thorough history, physical examination is important to help further identify the diagnosis. As noted in Table 30.2, up to 30% of patients may present with a palpable urethral mass. In addition, distal lesions may be grossly visible protruding through the meatus. These must be distinguished from benign lesions. Inguinal lymph nodes may be

**Table 30.2.** Presenting symptoms of 271 female patients with urethral carcinoma found in the recent literature

| Presenting symptoms | |
|---|---|
| Hematuria | 17 (6.3%) |
| Irritative voiding symptoms | 44 (16.2%) |
| Obstructive symptoms/urinary retention | 41 (15.1%) |
| Dysuria | 30 (11.1%) |
| Urethral bleeding | 81 (29.9%) |
| Perineal pain | 15 (5.5%) |
| Palpable mass | 29 (10.7%) |
| Fistula | 1 (0.4%) |
| Dyspareunia | 3 (1.1%) |
| Urinary incontinence | 7 (2.6%) |
| Incidental | 3 (1.1%) |

clinically evident in 20%–60% of patients at the time of presentation (JOYNER and McDOUGAL 1997). These palpable lymph nodes almost always represent metastatic spread rather than an inflammatory process (as is the case with penile cancer). Examination under anesthesia is necessary for adequate cystourethroscopy and biopsy of the suspicious lesion. As well, any palpable inguinal lymph node should be biopsied for appropriate staging (SKINNER and SKINNER 1988; AHLERING and LIESKOVSKY 1988).

Urethral carcinoma metastasizes primarily via hematogenous spread with little correlation between lymph node disease and distant metastasis. Metastases are primarily to the lung, liver, bones, and brain. However, less than 10% of patients have distant metastasis at the time of diagnosis (JOYNER and McDOUGAL 1997; SKINNER and SKINNER 1988; AHLERING and LIESKOVSKY 1988). Radiologic studies to assess metastatic disease should include CT scan of the abdomen and pelvis, radiographs of the chest, and bone scan. While suggested by some, a lymphangiogram is of limited value because of high false-negative and false-positive results (SKINNER and SKINNER 1988).

Recently in the literature, MRI has been noted to provide excellent anatomic detail of the pelvic structures, providing superior tissue contrast when compared to CT. While many have studied its use in female urinary incontinence (CARR et al. 1996), there are now reports of its usefulness in helping to stage urethral cancer (STROHBEHN et al. 1996; MORIKAWA et al. 1995). STROHBEHN et al. (1996) investigated the histologic detail of the urethra using high-resolution MRI and found an excellent correlation between the visible internal urethral anatomy and the gross histologic detail.

## 30.6
## Urethral Cancer Staging

Clinical stage is the most important prognostic factor in female urethral cancer. Currently, two staging systems are most commonly used. The first, that proposed by Grabstald, distinguishes the extent of tissue invasion without regard for tumor location, i.e., distal versus proximal (Table 30.3) (GRABSTALD et al. 1966). Depth of penetration does correlate well with overall survival, regardless of cell type. The reported 5-year survival rates by stage are as follows: stage A 45%, stage B 41%, stage C 26%, and stage D 18% (BRACKEN et al. 1976).

**Table 30.3.** Grabstald staging system for female urethral carcinoma

| | |
|---|---|
| Stage 0 | Carcinoma in situ |
| Stage A | Submucosal |
| Stage B | Muscular (invasion into periurethral tissues) |
| Stage C | Periurethral |
| Stage C1 | Invading muscular wall of vagina |
| Stage C2 | Invading muscle and mucosa of vagina |
| Stage C3 | Invading other adjacent structures (bladder, labia, clitoris) |
| Stage D | Metastases |
| Stage D1 | Inguinal nodes |
| Stage D2 | Pelvic nodes |
| Stage D3 | Para-aortic nodes |
| Stage D4 | Distant metastases |

**Table 30.4.** Prempree staging system for female urethral carcinoma

| | |
|---|---|
| I | Disease limited to distal half of urethra |
| II | Entire urethra, with extension to periurethral tissue, but not involving vulva or bladder neck |
| III a | Urethra and vulva |
| b | Urethra and vaginal muscle |
| c | Urethra and bladder neck |
| IV a | Parametrium or paracolpium |
| b | Metastases |
| 1 | Inguinal nodes |
| 2 | Pelvic nodes |
| 3 | Para-aortic nodes |
| 4 | Distant metastases |

Many investigators have shown that distal lesions have a far better prognosis than proximal lesions due to earlier diagnosis and more effective treatments for control of local disease. The Prempree system, modified from Chau, does distinguish tumor location as well as bladder neck involvement, which has been shown in the literature to be an important prognostic factor (Table 30.4) (PREMPREE et al. 1978). This staging system does not, however, provide a classification for superficial proximal lesions, which are quite infrequent.

## 30.7
## Treatment

Due to the rarity of urethral cancer, reported series in the literature are small, with marked variation in treatments based only on limited experiences. Thus it has been difficult for any single medical center to define a definitive therapeutic plan. In general, urethral carcinoma is a very malignant disease regardless of histologic type, and most would agree

each ureter and the ureters subsequently divided just proximal to the most distal clip. The proximal ureters are then carefully mobilized, taking caution to maintain their attachment with the infundibulopelvic ligament, which provides important collateral circulation to the ureters. The ureters are then tucked under the previously packed bowel until they are needed for the urinary diversion (SKINNER and SKINNER 1988).

A standard pelvic lymph node dissection is performed. The limits of dissection are the same as those used in standard radical cystectomy procedures; proximally to the level 1–2 cm above the aortic bifurcation; laterally to the genitofemoral nerve; distally (at the level of the external iliac artery) to the circumflex iliac vein; medially to Cooper's ligament; distally (at the level of the femoral canal) to the lymph node of Cloquet; posteriorly to the obturator fossa. Following the pelvic lymph node dissection, the lateral and posterior vascular pedicles are developed and divided as in a standard radical cystectomy procedure.

After the vagina has been opened distal to the cervix, the posterior pedicle is further divided by incising the lateral vaginal wall on each side approximately two-thirds distally so that the anterior vaginal wall remains with the anterior pelvic organs. The midline vertical incision is then extended distally over the pubis into the perineum (Figs. 30.2, 30.3) and then directed around the clitoris along the vulva on either side of the vagina until the 180° point of the vaginal circumference is reached. The incision is deepened with cautery down to the inferior ischial rim of the pubic ramus on either side. A periosteal elevator and cautery are then used to dissect the origins of the adductor muscles from off the anterior ischial rim and pubic ramus laterally to the obturator foramen. The lateral vaginal wall is then incised proximally on each side to join up with the vaginal incisions started from the abdomen (Fig. 30.3) (SKINNER and SKINNER 1988).

Avoiding the obturator nerve laterally and the previously ligated obturator vessels, a curved Kocher clamp is gently passed through the obturator foramen from the perineum to the pelvis. One end of a Gigli wire saw can then be clamped to the Kocher clamp and gently passed through the obturator foramen from the pelvis to the perineum. Another curved Kocher clamp is passed medial to the ischium from the perineum to the pelvis and the other end of the Gigli wire saw is clamped and passed from the pelvis to the perineum. A second Gigli wire saw is then positioned in the same manner around

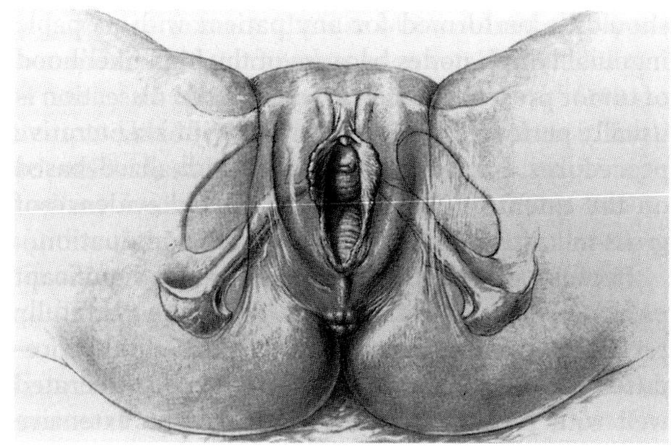

**Fig. 30.2.** Female perineum with underlying bone structures superimposed. [From SKINNER EC, SKINNER DG (1988) Management of carcinoma of the female urethra. In: SKINNER DG, LIESKOVSKY G (eds) Diagnosis and management of genitourinary cancer. Saunders, Philadelphia, pp 494–495]

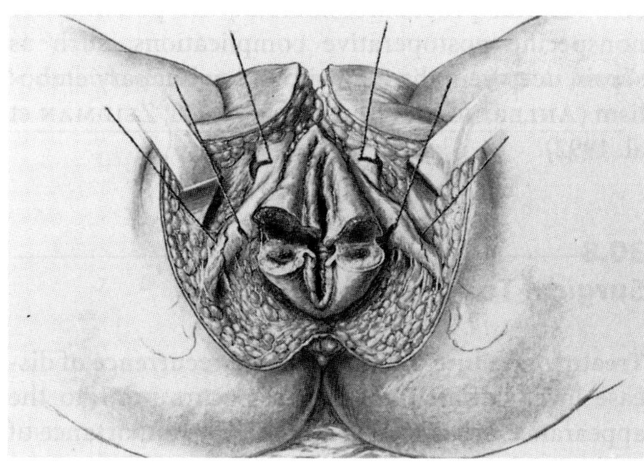

**Fig. 30.3.** View of perineum showing removal of the anterior vaginal wall and inferior rim of pubis using three Gigli saws which will allow en bloc removal of these structures with the bladder and pelvic lymph nodes. [From SKINNER EC, SKINNER DG (1988) Management of carcinoma of the female urethra. In: SKINNER DG, LIESKOVSKY G (eds) Diagnosis and management of genitourinary cancer. Saunders, Philadelphia, pp 494–495]

the opposite ischial rim of the pubic ramus. A third Gigli saw is then positioned in order to divide the pubis in half horizontally. A curved Kocher clamp is again passed through each obturator foramen and each end of this third Gigli saw is carefully passed through the right and left obturator foramen from the pelvis to the perineum. The three Gigli saws are in position to allow the lower rim of the pubis to be removed en bloc with the anterior pelvic organs once the remaining soft tissue between the lateral vaginal wall and the ischial rim of the pubic ramus is divided. This allows for excellent margins around the periurethral tissue and provides the best possible chance for local control of the disease. A urinary diversion of choice is then constructed (SKINNER and SKINNER 1988).

The perineum is closed by mobilizing the posterior vaginal wall, allowing the lateral walls to be sewn to the incised vulva. The wound is closed primarily in the area of the resected clitoris. A polyglycolic acid mesh can be used within the pelvis to further reinforce the pelvic floor and prevent a possible enterocele (SKINNER and SKINNER 1988). A large piece of mobilized greater omentum can serve this function as well. In the younger patients, consideration should be given to a vaginal reconstruction.

Complications include those following a standard radical cystectomy procedure, as well as some additional complications unique to this procedure. These include the development of osteitis pubis, resulting in pain and adductor spasms. In the author's experience, this occurs in approximately 18% of the patients, but can occur more frequently if more than 50 Gy of preoperative radiation has been administered. This complication can only be treated with palliative measures, but is usually self-limited. The rate of wound infections, occurring in approximately 1% of standard radical cystectomies, does not seem to be affected by the extended incision required for this procedure. However, any cosmetic reconstructive techniques can result in an increased wound complication rate, with either infection or dehiscence (SKINNER and SKINNER 1988).

# References


Ahlering T, Lieskovsky G (1988) Surgical treatment of urethral cancer in the male patient. In: Skinner DG, Lieskovsky G (eds) Diagnosis and management of genitourinary cancer. W.B. Saunders, Philadelphia, p 622

Benson R, Tunca J, Buchler D, Uehling D (1982) Primary carcinoma of the female urethra. Gynecol Oncol 14:313–318

Bolduan JP, Farah RN (1981) Primary urethral neoplasms: review of 30 cases. J Urol 125:198–200

Bracken RB, Johnson DE, Miller LS, et al. (1976) Primary carcinoma of the female urethra. J Urol 116:188–192

Carr L, Herschorn S, Leonhardt C (1996) Magnetic resonance imaging after intraurethral collagen injected for stress urinary incontinence. J Urol 155:1253–1255

Clayton M, Siami P, Guinan P (1992) Urethral diverticular carcinoma. Cancer 70:665–670

Desai S, Libertino J, Zinman L (1973) Primary carcinoma of the female urethra. J Urol 110:693–695

Elkon D, Kim J, Huddleston A, Constable W (1980) Primary carcinoma of the female urethra. South Med J 73:1439–1442

Evans K, McCarthy M, Sands J (1981) Adenocarcinoma of a female urethral diverticulum: a case report and review of the literature. J Urol 126:124–126

Gonzalez M, Harrison M, Boileau M (1985) Carcinoma in diverticulum of the female urethra. Urology 25:328–332

Grabstald H, Hilaris B, Henschke U, Whitmore W (1966) Cancer of the female urethra. JAMA 197:835–842

Hahn P, Krepart G, Malaker K (1991) Carcinoma of the female urethra. Urology 37:106–109

Hedden R, Husseinzadeh N, Bracken R (1993) Bladder sparing surgery for locally advanced female urethral cancer. J Urol 150:1135–1137

Johnson D, O'Connell J (1983) Primary carcinoma of female urethra. Urology 21:42–45

Johnson D, Kessler J, Ferrigni R, Anderson J (1989) Low dose combined chemotherapy/radiotherapy in the management of locally advanced urethral squamous cell carcinoma. J Urol 141:615–616

Joyner B, McDougal W (1997) Penile and urethral carcinoma – an overview. In: Crawford ED, Das S (eds) Current genitourinary cancer surgery. Williams & Wilkins, Baltimore, p 495

Katz J, Grabstald H (1976) Primary malignant melanoma of the female urethra. J Urol 116:454–457

Licht M, Klein E, Bukowski R, Montie J, Saxton J (1995) Combination radiation and chemotherapy for the treatment of squamous cell carcinoma of the male and female urethra. J Urol 153:1918–1920

Mayer R, Jackson FE, Clayton M (1987) Localized urethral cancer in women. Cancer 60:1548–1551

Mevorach R, Cos L, Di Saint 'Agnese P, Stoler M (1990) Human papillomavirus type 6 in grade I transitional cell carcinoma of the urethra. J Urol 143:126–127

Moinuddin M, Klein F, Hazra T (1988) Primary female urethral carcinoma. Cancer 62:54–57

Moore K (1985) Perineum and pelvis. In: Moore K (ed) Clinically oriented anatomy. Williams and Wilkins, Baltimore, p 298

Morikawa K, Togashi K, Minami S, Dodo Y, Imura T, Matsumoto M, Konishi J (1995) MR and CT appearance of urethral clear cell adenocarcinoma in a woman. J Comput Assist Tomogr 19:1001–1003

Narayan P, Konety B (1992) Surgical treatment of female urethral carcinoma. Urol Clin North Am 19:373–382

Pow-Sang J, Klimberg I, Hackett R, Wajsman Z (1988) Primary malignant melanoma of the male urethra. J Urol 139:1304–1306

Prempree T, Wizenberg M, Scott R (1978) Radiation treatment of primary carcinoma of the female urethra. Cancer 42:1177–1184

Shah A, Kalra J, Silber L, Molho L (1985) Squamous cell cancer of female urethra. Urology 25:284–286

Skinner E, Skinner DG (1988) Management of carcinoma of the female urethra. In: Skinner DG, Leiskovsky G (eds) Diagnosis and management of genitourinary cancer. W.B. Saunders, Philadelphia, p 490

Strohbehn K, Quit L, Prince M, Wojno K, Delancey J (1996) Magnetic resonance imaging anatomy of the female urethra: a direct histologic comparison. Obstet Gynecol 88:750–756

Tran L, Krieg R, Szabo R (1995) Combination chemotherapy and radiotherapy for a locally advanced squamous cell carcinoma of the urethra: a case report. J Urol 153:422–423

Turner A, Hendry W (1980) Primary carcinoma of the female urethra. Br J Urol 52:549–554

Weghaupt K, Gerstner G, Kucera H (1984) Radiation therapy for primary carcinoma of the female urethra: a survey over 25 years. Gynecol Oncol 17:58–63

Wiener J, Walther P (1994) A high association of oncogenic human papillomaviruses with carcinomas of the female urethra: a polymerase chain reaction-based analysis of multiple histological types. J Urol 151:49–53

Wiener J, Liu E, Walther P (1992) Oncogenic human papillomavirus type 16 is associated with squamous cell cancer of the male urethra. Cancer Res 52:5018–5023

Zeidman E, Desmond P, Thompson I (1992) Surgical treatment of carcinoma of the male urethra. Urol Clin North Am 19:359–372

# 31 Radiation Therapy for the Female Urethra

B. Micaily, M. Dzeda, J.E. Lahaniatis, and L.W. Brady

CONTENTS



## 31.1
## Introduction

Carcinoma of the female urethra is an uncommon tumor of the genitourinary tract. Few cases are being reported annually, and about 1500 cases have been reported in the literature (Grigsby 1992). Cancer of the female urethra represents 0.02% of all cancers in women and about 0.1% of all gynecologic malignancies (Johnson and O'Connell 1983; Weghaupt et al. 1984). A majority (85%) of cases of carcinoma of the urethra have been reported in white women while black women have been next (12%) in frequency (Hopkins and Grabstald 1986). The average age of diagnosis was 60 years of age, with the peak incidence between 50 and 80 years of age (Grabstald 1973). Squamous cell carcinoma is the most frequent histologic diagnosis, being reported in 70% of cases; transitional cell carcinoma is found in 15% followed by adenocarcinoma. The remaining cases include the following tumors: adenocystic carcinoma, clear cell adenocarcinoma, anaplastic tumors, Kaposi's sarcoma, lymphomas, and metastatic lesions. It is of interest to note a relatively frequent presence in the urethra of primary melanoma (Saileret et al. 1988).

Study of surgical specimens for the presence of human papillomavirus (HPV-16) revealed its presence in 59% of the 17 patients studied. Of the ten patients in whom HPV-16 was detected, 8 had invasive squamous cell carcinoma and 2 had a diagnosis of transitional cell carcinoma suggesting an association between HPV-16 and carcinoma of the female urethra (Weiner and Walther 1994).


B. Micaily, MD, Department of Radiation Oncology, Allegheny University of the Health Sciences, Allegheny University Hospitals, Hahnemann, 230 North Broad Street, Mail Stop 200, Philadelphia, PA 19102–1192, USA
M. Dzeda, MD, Department of Radiation Oncology, Allegheny University of the Health Sciences, Allegheny University Hospitals, Hahnemann, 230 North Broad Street, Mail Stop 200, Philadelphia, PA 19102–1192, USA
J.E. Lahaniatis MD, Department of Radiation Oncology, Allegheny University of the Health Sciences, Allegheny University Hospitals, Hahnemann, 230 North Broad Street, Mail Stop 200, Philadelphia, PA 19102–1192, USA
L.W. Brady, MD, Hylda Cohn/American Cancer Society Professor of Clinical Oncology, and Professor, Department of Radiation Oncology, Allegheny University of the Health Sciences, Allegheny University Hospitals, Hahnemann, 230 North Broad Street, Mail Stop 200, Philadelphia, PA 19102–1192, USA


## 31.2
## Tumor Behavior

### 31.2.1
### Anatomic Considerations

The female urethra is approximately 4 cm in length, extending from the bladder through the urogenital diaphragm to the vestibule, where it forms the urethral meatus. A small curve is formed with an anterior concavity because of the presence superiorly of the pubic ramus. The anterior vaginal wall abuts the urethra dorsally.

## 31.2.2
### Tumor Presentation and Spread

Bleeding is the most common presenting symptom, followed by pain and urinary difficulties (GRIGSBY 1992). Small tumors of the meatus may be misdiagnosed as a urethral caruncle which is a benign inflammatory lesion. With tumor progression it may ulcerate and extend to the perineum (PETERSON et al. 1973). Larger tumors of the distal urethra can be palpated during pelvic examination. More advanced tumors may present with urinary retention and overflow incontinence. In more than one-third of the patients, tumors are confined to the distal urethra with regional lymph node spread being uncommon (JOHNSON and O'CONNELL 1983; GRABSTALD 1973). The lymphatic drainage of the meatus parallels that of the vulva, which involves the superficial, deep inguinal, and external iliac lymph nodes. The entire urethra drains mainly to the obturator, internal and external iliac lymph nodes. Advanced stage II and III cases have been associated with up to a 50% incidence of inguinal or pelvic lymph node involvement. The incidence of bilateral lymph node involvement is about 30% in patients with any positive lymph nodes (GRIGSBY 1992). Distant metastases are found at the time of diagnosis in approximately 10% of patients. The most common metastatic sites include, in the order of decreasing frequency: the lung, liver, bone, and brain. Distant tumor spread is more common in adenocarcinoma and it does not seem to correlate with the presence of lymphatic involvement. Distant metastases are responsible for death in 30%–40% of patients (GRABSTALD 1973; PETERSON et al. 1973).

The two most significant prognostic factors affecting patient survival are the tumor stage and its location. GRIGSBY and CORN (1992) reported the actuarial 5-year progression-free survival to be 81%, 37%, and 7% for patients with tumors of <2 cm, 2–4 cm, and >4 cm, respectively. BRACKEN et al. (1976) noted a similar correlation between tumor size and survival. The reported 5-year survival rates were 60%, 46%, and 13% in patients with tumors of <2 cm, 2–4 cm, and >5 cm, respectively. Patients with early meatal tumors had an excellent 5-year survival rate of almost 90% (HOPKINS and GRABSTALD 1986). Involvement of the entire urethra, fixed lesions, infiltration of the adjacent organs, and lymph node metastases are well-documented poor prognostic factors. There was no statistically significant difference in treatment outcome in patients with different histologic diagnosis and presence or absence of adenopathy (GARDEN et al. 1993).

**Table 31.1.** Diagnostic workup for carcinoma of the female urethra

*General*
History
Physical examination, including detailed pelvic examination
    under anesthesia

*Special procedures*
Urine cytology
Punch biopsy
Urethroscopy
Cystoscopy
Rectosigmoidoscopy (advanced stages or if symptomatic)

*Radiographic evaluation*
Standard
    Chest radiographs
    Intravenous urography
    Computed tomography scan of abdomen and pelvis
    Barium enema (advanced stages or if symptomatic)
Complementary
    Urethrography
    Lymphangiography

*Laboratory evaluation*
Complete blood count
Chemistry profile
Urinalysis

Prior to selection of treatment, it is imperative to accurately define the tumor extent and complete diagnostic workup and tumor staging. Recommended diagnostic workup is shown in Table 31.1. The two commonly used staging systems are the TNM and Prempree systems. These staging systems are shown in Tables 31.2 and 31.3 (HENSON et al. 1992; PREMPREE et al. 1984).

## 31.3
### Treatment Selection and Outcome

### 31.3.1
### Early Stages (T15, T1N0, T2N0)

Tumors of the distal urethra limited to the mucosa can be treated either by surgery or by interstitial brachytherapy with similar excellent results. Treatment by surgery may involve the use of the following techniques: (1) laser, (2) local excision, (3) partial urethrectomy, or (4) total urethrectomy (NARAYAN and KONETY 1992). GRABSTALD et al. (1966) reported long-term survival in five of the seven patients treated with partial urethrectomy. The two remaining patients developed local recurrence and distant metastases 6 and 20 months after treatment,

**Table 31.2.** TNM classification for carcinoma of the urethra[a]

*Primary tumor* (T)

TX   Primary tumor cannot be assessed
T0   No evidence of primary tumor
Tis   Carcinoma in situ
Ta   Noninvasive papillary, polypoid, or verrucous carcinoma
T1   Tumor invades subepithelial connective tissue
T2   Tumor invades the periurethral muscle
T3   Tumor invades the anterior vagina or bladder neck
T4   Tumor invades other adjacent organs

*Regional lymph nodes* (N)

NX   Regional lymph nodes cannot be assessed
N0   No regional lymph node metastasis
N1   Metastasis in a single lymph node, 2 cm or less in greatest dimension
N2   Metastasis in a single lymph node, more than 2 cm but not more than 5 cm in greatest dimension, or multiple lymph nodes, not more than 5 cm in greatest dimension
N3   Metastasis in a lymph node more than 5 cm in greatest dimension

*Distant metastasis* (M)

MX   Presence of distant metastasis cannot be assessed
M0   No distant metastasis
M1   Distant metastasis

[a] Data from HENSON et al. (1992).


**Table 31.3.** Prempree modification staging for carcinoma of the female urethra[a]

| | |
|---|---|
| Stage I | Disease limited to the distal one-half of the urethra |
| Stage II | Disease involving the entire urethra, with extension to the periurethral tissues, but not involving the vulva or bladder neck |
| Stage III | |
| A | Disease involving the urethra and vulva |
| B | Disease invading the vaginal mucosa |
| C | Disease involving the urethra and bladder neck |
| Stage IV | |
| A | Disease invading parametrium or paracolpium |
| B | Metastases |
| 1 | Inguinal lymph nodes |
| 2 | Pelvic nodes |
| 3 | Para-aortic |
| 4 | Distant |

[a] Data from PREMPREE et al. (1983).


respectively. PETERSON et al. (1973) reported long-term tumor control in two patients with adenocarcinoma of the anterior urethra treated with surgical excision. The same investigators also reported another case where a patient with adenocarcinoma of the anterior urethra treated with local excision developed local and inguinal node recurrences 4 years after surgery. This tumor recurrence was controlled with salvage irradiation.

### 31.3.1.1
### Radiotherapy

Radiation therapy alone has been successful in treating distal urethral tumors. The reported cure rates with radiation therapy in early meatal tumors have ranged from 70% to 100%. ANTONIADES (1969) and PREMPREE et al. (1984) reported 100% 5-year survival in seven and three patients with meatal tumors, respectively. CHU (1973) reported the 5-year disease-free survival in 7 (64%) of 11 patients with distal urethral lesions treated with interstitial brachytherapy or brachytherapy in combination with external beam irradiation. WEGHAUPT et al. (1984) reported a 71% 5-year survival rate in 42 patients with anterior urethral tumors treated with a combination of intracavitary brachytherapy and external beam irradiation. Of the 42 patients treated, 40% had clinically positive lymph nodes. If these lymph nodes were >2 cm in diameter they were resected midway through the course of external beam radiotherapy.

### 31.3.1.2
### Brachytherapy Technique

Interstitial brachytherapy is well established as an effective alternative to surgery. Afterloading catheters using iridium-192 ($^{192}$Ir) are inserted to form a circular pattern around the urethral orifice. The treatment volume is defined with magnetic resonance imaging (MRI) and clinical evaluation (Fig. 31.1). Pretreatment planning is performed with a radiation physicist in attendance. This planning determines the number of radioactive sources along with their activity to best encompass the specified target volume and to deliver the desired dose rate. The patient, under spinal or general anesthesia, is placed in the lithotomy position and a Foley catheter is inserted into the bladder and its balloon inflated. The actual length of the urethra can be determined by gently pulling the balloon of the catheter toward the bladder neck, grasping the distal end of the catheter, deflating the balloon, and measuring the distance between the finger and the balloon. The Foley catheter is used as the carrier of the central source of the

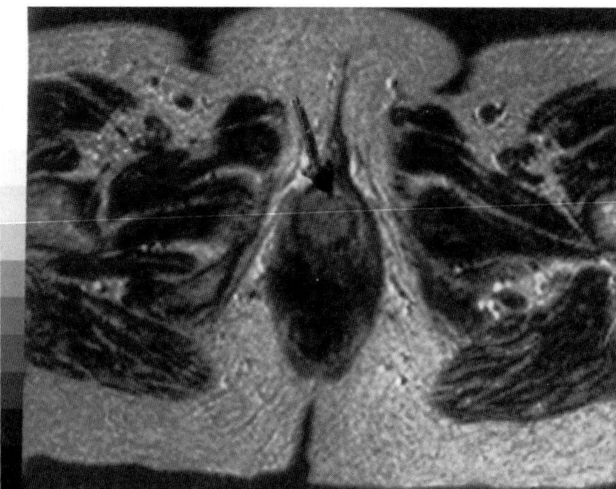

**Fig. 31.1.** Magnetic resonance image of a female pelvis. Cross-sectional view at urethral meatus, in a patient with squamous cell carcinoma of distal urethra. Note periurethral and anterior vaginal wall extension of the tumor (*solid arrow*)

implant. Stainless steel trocars spaced 1 cm apart, guided either by a template or by free hand, are inserted into the periurethral tissues in the circumferential pattern. Blind end plastic catheters are threaded into the trocars, and a metal stylet is used to keep the catheters in place as the trocars are removed. Metal buttons are placed over each catheter and crimped while the stylet remains in position. The stylet is then removed and the buttons are sutured to the skin to secure the afterloading catheters in place. Afterloading treatment planning is then carried out to determine the optimal loading of each catheter with $^{192}$Ir seeds so as to achieve a radiation dose distribution within the tumor volume that is as homogeneous as possible. After verification of source placement by radiography, a dose of 6000–7000 cGy is delivered at a dose rate of 60–120 cGy per hour to the periphery of the implant volume when brachytherapy is to be used alone (Figs. 31.2, 31.3).

### 31.3.2
### Advanced Stages (T3, T4, and Positive Nodes)

Tumor extension to the periurethral tissues, including the vagina and labia, or posteriorly into the bladder will usually require the use of multidisciplinary tumor management. The best results have been achieved with the use of preoperative irradiation followed by exenterative surgery and urinary diversion. KLEIN et al. (1983) reported on five female patients who received preoperative irradiation followed by anterior exenteration and inferior pubic rami resec-

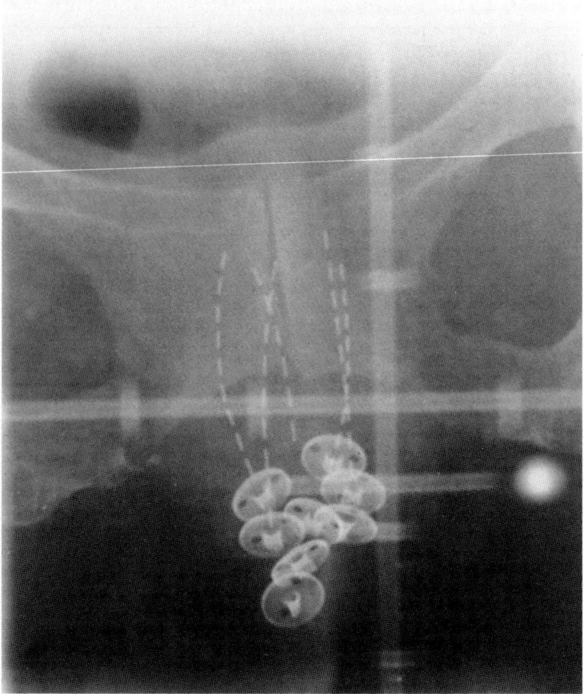

**Fig. 31.2.** Anteroposterior radiograph of an interstitial implant with $^{192}$Ir seeds using the afterloading technique. Forty-two seeds with an activity of 0.48 mg radium equivalent per seed were used in this patient

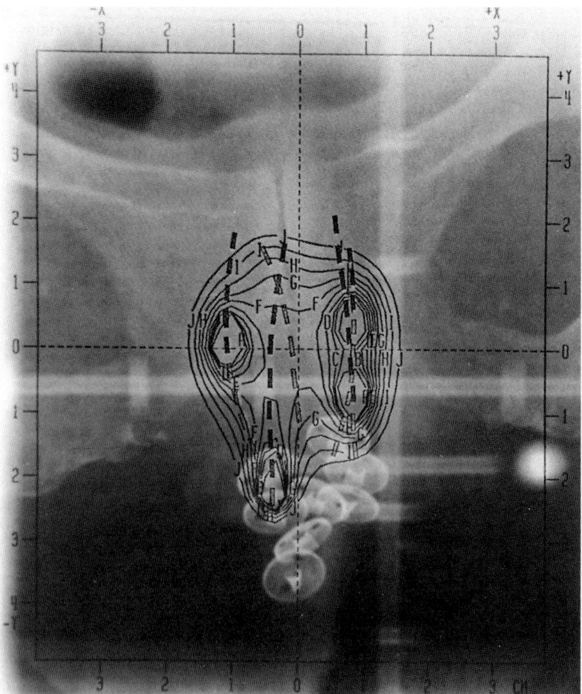

**Fig. 31.3.** Overlay of isodose distribution on the radiograph presented in Fig. 31.2. G line represents an isodose of 90 cGy per hour

tion. A 40% 5-year survival rate was obtained in this small group of patients.

### 31.3.2.1
### Surgical Treatment

Surgical management (see Chap. 30 for details) involves an anterior exenteration (cystourethrectomy) with an inguinal lymph node dissection. More advanced cases may require vaginal resection and reconstruction using gracilis-myocutaneous flaps. Involvement of the inferior pubic rami or symphysis pubis involves en bloc resection of the rami to ensure an adequate surgical margin (KLEIN et al. 1983). GRABSTALD et al. (1966) reported on the management of 15 patients with advanced carcinoma of the urethra treated by means of anterior or total exenteration. At 5 years post treatment, there were three survivors. BRACKEN et al. (1976) performed radical surgery in seven patients. Of the seven patients treated, four (57%) failed locally, with one of these four patients being salvaged by external beam irradiation for a perineal recurrence.

### 31.3.2.2
### Radiotherapy

In order to achieve adequate tumor volume coverage in patients with advanced carcinoma of the urethra, the use of external beam radiation therapy is required in addition to brachytherapy. Definitive treatment with radiation therapy consists in coverage of the whole pelvis with adequate width of the anterior and posterior portals to encompass the inguinal and external and internal iliac lymph nodes. This is followed by an interstitial brachytherapy boost. The pelvis is treated with a dose of 4500–5000 cGy in 4–5 weeks by external beam. A four-field pelvic technique is used to reduce treatment side-effects and allow adequate coverage of the medial inguinal lymph nodes (Figs. 31.4, 31.5). Care should be taken particularly when treating the perineum in the elderly patient to avoid confluent moist desquamation, which may interfere with treatment completion. This tissue reaction may be substantially reduced by eliminating the difference in tissue thickness by using either bolus or tissue compensators, or by treating the patient with the legs adducted to homogenize the radiation dose at the perineum. After a 1- to 2-week rest period, an additional 2000–3500 cGy is delivered by the afterloading interstitial implant (as

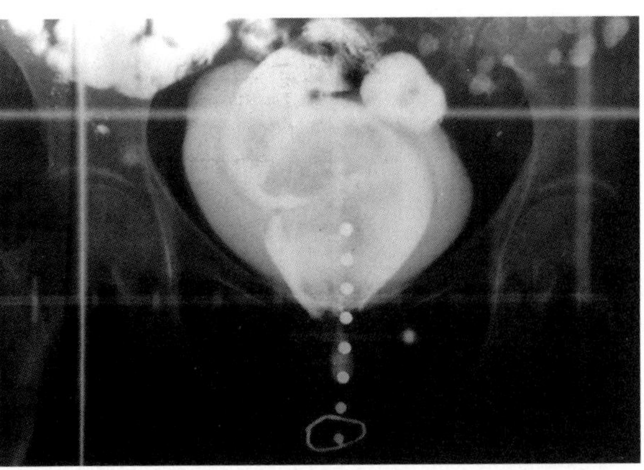

**Fig. 31.4.** Anteroposterior radiograph as a part of the treatment simulation process of the four-field pelvis technique for urethral cancer. The patient is in the prone position placed on a wedge-shaped sponge; the bladder and rectum are filled with contrast media. Note displacement of small bowel loops outside of the radiation fields. Markers on the urethral meatus and anus are shown on simulation radiographs. Note the inclusion in the radiation portal of the medial inguinal lymph nodes

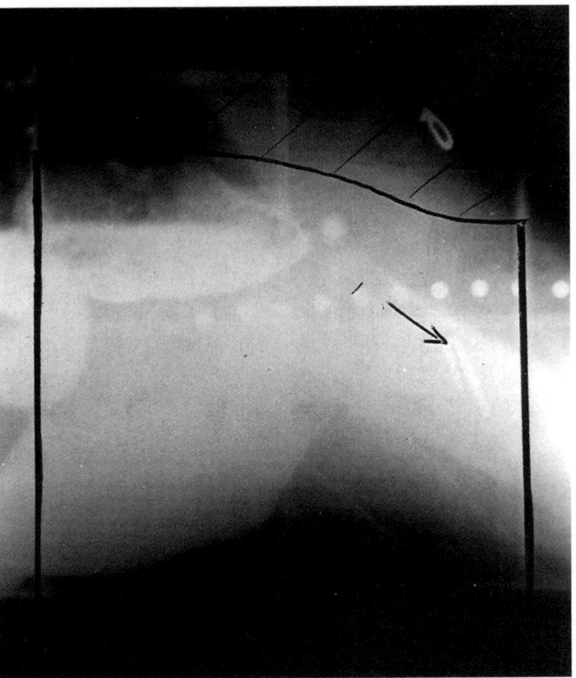

**Fig. 31.5.** Lateral simulation radiographs of the four-field pelvis technique for urethral cancer. The patient is in the prone position placed on a wedge-shaped sponge; the bladder and rectum are filled with contrast media. Note displacement of small bowel loops outside the radiation fields. Markers on the urethral meatus and anus are shown on simulation radiographs. Note the inclusion of the medial inguinal lymph nodes. The posterior wall of the rectum and the entire anus are excluded from the volume of interest

described in Sect. 31.3.1.2) for a cumulative tumor dose of 7000–8000 cGy. ANTONIADES (1969) reported a 36% 5-year survival rate in the 11 patients treated using external beam irradiation followed by brachytherapy. BRACKEN et al. (1976) reported a 25% 5-year survival for stage C and 20% 5-year survival for stage D lesions. PREMPREE et al. (1984) treated five patients with irradiation alone and two with preoperative irradiation. Four of the five patients treated had no evidence of disease at 5 years post treatment. One of the two patients receiving preoperative irradiation had no evidence of disease at 2 years and the other died of intercurrent disease. WEGHAUPT et al. (1984) reported a 50% 5-year survival rate in 20 patients with involvement of the posterior urethra or of its entire length, treated as previously described for the anterior urethral cases. Palliation with radiation therapy may provide local tumor control but it is usually of short duration (GARDEN et al. 1993).

## 31.4
## Treatment of Lymphadenopathy

Clinical involvement of inguinal lymph nodes warrants consideration of lymphadenectomy or radiotherapy. When the lymph nodes are clinically negative, prophylactic lymphadenectomy has not been proven to be superior to therapeutic node dissection (LEVINE 1980). Several investigators have recommended prophylactic inguinal lymph node irradiation (GARDEN et al. 1993; FOENS et al. 1991; HAHN et al. 1987). Those patients not receiving prophylactic inguinal node irradiation had a significantly higher (52%) inguinal failure rate than those who did (10%) receive this treatment. The use of elective inguinal lymph node irradiation has also resulted in a correspondingly higher survival rate as compared with those patients who did not receive this treatment, the 5-year survival rates being 60% and 18%, respectively (FOENS et al. 1991). Tables 31.4 and 31.5 provide a summary of reported treatment results for early and advanced-stage carcinoma of the urethra in females.

## 31.5
## Chemo-radiotherapy Combination

Several investigators have used concomitant chemotherapy and irradiation. Three medical centers have published case reports of patients with advanced

**Table 31.4.** Summary of treatment results for early female urethral carcinoma

| Reference | No. of patients | Treatment[a] | 5-year survival (%) |
|---|---|---|---|
| GRABSTALD et al. (1966) | 26 | R | 3/13 (23) |
|  |  | S | 8/10 (80) |
|  |  | R + S | 2/3 (67) |
| BRACKEN et al. (1976) | 30 | R (19) | (40–45)[b] |
|  |  | S (3) |  |
|  |  | R + S (8) |  |
| TAGGART et al. (1972) | 15 | R | 8/15 (53)[c] |
| ANTONIADES (1969) | 8 | R | 7/8 (87.5) |
| CHU (1973) | 11 | R | 7/11 (64) |
| PPREMPREE et al. (1984) | 7 | R | 5/7 (71) |
| WEGHAUPT et al. (1984) | 42 | R | 30/42 (71) |
| DESAI et al. (1973) | 10 | R | 4/10 (40) |

[a] R, Radiation therapy; S, surgery; R + S, radiation therapy plus surgery.
[b] Three-year survival estimated from survival curve.
[c] Two-year no evidence of disease.

**Table 31.5.** Summary of treatment results for advanced female urethral carcinoma

| Reference | No. of patients | Treatment[a] | 5-year survival (%) |
|---|---|---|---|
| GRABSTALD et al. (1966) | 48 | R | 1/14 (17) |
|  |  | S | 3/17 (18) |
|  |  | R + S | 5/17 (29) |
| BRACKEN et al. (1976) | 44 | R (35) | (20–25)[b] |
|  |  | S (8) |  |
|  |  | R + S (1) |  |
| TAGGART et al. (1972) | 22 | R (18) | 4/22 (18)[c] |
|  |  | S (4) |  |
| ANTONIADES (1969) | 11 | R | 4/11 (36) |
| CHU (1973) | 8 | R | 0/8 (0) |
| PREMPREE et al. (1984) | 7 | R (5) |  |
|  |  | R + S (2) | 4/5 (80) |
| WEGHAUPT et al. (1984) | 20 | R | 10/20 (50) |
| DESAI et al. (1973) | 6 | R | 1/6 (17) |

[a] R, Radiation therapy; S, surgery; R + S, radiation therapy plus surgery.
[b] Three-year survival estimated from survival curve.
[c] Two-year no evidence of disease.

squamous cell carcinoma of the female urethra treated with 5-fluorouracil, mitomycin C, and external beam irradiation with impressive results (JOHNSON et al. 1989; SHAH et al. 1985; TRAN et al. 1995). Another area of interest is the application of neoadjuvant chemotherapy with methotrexate, vinblastine, doxorubicin, and cisplatin (M-VAC) for transitional cell carcinoma of the female urethra. This treatment regimen has been successfully used in the management of transitional cell carcinoma of the bladder (SCHER et al. 1988).

## 31.6
## Treatment Complications

### 31.6.1
### Surgery

Surgical approaches such as anterior exenteration and inferior pubic rami resection have resulted in a substantial morbidity. Reported treatment complications of these procedures include: (1) rectovaginal fistula, (2) perineal herniation, (3) small bowel fistula, (4) abscess formation, and (5) fracture of the superior pubic ramus (KLEIN et al.1983; FOENS et al. 1991). These are in addition to the permanent ostomies necessitated by surgery.

### 31.6.2
### Radiotherapy

Reported complications of radiation therapy have been decreasing since the early 1980s due to adoption of the practice of treating multiple fields each day and using shrinking field techniques. Most medical centers report a complication rate of 12%–30% (ANTONIADES 1969; CHU 1973; GRIGSBY and CORN 1992; GARDEN et al. 1993; PREMPREE et al. 1984; FOENS et al. 1991). Previously reported complications include: (1) urethral strictures, (2) urinary incontinence, (3) cystitis, (4) osteomyelitis, (5) radiation enteritis, and (6) small bowel obstruction. Fistula formation is a severe complication of radiotherapy in patients with advanced disease. The existing tumor extension into adjacent organs undergoes necrosis following radiotherapy, resulting in fistula formation.

## 31.7
## Conclusions

Excellent results may be achieved with either surgery or radiotherapy for early distal urethral cancers (squamous and adenocarcinomas).

Early proximal or entire urethral cancers are best treated with a combination or external beam radiotherapy and brachytherapy with or without chemotherapy with excellent results and preservation of organ function. Surgery can be used for radiotherapy failures or persistent tumors.

Advanced carcinoma of the urethra requires a multimodality therapeutic approach, and a combination of radiation and chemotherapy appears to be the optimal way to treat these patients. Surgery should be used in biopsy-proven persistent tumors or recurrent tumors following radio-chemotherapy .

## References

Antoniades J (1969) Radiation therapy in carcinoma of the female urethra. Cancer 24:70–76

Bracken RB, Johnson DE, Miller LS, et al. (1976) Primary carcinoma of the female urethra. J Urol 116:188–192

Chu AM (1973) Female urethral carcinoma. Radiology 107:627–630

Desai S, Libertino JA, Zinman L (1973) Primary carcinoma of the female urethra. J Urol 110:693–695

Foens CS, Hussey DH, Staples JJ, et al. (1991) A comparison of the roles of surgery and radiation therapy in the management of carcinoma of the female urethra. Int J Radiat Oncol Biol Phys 21:961–968

Forman JD, Lichter AS (1992) The role of radiation therapy in the management of carcinoma of the male and female urethra. Urol Clin North Am 19:383–389

Garden AS, Zagars GK, Delclos L (1993) Primary carcinoma of the female urethra. Results of radiation therapy. Cancer 71:3102–3108

Grabstald H (1982) Commentary: urethral cancer. In: Johnson DE, Boileau MA (eds) Genitourinary tumors. Grune & Stratton, New York, p 287

Grabstald H (1973) Proceedings: tumors of the urethra in men and women. Cancer 32:1236–1256

Grabstald H, Hilaris B, Henschke U, Whitmore WF Jr (1966) Cancer of the female urethra. JAMA 197:835–842

Grigsby PW (1992) Female urethra. In: Perez CA, Brady LW (eds) Principles and practice of radiation oncology, 2nd edn Lippincott, Philadelphia, p 1059

Grigsby PW, Corn BW (1992) Localized urethral tumors in women: indications for conservative versus exenterative therapies. J Urol 147:1516–1520

Hahn P, Krepart G, Malaker K (1991) Carcinoma of female urethra. The Manitoba experience: 1958–1987. Urology 37:106–109

Henson DE, Hutter RV, Kennedy BJ (eds) (1992) Manual for staging of cancer, 4th edn. Lippincott, Philadelphia

Hopkins SC, Grabstald H (1986) Benign and malignant tumors of the male and female urethra. In: Walsh PC, Gittes RF, Perlmutter AD, Stamey TA (eds) Campbell's urology, 5th edn. Saunders, Philadelphia, p 1441

Johnson DE, O'Connell JR (1983) Primary carcinoma of the female urethra. Urology 21:42–45

Johnson DW, Kessler JF, Ferrigni RG, et al. (1989) Low dose combined chemotherapy/radiotherapy in the management of locally advanced urethral squamous cell carcinoma. J Urol 141:615–616

Klein FA, Whitmore WF Jr, Herr HW, et al. (1983) Inferior pubic rami resection with en bloc radical excision for invasive proximal urethral carcinoma. Cancer 51:1238–1242

Levine RL (1980) Urethral cancer. Cancer 45 (7 Suppl):1965–1972

Meis JM, Ayala AG, Johnson DE (1987) Adenocarcinoma or the urethra in women: a clinicopathologic study [published erratum appears in Cancer 1987; 60: 2900]. Cancer 60:1038–1052

Mostofi FK, Davis CJ Jr, Sesterhenn IA (1992) Carcinoma of the male and female urethra. Urol Clin North Am 19:347–358

Narayan P, Konety B (1992) Surgical treatment of female urethral carcinoma. Urol Clin North Am 19:373–382

Peterson DT, Dockerty MB, Utz DC, et al. (1973) The peril of primary carcinoma of the urethra in women. J Urol 110:72–75

Prempree T, Amonmarn R, Patanaphan V (1984) Radiation therapy in primary carcinoma of the female urethra. II. An update on results. Cancer 54:729–733

Rajan N, Tucci P, Mallouh C, Choudhury M (1993) Carcinoma in female urethral diverticulum: case reports and review of management. J Urol 150:1911–1914

Sailer SL, Shipley WU, Wang CC (1988) Carcinoma of the female urethra: a review of results with radiation therapy. J Urol 140:1–5

Scher HI, Yagoda A, Herr HW, et al. (1988) Neoadjuvant M-VAC (methotrexate, vinblastine, doxorubicin, and cisplatin) for extravesical urinary tract tumors. J Urol 139:475–477

Selch MT, Mark RJ, Fu YS, et al. (1993) Primary lymphoma of female urethra: long-term control by radiation therapy. Urology 42:343–346

Shah AB, Kalra JK, Silber L, Molho L (1985) Squamous cell cancer of the female urethra. Successful treatment with chemotherapy. Urology 25:284–286

Taggart CG, Castro JR, Rutledge FN (1972) Carcinoma of the female urethra. Am J Roentgen Radium Ther Nucl Med 114:145–151

Tran LN, Krieg RM, Szabo RJ (1995) Combination chemotherapy and radiotherapy for a locally advanced squamous cell carcinoma of the urethra: a case report. J Urol 153:422–423.

Weghaupt K, Gerstner GJ, Kocera H (1984) Radiation therapy for primary carcinoma of the female urethra: a survey over 25 years. Gynecol Oncol 17:58–63

Weiner JS, Walther PJ (1994) A high association of oncogenic human papillomaviruses with carcinomas of the female urethra: polymerase chain reaction-based analysis of multiple histologic types. J Urol 151:49

# Sarcoma of the Genito-Urinary Tract in Adults

# 32 Primary Retroperitoneal Sarcomas

A.J. Figueroa, J.P. Stein, and D.G. Skinner

CONTENTS



## 32.1
## Introduction

Retroperitoneal sarcomas are rare tumors that account for 10%–20% of all soft tissue sarcomas (Binder et al. 1978; Coran et al. 1970). Retroperitoneal sarcomas are responsible for only 0.1%–0.2% of all malignant lesions in the United States (Armstrong and Cohn 1965; Benmark et al. 1980; Binder et al. 1978; Bose 1979; Pack and Tabah 1954). Eighty-five percent of retroperitoneal tumors are malignant, and 35% are found to be sarcomas (Donnelly 1946; Melcow 1953; Pack and Tabah 1954). They can occur in patients of all ages, with a peak incidence in the sixth decade of life. The first description of a retroperitoneal tumor was reported

by Morgagni in 1761 (Morgagni 1969). The overall prognosis of patients with retroperitoneal sarcomas is poor; these tumors can become quite extensive, and invade adjacent organs prior to diagnosis. They are relatively resistant to chemotherapy and radiation therapy. Surgical intervention currently offers the best hope for cure, with the highest reported overall and disease-free survival and the lowest recurrence rates. However, these tumors can be difficult to completely resect en bloc (without positive surgical margins), resulting in a high incidence of local recurrence and poor survival rates.

## 32.2
## Clinical Presentation

Patients with retroperitoneal sarcomas present most commonly with abdominal or flank pain associated with a palpable abdominal mass which is associated with weight loss (Bose 1979; Braasch and Mon 1967; Cody et al. 1981; Oriana et al. 1977; Pack and Tabah 1954). Symptoms are related to the size, location, and associated organ involvement by the tumor. The average duration of symptoms to the time of presentation is 5 months. A nontender, palpable mass is found in 80%–90% of patients at initial presentation. Patients may give a history of increasing abdominal girth, while 40%–70% of patients describe vague, poorly localized discomfort. Nonspecific symptoms of nausea, vomiting, and back pain are uncommon. Neurologic signs and symptoms attributed to compression of the lumbar and sacral plexus nerve roots are present in 27%–33% (Cohan et al. 1988). Less commonly (15%), patients present with nonmalignant serous ascites secondary to external portal vein compression (Storm and Mahvi 1991). Gastrointestinal symptoms of a partially obstructed nature due to displacement or direct invasion by the mass are present in 10% of patients (Storm and Mahvi 1991). Acute or chronic gastrointestinal bleeding may occur if the tumor erodes into an adjacent portion of small or large intestine.


A.J. Figueroa, MD, Chief Resident, Department of Urology, University of Southern California, Kenneth Norris Jr. Comprehensive Cancer Center, 1441 Eastlake Ave., Suite 7414, Los Angeles, California 90033, USA
J.P. Stein, MD, Assistant Professor, Department of Urology, University of Southern California, Kenneth Norris Jr. Comprehensive Cancer Center, 1441 Eastlake Ave., Suite 7414, Los Angeles, California 90033, USA
D.G. Skinner, MD, Professor and Chairman, Department of Urology, University of Southern California, Kenneth Norris Jr. Comprehensive Cancer Center, 1441 Eastlake Ave., Suite 7414, Los Angeles, California 90033, USA

Urinary tract symptoms (dysuria and hematuria) are uncommon. Despite the proximity of the kidney and ureter to many of these retroperitoneal tumors, urinary tract obstruction is generally uncommon (Braasch and Mon 1967; Duncan and Evans 1977). Although rare, patients may present with hypoglycemia thought to be related to either the production of an insulin-like substance or the rapid utilization of glucose stores by some highly metabolically active sarcomas (Papaioannou 1966; Storm and Mahvi 1991). Other less common presenting symptoms may include lower extremity edema secondary to vena caval or lymphatic obstruction.

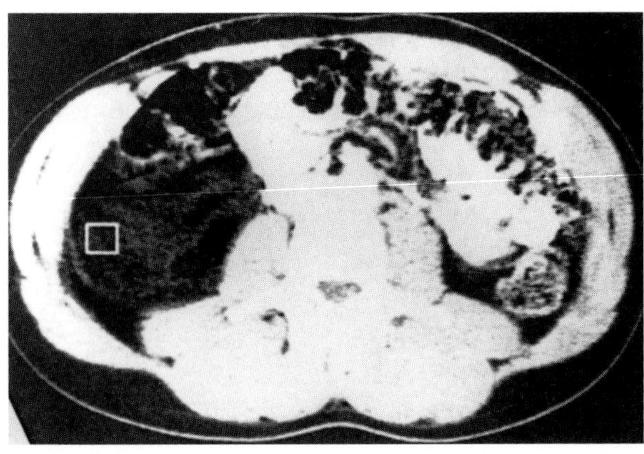

Fig. 32.1. Example of a CT scan of a primary retroperitoneal liposarcoma originating within Gerota's fascia around the right kidney

## 32.3
## Radiologic Evaluation

The most useful radiographic study in the evaluation of retroperitoneal sarcoma is computed tomography (CT) scan (de Santos et al. 1981; Kreel and Bydder 1981; Lindell et al. 1981; Neifeld et al. 1982). An abdominal CT scan can evaluate a retroperitoneal mass, and its relationship to adjacent structures. It can also identify lymph node involvement if greater than 1 cm in diameter and the presence of any locoregional metastases (see Chap. 4). Furthermore, CT scanning may help to distinguish sarcomas from other retroperitoneal malignancies, such as lymphomas or germ cell tumors (Dalton et al. 1989). However, CT scanning cannot distinguish the various sarcomatous cell types, with the exception of liposarcoma, which contains fat (Fig. 32.1). Additionally, it may provide a gross evaluation of renal function. Importantly, CT scanning plays a critical role in routine postoperative patient follow-up and detection of disease recurrence.

Magnetic resonance imaging (MRI) is being used with increasing frequency. It may prove useful in evaluating spinal cord involvement and determining whether the tumor extends along a spinal nerve root into the cord. MRI should be considered for all patients with neurologic symptoms. T1-weighted MRI images may better define the relationship of the tumor to other adjacent solid organs, including liver, spleen, and pancreas, than CT scanning. T2-weighted MR images may also provide better resolution of adjacent muscle invasion, and are particularly useful in determining the extent of tumor within the psoas or quadratus muscles and those tumors near the spinal foramina (Storm and Mahvi 1991). In cases where CT scan or clinical presenta-

tion suggests tumor thrombus involvement (inferior vena cava), MRI can be used to determine the extent of caval involvement. MRI is less invasive than venacavogram and provides better anatomic detail than CT scanning.

Angiography is reserved for those cases in which CT scan is inconclusive, or in which better definition of the vascular anatomy is needed prior to resection. It should not be used, however, to determine surgical resectability.

All patients with elevated serum alkaline phosphatase levels or bony pain should undergo a bone scan. Those patients considered for surgery should undergo a chest CT scan to evaluate for peripheral metastases of 1 cm or less in diameter. The standard chest radiographs will often miss small peripheral lung metastases associated with retroperitoneal sarcomas.

## 32.4
## Pathologic Evaluation

### 32.4.1
### Tumor Histology

Retroperitoneal sarcomas are derived from primary mesenchyme. The most common histologic type is liposarcoma (Cody et al. 1981; Coran et al. 1970; Fortner et al. 1981; Karakousis et al. 1995; McGrath et al. 1984; Oriana et al. 1977; Pack and Tabah 1954). Other histologic types include: leiomyosarcoma, fibrosarcoma, malignant fibrous histiocytoma, neurosarcoma, undifferentiated sarcomas, hemangiopericytoma, rhabdomyosarcoma, and other less common sarcomas (DALTON et al. 1989; McGRATH et al. 1984; STORM and MAHVI 1991).

## 32.4.2
### Tumor Grade

Determination of tumor grade depends on the degree of cytologic atypia, number of mitoses (5 per high power field), and the presence or extent of necrosis. Sarcomas are designated as grade 1 (G1 – well differentiated), grade 2 (G2 – intermediate grade, moderately differentiated), or grade 3 (G3 – poorly differentiated). The pathologic grade is one of the strongest predictors of clinical outcome and survival for patients with retroperitoneal sarcomas and is the basis of the American Joint Commission on Cancer (AJCC) staging system (Table 32.1) (BEARS et al. 1988). Of patients presenting with retroperitoneal sarcoma, 57% have histologically high tumor grade, and 43% have low grade (JAQUES et al. 1990).

## 32.4.3
### Tumor Stage

The histopathologic grade of the tumor determines the stage (I, II, and III) of the patient's disease. Stages a and b separate large and small sarcomas. Patients with a T1 tumor (less than 5 cm in diameter) are substage a; those with larger tumors (greater than 5 cm in diameter) are substage b. Tumors with local invasion (bone, nerves, vessels) are classified as T3. Tumors with lymph node metastases are classified as stage IVa while those with distant metastases are stage IVb.

## 32.5
### Management of Retroperitoneal Sarcomas

The optimal treatment for a retroperitoneal sarcoma is complete surgical extirpation. Every effort should be made toward complete en bloc excision of the tumor with adequate surgical margins. Different types of surgical approaches and incisions have been described, including the transperitoneal approach (through the midline), transverse incision (chevron), or thoracoabdominal incision. The ideal surgical incision should provide optimal exposure and visual-

**Table 32.1.** The American Joint Commission on Cancer (AJCC) staging system for retroperitoneal sarcomas

*Grade (G)*

| | |
|---|---|
| GX | Grade cannot be assessed |
| G1 | Well differentiated |
| G2 | Moderately differentiated |
| G3 | Poorly differentiated |
| G4 | Undifferentiated |

*Primary tumor (T)*

| | |
|---|---|
| TX | Primary tumor cannot be assessed |
| T0 | No evidence of tumor |
| T1 | Tumor size ≤5 cm |
| T2 | Tumor size >5 cm |
| T3 | Primary tumor grossly invading bone, major vessels, major nerves, or extensively infiltrating adjacent soft tissues with fixation |

*Regional lymph nodes (N)*

| | |
|---|---|
| NX | Regional nodes cannot be assessed |
| N0 | No regional lymph node metastases |
| N1 | Regional lymph node metastases |

*Distant metastases (M)*

| | |
|---|---|
| MX | Presence of distant metastases cannot be assessed |
| M0 | No distant metastases |
| M1 | Distant metastases |

*Stage grouping*

| | |
|---|---|
| Ia: | G1, T1, N0, M0 |
| Ib: | G1, T2, N0, M0 |
| IIa: | G2, T1, N0, M0 |
| IIb: | G2, T2, N0, M0 |
| IIIa: | G3, G4, T1, N0, M0 |
| IIIb: | G3, G4, T2, N0, M0 |
| IVa: | Any G, any T, N1, M0 |
| IVb: | Any G, any T, any N, M1 |

ization, and allow access for early vascular control of the tumor's principal blood supply. We are strong advocates (particularly for larger or vascular tumors) of the thoracoabdominal approach. The flank approach is suboptimal for large retroperitoneal tumors since it provides poor exposure, and early control of the major blood vessels is virtually impossible.

Resection of adjacent organs is often necessary to achieve complete excision. Up to 68% of the explorations require resection of adjacent organs to ensure negative margins (DALTON et al. 1989; JAQUES et al. 1990; McGRATH et al. 1984). The most frequently resected organs include: kidney (32%–46%), colon (25%), adrenal gland (18%), pancreas (15%), and spleen (10%) (JAQUES et al. 1990; McGRATH et al. 1984). Historically, incomplete surgical resection has been reported in 25%–65% of patients (ADAM et al. 1984; CODY et al. 1981; FORTNER et al. 1981; KARAKOUSIS et al. 1985; McGRATH et al. 1984; STORM and MAHVI 1991).

The most common cause of unresectability is adherence to the aorta, vena cava, pancreas, pelvic side wall, or peripheral nerve root. It should be emphasized that the ability to achieve a complete surgical excision affects overall outcome. Incomplete resection results in a high incidence of local recurrence and ultimate failure. Even in patients presumed to undergo complete resection, local recurrence rates ranging from 43% to 82% have been reported often in the absence of metastases (ADAM et al. 1984; CODY et al. 1981; FORTNER et al. 1981; GLENN et al. 1985; KARAKOUSIS et al. 1985, 1995; McGRATH et al. 1984; SOLLA and REED 1986). Patients with locally recurrent disease should be considered for salvage surgical therapy since complete resection can be achieved in more than a third of these patients.

The morbidity and mortality associated with surgical resection of retroperitoneal sarcomas has improved considerably. Most series report an operative mortality of 2%–7% and an operative morbidity of 6%–24% (CODY et al. 1981; JAQUES et al. 1990; McGRATH 1994). The most common complications following surgery are enterocutaneous fistula, intra-abdominal abscess, and intra-abdominal hemorrhage.

## 32.6
## Surgical Technique

Patient positioning is extremely important, and attention to detail facilitates all phases of the operation (Fig. 32.2). The patient should be positioned on the ipsilateral side of the operating table with the break of the table located immediately above the iliac crest. The contralateral leg is flexed 90° and the hips approximately 30°. The ipsilateral shoulder is then torqued approximately 20° off the horizontal, and the ipsilateral arm brought across the chest and placed in an adjustable arm rest. The pelvis remains nearly supine, perhaps rotated only 10° off the horizontal. A sheet roll is then placed longitudinally under the ipsilateral side of the back, and a similar roll is positioned under the contralateral side of the abdomen. The table is hyperextended, and the patient secured with wide adhesive tape at the shoulders, hips, and legs. The ipsilateral leg remains extended along the ipsilateral edge of the table and is supported by a pillow.

The incision generally begins at the mid-axillary line and extends over the eight or ninth rib. The precise rib incision depends on the extent and location of the retroperitoneal disease: the larger the

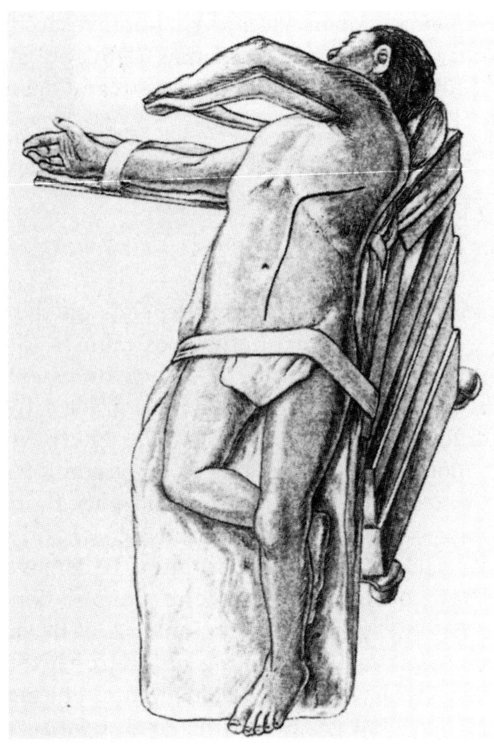

**Fig. 32.2.** Proper positioning of the patient for the modified thoracoabdominal approach. [From Skinner DG (1977) Considerations for management of large retroperitoneal tumors: use of the modified thoracoabdominal approach. J Urol 117:605]

mass, the higher the incision. The incision extends over the rib and across the costochondral junction into the epigastrium, where it courses inferiorly as a midline incision towards the pelvis. The incision may also be extended across the epigastrium to improve exposure to the contralateral retroperitoneum. A subperiosteal rib resection is performed, and the costochondral junction is divided. The rectus muscle is divided in the epigastrium and retracted laterally.

In the case of a large retroperitoneal tumor, the peritoneum is entered and the small bowel, ascending and transverse colon, duodenum, pancreas, and (on the left side) spleen must be mobilized completely on the superior mesenteric artery pedicle. The small bowel can be placed in a Lahey bag on the anterior chest wall (Figs. 32.3–32.6). It is essential that the superior mesenteric artery be identified at the point where it crosses over the left renal vein. This artery must not be injured, since it serves as the principal vascular pedicle for the small and large bowel. Care must also be taken to prevent excessive

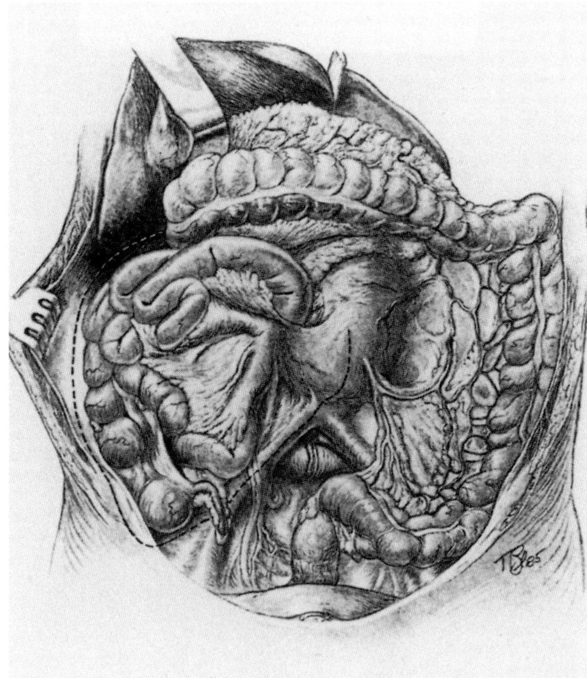

Fig. 32.3. Peritoneal incision necessary for complete mobilization of small bowel, ascending colon, duodenum, and pancreas. [From Skinner DG (1977) Considerations for management of large retroperitoneal tumors: use of the modified thoracoabdominal approach. J Urol 117:605]

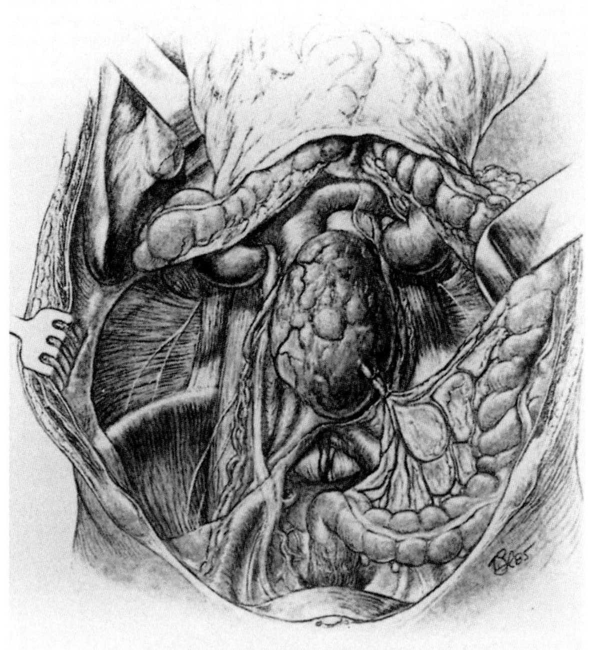

Fig. 32.4. Once the peritoneal attachments to the colon and small bowel mesentery have been incised, the entire retroperitoneum can be exposed through the right side of the chest by placing the intra-abdominal contents in a Lahey bag on the anterior chest wall. Care must be taken not to put too much tension on the superior mesenteric pedicle. [From Skinner DG (1977) Considerations for management of large peritoneal tumors: use of the modified thoracoabdominal approach. J Urol 117:605]

tension on this artery and to prevent injuring it with a retractor.

It is often necessary to ligate and divide the inferior mesenteric artery (at its aortal origin) to free the descending colonic mesentery. This is a safe maneuver if the marginal artery remains intact. If a portion of the colon does not appear viable at the end of the procedure, it should be resected. Occasionally, diarrhea or intermittent abdominal pain, usually associated with oral intake of food, may result from ischemia to the large bowel following ligation of the inferior mesenteric artery. This is a rare occurrence in particularly young patients and can usually be managed successfully and conservatively without long-term sequelae.

Generally, it is possible to mobilize the aorta and resect it free from the large retroperitoneal mass. Ligation and division of the lumbar arteries distal to the renal pedicle facilitates aortic mobilization. Troublesome bleeding from avulsed lumbar vessels may occur, but this can be avoided by individual ligation and division of each pair of vessels distal to the renal pedicle. The placement of hemoclips on the distal portion of the vessel facilitates this part of the operation, but it is best to ligate the lumbar vessels at the origin of the aorta and vena cava because the clips may be dislodged later in the procedure, causing bleeding behind the great vessels. Occasionally, troublesome bleeding from a torn lumbar vein or artery will develop despite all precautions. The use of an Allis clamp is helpful, and 4-0 arterial silk should be available in all cases. Only on rare occasions must the aorta be resected with the tumor mass and require replacement with a Dacron bypass graft.

Frequently, large retroperitoneal tumors will be intimately associated with the inferior vena cava and may obstruct this vessel. In such cases, it is best to resect the vena cava en bloc with the tumor. It may also be necessary to remove the ipsilateral kidney en bloc with the tumor. If the right kidney and vena cava are resected en bloc with the tumor, it is important to maintain the connection between the vena cava and the left renal vein, even when

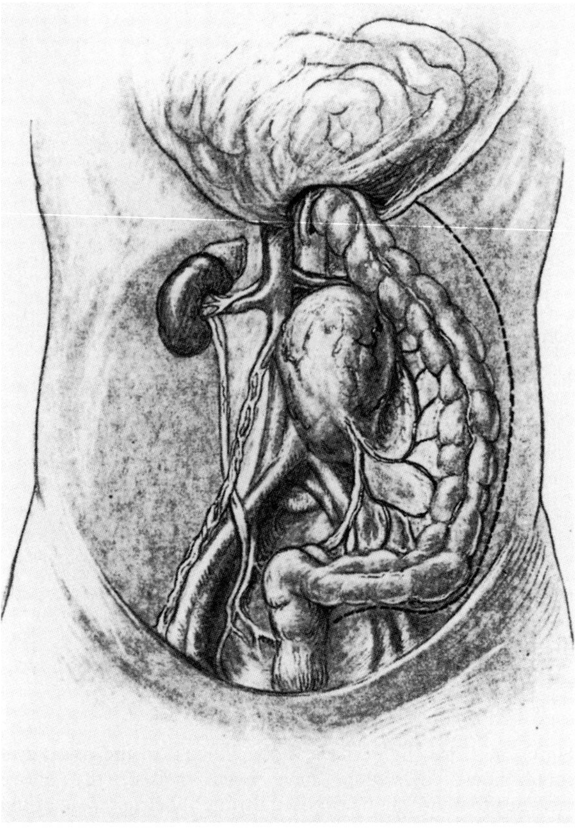

**Fig. 32.5.** Mobilization of the spleen, transverse colon, and descending colon for exposure of predominately left-sided lesions. For extensive tumors, the right colon and small bowel should be mobilized as illustrated in Fig. 32.4 and placed in a Lahey bag on the chest wall. [From Skinner DG (1977) Considerations for management of large retroperitoneal tumors: use other modified thoracoabdominal approach. J Urol 17:605]

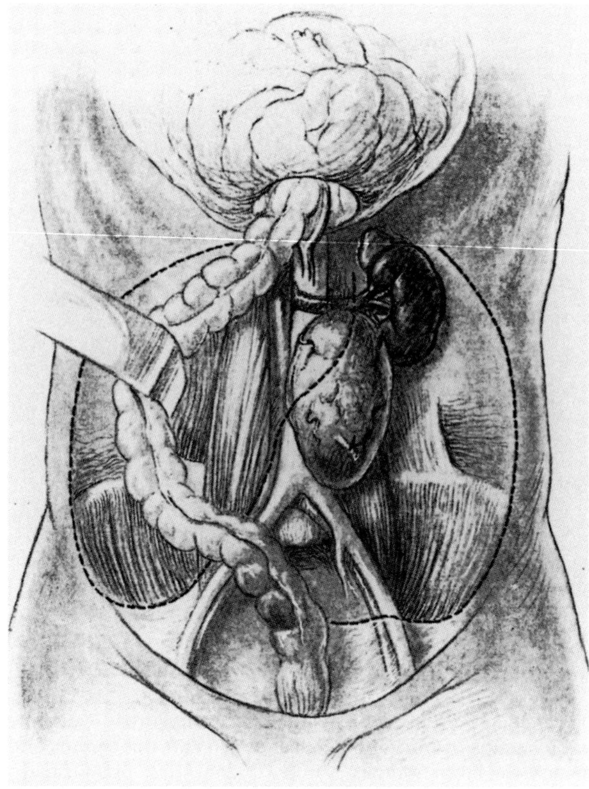

**Fig. 32.6.** Retroperitoneal exposure obtained through the left side of the chest following mobilization of the intra-abdominal contents. Note ligation of the inferior mesenteric artery necessary for mobilization of the descending colon. [From Skinner DG (1977) Considerations for management of large retroperitoneal tumors: use of the modified thoracoabdominal approach. J Urol 17:605]

preoperatively the vena cava had been obstructed completely.

It may be necessary to ligate or secure the cisterna chyli with a large hemoclip to prevent chylous ascites or the significant loss of protein following resection of retroperitoneal sarcomas. The cisterna chyli can be identified behind the right renal artery, medial to the right crus of the diaphragm, between the aorta and vena cava.

## 32.7
## Clinical Outcome

With a more aggressive surgical approach and improved perioperative care, patient survival has improved. Data combined from multiple series reported that the mean overall survival rates for all patients presenting with primary retroperitoneal sarcomas were 34% at 5 years and 18% at 10 years (Bramwell et al. 1985; Storm et al. 1981; Storm and Mahvi 1991; Wist et al. 1985). When analyzed according to the extent of resection, it is clear that complete resection provides the best hope for long-term survival. The overall survival rates for patients undergoing complete resection were 54% at 5 years and 45% at 10 years. More recent reviews reported overall 5-year survival rates of up to 70% and 5-year recurrence-free survival rates of 50% for patients undergoing complete resection with microscopically negative margins (Adam et al. 1984; Cody et al. 1981; Fortner et al. 1981; Glenn et al. 1985; McGrath et al. 1984; Solla and Reed 1986). Patients with grade 1 tumors have a 5-year survival rate ranging from 65% to 74% following complete surgical resection, compared to only a 25% 5-year survival rate in patients with grade 2 or grade 3 tumors, despite complete resection (JAQUES et al. 1990; STORM and MAHVI 1991).

Total surgical resection is not possible in 25%–65% of patients and the 5-year survival rates for patients undergoing partial resection ranges from 5% to 35% compared to 0%–15% for patients undergoing biopsy alone (CODY et al. 1981; DALTON et al. 1989; JAQUES et al. 1990; McGRATH et al. 1984; STORM et al. 1981). The 5-year survival rate for patients with unresectable tumors is dismal, ranging from 0% to 15% (KARAKOUSIS et al. 1985).

Local recurrence is an adverse prognostic factor in patients following resection of a retroperitoneal sarcoma (CODY et al. 1981; GLENN et al. 1985; POTTER et al. 1985). Patients with recurrent disease who undergo complete surgical resection of the recurrence have a median survival of 48 months, compared to a median survival of 22 months in patients whose recurrent disease is unresectable (JAQUES et al. 1990). The median time to recurrence is variable; however, in most series it is about 15 months (BEVILACQUA et al. 1991; DALTON et al. 1989). The first recurrence in up to 75% of patients is local; one-third of these patients will develop metastases. Even in patients without evidence of a recurrence in the first 5 years, 40% will ultimately present with recurrence within the next 5 years. When stratified according to tumor grade, the median time to recurrence in patients with high-grade primary retroperitoneal sarcomas is 15 months, compared to 44 months in patients with low-grade tumors (JAQUES et al. 1990).

The strongest predictors of clinical outcome (recurrence, survival) are the ability to perform a complete surgical resection and tumor grade (BEVILACQUA et al. 1991; DALTON et al. 1989; JAQUES et al. 1990; McGRATH et al. 1984). Other factors associated with improved clinical outcomes include: younger age of patient (less than 53 years of age) and absence of tumor fixation to adjacent retroperitoneal structures (T1 and T2 lesions) (DALTON et al. 1989; JAQUES et al. 1990). In one study, metastatic disease and T3 tumors were also associated with a poor clinical outcome (DALTON et al. 1989). Neither histologic type (BEVILACQUA et al. 1991) nor size of tumor nor gender of patient was found to be a predictor of outcome (BEVILACQUA et al. 1991; DALTON et al. 1989; JAQUES et al. 1990; McGRATH et al. 1984).

The most common sites of distant metastases are the liver and lungs (JAQUES et al. 1990). Distant metastases develop in 23% of patients during the course of follow-up. Risk factors for the development of distant metastases include: age (less than 50 years) and high-grade tumors (CODY et al. 1981). Jaques and associates reported that metastatic involvement of the lymph nodes is rare and occurs in only 0.8% of patients.

## 32.8
## Adjuvant Therapy

Although many investigators have been unable to demonstrate the effectiveness of adjuvant chemotherapy or radiotherapy (BEVILACQUA et al. 1991; CATTON et al. 1994; DALTON et al. 1989; ELIAS and ANTMAN 1988; GLENN et al. 1985; HESLIN et al. 1997; McGRATH et al. 1984), the use of adjuvant therapy may improve overall survival and decrease the incidence of recurrence particularly in patients with positive surgical margins or those with residual disease (GLENN et al. 1985; KINSELLA et al. 1988; SINDELAR et al. 1993).

In trials incorporating intraoperative radiotherapy (IORT), locoregional recurrences were significantly reduced; however, the median overall survival was similar in patients who received IORT and in those who underwent surgery alone (SINDELAR et al. 1993). In one trial, the combination of IORT and low-dose external beam irradiation therapy was found to be as effective as high-dose external beam radiation in preventing tumor recurrence following gross resection (KINSELLA et al. 1988). Although there was no significant improvement in long-term survival or freedom from relapse, it was suggested that the use of IORT plus low-dose external beam doses could be delivered with less morbidity than high-dose external beam alone (KINSELLA et al. 1988). These results are comparable to prior experience combining surgical resection and high-dose postoperative radiotherapy with or without adjuvant chemotherapy for retroperitoneal sarcomas (GLENN et al. 1985).

External beam irradiation to doses of 6000 cGy following partial resection of retroperitoneal sarcomas has been employed to treat a few patients with encouraging results (TEPPER et al. 1984; HARRISON et al. 1986). However, this high-dose irradiation (external beam, IORT) is associated with significant morbidity including: radiation enteritis, ureteral stenosis, and in the case of IORT, late development of femoral and lumbosacral neuropathy and radiation nephritis (GLENN et al. 1985; KINSELLA et al. 1988; SINDELAR et al. 1993).

## 32.9
## Conclusion

Primary retroperitoneal sarcomas are rare tumors that are very difficult to manage. They present significant problems for both the patient and the treating physician. Complete surgical resection at the time of initial presentation provides the best chance for long-term survival. Aggressive surgical resection of the tumor, adjacent involved organs, and soft tissue should be undertaken when it can be accomplished with an acceptable morbidity and mortality. The decision to operate must be based on the patient's overall medical condition, extent of tumor, the likelihood of complete resection, and the expertise and familiarity of the surgeon with this problem. Presently, there are no data to demonstrate a survival benefit or significant role for chemotherapy or radiation therapy other than investigational.

Recurrence rates remain high despite complete surgical resections and negative margins. It is clear that a 5-year survival is not a cure, and close follow-up is important to identify those patients who would benefit from surgical re-resection of recurrent disease. Follow-up should be diligent with a physical examination and routine serum laboratories every 2 or 3 months. Symptomatic patients with abdominal pain, an abdominal mass, or abdominal symptoms should undergo an abdominal CT scan or MRI and should have radiographs of the chest. Asymptomatic patients undergo an abdominal CT/MRI every 6 months for the first 5 years and then yearly thereafter. Ultimately, new strategies, trials, and anticancer modalities will be needed to improve survival rates in patients with retroperitoneal sarcomas.

## References


Adam YG, Oland J, Halevy A, Reif R (1984) Primary retroperitoneal soft-tissue sarcoma. J Surg Oncol 25:8–11

Armstrong JR, Cohn I Jr (1965) Primary malignant retroperitoneal tumors. Am J Surg 110:937–943

Bears OH, Henson DE, Hutter RUP, Myers MH (1988) American Joint Committee on Cancer Manual for Staging of Cancer, 3rd edn. Lippincott, Philadelphia, pp 127–129

Benmark S, Hafstrom L, Jonsson PE, et al. (1980) Retroperitoneal sarcoma treated by surgery. J Surg Oncol 14:307–314

Bevilacqua RG, Rogatko A, Hajdu SI, Bremnan MF (1991) Prognostic factors in primary retroperitoneal soft-tissue sarcomas. Arch Surg 126:328–334

Binder SC, Katz B, Sheridan B (1978) Retroperitoneal liposarcoma. Ann Surg 187:257–261

Bose B (1979) Primary malignant retroperitoneal tumors: analysis of 30 cases. Can J Surg 22:215–220

Braasch JW, Mon AB (1967) Primary retroperitoneal tumors. Surg Clin North Am 47:663–678

Bramwell VHC, Crowther D, Deakin DP, et al. (1985) Combined modality management of local and disseminated adult sarcomas. Br J Cancer 51:301–318

Catton CN, O'Sullivan B, Kotwall C, et al. (1994) Outcome and prognosis in retroperitoneal soft tissue sarcoma. Int J Radiat Oncol Biol Phys 29:1005–1010

Cody HS III, Turnbull AD, Fortner JG, Hajdu SI (1981) The continuing challenge of retroperitoneal sarcomas. Cancer 47:2147–2152

Cohan RH, Baker ME, Cooper C, et al. (1988) Computed tomography of primary retroperitoneal malignancies. J Comput Assist Tomogr 12:804–810

Coran AG, Crocker DW, Wilson RE (1970) A twenty-five year experience with soft-tissue sarcomas. Am J Surg 119:288–293

Dalton RR, Donohue JH, Mucha P, et al. (1989) Management of retroperitoneal sarcomas. Surgery 106:725–733

de Santos LA, Ginaldi S, Wallace S (1981) Computed tomography in liposarcoma. Cancer 47:46–54

Donnelly BA (1946) Primary retroperitoneal tumors: a report of 95 cases and a review of the literature. Surg Gynecol Obstet 83:705–717

Duncan RE, Evans AT (1977) Diagnosis of primary retroperitoneal tumors. J Urol 117:19–23

Elias AD, Antman KH (1988) Adjuvant chemotherapy for soft tissue sarcoma: a critical appraisal. Semin Surg Oncol 4:59–65

Fortner JG, Martin S, Hajdu S, Turnbull A (1981) Primary sarcoma of the retroperitoneum. Semin Oncol 8:180–184

Glenn J, Sindelar WF, Kinsella T, et al. (1985) Results of multimodality therapy of resectable soft-tissue sarcoma of the retroperitoneum. Surgery 97:316–324

Harrison LB, Gutierrez E, Fischer JJ (1986) Retroperitoneal sarcomas: the Yale experience and a review of the literature. J Surg Oncol 32:159–164

Heslin MJ, Lewis JJ, Nadler E, et al. (1997) Prognostic factors associated with long-term survival of retroperitoneal sarcoma: implications for management. J Clin Oncol 15:2832–2839

Jaques DP, Coit DG, Hajdu SI, Brennan MF (1990) Management of primary and recurrent soft-tissue sarcoma of the retroperitoneum. Ann Surg 212:51–59

Karakousis CP, Velez AF, Emrich LJ (1985) Management of retroperitoneal sarcoma and patient survival. Am J Surg 150:376–380

Karakousis CP, Gerstenbluth R, Kontzoglou K, Driscoll DL (1995) Retroperitoneal sarcomas and their management. Arch Surg 130:1104–1109

Kinsella TJ, Sindelar WF, Lack E, et al. (1988) Preliminary results of a randomized study of adjuvant radiation therapy in resectable adult retroperitoneal soft-tissue sarcomas. J Clin Oncol 6:18–25

Kreel L, Bydder GM (1981) Evaluation of retroperitoneal liposarcoma with computed tomography. J Comput Tomogr 5:111–116

Lindell MM Jr, Wallace S, de Santos LA, Bernardino ME (1981) Diagnostic technique for the evaluation of soft tissue sarcoma. Semin Oncol 8:160–171

McGrath PC (1994) Retroperitoneal sarcomas. Semin Surg Oncol 10:364–368

McGrath PC, Neifeld JP, Lawrence W Jr, et al. (1984) Improved survival following complete excision of retroperitoneal sarcoma. Ann Surg 200:200–204

Melcow MM (1953) Primary tumors of the retroperitoneum. J Int Coll Surg 19:401–449

Morgagni GB (1969) The seats and causes of diseases investigated by anatomy in five books, containing a great variety of dissections, with remarks. To which are added very accurate and copious indexes of the principal things and names therein contained. London: A. Miller and T. Cadell (Original published in Latin by Ex Typographia Remondiniana, 1761. Translation by Benjamin Alexander.)

Neifeld JP, Walsh JW, Lawrence W Jr (1982) Computed tomography in the management of soft tissue tumors. Surg Gynecol Obstet 155:535–540

Oriana S, Bonardi P, Preda F (1977) Primary retroperitoneal tumors. Tumori 63:397–405

Pack GT, Tabah EJ (1954) Primary retroperitoneal tumors: a study of 120 cases. Surg Gynecol Obstet 99:209–231, 313–341

Papaioannou AN (1966) Tumors other than insulinomas associated with hypoglycemia. Surg Gynecol Obstet 123:1093

Potter DA, Glenn J, Kinsella T, et al. (1985) Patterns of recurrence in patients with high-grade soft-tissue sarcomas. J Clin Oncol 3:353–366

Sindelar WF, Kinsella TJ, Chen PW, et al. (1993) Intraoperative radiotherapy in retroperitoneal sarcoma. Arch Surg 128:402–410

Solla JA, Reed K (1986) Primary retroperitoneal sarcomas. Am J Surg 152:496–498

Storm FK, Mahvi DM (1991) Diagnosis and management of retroperitoneal soft tissue sarcoma. Ann Surg 214:2–10

Storm FK, Eilber FR, Mirra J, Morton DL (1981) Retroperitoneal sarcomas: a reappraisal of treatment. J Surg Oncol 17:1–7

Tepper JE, Suit HD, Wood WC, et al. (1984) Radiation therapy of retroperitoneal soft tissue sarcomas. Int J Radiat Oncol Biol Phys 10:825–830

Wist E, Solheim OP, Jacobsen AB, Blom P (1985) Primary retroperitoneal sarcomas. Acta Radiol 24:305–310

Table 33.1. Staging system for soft tissue sarcomas as developed by the Memorial Sloan-Kettering Cancer Center (Russo et al. 1992)

| Stage | Grade | Size (cm) | Depth |
|---|---|---|---|
| 0 | Low | <5 | Superficial |
| 1 | Low | <5 | Deep |
| 2 | Low | >5 | Deep |
| 3 | High | <5 | Deep |
| 4 | High | >5 or evidence of metastasis | Deep |

Table 33.2. Immunocytologic stains available to distinguish epithelial tissues from mesenchymal tissues (Yao et al. 1988)

| Marker | Tissue |
|---|---|
| Cytokeratin | Epithelial |
| Epithelial membrane antigen | Epithelial |
| Vimentin | Mesenchymal |
| Desmin | Muscle |
| Myoglobin | Skeletal muscle |

ally, older reports may no longer be valid with the accessibility of more modern surgical techniques, newer delivery methods for radiation, and newer chemotherapeutic agents. Sarcomas, in general, remain a difficult therapeutic challenge due to their aggressive nature and their rarity. This chapter will review the latest in diagnosing and managing sarcomas of the bladder, prostate, and seminal vesicle.

## 33.2
## Bladder Sarcomas

Sarcomas of the bladder are thought to arise from pluripotent mesenchymal tissues of the bladder wall. Most bladder sarcomas tend to occur at or near the trigone, but may occur throughout the urinary bladder (Patterson and Barrett 1983). The histologic subtypes include: leiomyosarcoma, angiosarcoma, rhabdomyosarcoma, liposarcoma, chondrosarcoma, osteosarcoma, and malignant fibrous histiocytoma. The rarest types (liposarcoma, chondrosarcoma, and osteosarcoma), may occur with malignant epithelial cell types (transitional cell carcinoma, squamous cell carcinoma or adenocarcinoma), referred to as carcinosarcomas. In general, patients with bladder sarcomas tend to fare better than those arising from the prostate or seminal vesicle. This is possibly due to earlier detection as most patients

with bladder sarcomas present with gross hematuria (Russo et al. 1992).

### 33.2.1
### Bladder Leiomyosarcoma

Leiomyosarcoma of the bladder is the most common sarcoma of the urinary bladder. It occurs two times more frequently in men than in women and usually presents during the sixth decade of life (Swartz et al. 1985). Patients present most commonly with painless gross hematuria (Swartz et al. 1985; Ahlering et al. 1988). Other presenting symptoms may include urinary frequency, dysuria, urgency, lower abdominal pain, lower back pain, and a palpable mass (Swartz et al. 1985; Ahlering et al. 1988).

Grossly, leiomyosarcomas of the bladder appear as a submucosal nodule or as an ulcerating mass and are usually well circumscribed, although they are not encapsulated. Their color varies from a gray-white to a yellow-tan (Swartz et al. 1985). Microscopically, spindle cells are seen arranged in parallel bundles and usually involve the lamina propria and the muscularis (Alabaster et al. 1981). These malignant tumors have nuclear abnormalities which are distinguished from their benign counterparts (leiomyomas). It is critical to distinguish between a leiomyoma and leiomyosarcoma because the treatment for a leiomyoma of the bladder is simple enucleation (Kabalin et al. 1990).

Leiomyosarcomas are generally chemo- and radioresistant tumors and wide surgical extirpation remains the treatment of choice. Radical cystectomy for leiomyosarcomas has resulted in a 5-year survival rate of 65% (Tsukamoto and Leiber 1991). Prophylactic urethrectomy is not indicated, with only one reported case of a bladder sarcoma developing a urethral recurrence (Mackenzie et al. 1968). Ahlering et al. (1988) reported their surgical results on seven patients with leiomyosarcoma of the bladder. Of the seven patients undergoing surgical exenteration, three underwent neoadjuvant chemotherapy, one received preoperative radiation therapy, and three received adjuvant chemotherapy. All seven patients were free of disease at an average length of follow-up of 48 months. Sen et al. (1985) also achieved excellent control for two patients with localized leiomyosarcoma of the bladder using radical cystectomy; both patients were free of disease at 78 and 86 months. Although we do not advocate its use, partial cystectomy can be performed in a carefully selected group of patients when the size and location of the tumor allow for adequate surgical margins (Swartz et al. 1985; Mackenzie et al. 1971). In a review of ten patients with leiomyosarcomas of the bladder, Swartz et al. (1985) successfully treated four patients with partial cystectomies (free of disease at 5, 6, 6, and 9 years); one patient received adjuvant chemotherapy and one received adjuvant radiotherapy. The longest reported survival following segmental resection for a leiomyosarcoma of the bladder is 11 years (Smith and Kellert 1944). Russo et al. (1992) treated two patients with small bladder leiomyosarcomas (2 cm) using transurethral resection alone. Both patients are free of disease at 7 years.

Due to the limited number of reported cases, the role for neoadjuvant or adjuvant chemotherapy and radiotherapy has not been firmly established. It has been suggested that chemotherapy be reserved for those patients with metastatic disease. Chemotherapy agents that have been used with limited success include doxorubicin, vincristine, cyclophosphamide, and actinomycin D (Swartz et al. 1985; Ahlering et al. 1988). Ahlering et al. (1988) used neoadjuvant and adjuvant chemotherapy for three patients with bulky bladder leiomyosarcomas resulting in freedom from disease for 40, 65, and 97 months, respectively. They reported the histologic changes that occurred after two and three cycles of preoperative cisplatinum and doxorubicin, noting 95% and 98% cystic necrosis in the primary tumor, respectively. While their numbers are small, these authors recommend two cycles of chemotherapy for patients with histologic evidence of chemosensitivity or for those with pathologic stage P3A or greater.

## 33.2.2
## Bladder Rhabdomyosarcoma

Because skeletal muscle is not a normal component of the bladder wall, rhabdomyosarcoma of the bladder is thought to arise from mesenchymal pluripotent cells. This cell type is distinctly more common in children than adults, but is an aggressive tumor at any age. Rhabdomyosarcomas of the bladder present most frequently with gross painless hematuria, as do most malignant tumors of the bladder. Rhabdomyosarcomas present with metastatic disease in 20% to 40% of cases, which is the highest metastatic rate among all bladder sarcomas. Russo et al. (1992) reported that of nine (21%) patients with GU sarcomas that presented with metastatic disease,

eight had rhabdomyosarcoma. These aggressive tumors can spread by lymphovascular and hematogenous routes to distant sites, most commonly to the liver and lung.

Rhabdomyosarcomas are histologically distinct tumors characterized by primitive muscle cells called eosinophilic rhabdomyoblasts and muscle fibers with cytoplasmic cross striations. In adults, three cell types of rhabdomyosarcoma are described: spindle, alveolar, and giant cell. All are associated with a poor prognosis. This malignant tumor must be distinguished from its benign counterpart, rhabdomyoma, which is treated with conservative excision only.

Treatment is limited in adults unlike the multimodality treatments used in children. In adults, rhabdomyosarcomas are generally resistant to chemotherapy and radiation therapy. Aggressive surgical extirpation is the treatment of choice for those patients with localized disease. Ahlering et al. (1988) treated a large bladder rhabdomyosarcoma with neoadjuvant chemotherapy and radiation therapy, followed by cystectomy. Pathologic evaluation revealed no significant histologic changes from the neoadjuvant treatments. Despite aggressive efforts, the reported overall 5-year survival is only 40% (Tsukamoto and Leiber 1991).

## 33.2.3
## Bladder Liposarcoma, Chondrosarcoma, and Osteosarcoma

Of all bladder sarcomas, the rarest cell types are liposarcomas, chondrosarcomas, and osteosarcomas. These cell types are thought to arise from pluripotent mesenchymal tissue and not from structures normally present within the bladder wall. The chondrosarcoma and osteosarcoma cell types occur more commonly as the mesenchymal counterpart in a carcinosarcoma and are generally very malignant (Young and Rosenberg 1987).

Primary osteosarcoma of the urinary bladder is extremely rare, with only 22 cases reported in the literature (Young and Rosenberg 1987). Most extraosseous osteosarcomas occur in the older age groups, whereas osteosarcoma of the bone occurs in a much younger age group. In a review of the literature by Young and Rosenberg (1987), 18 of the 22 patients were male, with an average age of 62 years (range of 41–83). The etiology of this sarcoma is not clear, though radiation-induced osteosarcoma has been described. Presenting symptoms are similar to other bladder sarcomas and include gross hematuria and irritative voiding symptoms (BERENSON et al. 1986; YOUNG and ROSENBERG 1987; NICOLAI and SPJUT 1959).

The pathologic diagnosis of osteosarcoma is difficult and must be distinguished from transitional cell carcinoma with osseous metaplasia and carcinosarcoma with an osteosarcoma component. This differentiation is important due to the worse prognosis associated with osteosarcoma (YOUNG and ROSENBERG 1987). Immunohistochemical stains may be helpful in identifying malignant epithelial components within the tumor, such as carcinoembryonic antigen and cytokeratins (ESPINOZA and AZAR 1982).

Osteosarcoma of the bladder is associated with a poor prognosis. Of the patients reported in the literature, 82% died of their disease within 6 months of diagnosis (YOUNG and ROSENBERG 1987). Treatment should be applied on an individual basis. Because of the aggressive nature of this tumor, most patients can only be offered chemotherapy. Surgical resection for very large, symptomatic tumors may be beneficial for palliation.

Liposarcomas of the bladder present primarily in middle-aged patients with no sex predilection (ROSI et al. 1983). While they occur very infrequently in the bladder wall, only three cases in the literature describe a perivesical location (EDSON et al. 1961; POLSKY et al. 1974; DAS 1980). Patients may present with hematuria. When this tumor arises in a perivesical location the presenting symptoms may include prostatitis and suprapubic discomfort (EDSON et al. 1961).

Liposarcomas have a varied histologic appearance, including normal appearing adipocytes; large anaplastic cells with vacuolated cytoplasm and large nuclei; anaplastic fibroblasts; and variable amounts of myxoid tissue (ROSI et al. 1983). Myxoid varieties have a better prognosis (ENZINGER and WINSLOW 1962; DAS 1980). Prognosis is strongly associated with tumor grade. The more poorly differentiated the tumor, the more aggressive the behavior, with deeper infiltration and increasing probability of metastasis. These tumors grow very rapidly and are known for reaching an enormous size.

Liposarcomas are easy to shell out, but have fine tumorous extensions which are impossible to dissect out (EDSON et al. 1961). The recommended treatment for adult bladder liposarcoma is extirpative surgery. Radiotherapy may play an important role for more anaplastic tumors by decreasing the risk of

local recurrence (KINNE et al. 1973; SUIT et al. 1975; CELIK et al. 1980).

## 33.2.4
## Bladder Angiosarcoma

Angiosarcoma of the urinary bladder is an exceedingly rare tumor, with only a few cases reported in the literature. This sarcoma is associated with many possible etiologic factors, although it has occurred spontaneously (RAVI 1993). Suggested etiologic risk factors include exposure to thorium dioxide, arsenic, polyvinyl chloride, radiation, chemotherapy, and retained foreign body material (RAVI 1993; MORGAN et al. 1989). Presenting symptoms are typical of bladder tumors in general, such as gross hematuria and irritative voiding complaints. Despite the aggressive nature of this tumor, conservative surgical resection followed by postoperative radiation treatment has been successful in one reported case (RAVI 1993). Pathologic diagnosis is aided by the use of immunohistochemical markers. Both factor VIII-related antigen and Ulex lectin are markers for endothelial cells, the latter being thought to be more sensitive (ARAGONA et al. 1991).

## 33.2.5
## Bladder Carcinosarcoma

Carcinosarcomas contain both a malignant epithelial and a mesenchymal component and rarely occur in the urinary bladder. The age range and presenting symptoms are similar to those of transitional cell carcinoma. This tumor is more common in males, with a male to female ratio of 4:1. Grossly, this tumor most commonly occurs around the trigone. Carcinosarcomas present a challenge to the pathologist because of the difficulty in diagnosing these tumors. The differential diagnosis includes a pure epithelial tumor with surrounding sarcomatous changes and transitional cell induction of ossification in the underlying stroma resembling osteogenic sarcoma. The presence of true heterotopic tissue as well as immunohistochemical markers may help secure the pathologic diagnosis. A possible etiology to carcinosarcoma of the bladder is a history of pelvic irradiation, as has been reported in a few cases (SCHOBORG et al. 1980). The therapeutic decision on the management of this tumor should be based on its most malignant component. Depending on the histology, treatment should include extirpative surgery with adjuvant radiation and chemotherapy (SCHOBORG et al. 1980).

## 33.2.6
### Malignant Fibrous Histiocytoma of the Bladder

Malignant fibrous histiocytoma (MFH) is the most common adult soft tissue sarcoma, but is rarely found in the bladder. This sarcoma is almost exclusively a disease of adults and usually presents in the sixth or seventh decade. Epidemiological data demonstrate a male to female ratio of 3:2, with Caucasians affected more often than blacks or Orientals (OESTERLING et al. 1990). The most frequent site of involvement is the deep fascia or skeletal muscles of the lower extremity (the thigh), with involvement of the genitourinary tract being the least frequent site. A review of 59 MFH cases in the literature revealed an incidence of lung metastasis of 49%, liver metastasis of 12%, and regional lymph node metastasis of 22%. While MFH has been reported throughout the genitourinary tract, the kidney is the most common site. There are only 15 well-documented cases of MFH occurring in the bladder (OESTERLING et al. 1990; EGAWA et al. 1994). Presenting symptoms are similar to those of other bladder tumors, and include gross hematuria, bladder outlet obstructive complaints, and irritative voiding symptoms (OESTERLING et al. 1990).

Pathology of MFH reveals a pleomorphic tumor with both fibroblast-type cells and histiocyte-like cells. The quantity of each cell type varies, defining a histologic categorization into five subtypes: myxoid, giant cell, angiomatoid, storiform-pleomorphic, and inflammatory (WEISS 1982). The pleomorphic variety is the most common, accounting for 70% of all cases, while the inflammatory variety is the least common (HOLLOWOOD and FLETCHER 1995). The most aggressive form is the inflammatory type, which may be associated with a fever and leukocytosis (ANGERVALL et al. 1981). The types of bladder MFH reported in the literature include myxoid and inflammatory subtypes.

While radiation and chemotherapy have been used for MFH, surgery remains the best treatment for an attempt at local cure. Even after aggressive resections, local recurrence is high, occurring in up to 50% of treated cases (OESTERLING et al. 1990; WEISS and ENZINGER 1977). Adjunctive therapy has included both radiation and chemotherapy. MFH has been shown to be very radiosensitive. It has been suggested that radiation therapy be used immedi-

ately after surgical resection in order to decrease the risk of local recurrence (REAGAN et al. 1981). Despite adjuvant treatment with radiation, the rate of metastatic spread ranges from 23% to 43% (OESTERLING et al. 1990). The use of adjuvant chemotherapy is therefore warranted. Doxorubicin has been shown to be the most effective in the treatment of soft tissue sarcomas in general, and is the chemotherapeutic drug of choice for MFH (OESTERLING et al. 1990). Furthermore, there is a known synergistic effect between doxorubicin and radiation (BELLI and PIRO 1977). Others have tried cyclophosphamide, vincristine, and actinomycin D with limited success (LEITE et al. 1977).

There is no uniform treatment plan due to the rarity of this tumor. In general, tumors that are surgically resectable are approached in an aggressive manner with wide local excision, followed by radiation to the tumor bed and adjuvant doxorubicin-based chemotherapy. If the tumor is unresectable, or the patient is a poor surgical candidate, then radiation to the primary tumor followed by doxorubicin chemotherapy may provide a chance for prolonged survival (OESTERLING et al. 1990).

## 33.3
### Prostate Sarcomas

Sarcomas of the prostate gland are quite uncommon, accounting for less than 0.5% of all prostatic tumors (NGHIEM et al. 1995; TANNENBAUM 1975; TRIPATHI and DICK 1969). The reported histologic subtypes are not as extensive as those described for the bladder and include leiomyosarcoma, rhabdomyosarcoma, carcinosarcomas, and lymphomas. While rhabdomyosarcomas of the prostate occur more commonly in children, leiomyosarcomas are the most common sarcomas that occur in the adult prostate (RUSSO et al. 1992). Prostatic sarcomas generally present with obstructive symptoms rather than gross hematuria. Most prostate sarcomas are of significant tumor size and have poorly differentiated histology resulting in a poor prognosis (RUSSO et al. 1992). Sarcomas of the prostate tend to be locally aggressive with invasion into the surrounding structures often making it difficult to determine the exact tissue of origin during the diagnostic workup. The use of a CT scan and magnetic resonance imaging (MRI) preoperatively can help define the tissues of origin in the pelvis. Additionally, using both T1- and T2-weighted MRI can help delineate the histologic diagnosis (RUSSO et al. 1993; NGHIEM et al. 1995).

Prostate sarcomas must be distinguished from adenocarcinoma as well as from benign tumors (OLSON et al. 1994). Cystosarcoma phylloides of the prostate is one such benign tumor; a rare tumor of hyperplastic and neoplastic glandular-stromal proliferations (OLSON et al. 1994). While the etiology of prostate sarcomas is not known, there have been two reports of radiation-induced sarcomas of the prostate, including one undifferentiated and one leiomyosarcoma (NGHIEM et al. 1995; SCULLY et al. 1990). Treatment usually requires aggressive surgical extirpation, though up to 40% of prostate sarcomas may be unresectable (RUSSO et al. 1992). Overall, prostate sarcomas are associated with a poor prognosis.

### 33.3.1
### Prostate Leiomyosarcoma

Leiomyosarcoma is the most common sarcoma type to occur in the prostate, but it represents less than 0.1% of all prostate malignancies (CHEVILLE et al. 1995). The largest series is from the Mayo clinic by CHEVILLE et al. (1995), who reported on the clinical outcome of 23 patients and compared this with immunohistological data. They noted marked variability in the histologic appearance of leiomyosarcomas and found most tumors to be reactive with antibodies to vimentin and actin and some to be reactive with antibodies to keratin. In addition, some tumors were found to be reactive with cytokeratin, once believed to be exclusive to tumors of epithelial origin. Most patients present with urinary obstructive symptoms, including decreased force of stream, urinary frequency, and urgency. Perineal pain occurs in approximately 25% of patients. There is no elevation in serum prostate specific antigen associated with these sarcomas (CHEVILLE et al. 1995).

The pathology of prostate leiomyosarcomas can vary widely, from almost normal-appearing smooth muscle to sclerotic stroma and those with epithelioid features. Most are found to be high grade at the time of diagnosis, though length of survival is unpredictable (CHEVILLE et al. 1995). Despite aggressive therapeutic measures, local recurrence is frequent; distant metastases are less common (AHLERING et al. 1988). The lung is the most common site of metastatic spread; spread to the brain, liver, kidney, bones, and lymph nodes has also been reported (CHEVILLE et al. 1995). CHEVILLE et al. reported a

prolonged survival in two patients at 67 and 72 months using multimodality treatments. As well, AHLERING et al. (1988) reported on four patients with leiomyosarcoma of the prostate with no evidence of recurrent disease in three of the patients at 60, 87, and 73 months using combined therapy, including surgery, radiation, and chemotherapy. While the numbers at individual institutions are too small to define a definitive treatment plan for these tumors, an aggressive approach appears warranted. A reasonable treatment plan may include radical surgical resection followed by adjuvant radiation (30–45 Gy) for residual disease, and chemotherapy (doxorubicin and cisplatinum) for disseminated disease (AHLERING et al. 1988).

### 33.3.2
### Prostate Carcinosarcoma

Carcinosarcoma of the prostate is a rare malignancy involving both adenocarcinoma and a sarcoma cell type. The largest reported series is from the Mayo Clinic with retrospective data collected on 21 patients over a period of nearly 50 years (DUNDORE et al. 1995). This type of tumor occurs primarily in the sixth to seventh decade, with an average age of 68 years in the Mayo Clinic series. In this series, the majority of the carcinosarcomas had osteosarcoma as the sarcoma element (69%), with leiomyosarcoma being the second most common (25%) and rhabdomyosarcoma found in one patient (6%) (DUNDORE et al. 1995). Others have reported chondrosarcoma, malignant fibrous histiocytoma, myosarcoma, fibrosarcoma, and angiosarcoma. When data were available, only one of five patients was found to have an abnormal prostate specific antigen value preoperatively. In a review of the literature, WICK et al. (1989) noted that prostatic acid phosphatase was usually normal or only slightly elevated. Most patients presented with urinary obstructive symptoms and were subsequently diagnosed following a transurethral resection of the prostate. While all of the patients presented with advanced disease (stage C–D), only one was found to have an abnormal rectal examination (DUNDORE et al. 1995).

The pathology typically reveals the adenocarcinoma areas to be moderate to poorly differentiated with an abrupt transition to the sarcoma cell type. The immunohistochemistry of these carcinosarcomas is quite predictable. In the Mayo Clinic series, the adenocarcinoma regions showed reactivity with keratin (100%), and positivity for PSA (75%), whereas the sarcoma regions of the tumor showed reactivity with vimentin (100%) (DUNDORE et al. 1995).

The treatment approach in the Mayo Clinic series is similar to that used for prostate adenocarcinoma in general. Again many patients had undergone a TURP prior to any formal treatment, with a few patients undergoing a radical prostatectomy, cystoprostatectomy, or anterior exenteration. Several patients received radiation therapy and several underwent hormonal treatment. Interestingly, approximately half of all reported patients with carcinosarcoma of the prostate had a diagnosis of acinar adenocarcinoma previously. It is possible that the treatment of an adenocarcinoma with hormonal or radiation therapy may result in the development of a carcinosarcoma. Additionally, it is important to note that estrogen therapy can result in a desmoplastic reaction in the stroma, which must be distinguished histologically from a true carcinosarcoma. Electron microscopy and immunohistochemistry may help to differentiate a prostate carcinoma with sarcomatous elements from a true carcinosarcoma (ORDONEZ et al. 1982; ZENKLUSEN et al. 1990). For instance, noting intercellular junctions or well-developed desmosomes helps support the finding of a carcinoma. Immunohistochemical stains to keratin, vimentin, desmin, epithelial membrane antigen, prostate-specific antigen, myoglobin, muscle-specific antigen, and S-protein may also be very beneficial in determining the diagnosis (WICK et al. 1989).

In the Mayo Clinic series, 24% of patients presented with metastatic disease at the time of diagnosis and 81% of the patients eventually developed metastatic disease, primarily to the lung (48%), bone (33%), and brain (19%). The 5-year cancer-specific survival was 41% and 7-year survival was 14%. Throughout the literature, results of outcome are uniformly poor with only one long-term survivor out to 85 months after pelvic exenteration, hormonal therapy, and resection of a pulmonary metastatic lesion (DUNDORE et al. 1995). In two large series, no predictors of outcome were identified, including age, history of radiation or hormonal treatment, histologic subtype, percentage of necrosis, percentage of sarcomatous elements, subtype grade, number of mitotic figures, and degree of pleomorphism (DUNDORE et al. 1995; SHANNON et al. 1992).

### 33.3.3
### Prostate Rhabdomyosarcoma

While rhabdomyosarcoma is the most common sarcoma to occur in the prostate, it is extremely rare to find it in the adult. The average age of occurrence is 5 years overall, with an average age of 39 years in the adult literature, ranging from 18 to 68 (WARING and NEWLAND 1992). With less than ten adult cases reported in the literature, recommendations on treatment are limited, as opposed to the pediatric literature. These tumors are typically of the embryonal type, are rapid growing and present with large pelvic or abdominal masses (WARING and NEWLAND 1992). Different from other sarcoma types, rhabdomyosarcomas tend to spread via the lymphatics with the development of subsequent widespread metastatic disease. Presenting symptoms in adults are those of urinary obstruction and dysuria, while rectal discomfort is more common in the pediatric population. On digital rectal examination the prostate is firm and smooth, compared with the hard, nodular feel of prostatic carcinoma. Serum studies of PSA and PAP are normal. Metastatic disease is most commonly to the lung, bone, and liver; however, the bone lesions are osteoclastic and found throughout the skeleton structure, as opposed to metastasis from adenocarcinoma of the prostate.

Of the nine cases found in the literature, two were not grossly described and six of the remaining seven were found to be infiltrating the surrounding structures (WARING and NEWLAND 1992). Clinically rhabdomyosarcoma in the adult prostate is quite distinct from adenocarcinoma with no change in serum markers, and a different pattern of spread. The pathologic diagnosis, however, may be quite difficult. The appearance of the embryonal type of rhabdomyosarcoma may be similar to other myxoid, spindle cell, or small cell tumors, making the differential diagnosis extensive (WARING and NEWLAND 1992). As for other sarcomas, electron microscopy and immunohistochemistry help to secure the diagnosis. Specific markers for rhabdomyosarcoma are to myoglobin, skeletal muscle actin, and myosin.

Treatment of these aggressive tumors is formulated on an individual basis and involves the use of surgery, radiation, and chemotherapy. The pediatric population has enjoyed a significant improvement in survival due to the advances in multimodality treatment; however the adult population has continued to display an extremely poor prognosis. Of the nine cases reported in the literature, eight had adequate follow-up; all eight were dead from their disease during their follow-up of approximately 17 months from diagnosis (WARING and NEWLAND 1992).

## 33.4
## Retrovesical/Seminal Vesicle Sarcomas

Tumors of the seminal vesicle are quite rare and also tend to present with large sizes, making it difficult to determine the exact tissue of origin (CHIOU et al. 1985; LAZARUS 1946). Many of these tumors are simply referred to as retrovesical. Criteria have been described by DALGAARD and GIERTSEN (1956) for determining whether a tumor is truly seminal vesicle in origin and they include: histology confirmed by biopsy, tumor confined to or centered in the seminal vesicle, and no other primary tumor(s). As is true throughout the genitourinary tract, mesenchymal tumors in this region are very uncommon. They occur in the older age groups, with a range of 25 to 77 (SCHNED et al. 1986). The histologic varieties of malignant mesenchymal tumors that occur in the retrovesical region are similar to those found in the prostate, but are more often poorly defined. They include pleomorphic cell sarcoma, primary sarcoma, granular cell tumor, round cell sarcoma, and hemangiosarcoma, along with the more typical liposarcoma, leiomyosarcoma, and fibrosarcoma (SCHNED et al. 1986). Most patients present with symptoms related to metastatic disease or to invasion into surrounding structures (rectum, pelvis, bladder, or prostate), often causing delay in diagnosis. Pain in the rectum or anus, pelvis, or low back is not uncommon, along with urinary obstructive symptoms (CHIOU et al. 1985; WILLIAMSON 1978). There have been a few reports of patients with no symptoms, the tumor being found incidentally (DALGAARD and GIERTSEN 1956; SCHNED et al. 1986; RUSSO et al. 1992).

Treatment of these tumors has largely been by surgical extirpation. RUSSO et al. (1992) treated two patients with leiomyosarcomas of the seminal vesicle with surgical resection only. Both patients are free of disease at 24 and 29 months, respectively. The longest documented follow-up after successful surgical excision of a seminal vesicle sarcoma is 3 years for a round cell type (SCHNED et al. 1986). There has been one prior report of combined surgery and radiation therapy using both external beam (20 Gy) and radon seed implants for a pleomorphic cell type occurring in the seminal vesicle. That patient was alive with disease at 18 months' follow-up. There has been one prior report of surgery combined with chemotherapy that was successfully used for a sarcoma in this region for an extraskeletal pelvic Ewing's sarcoma contiguous with the right seminal vesicle (JOHANSEN et al. 1988). Hormonal therapy using estrogens and bilateral orchiectomy has been attempted with no significant advantage (SCHNED et al. 1986; BENSON et al. 1984). Because sarcomas arising in the retrovesical or seminal vesicle region are rare, no definite treatment recommendations can be made. Each patient must be evaluated thoroughly and therapy decided on an individual basis.

## References


Ahlering TE, Weintraub P, Skinner DG (1988) Management of adult sarcomas of the bladder and prostate. J Urol 140:1397–1399

Alabaster AM, Jordan WP, Soloway MS, Shippel RM, Young JM (1981) Leiomyosarcoma of the bladder and subsequent urethral recurrence. J Urol 125:583–585

Angervall L, Hagmar B, Kindblom L-G, et al. (1981) Malignant giant cell tumor of soft tissues: a clinicopathologic, ultrastructural, angiographic and microangiographic study. Cancer 47:736–747

Aragona F, Ostardo E, Prayer-Galetti T, Piazza R, Capitanio G (1991) Angiosarcoma of the bladder: a case report with regard to histologic and immunohistochemical findings. Eur Urol 20:161–163

Belli JA, Piro AJ (1977) The interaction between radiation and adriamycin damage in mammalian cells. Cancer Res 37:1624–1630

Benson RC, Clark WR, Farrow GM (1984) Carcinoma of the seminal vesicle. J Urol 132:483–485

Berenson RJ, Flynn S, Freiha FS, Kempson RL, Torti FM (1986) Primary osteosarcoma of the bladder. Cancer 57:350–355

Celik C, Karakousis CP, Moore R, Holyoke ED (1980) Liposarcomas: prognosis and management. J Surg Oncol 14:245

Cheville JC, Dundore PA, Nascimento AG, Meneses M, Kleer E, Farrow GM, Bostwick DG (1995) Leiomyosarcoma of the prostate. Cancer 76:1422–1427

Chiou RK, Limas C, Lange PH (1985) Hemangiosarcoma of the seminal vesicle: case report and literature review. J Urol 134:371–373

Dalgaard JB, Giertsen JC (1956) Primary carcinoma of the seminal vesicle; case and survey. Acta Pathol Microbiol Scand 39:255–257

Das S (1980) Retrovesical liposarcoma. Br J Urol 52:163

Dundore PA, Cheville JC, Nascimento AG, Farrow GM, Bostwick DG (1995) Carcinosarcoma of the prostate. A report of 21 cases. Cancer 76:1035–1042

Edson M, Friedman J, Richardson JF (1961) Perivesical liposarcoma: a case report. J Urol 85:767–770

Egawa S, Uchida T, Koshiba K, Kagata Y, Iwabuchi K (1994) Malignant fibrous histiocytoma of the bladder with focal rhabdoid tumor differentiation. J Urol 151:154–156

Enzinger FM, Winslow DJ (1962) Liposarcoma. A study of 103 cases. Virchows Arch A Pathol Anat Histopathol 335:367

Espinoza CG, Azar HA (1982) Immunohistochemical localization of keratin-type proteins in epithelial neoplasms:

correlation with electron microscopic findings. Am J Clin Pathol 78:500–507

Hollowood K, Fletcher CDM (1995) Malignant fibrous histiocytoma: morphologic pattern or pathologic entity. Semin Diag Pathol 12:210–220

Johansen TEB, Huseby A, Stenwig JT (1988) Extraskeletal Ewing's sarcoma contiguous with the seminal vesicle. Scand J Urol Nephrol 22:237–239

Kabalin JN, Freiha FS, Niebel JD (1990) Leiomyoma of bladder. Urology 35:210–212

Kinne DW, Chu FC, Huvos AG, Yagoda A, Fortner JG (1973) Treatment of primary and recurrent retroperitoneal liposarcoma. Twenty-five year experience at Memorial Hospital. Cancer 31:53

Lazarus JA (1946) Primary malignant tumors of the retrovesical region with special reference to malignant tumors of the seminal vesicle; report of a case of retrovesical sarcoma. J Urol 55:190

Leite C, Goodwin JW, Sinkovics JG, Baker LH, Benjamen R (1977) Chemotherapy of malignant fibrous histiocytoma: a Southwestern Oncology Group report. Cancer 40:2010

Mackenzie AR, Whitmore WF, Melamed MR (1968) Myosarcomas of the bladder and prostate. Cancer 22:833–844

Mackenzie AR, Sharma TC, Whitmore WF, Melamed MR (1971) Non-extirpative treatment of myosarcomas of the bladder and prostate. Cancer 28:329–334

Morgan MA, Moutos DM, Pippitt CH, Suda RR, Smith JJ, Thurnau GR (1989) Vaginal and bladder angiosarcoma after therapeutic irradiation. South Med J 82:1434–1436

Nghiem HV, Sommer FG, Moretto JC (1995) MRI of radiation-induced prostate sarcoma. Clin Imag 19:54–56

Nicolai CH, Spjut HJ (1959) Primary osteogenic sarcoma of the bladder. J Urol 82:497–499

Oesterling JE, Epstein JI, Brendler CB (1990) Myxoid malignant fibrous histiocytoma of the bladder. Cancer 66:1836–1842

Olson EM, Trambert MA, Mattrey RF (1994) Cystosarcoma phylloides of the prostate: MRI findings. Abdom Imag 19:180–181

Ordonez NG, Ayala AG, von Eschenbach AC, Mackay B, Hanssen G (1982) Immunoperoxidase localization of prostatic acid phosphatase in prostatic carcinoma with sarcomatoid changes. Urology 19:210–214

Patterson DE, Barrett DM (1983) Leiomyosarcoma of the urinary bladder. Urology 21:367–369

Polsky MS, Vitenson JH, Wilson JM, Woodhead DM, Weber CH (1974) Retrovesical liposarcoma. Urology 3:226

Powers JH, Van Zandt Hawn C, Carter RD (1956) Osteogenic sarcoma and transitional cell carcinoma occurring simultaneously in the urinary bladder: report of a case. J Urol 76:263–269

Ravi R (1993) Primary angiosarcoma of the urinary bladder. Arch Esp Urol 46:351–353

Reagan MT, Clowry LJ, Cox JD, Rongala N (1981) Radiation therapy in the treatment of malignant fibrous histiocytoma. Int J Radiat Oncol Biol Phys 7:311–315

Ro JY, El-Naggar AK, Amin MB, Sahin AA, Ordonez NG, Ayala AG (1993) Pseudosarcomatous fibromyxoid tumor of the urinary bladder and prostate. Hum Pathol 24:1203–1210

Rosi P, Selli C, Carini M, Rosi MF (1983) Myxoid liposarcoma of the bladder. J Urol 130:560–561

Russo P, Brady MS, Conlon K, Hajdu SI, Fair WR, Herr HW, Brennan MF (1992) Adult urologic sarcoma. J Urol 147:1032–1037

Russo P, Demas B, Reuter V (1993) Adult prostatic sarcoma. Abdom Imag 18:399–401

Schned AR, Ledbetter JS, Selikowitz SM (1986) Primary leiomyosarcoma of the seminal vesicle. Cancer 57:2202–2206

Schoborg TW, Saffos RO, Rodriquez AP, Scott C (1980) Carcinosarcoma of the bladder. J Urol 124:724–727

Scully JM, Uno JM, McIntyre M, Mosely S (1990) Radiation-induced prostatic sarcoma: a case report. J Urol 144:746–748

Sen SE, Malek RS, Farrow GM, Lieber MM (1985) Sarcoma and carcinosarcoma of the bladder in adults. J Urol 133:29–30

Shannon RL, Ro JY, Grignon DJ, Ordonez NG, Johnson DE, Mackay B, Tetu B, Ayala AG (1992) Sarcomatoid carcinoma of the prostate. Cancer 69:2676–2682

Smith G, Kellert E (1944) Leiomyosarcoma of the urinary bladder. Urol Cutan Rev 48:564–566

Suit HD, Russel WO, Martin RG (1975) Sarcoma of soft tissue: clinical and histopathologic parameters and response to treatment. Cancer 35:1478

Swartz DA, Johnson DE, Ayala AG, Watkins DL (1985) Bladder leiomyosarcoma: a review of 10 cases with 5-year follow-up. J Urol 133:200–202

Tannenbaum M (1975) Sarcomas of the prostate gland. Urology 5:810–814

Torenbeek R, Blomjous CEM, de Bruin PC, Newling DWW, Meijer CJLM (1994) Sarcomatoid carcinoma of the urinary bladder. Am J Surg Pathol 18:241–249

Tripathi VNP, Dick VS (1969) Primary sarcoma of the urogenital system in adults. J Urol 101:898–904

Tsukamoto T, Leiber MM (1991) Sarcomas of the kidney, urinary bladder, prostate, spermatic cord, paratestis and testis in adults. In: Raaf JH (ed) Management of soft tissue sarcomas. Year Book Medical Publishers, Chicago

Waring PM, Newland RC (1992) Prostatic embryonal rhabdomyosarcoma in adults. Cancer 69:755–762

Weiss SW (1982) Malignant fibrous histiocytoma. A reaffirmation. Am J Surg Pathol 6:773–784

Weiss SW, Enzinger FM (1977) Myxoid variant of malignant fibrous histiocytoma. Cancer 39:1672–1685

Wick MR, Young RH, Malvesta R, Beebe DS, Hansen JJ, Dehner LP (1989) Prostatic carcinosarcomas. Clinical, histologic and immunohistochemical data on two cases, with a review of the literature. Am J Clin Pathol 92:131–139

Williamson RCN (1978) Seminal vesicle tumours. J R Soc Med 71:286–288

Yao JCT, Wang WCC, Tseng HH, Hwang WS (1988) Primary rhabdomyosarcoma of the prostate. Acta Cytol 32:509–512

Young RH, Rosenberg AE (1987) Osteosarcoma of the urinary bladder. Cancer 59:174–178

Zenklusen HR, Weymuth G, Rist M, Mihatsch MJ (1990) Carcinosarcoma of the prostate in combination with adenocarcinoma of the prostate and adenocarcinoma of the seminal vesicles: a case report with immunohistochemical analysis and review of the literature. Cancer 66:998–1001

# 34 Hematologic Malignancies Involving the Genitourinary System

A. MOHRBACHER

CONTENTS



## 34.1 Introduction

Hematologic malignancies can infiltrate any organ system in the body, including the genitourinary (GU) system. Leukemias involving solid organs in general are already widespread throughout many organ systems, and with rare exceptions do not have primary presentations in the GU tract. Lymphomas are more likely to have primary or focal involvement of the GU tract. This involvement of the GU system can be conceptualized in the following manifestations: (1) primary lymphoma presentations in the GU tract; (2) secondary tumor spread of a systemic lymphoma to the GU tract; or (3) extrinsic compression of the GU system from adenopathy in the abdomen or pelvis.


A. MOHRBACHER, MD, Department of Hematology, USC School of Medicine, 1441 Eastlake Ave., Los Angeles, CA 90033, USA


## 34.2 Lymphoma of the Genitourinary System: Kidney

The most common site of involvement of non-Hodgkin's lymphoma (NHL) in the GU tract is the kidney. Several hundred cases of lymphoma involving the kidneys have been reported in the literature, but only 10% or less of these cases actually appear to be primary lymphoma of the kidney. These sometimes display remarkable similarity to the presentation of primary renal cell carcinoma, with a solitary lesion of the renal parenchyma. There may even be tumor extension into the inferior vena cava producing a tumor thrombus, with clinical findings of bilateral lower extremity edema (WAGNER et al. 1993). Renal lymphoma may present with a massively enlarged kidney without a discernible specific solitary lesion (REZNEK and RICHARDS 1990). Remarkably, these kidney primaries uncommonly cause actual renal dysfunction (MOREL et al. 1994).

More common is secondary involvement of the kidney in a systemically widespread lymphoma. Lymphoma is one of the few malignancies that specifically metastasize to kidneys. Initial computed tomographic (CT) findings may be misleading, with the appearance of small round hypodensities in renal parenchyma often attributed to simple cysts (see Chap. 4). Systemic lymphoma involving kidneys is commonly bilateral (COHAN 1990). Generalized lymphoma involving kidneys is considered stage IV by the Ann Arbor staging system, in contradistinction to a primary solitary lymphoma of one kidney, which is termed stage IE (for "extranodal"). Again, secondary involvement of the kidney rarely leads to alteration of renal function or hematuria. At autopsy series, incidental involvement of kidneys is noted in a much greater (13%–38%) proportion of patients than seen clinically (RICHARDS et al. 1990).

The two largest institutional studies of renal involvement in patients with NHL were reported in 1994 by Morel from France and in 1995 from the Mayo Clinic (MOREL et al. 1994; OKUNO et al. 1995).

The French series reviewed nearly 2000 cases of aggressive lymphoma treated in two prospective trials. Of the 2000 patients treated, renal involvement was noted in 48, of whom only four had primary (stage IE) kidney lymphoma. Therefore renal involvement by systemic aggressive lymphoma was found in approximately 3% of cases, and the primary renal cases were less than 10% of these cases (therefore 0.25% of all aggressive lymphoma cases). The majority of the 48 cases were large cell lymphoma (60%), with less than 10% each of immunoblastic, lymphoblastic, or diffuse mixed cell, and less than 5% each of follicular large and diffuse small cell lymphomas; 8% of cases were unclassified. Poor prognostic features of increased lactate dehydrogenase (LDH), bulky tumor mass >10 cm, and poor performance status (ECOG > 2) were present in 76%, 69%, and 20% of patients, respectively. Patterns of renal involvement were quite varied; 43% of patients had bilateral involvement of kidneys, 31% had multiple intraparenchymal nodules, 29% had direct invasion into the kidney from a perirenal mass, 21% had a single intraparenchymal mass, and 19% had diffuse infiltration of the kidney(s). Mild elevation of creatinine (>120 µml/l was noted in 21% of patients, and 6% had acute renal failure. In all except one patient renal dysfunction resolved after administration of chemotherapy. Treatment with varied chemotherapy regimens resulted in a complete remission rate of 57%. Disease-free survival and overall survival at 4 years were 39% and 58%, respectively. Renal involvement by lymphoma and renal failure did not prove to be significant prognostic factors. The standard prognostic factors consisting of tumor bulk and poor performance status were predictive of likelihood of survival. Other poor prognostic clinical features tended to accompany these stage IV cases with renal involvement including: B symptoms in 65%, bulky tumor (>10 cm) in 69%, elevated LDH in 76%, and other extranodal disease in 42%. This included marrow involvement in one-third, gastrointestinal involvement in one-third, and liver involvement in one-quarter; lung, CNS, bone, pleura, pancreas, skin, orbit, testes, ovary, and thyroid were less commonly involved (MOREL et al. 1994).

The second large series, published in 1995 from the Mayo Clinic (OKUNO et al. 1995), reviewed several hundred cases of NHL lymphoma treated over a 6-year period. A total of 176 patients were identified to have renal involvement; five of these cases appeared to be primary renal NHL. Of these five patients, all presented with flank pain and had B cell type; 60% had elevation of serum creatinine.

Tumor histology was diffuse large cell in four of the five patients, and small non-cleaved non-Burkitt's lymphoma in the remaining patient. Two of the five patients achieved durable (>2 years) complete response after chemotherapy and consolidation radiation therapy, but the remaining three patients had short survival. The authors speculated about a role for surgical debulking of renal lymphoma, although the data on treatment outcomes from other sites of lymphoma involvement did not support this hypothesis. It is difficult to justify a surgical intervention based on the outcome in these few patients.

## 34.3
## Patterns of Renal Involvement

Several radiologic series have reviewed the distribution of renal lesions of lymphoma. COHAN (1990) reported on 29 patients with renal or perirenal lymphoma. Bilateral lesions were present in 59%, and 42% of these patients had accompanying retroperitoneal adenopathy. Approximately one-quarter of the 29 patients had a single renal or perirenal lesion adjacent or contiguous with bulky retroperitoneal adenopathy. This was suggestive that the renal involvement was secondary spread from the adjacent perirenal disease. No patients in this series had diffuse involvement or kidney enlargement, and only one had a solitary mass. REZNEK and RICHARDS (1990) reported on 26 cases of lymphoma involving kidney. Two of these patients had Hodgkin's disease; 43% developed renal involvement of systemic lymphoma only at relapse, and 43% had no retroperitoneal adenopathy. As in the French series by Morel et al., most patients had other sites of extranodal disease at the time of presentation, commonly the bone. Renal involvement was noted in 3% of all lymphoma patients undergoing routine CT staging. Another series of 23 cases from St. Bartholomew's Hospital showed concordant patterns: 73% of patients had high-grade histologies, 37% had no associated retroperitoneal adenopathy, and 86% had other concurrent extranodal sites of involvement, again a poor prognostic feature (RICHARDS et al. 1990). As in MOREL's report, renal involvement per se was not an independent adverse prognostic factor.

## 34.4
## Workup and Staging

### 34.4.1
### Workup

Because lymphoma involvement of the GU tract is frequently secondary to systemic disease, and associated with other extranodal disease, thorough workup is critical in the initial evaluation of lymphoma. Patients should have CT scans of the neck, chest, abdomen, and pelvis, a gallium scan, and bilateral bone marrow biopsies. The gallium scan may be confirmatory if large (>2 cm) hypolucent lesions are seen in the kidney, demonstrating increased uptake of radiotracer. Lumbar puncture is not routinely performed unless a patient demonstrates neurologic symptoms, is HIV positive, or has a high-grade lymphoma.

Prognosis and treatment are directly related to pathologic subtype of lymphoma. Pathologic classification is usually based on the histologic appearance of individual lymphoma cells, i.e., small vs large cells, with or without cleaved nuclei, as well as the organization of cells in the lymphoma lesion, i.e., in a follicular or diffuse pattern. Therefore fine-needle aspiration (FNA), which disperses cells into a suspension, is generally inadequate for precise definition of lymphoma subtype. FNA, however, may permit staining for lymphoma surface markers such as CD20 or CD19, and staining for kappa or lambda light chain monoclonality to confirm malignant B cell proliferation. Therefore FNA may offer some preliminary assistance in distinguishing carcinomas (which usually stain positively for keratin) from lymphomas (which should stain positive for CD19 or CD20), to avoid, for example, an unnecessary nephrectomy in a patient with a primary renal lymphoma.

There are no specific serum markers of lymphoma, although large cell and other high-grade lymphomas of significant bulk or extent may be associated with an elevated LDH. Serum $\beta_2$-microglobulin is frequently elevated in aggressive lymphomas, but has not been demonstrated as a significant independent risk factor in the widely accepted International Prognostic Scoring System.

Small radiologic series of assessment of renal lesions by magnetic resonance imaging (MRI) or ultrasound have failed to demonstrate sensitive or specific performance of either modality to distinguish lymphoma from other malignancies involving the kidneys or sites of the GU tract. One large retrospective study (Hauser et al. 1995) assessed the relative value of CT, ultrasound, and MRI in 560 bilateral solid multifocal intrarenal and perirenal lesions. The authors concluded that lymphoma, renal cell carcinoma, and adenomas could not be distinguished by the use of these imaging techniques. Lymphoma was somewhat more likely in bilateral lesions and more likely to infiltrate perinephric fat.

### 34.4.2
### Biopsy

In light of the above, tissue core biopsies are preferable to FNA, and full surgical biopsy more desirable yet in cases of suspected lymphoma. In cases of suspected GU tract or renal lesions with associated adenopathy, a full lymph node biopsy through a surgical or laparoscopy approach is often the procedure of choice, as follicular lymphomas are best defined from histology of a full lymph node. Confirmation that an associated renal mass is lymphoma and not a separate primary may then be relegated to a fine-needle or CT-guided needle biopsy if this information will change therapeutic managment. There have been reports of synchronous diagnoses of renal carcinoma and lymphoid malignancies in the literature.

## 34.5
## Other Sites of Involvement

### 34.5.1
### Bladder

While kidney is the most frequent site of primary or secondary extrarenal involvement of NHL, at least 70 case reports of lymphoma involving the urinary bladder are found in the literature (Fernandez-Acenero et al. 1996). Clinical presentations of bladder involvement of NHL are rare (0.1%), although postmortem series report an incidence of bladder involvement of up to 13% (Racioppi et al. 1996). It is to be noted that this presentation of lymphoma has been predominantly reported in middle-aged females and may be related to prior history of cystitis in 20% (Ohsawa et al. 1993). It is described as a submucosal lesion, edematous and smooth on cystoscopy, at times friable or hemorrhagic (Downs 1997). One case was reported with the first presentation being suspicious malignant cells on urine cytology. A clinical review of 30 cases of NHL of the bladder noted gross hematuria in the majority of patients, a solitary mass in two-thirds, multiple masses in a quarter, and diffuse involvement in the remainder (Ohsawa et al. 1993).

In contrast to the predominance of aggressive histologies in the reported cases of renal lymphoma, low-grade histology is often seen in lymphomas of the bladder, which are included in the spectrum of mucosa-associated lymphoid tissue, or MALT lymphomas (Pawade et al. 1993). Biopsies from four patients in one series of these MALT type lesions confirmed reactive germinal centers with follicular colonization by malignant cells in two cases. One unusual case reported described a Burkitt's lymphoma of the bladder occurring after treatment and remission of lymphocyte-predominant Hodgkin's disease, with molecular clonotypic analysis showing both lesions to be of similar origin (Yoshinaga et al. 1996). Several reports of lymphoepithelial malignancies of the bladder have emphasized the importance of scrupulous pathology review and immunohistochemistry to verify whether malignant cells are truly of lymphoid origin (Amin 1995). In these cases, keratin-positive and leukocyte common antigen-negative staining confirmed carcinoma, and B and T cell markers showed a predominance of T cells, presumably reactive in nature. An intense lymphoid or plasma cell infiltrate of a bladder carcinoma can be mistaken for malignant lymphoma. A case of granulocytic sarcoma, an isolated soft tissue variant biologically similar to the cells of acute myelogenous leukemia, has been reported involving the bladder and causing obstructive uropathy (Martinelli et al. 1997). Again, appropriate suspicion for these unusual entities and immunohistochemical verification of malignant cell type is mandatory.

## 34.5.2
## Testes

Testicular involvement with NHL has been reported uncommonly in the adult literature (Mazzu et al. 1995). However, the testes are a relatively frequent site of involvement of childhood acute lymphocytic leukemia, and are thought to be an immunologically privileged site. In adults, lymphoblastic lymphoma, a variant of similar cell biology to acute lymphocytic leukemia (ALL), has been reported with testicular presentations. The testes may also be a sanctuary for leukemic cells with relatively poor chemotherapy penetration, prompting various therapeutic approaches to prevent relapse at this site. Testicular

biopsies and radiation were advocated in the past but are now generally reserved for cases of suspected active involvement, as current ALL regimens are associated with a lower incidence of testicular relapses than in the past (Gutjahr and Humpl 1995).

A radiologic report noted that testicular sonograms on patients with involvement by leukemia or lymphoma could show either homogeneous hypoechogenicity or multifocal hypogenic lesions, increased intralesional flow on Doppler sonography, and in virtually all cases, enlarged testes (Mazzu et al. 1995). Another urologic report described three cases of asynchronous recurrence of a primary testicular lymphoma occurring in the contralateral testicle at a mean of 6 months since diagnosis (Selli 1994). These three cases and others reported in the literature have confirmed a poor prognosis for patients presenting with testicular lymphoma (Economopoulos 1996). One unusual report described three cases of an extremely unusual entity, T/NK cell lymphoma, involving the testes (Chan et al. 1996). This lymphoproliferative disorder is thought to be associated with Epstein-Barr Virus (EBV) infection, and in situ hybridization for EBV was positive in these clinically aggressive testicular cases. All three of these patients died within 5 months of diagnosis.

## 34.5.3
## Other Genitourinary Sites

Non-Hodgkin's lymphoma of other genitourinary sites, including the uterus, cervix, prostate, urethra, and ureters, are extremely rare, with only a few reports of each site of involvement found in the literature (Claikens et al. 1997; Kawakami and Mori 1995; Curry et al. 1993; Simpson et al. 1990). Cases of prostate involvement have been seen in young males, and, in one case, as an incidental concurrent finding during lymph node dissection for locally invasive prostate cancer, as secondary extension of Stage I large cell lymphoma from an adjacent iliac node (Mohrbacher A.F., personal communication). Gynecologic presentations have included four cases of lymphoma of the uterus or cervix diagnosed by MRI studies, showing an unusual diffuse enlargement and thickening of the uterine corpus or cervix (Kawakami and Mori 1995). Although these sites are too uncommon to permit much epidemiologic analysis, the association of HIV infection with unusual extranodal presentations of NHL should be kept in mind in evaluation and workup of such patients.

## 34.6
## Genitourinary Lymphoma Following Renal Transplantation

A now well-recognized complication of renal transplantation is risk of secondary malignancies, especially NHL (MORRISON et al. 1994; PENN 1993; WONG and HARRISON 1992; HONDA et al. 1990). This association is attributed to the immunosuppressive agents used to prevent rejection of the transplant. It is consistent with the markedly increased incidence of NHL in patients with AIDS, where T cell immune surveillance of early malignancies is presumably depressed. These post-transplantation lymphoproliferative disorders range from polyclonal lymphoproliferative processes of questionable malignant potential, to aggressive B cell immunoblastic lymphomas. In a review of 26 cases of post-transplantation lymphoproliferative disorder, 12/17 were monoclonal B cell, 2/17 were T cell, and 3/17 were polyclonal B cell neoplasms (MORRISON et al. 1994). Particularly noteworthy is the remarkable predominance of primary CNS lymphoma, again parallel to advanced AIDS-associated NHL, and the 22% incidence of lymphoma involving the renal allograft itself (MORRISON et al. 1994; PENN 1993). Hodgkin's disease has been reported in renal transplant patients as well, developing at a mean of 49 months post-transplantation (GARNIER et al. 1996). These cases were notable for the predominance of mixed cellularity subtype, six of seven cases, with one case of lymphocyte depletion subtype.

Radiation of bladder, uterine cervix, testicle, and prostate cancers has rarely been associated with subsequent development of hematologic malignancies, i.e., lymphoma, myeloma, and acute myeloid leukemia, or myelodysplastic syndrome (WERNER-WASIK 1995; HELLBARDT et al. 1990). Conversely, treatment of lymphomas and leukemias has been associated with an increased frequency of bladder cancer (TRAVIS et al. 1993).

## 34.7
## AIDS-Related Lymphomas

B cell NHL occurs at a much higher frequency in HIV positive individuals, with relative risk ratio of over a hundred to one. Non-Hodgkin's lymphoma is considered an AIDS defining illness (LEVINE 1992). In a series of 112 HIV-positive patients with newly diagnosed NHL, RADIN et al. (1993) noted this was the AIDS-defining illness in 79%. Mechanisms for this predisposition include loss of tumor surveillance by T cells, disregulation of B cells in the absence of T cells, and uncontrolled Epstein-Barr virus infection. HIV-related lymphomas differ from non-HIV-related cases by virtue of the extremely high proportion of high-grade histology; 90% are large cell, immunoblastic or small noncleaved (non-Burkitt's). In addition, an extremely high proportion of HIV-related lymphomas arise in extranodal sites, including kidney and testes, at a higher frequency than seen in historical non-HIV lymphoma series. Staging and treatment issues are similar to those in non-HIV patients, with two important additional considerations. HIV patients more frequently have extensive or stage IV disease, with the need for particularly careful staging by CT, gallium, scans, bone marrow biopsy, and, due to the high rate of CNS involvement, also a lumbar puncture. Because of the unusual extranodal presentation of AIDS-related lymphomas, conversely, any patient presenting with lymphoma of the genitourinary system should be considered for HIV testing.

## References


Amin R (1995) Case report: primary non-Hodgkin's lymphoma of the bladder. Br J Radiol 68:1257–1260

Chan JK, Tsang WY, Lau WH, Cheung MM, Ng WF, Yuen WC, Ng CS (1996) Aggressive T/natural killer cell lymphoma presenting as testicular tumor. Cancer 77:1198–1205

Claikens B, Oyen R, Goethuys H, Boogaerts M, Baert AL (1997) Non-Hodgkin's lymphoma of the prostate in a young male. Eur Radiol 7:238–240

Cohan RH (1990) Computed tomography of renal lymphoma. J Comput Assist Tomogr 14:933–938

Curry NS, Chung CJ, Potts W, Bissada N (1993) Isolated lymphoma of genitourinary tract and adrenals. LA – Eng Urol 41:494–498

Downs TM (1997) Non-Hodgkin's lymphoma can mimic renal adenocarcinoma with inferior vena caval involvement. Urology 49:276–278

Economopoulos T (1996) Primary extranodal non-Hodgkin's lymphoma in adults: clinicopathological and survival characteristics. Leuk Lymphoma 21:131–136

Fernandez-Acenero MJ, Martin-Rodilla C, Lopez-Garcia-Asenjo J, Coca-Menchero S, Sanz-Esponera J (1996) Primary malignant lymphoma of the bladder. Report of three cases. Pathol Res Pract 192:160–163

Garnier JL, Lebranchu Y, Dantal J, et al. (1996) Hodgkin's disease after transplantation. Transplantation 61:71–76

Gutjahr P, Humpl T (1995) Testicular lymphoblastic leukemia/lymphoma. World J Urol 13:230–232

Hauser M, Krestin GP, Hagspiel KD (1995) Bilateral solid multifocal intrarenal and perirenal lesions: differentiation with ultrasonography, computed tomography and magnetic resonance imaging. Clin Radiol 50:288–294

Hellbardt AM, Mirimanoff RO, Obradovic M, Mermillod B, Paunier JP (1990) The risk of second cancer (SC) in patients treated for testicular seminoma. Int J Radiat Oncol Biol Phys 18:1327–1331

Honda H, Barloon TJ, Franken EA Jr, Garneau RA, Smith JL (1990) Clinical and radiologic features of malignant neoplasms in organ transplant recipients: cyclosporine-treated vs untreated patients. AJR 154:271–274

Kawakami S, Mori T (1995) MR appearance of malignant lymphoma of the uterus. J Comput Assist Tomogr 19:238–242

Levine AM (1992) AIDS associated malignant lymphoma. Med Clin North Am 76:253–268

Martinelli GV, Vianelli N, De Vivo A, et al. (1997) Granulocytic sarcomas: clinical, diagnostic and therapeutical aspects. Leuk Lymphoma 24:349–353

Mazzu D, Jeffrey RB Jr, Ralls PW (1995) Lymphoma and leukemia involving the testicles: findings on gray-scale and color Doppler sonography. AJR Am J Roentgenol 164:645–647

Morel P, Dupriez B, Herbrecht R, et al. (1994) Aggressive lymphomas with renal involvement: a study of 48 patients treated with the LNH-84 and LNH-87 regimens. Groupe d'Etude des Lymphomes de l'Adulte. Br J Cancer 70:154–159

Morrison VA, Dunn DL, Manivel JC, Gajl Peczalska KJ, Peterson BA (1994) Clinical characteristics of post-transplant lymphoproliferative disorders. Am J Med 97:14–24

Ohsawa M, Aozasa K, Horiuchi K, Kanamaru A (1993) Malignant lymphoma of bladder. Report of three cases and review of the literature. Cancer 72:1969–1974

Okuno SH, Hoyer JD, Ristow K, Witzig TE (1995) Primary renal non-Hodgkin's lymphoma. An unusual extranodal site. Cancer 75:2258–2261

Pawade J, Banerjee SS, Harris M, Isaacson P, Wright D (1993) Lymphomas of mucosa-associated lymphoid tissue arising in the urinary bladder. Histopathology 23:147–151

Penn I (1993) Incidence and treatment of neoplasia after transplantation. J Heart Lung Transpl 12:S328–S336

Racioppi MM, Matei DV, Sica S, Pizzo M, Destito A, Alcini A, Alcini E (1996) Non-Hodgkin's lymphoma: a case report of a secondary bladder involvement. Scand J Urol Nephrol 30:429–431

Radin DR, Esplin JA, Levine AM, Ralls PW (1993) AIDS-related non-Hodgkin's lymphoma: abdominal CT findings in 112 patients. AJR Am J Roentgenol 160:1133–1139

Reznek RH, Richards MA (1990) CT in renal and perirenal lymphoma: a further look. Clin Radiol 42:233–238

Richards MA, Mootoosamy I, Reznek RH, Webb JA, Ta L (1990) Renal involvement in patients with non-Hodgkin's lymphoma: clinical and pathological features in 23 cases. Hematol Oncol 8:105–110

Selli CA (1994) Asynchronous bilateral non-Hodgkin's lymphoma of the testis: report of three cases. Urology 44:930–932

Simpson RH, Bridger JE, Anthony PP, James KA, Jury I (1990) Malignant lymphoma of the lower urinary tract. A clinico-pathological study with review of the literature. Br J Urol 65:254–260

Travis LB, Curtis RE, Glimelius B, et al. (1993) Second cancers among long-term survivors of non-Hodgkin's lymphoma. J Natl Cancer Inst 85:1932–1937

Wagner JR, Honig SC, Siroky MB (1993) Non-Hodgkin's lymphoma can mimic renal adenocarcinoma with inferior vena caval involvement [see comments]. LA – Eng Urol 42:720–723; discussion 723–724

Werner-Wasik M (1995) Increased risk of second malignant neoplasms outside radiation fields in patients with cervical carcinoma. Cancer 75:2281–2285

Wong RC, Harrison P (1992) NonEBV-related B-cell lymphoma in a renal transplant patient responding to acyclovir and reduction in immunosuppression. Postgrad Med J 68:145–146

Yoshinaga H, Miyasaka N, Kamiyama R, et al. (1996) Clonal identification of Burkitt's lymphoma arising from lymphocyte-predominant Hodgkin's disease. Br J Hematol 95:380–382

# 35 Rhabdomyosarcoma of the Genitourinary Tract in Pediatric Patients

R. LAVEY

CONTENTS



## 35.1 Introduction

Rhabdomyosarcoma accounts for the vast majority of sarcomas of the genitourinary (GU) system in children and approximately 4% of all pediatric solid malignancies, totalling about 250 cases per year in the United States. Twenty-six percent of all rhabdomyosarcoma cases enrolled in the Intergroup Rhabdomyosarcoma Study (IRS)-III from 1984 to 1991 arose from organs of the GU system (CRIST et al. 1995). Of 353 patients with rhabdomyosarcoma of GU sites enrolled in IRS-I or IRS-II between 1972 and 1984, the site of origin was paratesticular in 35%, bladder in 25%, prostate in 24%, vagina in 7%, and other sites, including cervix, vagina, and vulva, in 8% (NEWTON et al. 1988; LOBE et al. 1996). As suggested by the high proportion of paratesticular and prostate primary sites, rhabdomyosarcoma oc-


R. LAVEY, MD, Department of Radiation Oncology, Children's Hospital Los Angeles, 4650 Sunset Blvd., Los Angeles, CA 90027, USA


curs more frequently in boys than girls. The male to female ratio of incidence in all sites is 1.4 : 1. Rhabdomyosarcoma occurs over 3 times more frequently among Caucasians (4.4 per million children) than blacks (1.3 per million children). Overall, the peak incidence of rhabdomyosarcoma is at 2–5 years of age. Seventy percent of cases occur before age 10. Rhabdomyosarcoma patients have a disproportionately high rate of congenital anomalies, usually involving the gastrointestinal, genitourinary, cardiovascular, or central nervous system (RUYMAN et al. 1988). Children with neurofibromatosis have an elevated risk for rhabdomyosarcoma (McKEEN 1987). Rhabdomyosarcoma has also been associated with paternal cigarette smoking and chemical exposure (GRUFFERMAN et al. 1982).

## 35.2 Pathology

Rhabdomyosarcoma is a highly malignant neoplasm that arises from embryonal mesenchyme with the potential for differentiating into striated muscle. The myogenic origin of the tumor is demonstrated by positive staining for desmin or muscle-specific actin (PARHAM et al. 1991). Recent IRS studies categorize rhabdomyosarcoma into two prognostically significant histologic categories: favorable and unfavorable. The alveolar and undifferentiated subtypes are considered unfavorable and the other subtypes (embryonal, pleomorphic, and mixed) are favorable. Whether the histology is favorable or unfavorable, diploid tumors were found on multivariate analysis to have a worse prognosis than hyperdiploid tumors (SHAPIRO et al. 1991).

In the IRS-I and IRS-II studies, 91% of patients with GU rhabdomyosarcoma had the embryonal subtype (20% of which were sarcoma botryoides), 2% had the alveolar subtype, 1% had the pleomorphic subtype, and 6% were indeterminate or not classifiable (NEWTON et al. 1988). Embryonal tumors consist of primitive mesenchymal cells that show a spectrum of differentiation of rhabdomyoblasts. The more mature malignant cells tend to be elongated or spindle-shaped, while the less mature cells are round. The embryonal subtype resembles normally developing skeletal muscle in the 7- to 10-week old fetus. It is associated with overexpression of the oncogenes *n-myc*, *n-ras*, and *k-ras* (DIAS et al. 1990). The sarcoma botryoides variant of embryonal rhabdomyosarcoma occurs most commonly in sites having an open lumen into which the tumor can grow, such as the bladder, vagina, and nasopharynx. It is characterized by a subepithelial cambium layer of condensed cells producing polypoid masses resembling a cluster of grapes and carries a particularly favorable prognosis. Alveolar tumors are characterized by interconnecting strands of anastomosing fibrovascular connective tissue septa, which form spaces similar to pulmonary alveoli. Small, round malignant cells with scanty eosinophilic cytoplasm lie free in these spaces. The alveolar subtype resembles developing skeletal muscle in the 10- to 20-week old fetus. It is associated with the t(2;13) and t(1;13) chromosome translocations, the PAX 3-FKHR and PAX 7-FKHR gene fusion products, and overexpression of the oncogene *c-myc* (DIAS et al. 1990; DOUGLAS 1987). The t(2;13) translocation carries a dismal prognosis (DOUGLAS et al. 1993). Fortunately, the unfavorable alveolar and undifferentiated subtypes are rare in GU primary tumors. The pleomorphic subtype contains giant anaplastic cells with single large nuclei. It accounts for less than 1% of rhabdomyosarcomas. Prognosis is inversely associated with the number of anaplastic cells present (KODET et al. 1993).

## 35.3
## Staging

Rhabdomyosarcoma is both locally invasive and prone to metastasize. The most common sites of disease dissemination are regional lymph nodes, lungs, bone, and bone marrow. Computerized tomography (CT) of the chest is performed to evaluate for pulmonary metastases, of the abdomen to evaluate for retroperitoneal lymph node involvement, and of the pelvis to examine extent of the primary tumor and presence of pelvic or inguinal adenopathy. The bones and bone marrow are evaluated by nuclear medicine bone scan and bone marrow aspirate and biopsy.

There are two staging systems for rhabdomyosarcoma in current use. The TNM-UICC system is based on clinical criteria and the IRS grouping system is based on surgical findings and the extent of resection. The genitourinary tract is generally a favorable location for rhabdomyosarcoma, with paratesticular and genital tumors having a better prognosis for cure than tumors arising from the bladder or prostate (Fig. 35.1).

### 35.3.1
### TNM-UICC System

The TNM-UICC system (Table 35.1) classifies all genitourinary tumors without hematogenous dissemination, except those arising from the bladder or prostate, as stage I. Bladder and prostate primaries 5 cm or less in diameter and without nodal or hematogenous spread are classified as stage II. Bladder and prostate primaries greater than 5 cm in diameter and/or with nodal or hematogenous spread are classified as stage III. Hematogenous dissemination places any tumor in stage IV. Multivariate analysis of data from cooperative group studies from the IRS, International Society of Pediatric Oncology (SIOP), and Germany and Italy found that primary site and

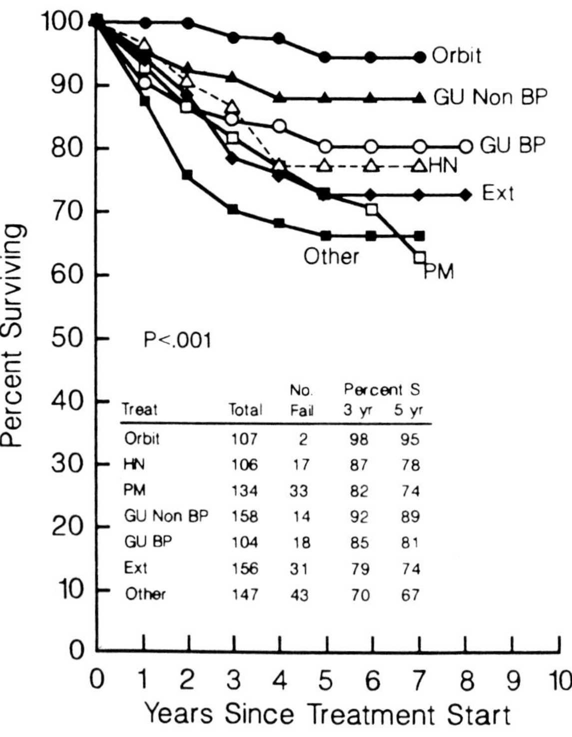


Fig. 35.1. Survival among patients with rhabdomyosarcoma enrolled in the IRS-III study according to tumor site and years since treatment (CHRIST et al. 1995)

**Table 35.1.** Pretreatment TNM clinical staging system for genitourinary rhabdomyosarcoma (UICC)

| Stage | GU site | Diameter | Involved nodes | Distant metastases |
|---|---|---|---|---|
| 1 | Paratesticular or genital | Any | Yes or no | No |
| 2 | Bladder or prostate | ≤5 cm | No | No |
| 3 | Bladder or prostate | ≤5 cm | Yes | No |
|   |   | >5 cm | Yes or no | No |
| 4 | Any | Any | Yes or no | Yes |

**Table 35.2.** The Intergroup Rhabdomyosarcoma Study (IRS) clinical group staging system

| | |
|---|---|
| Group I | Completely resected localized disease without lymph node involvement. No distant metastasis. |
| Group II | Grossly resected tumor with microscopic residual disease at the primary site or in regional lymph nodes. No distant metastasis. |
| Group III | Incompletely resected tumor with gross residual disease at the primary site or in regional lymph nodes. No distant metastasis. |
| Group IV | Distant metastatic disease present at diagnosis. |

infiltration outside the site of origin were independent prognostic factors for survival (RODARY et al. 1991). In the IRS-II study, 10-year overall survival among patients with bladder or prostate primaries was 70% compared to 80% among patients with other GU primary sites (MAURER et al. 1993; LAWRENCE et al. 1987a). Although the TNM-UICC system distinguishes between primary tumor confinement to its site of origin (T1) and infiltration beyond its origin (T2), it does not separate the T1 and T2 tumors into different stages.

## 35.3.2
## IRS Grouping System

The IRS grouping system (Table 35.2) has been in use since 1972. Unlike the TNM-UICC system, it takes into account the prognostically important extent of surgical resection, but fails to consider the site of primary tumor. Briefly, IRS group I includes localized tumors that have been completely resected. Group II includes tumors with residual microscopic disease, evidenced by either positive resection margins at the primary site or regional lymph node involvement that has been grossly resected. Group III includes tumors with residual gross disease at the primary site or in regional lymph nodes postoperatively. Group IV includes all tumors with distant spread of disease. The TNM-UICC system, which takes into account the site and size of the primary tumor, is currently used to determine the chemotherapy regimen to be used postoperatively. The IRS system, which is based on the extent of locoregional disease remaining postoperatively, is currently used to determine whether radiation therapy is to be used, and to what site and dose it should be given. Neither system takes into account histologic subtype, which is also a strong prognostic factor that currently influ-

ences the selection of both chemotherapy and radiation therapy.

## 35.4
## Paratesticular Tumors

### 35.4.1
### Tumor Behavior

Paratesticular rhabdomyosarcomas accounted for 12% of childhood scrotal tumors and 8% of all rhabdomyosarcoma cases in the IRS-I and IRS-II studies (WIENER 1993). Rhabdomyosarcoma of the paratesticular region usually arises from the distal spermatic cord and presents as a painless, unilateral scrotal swelling or mass above the testis, sometimes associated with a hydrocele. Physical examination and ultrasonography reveal a solid, firm mass that is usually distinct from the testis. It is uncommon to have either fixation of the mass to the scrotal skin or inguinal adenopathy upon presentation. Unlike other sites of rhabdomyosarcoma, the paratesticular region has an almost equal likelihood of presentation at each 5-year period between 0 and 20 years of age (RANEY et al. 1987). The most common site of metastasis is the para-aortic node chain, as malignant cells may follow the course of the spermatic cord into the renal hilar retroperitoneal space. Twenty-six to 27% percent of patients had para-aortic nodal metastasis at presentation in the IRS-II and IRS-III studies (LAWRENCE et al. 1987b; WIENER et al. 1994). The ipsilateral inguinal lymph nodes were involved in 16% of cases in IRS-I and IRS-II. Contralateral inguinal node involvement is rare, as is iliac node involvement in the absence of para-aortic adenopathy (RANEY et al. 1978, 1987). Distant hematogenous metastasis is detected at presentation in about 15% of cases (RANEY et al. 1987; LAQUAGLIA et al. 1989). The histologic subtype has been found to be embryonal in 90% of cases and alveolar in the other 10%. An analysis of 173 paratesticular rhabdomyosarcoma cases enrolled in IRS-I, II, or III found that the one-third of patients whose tumor consisted almost exclusively of spindle-shaped cells with only sparse amounts of intercellular collagen (the spindle-cell variant) had a 5-year survival rate of 95%, compared to a 5-year survival of 80% among the non-spindle-cell embryonal cases (LEUSCHNER et al. 1993).

The paratesticular location carries a favorable prognosis, warranting its classification as stage 1 in the IRS staging system. Among the favorable characteristics of the paratesticular tumors are the preponderance of the embryonal histology, their superficial location leading to early diagnosis and uncomplicated resection, and a relatively low propensity to metastasize. The 5-year progression-free survival of patients in the IRS-I and IRS-II studies with paratesticular rhabdomyosarcomas was 93% if there was no evidence of metastasis on staging CT scan, 69% if the CT scan was positive for para-aortic node metastasis, and 57% if there was hematogenous metastasis on presentation. With salvage treatment, overall survival approached 90% (RANEY et al. 1987). Among clinical group I patients entered in all three reported IRS studies, only 8 of 128 (6%) relapsed after either postoperative VA or VAC chemotherapy. In the IRS-III study, the 5-year survival was 91% among all patients without hematogenous metastasis. Although histologic subtype, primary tumor size, and completeness of resection were not prognostic in IRS-III, age and para-aortic node positivity on abdominal CT scan were independent, statistically significant prognostic factors. The 5-year survival was 96% among patients with clinically negative nodes compared to 69% among patients with clinically positive nodes ($P < 0.001$), and 97% among patients below 10 years of age compared to 84% among patients above age 10 ($P = 0.03$) (WIENER et al. 1994).

## 35.4.2
## Treatment

*Surgery.* The initial treatment for solid paratesticular masses in children should be inguinal orchiectomy with complete resection of the spermatic cord structures to the level of the inguinal ring. A trans-scrotal procedure increases the incidence of local recurrence and nonregional lymph node me-

tastasis. If the tumor was inappropriately biopsied or removed by a trans-scrotal approach, removal of the remaining spermatic cord using an inguinal approach and a partial hemiscrotectomy including the prior scrotal incision is indicated. Retroperitoneal lymph node dissection was a standard part of the staging evaluation in IRS studies I–III, but was eliminated from IRS-IV and IRS-V except in patients with suspicious abdominal CT scans due to its morbidity. In the IRS-I study, retroperitoneal node dissection resulted in a 10% incidence of intestinal obstruction, 8% incidence of ejaculatory dysfunction, and 5% incidence of lower extremity edema (HEYN et al. 1992).

An analysis of the need for retroperitoneal lymph node biopsy or sampling in patients with stage 1, clinical group I disease was conducted in 1992 utilizing the combined results of the IRS-III, German Oncology Group CWS-81, and Italian Oncology Group Italy-79 studies. Retroperitoneal adenectomy uncovered lymph node involvement in only 3 of 88 (3%) patients with negative clinical lymph node evaluation in these studies. Lymph node relapse occurred in only two patients, both of whom had negative staging lymphadenectomies (RODARY et al. 1992b). Another evaluation of the need for para-aortic adenectomy analyzed results in the 110 IRS-III patients with paratesticular rhabdomyosarcoma who underwent abdominal CT scanning (95%) or ultrasound evaluation (5%) followed by retroperitoneal lymph node sampling. It found that clinical evaluation detected only 17 of the 30 pathologically positive cases, a 57% sensitivity rate. Seventy-nine of the 80 pathologically negative cases were also clinically negative, a specificity rate of 99%. The false-positive rate of abdominal CT scanning or ultrasound was only 6% (1/18) and the false-negative rate was 14% (13/92) (WIENER et al. 1994). The para-aortic nodal relapse rate was 1% (1/110), even lower than in the multigroup analysis cited above (OLIVE et al. 1984). As in the multigroup study, the nodal relapse occurred in a patient who had negative findings from an extensive retroperitoneal node dissection and did not receive postoperative radiation therapy (WIENER et al. 1994).

Two cooperative groups outside the United States, the International Society of Pediatric Oncology and the Children's Solid Tumor Group, have reported low rates of nodal relapse in prospective trials in which node sampling and radiation therapy was omitted in patients with complete primary tumor resection and negative abdominal CT scans (OLIVE et al. 1984; PLOWMAN 1988). Disease recurred in only 2 of 19 patients (11%), one of whom had not received chemotherapy. Both patients recurred in the para-aortic nodes and were rendered disease-free by salvage therapy (OLIVE et al. 1984). Six patients in the IRS-III study did not undergo node sampling or para-aortic nodal irradiation after negative abdominal CT scanning. One relapsed simultaneously in the bone marrow and para-aortic nodes; the other five remained disease-free. Because of the potential for complications following retroperitoneal lymph node dissection, low rate of retroperitoneal node relapse, and success in salvaging relapsed pateints, the IRS-IV and IRS-V studies include exploratory laparotomy and retroperitoneal node dissection or sampling only for patients with positive CT or MRI scanning or palpable adenopathy (RODARY et al. 1992b). Preliminary analysis of the results from IRS-IV shows no difference in nodal relapse rate or failure-free survival compared to IRS-III. However, some experts still advocate surgical staging for all patients, in consideration of the low sensitivity of abdominal CT scanning in IRS-III, insufficient experience without surgical staging and irradiation of pathologically node-positive patients, and reduced surgical morbidity with the use of laparoscopy and/or limited unilateral node dissection (WIENER et al. 1994).

Appropriate surgery should render all paratesticular rhabdomyosarcoma cases group I (completely resected) locally. The chance of local relapse following complete resection and postoperative chemotherapy is less than 5%. Patients with no evidence of nodal and/or hematogenous spread of disease therefore do not receive radiation therapy unless there has been local tumor spillage. In the unusual case in which the scrotal skin contains malignant cells, radiation therapy should be given to the scrotum. The contralateral testicle should be transposed or abdomen into the thigh prior to scrotal irradiation to avoid sterilization, then reimplanted into the scrotum following radiation therapy (RANEY et al. 1987). Radiation therapy to the para-aortic and ipsilateral iliac nodes, in combination with chemotherapy, is indicated if node dissection has demonstrated the presence of tumor (clinical group II) or there is unresectable adenopathy (clinical group III). With this treatment, the risk of nodal relapse is only 1% (WIENER et al. 1994). The inguinal nodes are irradiated only in patients with demonstrated inguinal node involvement.

*Chemotherapy.* Multiagent cytotoxic chemotherapy given for a period of 10–12 months is part of the standard treatment of all stages and groups of rhabdomyosarcoma. Prior to the introduction of chemotherapy for rhabdomyosarcoma in the mid-1960s, only 10%–20% of children with rhabdomyosarcoma of the genitourinary organs survived long term (FLEMING et al. 1984; TEFFT and JAFFE 1973; GROSFELD et al. 1972). In the 1980s, with the combined use of intensive chemotherapy with surgery and/or radiation therapy for local control, the proportion surviving rose to over 70% (LOUGHLIN et al. 1989). The IRS-V study for localized tumors without nodal or hematogenous spread (Low-Risk Protocol) that opened in 1997 includes 46 weeks of chemotherapy, using vincristine and actinomycin D (VA) for patients with favorable histology tumors and vincristine, actinomycin D, and cyclophosphamide (VAC) for patients with unfavorable histology tumors.

*Radiation Therapy.* Radiation therapy in the IRS-V study is given starting after 3 weeks of chemotherapy only to patients with tumor spillage at the primary site. Radiation therapy is given earlier than in IRS-IV, in which irradiation was begun after 9 weeks of chemotherapy. The irradiated volume is the region of tumor spillage with 2-cm margins. Patients are given a total dose of 3600 cGy in 20 fractions of 180 cGy. The radiation dose was reduced from the 4140 cGy given for microscopic disease in prior IRS studies in an attempt to reduce radiation-related morbidity in a group of patients with an expected 95% long-term survival rate. The local control rate among 204 IRS-III patients treated with 4140 cGy for microscopic residual disease was 91%. Justification for the dose reduction comes from two reports of good local control in small series of patients treated with 3000–3650 cGy for microscopic rhabdomyosarcoma at Memorial Sloan-Kettering Cancer Center and St. Jude Children's Research Hospital (ETCUBANAS et al. 1987; MANDELL et al. 1990).

Patients with nodal metastasis or residual disease at the primary site should receive radiation therapy in combination with chemotherapy. Three chemotherapy regimens for this "intermediate-risk" patient group are being compared in the IRS-IV study, the standard VAC, vincristine-actinomycin D-ifosfamide (VAI), and vincristine-ifosfamide-etoposide (VIE). Patients in IRS-IV, which was opened in 1991, are randomized to receive eight courses of one of these three regimens followed by four courses of VAC over a total treatment period of 44 weeks. Radiation therapy is given starting on week 9 of chemotherapy. Actinomycin D and etoposide are withheld from the chemotherapy courses administered during radiation therapy. The target volume for incompletely resected tumors is the extent of tumor at diagnosis with a 2-cm margin. Patients with nodal metastasis receive radiation to the entire para-aortic and ipsilateral iliac node chains. All patients with postoperative microscopic residual disease are given a total dose of 4140 cGy in daily fractions of 180 cGy. This treatment is expected to achieve a 90% locoregional control rate. Patients with postoperative gross residual disease are randomized to receive 5040 cGy in once daily fractions of 180 cGy or 5940 cGy in twice daily fractions of 110 cGy. In the IRS-II study, patients with gross residual disease who were given 4000–5500 cGy in once daily fractions had a local relapse rate of 16% and a locoregional relapse rate of 32%. A dose of 6000 cGy given in once daily fractions of 200 cGy has been reported to result in higher rates of both local control and permanent morbidity (DONALDSON et al. 1973; HEYN et al. 1976; TEFFT et al. 1986). Hyperfractionated radiation therapy with concurrent multiagent chemotherapy has been shown to be feasible for rhabdomyosarcoma patients without undue toxicity, first at Memorial Sloan-Kettering Cancer Center (MANDELL et al. 1988), then in 284 patients treated on the IRS-IV pilot study (DONALDSON et al. 1995). It is hoped that hyperfractionation will provide the benefits of an increased cumulative radiation dose without the accompanying morbidity.

## 35.5
## Bladder Tumors

### 35.5.1
### Tumor Presentation

Rhabdomyosarcomas account for approximately 90% of all bladder malignancies in children. The bladder was the site of 5% of all rhabdomyosarcomas entered into the IRS-I and IRS-II studies (NEWTON et al. 1988). Tumors generally arise from the submucosa of the trigone or dome of the bladder and protrude into the bladder lumen. In boys, bladder tumors often invade the prostate, making it difficult to determine which is their organ of origin. The tumor commonly presents with pelvic pain and dysuria, polyuria, hematuria, and urinary retention. Tumors located in the dome of the bladder may produce a palpable low abdominal mass. Ultrasonography usually delineates the mass well (BAHNSON et al. 1989). A histologic diagnosis can often be made

by cystoscopy. The histologic subtype was embryonal in 55% and botryoid in 40% of cases in the IRS-I and IRS-II studies. Dissemination into regional lymphatics, usually the hypogastric and external iliac and less commonly the para-aortic nodes, was detected in 21% of IRS-I and IRS-II patients (LAWRENCE et al. 1987b). Distant metastasis is unusual, occurring in only 6% of patients in the IRS-I study. Reported sites of distant metastasis include the lung, pleura, bone marrow, and liver (HAYS et al. 1982).

### 35.5.2
### Treatment

Local control of the primary bladder tumor is strongly associated with complete resection of the primary tumor. Surgical therapy ideally is a partial cystectomy resulting in complete resection with preservation of bladder function. This is more feasible with tumors located in the bladder dome than in the trigone or neck. Only rarely can the tumor be completely resected at presentation with preservation of bladder and urethral function. The initial operative procedure is therefore generally limited to a biopsy for diagnostic purposes. Chemotherapy and radiation therapy are then employed prior to definitive surgical resection.

The IRS-I study demonstrated that pelvic exenteration is not required for cure. All five patients in whom negative surgical margins were obtained by partial cystectomy remained free from relapse after postoperative adjuvant radiation and chemotherapy (HAYS et al. 1990). However, 42% of patients underwent exenteration at diagnosis. Overall, 70% of patients remained free of disease at 3 years, but only 23% were alive with bladder function. In an attempt to increase the bladder retention rate, the IRS-II study utilized primary triple-agent (VAC) chemotherapy followed at week 16 by radiation therapy. This resulted in initial bladder conservation in 97% of patients, but within 3 years 50% of patients relapsed and only 22% remained alive with bladder function (RANEY et al. 1990). Both bladder preservation and survival improved in the IRS-III study, in which radiation therapy was moved forward from week 16 to week 6, vincristine was administered weekly, and cisplatin and doxorubicin were added to the VAC regimen. Surgery was performed after radiation therapy to document a complete response to treatment or perform a conservative resection of residual disease, if possible. The 4-year results for 83 bladder or prostate rhabdomyosarcomas treated in IRS-III were an overall survival of 85% and survival with bladder function of 60% (HAYS et al. 1995; CRIST et al. 1995). Of the 40 patients who underwent partial cystectomy on IRS studies I–III, 78% have survived and 75% of the survivors have no bladder-related symptoms (HAYS et al. 1995). Because none of the IRS studies found a survival benefit from the addition of doxorubicin with or without cisplatin to the VAC regimen, these drugs are not being used in the IRS-IV or IRS-V studies.

The vast majority of patients with bladder rhabdomyosarcoma have unresected primary tumors at the start of chemotherapy. In IRS-III these patients underwent intensive chemotherapy for 20 weeks with or without radiation therapy prior to definitive surgery. For tumors in the neck or trigone of the bladder, pelvic radiation therapy was incorporated starting after 6 weeks of chemotherapy. For tumors of the dome of the bladder, radiation therapy was utilized only if there was residual disease after chemotherapy and second-look surgery. Bladder tumors greater than 5 cm in maximum diameter or not completely resected at diagnosis but without hematogenous metastasis are categorized as "intermediate risk" by the IRS. Treatment of these tumors on the IRS-V pilot study involves 13 courses of VAC chemotherapy given over 38 weeks with definitive surgery or radiation therapy performed after 12 weeks of chemotherapy. The pilot includes escalation of the dose of cyclophosphamide that is given during the first four (induction) courses prior to surgery and/or radiation therapy. Radiation therapy is used if conservative surgery is not feasible or there is residual disease after surgery. The target volume is the initial tumor with a 2-cm margin and the dose is the standard used in IRS-III and IRS-IV, 4140 cGy in 23 daily factions for microscopic disease and 5040 cGy in 28 daily fractions for gross disease. A few bladder rhabdomyosarcoma patients are categorized as "low-risk" by the IRS. These children had a primary tumor no greater than 5 cm in maximum diameter that was completely resected at diagnosis and no nodal or hematogenous disease spread. Their chemotherapy is as described for low-risk paratesticular tumors above, 46 weeks of VA for favorable histology or VAC for unfavorable histology tumors. No radiation therapy is given for this patient group in the absence of postoperative residual disease.

## 35.6
## Prostate Tumors

### 35.6.1
### Tumor Behavior

The prostate was the site of 5% of all rhabdomyosarcomas entered into the IRS-I–III studies (NEWTON et al. 1988; MAURER et al. 1993; CRIST et al. 1995). These tumors usually present with dysuria, polyuria, and urinary retention caused by compression of the base of the bladder and infiltration of the bladder neck and urethra. Invasion of the bladder by prostate tumors often makes determination of the organ of origin difficult. Tumors from the prostate and bladder are usually categorized together and treated in like manner. The histologic subtype was embryonal in 85% of cases, botryoid in 7%, and alveolar in 5% in the IRS-I and IRS-II studies. The IRS-III study included 51 tumors of prostate origin, of which 82% were embryonal, 6% undifferentiated, 6% sarcoma not otherwise specified, and 4% extraosseous Ewing's sarcoma (LOBE et al. 1996). Dissemination into regional lymphatics, usually the hypogastric and external iliac and less commonly the para-aortic nodes, was detected in 42% of IRS-I and IRS-II patients (LAWRENCE et al. 1987b). Distant metastasis was detected at presentation in 10% of patients in the IRS-III study (LOBE et al. 1996).

### 35.6.2
### Treatment

Prostate rhabdomyosarcomas, like bladder primaries, generally cannot be completely resected at presentation with preservation of bladder and urethral function. The initial operative procedure is therefore generally limited to a biopsy for diagnostic purposes. Only 2 of 46 (4%) patients with nonmetastatic disease entered in IRS-III had initial gross resection of their primary tumor. The other 44 patients underwent intensive chemotherapy for 20 weeks concurrently with radiation therapy prior to definitive surgery.

External beam radiation therapy to the primary tumor site, either 5040 cGy given in once-daily fractions of 180 cGy or 5940 cGy given in twice daily fractions of 110 cGy, is incorporated starting after 8 weeks of chemotherapy in the IRS-IV study. In IRS-III, 4500 cby was given in once-daily fractions of 180 cby starting after 6 weeks of chemotherapy. The earlier use of radiation and more intensive chemotherapy in IRS-III compared with IRS-II was associated with an improvement in overall survival from 49% to 82%. Sixty-four percent of the surviving patients retained bladder function (LOBE et al. 1996). Treatment of prostate and bladder rhabdomyosarcomas using intensive chemotherapy with or without concurrent radiation therapy followed by conservative surgery also produced a good chance of survival with bladder preservation in several smaller series. At Memorial Sloan-Kettering Cancer Center, overall survival among 25 patients was 72%, with 50% of survivors retaining bladder function (GHAVINI et al. 1984). In 15 patients treated at St. Jude Children's Research Hospital, 11 survived (73%), nine with functional bladders (PRATT 1984). All ten survivors among 12 (83%) patients reported from Europe retained their bladders (VOUTE et al. 1981). The desire to preserve organ function should not overshadow the need to completely resect the primary tumor. Prostatectomy without cystectomy has been reported to result in a 40% local relapse rate (MCLORIE et al. 1989).

Brachytherapy, consisting in the temporary implantation of radioactive iodine-125 seeds into the tumor, provides a means of administering a large radiation dose to the target with rapid dose falloff in the surrounding normal tissues. The Institute Gustav-Roussy reported on 12 selected prostate or bladder tumors treated with chemotherapy followed by conservative surgery and postoperative brachytherapy to the tumor bed. External beam radiation was not used. The 5-year relapse free survival with functional bladder was 75%. The investigators recommended this approach for primary tumors smaller than 4 cm in maximum diameter (HAIE-MEDER et al. 1994). This limits the applicability of brachytherapy, as the mean prostatic tumor entered in IRS-III was 7.2 cm in diameter (LOBE et al. 1996).

## 35.7
## Female Genital Tract Tumors

### 35.7.1
### Tumor Characteristics

Tumors of the female genital tract accounted for 12% of all rhabdomyosarcomas entered in the IRS-I and IRS-II studies. Seventy-six percent of the female genital tumors were vaginal or vulvar in origin, with others originating from the cervix or uterus. The histologic subtype was botryoid in two-thirds of cases

and standard embryonal in one-third (NEWTON et al. 1988). In the IRS-III study, 92% of vaginal tumors were of the botryoid histology (ANDRASSY et al. 1995). Dissemination into regional lymph nodes was detected at presentation in only 6% of patients in IRS-I and IRS-II (LAWRENCE et al. 1987b).

Girls with vulvar or vaginal tumors usually present with a foul-smelling vaginal discharge, difficulty with urination, bleeding, and a firm vulvar nodule or protruding polypoid mass (HAYS 1980; HAYS et al. 1981; ANDRASSY et al. 1995). The tumor is usually located on the anterior wall of the middle or lower vagina. In IRS-III, 89% (24 of 27) of patients with vulvar or vaginal tumors were under age 4 years at presentation (ANDRASSY et al. 1995).

Tumors of the cervix and uterus usually occur at a later age, with a peak incidence in the second decade of life in most series (HAYS et al. 1981, 1985, 1988; BRAND et al. 1987; DAYA and SCULLY 1988) and a mean age at diagnosis of 5.5 years in the IRS-III and pilot IRS-IV studies (CORPRON et al. 1995). Cervical tumors present with a vaginal mass and discharge or bleeding. Tumors of the uterine corpus present with menstrual irregularity and/or an abdominal mass and pain (HAYS et al. 1985, 1988). Tumors of the cervix or uterus are rare, with only 13 cases registered in IRS-I and IRS-II (HAYS et al. 1988) and 14 cases in IRS-III and pilot IRS-IV. The histology of the 14 cervix or uterine tumors in IRS-III and pilot IRS-IV was standard embryonal in ten, botryoid in three, and alveolar in one (CORPRON et al. 1995). Staging evaluation of all female genital tumors should include cystoscopy and vaginoscopy.

### 35.7.2
### Treatment

*Vulvar and Vaginal Tumors.* The traditional surgical treatment for vaginal tumors, anterior exenteration and urinary diversion, was used in the IRS-I study. Later IRS studies have emphasized primary chemotherapy to diminish the size of the tumor, followed by less mutilating surgery and/or radiation therapy. Most vulvar or vaginal patients in the IRS-II and IRS-III studies had initial surgery limited to biopsy only. Chemotherapy was then given, with partial responders undergoing conservative surgery (partial vaginectomy with or without hysterectomy, wide local excision, or biopsy only) or radiation therapy after either 16 (IRS-II) or 20–28 (IRS-III) weeks of chemotherapy. If surgery was chosen as the local control modality, radiation therapy was only administered to patients with positive margins or gross residual disease. Target volume and doses were as described above for bladder and prostate tumors. The 3-year survival using this approach in IRS-II was 86% (18 of 21 patients) (RANEY et al. 1990). The IRS-III study included 24 patients with vaginal primaries, 23 of whom (96%) had localized disease, and three patients with vulvar primaries, all localized. All three vulvar tumors were cured, two by wide local excision followed by chemotherapy, the other with 4140 cGy postoperative external beam radiation therapy added due to positive surgical margins. Among the 23 patients with localized vaginal tumors, none had recurrence of disease and 20 (87%) remained alive and relapse-free for a minimum of 5 years after diagnosis. There were two chemotherapy-related deaths and one death of unknown cause. Fifty percent of the survivors did not undergo surgical resection of their tumor; six (30%) had chemotherapy only and four (20%) underwent chemotherapy with local radiation therapy (ANDRASSY et al. 1995).

The IRS-IV study recommends biopsy for diagnosis, 9 weeks of triple-agent induction chemotherapy (VAC, VAI, or VIE), then definitive conservation surgery followed by continuation chemotherapy for vaginal tumors. Postoperative brachytherapy or external beam radiation therapy to 4140 cGy in 23 daily fractions is given to patients with positive surgical margins. In the unusual situation of gross residual disease, external beam radiation is given to 5040 cGy in 28 daily fractions. Brachytherapy has the attractive feature of limiting the volume of radiation exposure, but must be performed with care, as it resulted in a rectal-vaginal-vesical fistula in the one patient given brachytherapy on IRS-III (ANDRASSY et al. 1995). Vaginal intracavitary brachytherapy is used as standard treatment in place of vaginectomy at Memorial Sloan-Kettering Cancer Center and the Institute Gustave-Roussy (ANDRASSY et al. 1995; FLAMANT et al. 1990). The Institute Gustave-Roussy reported excellent local control with minimal long-term morbidity using this approach. Of 12 patients followed for at least 10 years, 11 (92%) have normal menses and six (50%) have normal sexual intercourse (FLAMANT et al. 1990).

*Cervix and uterus tumors.* Rhabdomyosarcomas of the cervix and uterus have a greater tendency to metastasize than do vaginal and vulvar tumors. Three of 14 patients with cervical or uterine tumors (21%) in the IRS-III and pilot IRS-IV studies presented with distant metastases. Among the remaining 11 patients, four (36%) died of sepsis during chemotherapy, one died of progressive local and distant disease, and six (55%) remain without evidence of disease. The only girl having an unfavorable (alveolar) histology tumor was the sole patient to die of disease. All three patients who presented with metastatic disease and responded completely to chemotherapy remain relapse-free at 1.5–6 years after diagnosis. Of the seven surviving patients, only two underwent hysterectomy and vaginectomy and two received radiation therapy (CORPRON et al. 1995). In published series of sarcoma botryoides of the cervix treated outside the IRS, 29 of 34 patients (85%) were long-term survivors (BRAND et al. 1987; DAYA and SCULLY 1988). Many of the patients had biopsy only or organ-conserving surgery. These results indicate that the response to chemotherapy is better in the uterine corpus and cervix tumors than suggested by the IRS-I and IRS-II studies and that an approach based on primary chemotherapy and delayed conservative surgery is reasonable.

*IRS-IV Protocol.* Patients with female genital tumors are treated on the IRS-IV study as described above for paratesticular tumors with postoperative residual disease. After biopsy for diagnosis, patients are randomized to receive eight courses of VAC, VAI, or VIE followed by four courses of VAC over a total treatment period of 44 weeks. Radiation therapy is started after 9 weeks of chemotherapy. Uterine cervix or corpus tumors are randomized to receive standard or hyperfractionated external beam irradiation to 5040 or 5940 cGy. None of the vulvar and vaginal tumor patients receive more than 5040 cGy, as this dose was sufficient to produce excellent local control in prior IRS studies. Second-look surgery is performed after completion of the entire course of chemotherapy. Resection is done only if residual disease is identified.

## 35.8
## Metastatic Disease

The survival rate using standard chemotherapy for patients having metastatic disease with bone marrow involvement is 7% and without bone marrow involvement it is 23% (MAURER et al. 1993). Two IRS-V studies are currently investigating newer strategies. One alternates VAC with VCT (vincristine-cyclophosphamide-topotecan) chemotherapy for 44 weeks. Radiation therapy is given starting after 15 weeks of chemotherapy. The other study uses alternating VAC and IE chemotherapy and radiation therapy prior to conditioning with carboplatin-etoposide-melphalan and autologous bone marrow transplantation. Radiation is administered to the primary tumor as well as all sites of metastatic disease. Radiation therapy is emphasized in place of surgery for local control to minimize morbidity in this poor prognosis group of patients. It is hoped that new agents and more intensive chemotherapy will improve their chance of survival.

## 35.9
## Conclusions

Pediatric rhabdomyosarcoma is a model of rapid clinical progress occurring from creative cooperative group protocol development and high rates of accession onto the protocols. Cure rates have increased from approximately 20% to 75% in the past two decades. Multiagent chemotherapy is given to all patients. Surgery and/or radiation therapy are used for local control of the primary tumor and involved regional lymph nodes. Current protocols emphasize decreasing long-term morbidity due to treatment in the low-risk group of patients, increasing cure rates while preserving organ function in the intermediate-risk group of patients, and developing more effective chemotherapy regimens for those with metastatic disease.

## References


Andrassy RJ, Hays DM, Raney B, et al. (1995) Conservative surgical management of vaginal and vulvar pediatric rhabdomyosarcoma: a report from the Intergroup Rhabdomyosarcoma Study III. J Pediatr Surg 30:1034–1037

Bahnson RR, Zaonts MR, Maizels M, Shkolnik AA, Firlit CF (1989) Ultrasonography and diagnosis of pediatric genitourinary rhabdomyosarcoma. Urology 33:64–68

Brand E, Berek JS, Nieberg RK, Hacker NF (1987) Rhabdomyosarcoma of the uterine cervix: sarcoma botryoides. Cancer 60:1552–1560

Corpron CA, Andrassy RJ, Hays DM, et al. (1995) Conservative management of uterine pediatric rhabdomyosarcoma: a report from the Intergroup Rhabdomyosarcoma Study III and IV Pilot. J Pediatr Surg 30:942–944

Crist W, Gehan EA, Ragah AH, et al. (1995) The Intergroup Rhabdomyosarcoma Study III. J Clin Oncol 13:610–630

Daya DA, Scully RE (1988) Sarcoma botryoides of the uterine cervix in young women: a clinicopathological study of 13 cases. Gynecol Oncol 29:290–304

Dias P, Kuma P, Marsden H, et al. (1990) N-*myc* gene is amplified in alveolar rhabdomyosarcomas (RMS) but not in embryonal RMS. Int J Cancer 45:593–596

Donaldson SS, Castro JR, Wilbur JR, Jesse RH Jr. (1973) Rhabdomyosarcoma of the head and neck in children: combination treatment by surgery, irradiation and chemotherapy. Cancer 31:26–35

Donaldson SS, Asmar L, Breneman J, et al. (1995) Hyperfractionated radiation in children with rhabdomyosarcoma – results of an Intergroup Rhabdomyosarcoma Pilot Study. Int J Radiat Oncol Biol Phys 32:903–911

Douglass EC, Valentine M, Etcubanas E et al. (1987) A specific chromosomal abnormality in rhabdomyosarcoma. Cytogenet Cell Genet 45:148

Douglass E, Shapiro D, Valentine M, et al. (1993) Alveolar rhabdomyosarcoma with the t(2;13): cytogenetic findings and clinicopathologic correlations. Med Pediatr Oncol 1:83–87

Etcubanas E, Rao BN, Kun LE, et al. (1987) The impact of delayed surgery on radiotherapy dose and local control of rhabdomyosarcoma. Arch Surg 122:1451–1454

Flamant F, Gerbaulet A, Nihoul-Fekete C, Valteau-Couanet D, Chassagne D, Lemerle J (1990) Long-term sequelae of conservative treatment by surgery, brachytherapy, and chemotherapy for vulval and vaginal rhabdomyosarcoma in children. J Clin Oncol 8:1847–1853

Fleming KD, Etcubarias E, Patterson R, et al. (1984) The role of surgical resection when combined with chemotherapy and radiation in the management of pelvic rhadomyosarcoma. Ann Surg 199:509–514

Ghavini F, Herr H. Jereb B, et al. (1984) Treatment of genitourinary rhabdomyosarcoma in children. J Urol 132:313–319

Grosfeld JL, Smith JP, Clatworthy HW (1972) Pelvic rhabdomyosarcoma in infants and children. J Urol 107:673–675

Grufferman S, Wang H, Delong E, Kimm S, Delzell E, Falletta J (1982) Environmental factors in the etiology of rhabdomyosarcoma in childhood. J Natl Cancer Inst 68:107–113

Haie-Meder C, Flamant F, Revillon Y, et al. (1994) Brachytherapy in the multidisciplinary therapy of prostate and/or bladder rhabdomyosarcomas in children (abstract). Med Pediatr Oncol 23:188

Hays DM (1980) Pelvic rhabdomyosarcoma in childhood: diagnosis and concepts of management reviewed. Cancer 45:1810–1814

Hays DM, Raney RB, Lawrence W, et al. (1981) Rhabdomyosarcoma of the female urogenital tract: J Pediatr Surg 16:828–834

Hays DM, Raney RB Jr, Lawrence W Jr, Soule EH, Gehan EA, Tefft M (1982) Bladder and prostatic tumors in Intergroup Rhabdomyosarcoma Study (IRS-I): results of therapy. Cancer 50:1472–1482

Hays DM, Shimada H, Raney RB Jr, et al. (1985) Sarcomas of the vagina and uterus: the Intergroup Rhabdomyosarcoma Study. J Pediatr Surg 20:718–724

Hays DM, Shimada H, Raney RB Jr, et al. (1988) Clinical staging and treatment results in rhabdomyosarcoma of the female genital tract among children and adolescents. Cancer 61:1893–1903

Hays D, Lawrence W Jr, Crist W, et al. (1990) Partial cystectomy in the management of rhabdomyosarcoma of the bladder: a report from the Intergroup Rhabdomyosarcoma Study. J Pediatr Surg 25:719–723

Hays D, Raney R, Wharam MD, et al. (1995) Children with vesical rhabdomyosarcoma (RMS) treated by partial cystectomy with neoadjuvant or adjuvant chemotherapy, with or without radiotherapy. A report from the Intergroup Rhabdomyosarcoma Study (IRS) Committee. J Pediat Hemat Oncol 17:46–52

Heyn R, Ragab A, Raney RB Jr, et al. (1976) Late effects of therapy in orbital rhabdomyosarcoma in children: a report from the Intergroup Rhabdomyosarcoma Study. Cancer 57:1738–1743

Heyn R, Raney RB, Hays DM, et al. (1992) Late effects of therapy in patients with paratesticular rhabdomyosarcoma: for the Intergroup Rhabdomyosarcoma Study Committee. J Clin Oncol 10:614–623

Kodet R, Newton WA, Hamoudi AB, Asmar L, Jacobs DL, Maurer HM (1993) Childhood rhabdomyosarcoma with anaplastic (pleomorphic) features: a report of the Intergroup Rhabdomyosarcoma Study. Am J Surg Pathol 17:443–453

LaQuaglia MP, Ghavini F, Heller G, et al. (1989) Mortality in pediatric paratesticular rhabdomyosarcoma: a multivariate analysis. J Urol 142:173–178

Lawrence W, Gehan EA, Hays DM, et al. (1987a) Prognostic significance of staging factors of the UICC staging system in childhood rhabdomyosarcoma: a report from the Intergroup Rhabdomyosarcoma Study (IRS-II). J Clin Oncol 5:46–54

Lawrence W Jr, Hays D, Heyn R, et al. (1987b) Lymphatic metastases with childhood rhabdomyosarcoma: a report from the Intergroup Rhabdomyosarcoma Study. Cancer 60:910–915

Leuschner I, Newton WA Jr, Schmidt D, et al. (1993) Spindle cell variants of embryonal rhabdomyosarcoma in the paratesticular region: a report of the Intergroup Rhabdomyosarcoma Study. Am J Surg Pathol 17:221–230

Lobe TE, Wiener E, Andrassy RJ, et al. (1996) The argument for conservative, delayed surgery in the management of prostatic rhabdomyosarcoma. J Pediatr Surg 31:8:1084–1087

Loughlin KR, Retik AB, Weinstein HJ, et al. (1989) Genitourinary rhabdomysarcoma in children. Cancer 63:1600–1606

Mandell LR, Ghavimi F, Exelby P, Fuks Z (1988) Preliminary results of alternating multi-agent chemotherapy (CT) and hyperfractionated radiotherapy (HART) in advanced rhabdomyosarcoma (RMS): the Memorial Hospital (MSKCC) experience. Int J Radiation Oncol Biol Phys 15:197–203

Mandell L, Ghavimi F, Peretz T, et al. (1990) Radiocurability of microscopic disease in childhood rhabdomyosarcoma with radiation doses less than 4000 cGy. J Clin Oncol 8:1536–1542

Maurer H, Gehan E, Beltangady M, et al. (1993) The Intergroup Rhabdomyosarcoma Study-II. Cancer 71:1904–1923

McKeen E (1987) Rhabdomyosarcoma complicating multiple neurofibromatosis. J Pediatr 93:992–993

McLorie GA, Abara OE, Churchill BM, et al. (1989) Rhabdomyosarcoma of the prostate in childhood: current challenges. J Pediatr Surg 24:977–981

Newton WA Jr, Soule EH, Hamoudi AB, Reiman HM, Shimada H, Beltangady M, Maurer H (1988) Histopathology of childhood sarcomas, Intergroup Rhabdomyosarcoma Studies I and II: clinicopathologic correlation. J Clin Oncol 6:67–75

Olive D, Flamant F, Zucker JM, et al. (1984) Periaortic lymphadenectomy is not necessary in the treatment of localized paratesticular rhabdomyosarcoma. Cancer 54:1283–1287

Parham E, Webber B, Holt H, Williams W, Maurer H (1991) Immunohistochemical study of childhood rhabdomyo-

sarcomas and related neoplasms: results of an Intergroup Rhabdomyosarcoma Study Project. Cancer 67:3072–3080

Plowman PN (1988) Radiotherapy of pediatric genitourinary tumors. In: Broecker BH, Klein FA, eds. Pediatric tumors of the genitourinary tract. Liss, New York, pp 263–281

Pratt C (1984) Rhabdomyosarcoma of bladder, prostate and vagina. Dialogue Pediatr Urol 7:6–7

Raney RB, Hays DM, Lawrence W Jr, et al. (1978) Paratesticular rhabdomyosarcoma in childhood. Cancer 42:729–736

Raney RB Jr, Tefft M, Lawrence W Jr, et al. (1987) Paratesticular sarcoma in childhood and adolescence: a report from the Intergroup Rhabdomyosarcoma Studies I and II, 1973–1983. Cancer 60:2337–2343

Raney R Jr, Gehan E, Hays D, et al. (1990) Primary chemotherapy with or without radiation therapy and/or surgery for children with localized sarcoma of the bladder, prostate, vagina, uterus, and cervix. Cancer 65:2787–2792

Rodary C, Gehan E, Flamant F, et al. (1991) Prognostic factors in 951 non-metastatic rhabdomyosarcoma in children: a report from the International Rhabdomyosarcoma Workshop. Med Pediatr Oncol 19:89–95

Rodary C, Flamant F, Maurer H, Gehan E, Carli M, Treuner J (1992a) For the SIOP 6th International Workshop, Paris, 1992; Internat. Soc. of Pediatr. Oncol., October 12–16, Hanover, Germany

Rodary C, Flamant F, Maurer H, et al. (1992b) Initial lymphadenectomy is not necessary in localized and completely resected paratesticular rhabdomyosarcoma. Med Pediatr Oncol 20:430

Ruyman FB, Maddux HR, Ragab A, et al. (1988) Congenital anomalies associated with rhabdomyosarcoma: an autopsy study of 115 cases. A report from the Intergroup Rhabdomyosarcoma Study Committee (representing the Children's Cancer Study Group, the Pediatric Oncology Group, the United Kingdom Children's Cancer Study Group, and the Pediatric Intergroup Statistical Center). Med Pediatr Oncol 16:33–39

Shapiro E, Parham D, Douglass E, et al. (1991) Relationship of tumor-cell ploidy to histologic subtype and treatment outcome in children and adolescents with unresectable rhabdomyosarcoma. J Clin Oncol 9:159–166

Tefft M, Jaffe N (1973) Sarcoma of the bladder and prostate in children. Rationale for the role of radiation therapy based on a review of the literature and a report of fourteen additional patients. Cancer 32:1161–1177

Tefft M, Lattin PB, Jereb B, et al. (1986) Acute and late effects on normal tissues following chemo- and radiotherapy for childhood rhabdomyosarcoma and Ewing's sarcoma. Cancer 37:1201–1217

Voute PA, Vos A, deKraker J, et al. (1981) Rhabdomyosarcomas: chemotherapy and limited supplemental treatment programme to avoid mutilation. NCI Monogr 56:121–125

Wiener ES (1993) Rhabdomyosarcoma: new dimensions in management. Semin Pediatr Surg 2:47–58

Wiener ES, Lawrence W, Hays D, et al. (1994) Retroperitoneal node biopsy in paratesticular rhabdomyosarcoma. J Pediatr Surg 29:171–178

# 36 Measures to Optimize Quality of Life in Patients Treated for Genitourinary Tumors

S.C. FORMENTI

CONTENTS



## 36.1 Introduction

The development of more effective cancer treatments is ideally reflected by longer patient survival. However, concomitant with progress in lengthening cancer-related survival, questions about the quality of life (QOL) associated with a longer survival have arisen. This has led to the development of a new discipline that specifically deals with the assessment of QOL. Furthermore, during the past decade the continuous growth of managed care has generated new interest in measuring various parameters of treatment outcome. While disease-free and overall survival remain central measures of outcome, the patient's QOL during the course of the disease or after recovery is also a very important parameter that deserves precise recording and measuring.

Measuring health-related QOL is a challenging task since "normal health" is an abstract concept. The World Health Organization defines health as "a state of complete physical, mental and social well-being." Generally, studies on QOL refer to this definition as "health-related quality of life." Any "cancer diagnosis" has in itself a profound impact on a patient's QOL: it inevitably elicits fears about death and loss of control. However, the anatomical site and the peculiar pattern of spread of different cancers are associated with a diverse range of symptoms and impairments, making the objective and subjective experience of cancer "site specific."

Patients with genitourinary malignancies characteristically suffer compromise of urinary and sexual function in the course of their disease, either as a direct effect of their cancer or, more often, as a side-effect of cancer treatment. Progress in the management of these tumors has made it possible to restore or preserve urinary and sexual function in an increasing number of patients. This restoration of function has a great impact on the self-image and self-confidence of cancer patients. OFMAN (1995) has recently reviewed the sexual implications for patients with a diagnosis of a genitourinary malignancy. Noticeably, the experience of having had surgery in the area of the genitals may generate functional impairment for psychological reasons. This is in addition to the objective impairment incurred as a result of the treatment. In an interesting study comparing patients who underwent inguinal hernia repair with those who had transurethral prostatectomy, it was found that both surgical procedures frequently had minor negative sexual consequences (LIBMAN et al. 1991). It is of interest to note the study's important conclusion that the psychosexual consequences of the two procedures were not very different.

## 36.2 Pitfalls in Evaluating Quality of Life Issues

The process of adjustment by the patient to functional changes resulting from a diagnosis of genitourinary malignancy is often more complicated than predicted by either the patient or the doctor. The latter is likely to underestimate treatment complications, as documented in several studies in different types of cancer (MCNEAL et al. 1978).

S.C. FORMENTI, MD, Associate Professor, Department of Radiation, Oncology, and Medicine, University of Southern California, School of Medicine, 1441 Eastlake Avenue, Los Angeles, CA 90033-0804, USA

Among genitourinary malignancies, prostate cancer has served as an excellent model to illustrate this important problem. The work of Litwin and co-workers can be considered as an elegant example of the inadequacy of doctors in measuring QOL parameters. Their study, reported at the 1997 Annual Meeting of the American Urological Association, evaluated more than 2000 patients from the Cancer of the Prostate Strategic Urological Research Endeavor database (CaPSURE). CaPSURE is a national observational longitudinal database started in 1995 which enrolls prostate cancer patients from 27 sites in the United States. For each patient observed the database accrues information obtained from the treating urologist and the patient. The urologist provides complete medical history and the records of each subsequent follow-up office visit, and the patient provides data through a quarterly questionnaire package on health-related QOL. Litwin and co-workers found that in each of the QOL areas examined, the doctors' assessment significantly differed from the patients' assessment ($P = 0.002$), with physicians consistently underestimating the magnitude of patients' impairment. The investigators concluded that QOL outcomes in prostate cancer are probably best measured by patients themselves.

Assessment of QOL is exquisitely subjective, making it literally impossible for anybody else but the patient to accurately assess it. Several studies have reported that for many individuals the advantage of preserving important function outweighs the benefit of longer survival (MCNEAL et al. 1981). SINGER et al. (1991) reported a study of 50 men aged 45–70 years without known prostate cancer. Sixty-eight percent of the respondents were willing to trade off a 10% or greater chance for 5 years' survival in order to maintain sexual potency. Most importantly, even men who were impotent at the time of the study were willing to consider trading off longevity in an effort to preserve the possibility of return of erectile function.

Due to major differences in QOL issues in patients with different genitourinary tumors, each major primary site of cancer warrants separate discussion. For instance, with the exception of renal, bladder, and urethral cancer, genitourinary malignancies affect mostly men. As compared to female patients, male patients tend to more frequently cope with their disease by using denial. Denial is a defense mechanism in addition to the patient's avoidance of discussion of feelings about the cancer and the treatment. Conversely, female patients more frequently tend to adopt coping mechanisms based on communicating thoughts and feelings about their condition (OFMAN 1995).

It is of importance also to recognize that QOL issues vary according to the age of patients. The age at diagnosis differs among genitourinary malignancies, e.g., testicular cancer is typically diagnosed in young men while prostate cancer is diagnosed in older men.

## 36.3
## Bladder Cancer

Carcinoma of the bladder arises in older men and in postmenopausal women. When diagnosed with bladder cancer, patients' major concern is usually whether they will lose their bladder and consequently lose their voiding function. Patients with early stages of bladder cancer are initially managed by surgical removal of the tumor (TURB), followed by adjuvant intravesical treatment with BCG or chemotherapy. These treatments are generally quite well tolerated (BOHLE et al. 1996) even if at careful self-assessment patients tend to report decreased sexual desire and painful intercourse (SCHOVER 1987).

Approximately 50% of the patients with originally superficial bladder cancer eventually suffer local recurrences that evolve into muscle-invasive tumors, necessitating cystectomy. Originally, the surgical procedure for reconstruction after cystectomy consisted in ileal conduit or Kock pouch with diversion of the urine to a stoma on the abdominal wall. The change in body image and the problems associated with the process of adjusting to these neobladders are well documented by the studies of SCHOVER et al. (1986) in both male and female patients who underwent cystectomy followed the above reconstructions. Similarly, prior to cystectomy FOSSA et al. (1987) evaluated 59 patients who answered a questionnaire about their QOL expectations following radical cystectomy. Forty-nine relapse-free patients filled in a comparable questionnaire after a median of 36 months following cystectomy. Most responders reported that they had to make significant adjustments in their professional and social lives. This study could be biased by the fact that original assessment of QOL was undertaken at the time of cancer diagnosis and discussion about cystectomy. Since in most individuals such a diagnosis represents a very stressful time it might not be representative of the patient's baseline QOL assessment. Interestingly, OISHI et al. (1993) studied 60 Japanese patients with a continent urinary reservoir and found that approximately one out of five had stopped working as a consequence of their surgery. In addition, while 80% reported not to be bothered by having a stoma, they were nonetheless embarrassed to show their stoma to their family members. Especially during the first few months after cystectomy incontinence is the main concern for most patients. In spite of the fact that incontinence is a side-effect of surgery, it tends to have a profound impact on patients' self-esteem, and it dramatically influences the extent of the patient's participation in social activities. Concern about incontinence may induce the patient's withdrawal and depression (OFMAN 1995).

Probably independently from any other associated dysfunction, patients are very concerned about their partner's reaction to their ileostomy. As a measure to help to prevent some of the problems associated with a urinary stoma, SCHOVER and FIFE (1985) suggested encouraging the partner to see the ostomy right after surgery, while the patient is still in the hospital. Sharing the experience with the partner from the outset helps both partners to improve the adjustment. OFMAN (1995) suggests that brief sexual counseling for men and their partners on how to adjust love making to the presence of the ostomy may prevent more severe damage to the couple's sexual life.

These concerns and restraints inevitably impact on a patient's sexual life. In this respect female patients appear to cope better than their male counterparts. SMITH and BABAIAN (1989), in a study of 128 consecutive bladder cancer patients undergoing radical cystectomy with ileal conduit, reported that women's adjustment after surgery was significantly better than men's. They identified several possible factors contributing to this difference, with women being found to be more independent in caring for the stoma and to have less change in self-image, level of activity, or response of friends. NORDSTROM and NYMAN (1992) studied sexual function after cystectomy in women and found that five of the six women reported either ceased or decreased sexual activity. Their main complaints were inhibited sexual desire, dyspareunia, and vaginal dryness. Radical cystectomy in female patients includes the removal of the bladder and urethra, uterus with ovaries and fallopian tubes, and anterior wall of the vagina. As a consequence of this surgical procedure the patient is often left with a narrowed or shortened vagina, with possible pain, numbness, or loss of sensation at intercourse. To prevent scarring and foreshortening of the vagina it is important to stress

to the patient the necessity for regular daily use of vaginal dilators. Lubricants during sexual activity are often needed to compensate for the loss of natural lubrication. Loss of lubrication is multifactorial, since it is caused both by reduced blood flow in the reconstructed vagina and by treatment-induced menopause, given that both ovaries are also removed during surgery.

Radical cystectomy in men includes the removal of the prostate. As a consequence male patients commonly face erectile dysfunction due to transection of the nerves governing erection and loss of ejaculation. Erectile dysfunction was reported by 91% of patients in a study of sexual function in men following standard radical cystectomy. Approximately half of the patients remained sexually active and were able to achieve orgasm. Probably because the orgasm was not accompanied by ejaculation, a diminished intensity of the orgasm was reported by 53% of the respondents of this study (SCHOVER et al. 1986).

During the past decade progress in urological surgical techniques has dramatically affected the QOL of both female and male patients with bladder cancers. It is now possible to anastomose the neobladders to the patient's urethra in most male patients. More recently the use of this important procedure was also successfully applied in selected female patients (STEIN et al. 1997).

In selected male patients the introduction of nerve-sparing surgical techniques has opened a possibility of performing cystectomies while sparing one or both of the neurovascular bundles (WALSH and MOSTWIN 1984). This important modification of the original procedure has been reported to permit maintenance of potency in 60%–70% of patients (MARSHALL et al. 1991). Consequently, following cystectomy for carcinoma of the bladder more and more patients are able to maintain both continence and potency.

## 36.4
## Prostate Cancer

Prostate cancer is the most commonly diagnosed cancer in men. Approximately 80% of all prostate cancers are diagnosed in men aged 65 years or older. Urinary continence and sexual potency are the areas of function most commonly affected by prostate cancer treatment. Generally, management of localized prostate cancer is by radical prostatectomy, or definitive radiation therapy, or a combination of surgery and postoperative radiotherapy.

Nerve-sparing prostatectomy, originally introduced by WALSH (1988), has allowed preservation of potency in the majority of selected patients who were potent prior to surgery. QUINLAN et al. (1991), in a study of 500 men treated with nerve-sparing surgery, reported erectile dysfunction in 32% of patients. This was compared with an 85% incidence of erectile dysfunction after conventional radical prostatectomy (MYERS and FLEMING 1983). Noticeably, recovery of erectile function occurs significantly more often in younger men and in those who have undergone bilateral nerve-sparing surgery. The process of postsurgical recovery of this function, however, may exceed 6 months in some patients.

Following the administration of definitive pelvic radiotherapy for management of prostate cancer there has been wide variation in the reported incidence of erectile impotence, ranging from 14% to 50% (BANKER 1988).

This reported wide range in the incidence of impotence following pelvic irradiation most probably reflects differences in patient selection in different series. In fact, it is essential to evaluate sexual function prior to radiation treatment since the rate of preexisting impotence among patients receiving definitive radiotherapy for prostate cancer has been shown to be as high as 69% (ZINREICH et al. 1990). Unfortunately, most series have failed to report the baseline evaluation of patients' pretreatment potency status. There is an obvious need for prospective studies in patients undergoing definitive pelvic irradiation for carcinoma of the prostate. Such studies would be required to have a well-documented quantitative assessment of erectile function prior to the administration of radiotherapy. The mechanism underlying radiation-induced impotence is not completely understood. Vascular origin of impotence as a part of the normal aging process, or as a consequence of chronic hypertension and diabetes mellitus, has been shown to increase the risk of postradiation impotence (PEREZ and EISBRUCH 1993). The studies reporting on the incidence of impotence among irradiated prostate cancer patients have analyzed series in which a total dose of 60–75 Gy was delivered to the prostate, usually as a part of definitive treatment (PEREZ et al. 1993; VAN HERRINGS et al. 1988).

### 36.4.1
### The USC Experience

To our knowledge no other reports are available on the effect on potency of lower doses of radiation, in the range of 45–55 Gy, given in the postoperative setting. As already mentioned, the surgical management of prostate cancer has been changing over the past 10 years since the introduction of Walsh's nerve-sparing prostatectomy, which aims at preserving erectile potency. This surgical option is generally offered to potent men with clinical stage A and B prostate cancer. However, it is well known that up to 50% of patients with clinical stage B disease are found at surgery to have extracapsular tumor extension and up to 45% of operated patients are left with positive surgical margins (CATALONA and BIGG 1990; ROSEN et al. 1992; WHITMORE and MACKENZIE 1959). Retrospective studies have reported that postoperative radiotherapy given to pathologic stage C patients is capable of reducing the incidence of local recurrence from 28%–68% to 0%–8% (SHEVLIN et al. 1989; GIBBONS et al. 1986; ANSCHER and PROSNITZ 1991). Furthermore, better 10-year disease-free survival rates are achieved when radiotherapy is used adjuvantly, compared with its elective use at the time of palpable local recurrence. The findings suggest that, at least in some patients, the local effect of adjuvant radiation may be to influence the pattern of metastatic spread (PETROVICH et al. 1991, 1995, 1998). At USC we have been systematically using moderate doses (45–54 Gy) of postoperative irradiation to the prostatic bed in patients who are found at radical prostatectomy to have extracapsular disease, residual microscopic positive margins, and/or seminal vesicle involvement (FREEMAN et al. 1993; PETROVICH et al. 1998). The use of this treatment program in 201 unselected pathologic stage C (T3) patients with median follow-up of 5 years resulted in 5- and 10-year overall survival rates of 92% and 83%, respectively, and 5- and 10-year disease-free (clinical and prostate-specific antigen) survival rates of 67% and 53%, respectively. There was also a 4% incidence of local recurrence (PETROVICH et al. 1998). The treatment was very well tolerated by the study patients, who maintained good quality of life during and after the treatment. This was accomplished with the use of modified radiotherapy techniques and change of patients' diet for the duration of the radiation treatment course.

We have analyzed the morbidity of adding radiotherapy in the subset of prostate cancer patients who were treated at our institution with nerve-sparing prostatectomy (FORMENTI et al. 1996). Specifically, the rate of recovery of urinary continence and potency at 1 year posttreatment was studied among 84 patients who received adjuvant radiotherapy and compared with the 160 patients who did not receive adjuvant radiotherapy. With the limitation of retrospective data collected by subjective reports from the patients, our study suggests that at 1 year from treatment, moderate doses of postoperative radiotherapy did not have a significant impact on the recovery of urinary continence and potency after nerve-sparing prostatectomy. This was despite the fact that patients in the surgery-radiotherapy group had more advanced disease and conceivably may have also received more extensive surgery. Whether the radiation protocol as used in our study impacts on the long-term preservation of recovered potency needs to be assessed at longer follow-up. Such a study to determine the state of sexual potency and urinary continence at 4-year follow-up is currently underway at USC.

## 36.4.2
### Metastatic Prostate Cancer

Patients with locally advanced and those with metastatic prostate cancer may survive with their disease for a long period of time. QOL issues are often central to their existence. Advanced stage prostate cancer is commonly treated by hormonal manipulation. Testosterone deprivation, accomplished either by bilateral orchiectomy or by androgen blockade, is usually the first-line therapy. Androgen blockade can be achieved by the administration of estrogen, flutamide, or LH-RH analogs. All these treatments produce sexual side-effects, like loss of desire for sexual activity and impaired erectile function. Moreover, because of the psychological implications associated with it, bilateral orchiectomy can have negative effects on body image. Objective changes such as loss of body hair and gynecomastia may occur and are accompanied by subjective symptoms like fatigue and hot flashes. KARLING et al. (1994) surveyed 63 men after androgen deprivation therapy and found that after 5 years 48% of patients still had hot flashes.

Flutamide alone seems to cause fewer sexual side-effects than the other therapies (SOGANI and WHITMORE 1988). However, RUSSEAU et al. (1988) found that the combination of flutamide and medical or surgical castration abolished sexual activity in 80% of the 44 patients whose sexual function the authors assessed before and during therapy.

## 36.5
### Penile Cancer

Cancer of the penis carries the most devastating psychological significance of castration. When detected earlier, local excision and/or laser beam therapy are available treatment options. Radiation therapy can also be successfully used in these patients. Unfortunately, men frequently seek treatment late, and in advanced stages of the disease conservative surgical management or radiotherapy cannot be offered. Required treatment in these patients consists in partial or total penectomy (SCHOVER et al. 1994).

OPJORDSMOEN and FOSSA (1994) have reported the long-term psychosocial and sexual effects of treatment for penile cancer in 30 Norwegian men. Patients treated with partial or total penectomy had a worse outcome with regard to sexual function than patients treated conservatively by local excision/laser beam or radiation therapy. However, when tested by a semistructured interview and by the several validated questionnaires no differences in the other domains of QOL were detected among the different subsets of patients. Noticeably, seven (23%) of the study patients reported that if asked again they would trade lower long-term survival to increase the odds of remaining potent. The authors concluded that it is extremely important to thoroughly discuss with patients with carcinoma of the penis all of the available treatment options and their consequences (OPJORDSMOEN and FOSSA 1994). WITKIN and KAPLAN (1983) have reported on the role of sex therapy to support and train patients to cope with penile cancer and on the favorable consequences of treatment.

## 36.6
### Testicular Cancer

Because of the high recovery rate in testicular cancer patients, QOL issues are of particular importance. The prognosis of patients with seminoma treated with radiotherapy has been good for many years, with long-term survival rates greater than 90% (JAVADPOUR 1980). Combination chemotherapy and tumor-reducing surgery have dramatically affected the outcome in nonseminoma testicular tumors (EINHORN and DONOHUE 1977). Moreover, survivors of testicular cancer, particularly nonseminoma germ cell tumors, represent an ideal subset of patients to study QOL issues. In fact, the disease is relatively age-specific, affecting men primarily between 20 and 35 years of age. In addition, the psychological implications of testicular cancer and its treatment have rendered it a classic paradigm to study psychosexual problems associated with cancer.

Similar to penile cancer, in testicular cancer the time of diagnosis can be delayed because of embarrassment related to the site of disease and frequent relative paucity of symptoms. Once diagnosed, men are further challenged in their self-esteem because of the effects of treatment on sexuality and masculinity. In patients with seminoma, treatment includes ipsilateral orchiectomy, followed either by bilateral retroperitoneal lymphadenectomy (RPLND) or by radiation therapy. In patients with metastatic spread, chemotherapy is added to the treatment regimen. For nonseminoma tumors, retroperitoneal lymphadenectomy may be followed by several courses of chemotherapy. More recently, a policy of observation only is being advised in carefully selected patients with localized germ cell tumors. This policy is sound with a routine use of computerized tomography during follow-up. The no-treatment policy permits the preservation of ejaculation and fertility among these carefully selected patients, but stress and anxiety associated with no treatment and the policy of observation must not be underestimated.

Fertility impairment is probably the main side-effect of the treatments of this disease. The causes are multifactorial and reflect the type of treatment received. As already mentioned, patients undergoing RPLND are usually unable to ejaculate postoperatively.

Some patients experience retrograde ejaculation, while others have total paralysis of the reflex due to the damage to the para-aortic sympathetic nervous system pathways controlling emission. In some cases, anterograde ejaculation returns with passage of time. Sympathomimetic and anticholinergic drugs have been used to help restore ejaculatory function (NIJMAN et al. 1992).

A nerve-sparing lymph node dissection technique introduced in 1984 has reduced the incidence of postoperative ejaculatory dysfunction from 36% to 16% (JONES et al. 1993). Moreover, the addition of chemotherapy has enabled patients with stage A and stage B disease to undergo unilateral RPLND with the aim of retaining ejaculatory function (DOERR et al. 1993). Recent advances in the treatment of this disease have resulted in a strategy of withholding RPLND for selected patients since the majority of patients who previously received RPLND were found to have uninvolved lymph nodes and therefore

would not have needed this surgery (NIJMAN et al. 1987; DONOHUE and FOSTER 1990).

Other threats to fertility (often interacting in patients managed by a multimodality approach) come from chemotherapy and suppressed spermatogenesis after radiation therapy. The latter complication can be prevented by careful planning and delivery of radiation treatment, with protection of the contralateral testis by multiple blocking devices (KUBO and SHIPLEY 1982).

Interestingly, hypofertility has been speculated to predate the diagnosis of testicular cancer, possibly due to genetic or environmental factors. However, most investigators agree that the contribution of therapy is predominant in determining fertility disturbances among these men (BERTHELSEN and SKAKKEBAEK 1983).

Adjustment to treatment side-effects is a complex process that begins at diagnosis and extends long after treatment has been completed. Furthermore, response to fertility impairment is affected by the sociodemographic and clinical profile of the patient. RIEKER et al. (1990) identified five fertility adjustment responses among 153 testicular cancer patients studied. She classified them as: sperm banking awareness, adoption awareness, fertility testing, trying to father children, and fertility distress. At multivariate analysis younger men (<35 years of age), without children and with college education were more likely to select sperm banking if their relationship was under stress. Men seeking fertility testing were patients with preserved ejaculatory capacity and the same group was trying to father children. Only the condition of childlessness significantly predicted for propensity toward considering adoption. The study identified a subset of men at greatest risk for infertility-related distress. This high-risk group includes childless patients with posttreatment ejaculatory dysfunction. Consistently, long-term infertility distress was also significantly associated with previous RPLND.

Fertility, the ability to procreate, contributes to the individual's understanding of him- or herself. Since it contributes to differentiating male from females its importance includes self-image and self-esteem. Physiologically loss of fertility in women is age related and is associated with the emergence of menopause. Men do not usually lose fertility even in advanced age. Therefore, its loss can be experienced as a severe threat to a man's identity as a youthful, capable person and may trigger a period of depression and mourning. Health care providers must be aware of these strong psychological implications associated with loss of fertility due to any cause and in patients at any age.

In genitourinary malignancies education about treatment effects on fertility is crucial. Discussion at the time of diagnosis is the most critical tool available to help patients adjust to this loss. Testicular cancer is an excellent paradigm to learn the far-reaching implications of fertility for QOL. In fact, while absence of ejaculation and fertility concerns are the most prominent sexual side-effects of treatment for testicular cancer, a number of reports document additional sexual difficulties among this patient population. For instance, SCHOVER and VON ESCHENBACH (1985a) reported in a survey of 121 patients treated for nonseminoma testicular cancer that 11% were not sexually active at all, 9% had sexual activity less than once a month, 10% had erectile dysfunction, and 38% reported a decrease in their pleasure at orgasm. At 1 year from diagnosis of cancer of the testis, RIEKER et al. (1989) found that among 223 patients, 30% experienced overall sexual performance distress, 10% had erectile difficulties, and 6% were anorgasmic. In a retrospective study of 34 married couples, GRITZ et al. (1989) documented that 23.5% of the men reported still feeling less attractive as a result of treatment undergone 4 years earlier. Similarly, AASS et al. (1993) performed a pretreatment and posttreatment follow-up study of 76 testicular cancer patients and documented that even 3 years posttherapy 30% of the men reported some degree of sexual difficulty compared with their lives before cancer treatment. Long-term physical, sexual, and emotional sequelae of non-germ cell testicular cancer were measured in a study of 109 survivors interviewed an average of 9 years after treatment (DOUCHEZ et al. 1993). The study compared the survivors with an age-matched control group of men without cancer. Physical sequelae among survivors were consistently predictable by analyzing the type of treatment the patient had received. Surgically treated patients had incisional hernias and ejaculatory dysfunction, while patients who had both surgery and radiation therapy reported additional gastrointestinal symptoms. During cancer therapy 57% of patients had sexual problems but residual problems persisted long after completion of treatment in 38% of the survivors, compared to 11% of those in the control group ($P < 0.001$).

Finally, in a study of long-term cancer survivors including mostly patients with Hodgkin's disease and germ cell tumors, Olweny et al. (1993) found that such patients enjoyed a QOL similar to that of their neighbors when subjective measures of well-being were analyzed. The control group, however, was not cancer controlled or matched to the index case based on sex, age, and address. In spite of this, the index cases reported more sexual dysfunctions, confirming the hypothesis that sexual dysfunction is a symptomatic long-term sequela of cancer treatment.

## 36.7
## Conclusions

As more effective therapies are developed for a variety of human cancers, issues related to the experience of facing and conquering a malignancy become more and more of interest. Cancer cure has been defined as the attainment of normal life expectancy and has been characterized by three main components: (1) the attainment of a complete remission, (2) a stage of survival where there is minimal or no risk of recurrence, and (3) the restoration of physical, developmental, functional, and psychosocial aspects of health (HAMMOND 1986). Measures to optimize QOL are necessary to achieve the global restoration of patient's functions.

Adjustments to surgical consequences and functional impairments are a common challenge for patients affected by genitourinary malignancies. Treatment toxicity that affects the patient's sexual life is common and can improve with time and proper support. Health care providers have an important duty to maintain open communication with the patient before, during, and after treatment completion. Preventive discussion of sexual concerns and expected sexual side-effects of treatment should start at diagnosis and continue during the time of treatment decision. During and after treatment, instructions and advice must be provided on how function can be at least partially restored and treatment side-effects managed.

Clinical research must continue to explore measures to limit side-effects of treatment. Physicians need to be more proactive in discussing and addressing functional and psychosexual issues with genitourinary cancer patients. In this process, they need to be aware and respectful of the exquisitely subjective nature of their patients' choices regarding QOL.

## References

Aass N, Grunfeld B, Kaalhus O, Fossa SD (1993) Pre- and post-treatment sexual life in testicular cancer patients: a descriptive investigation. Br J Cancer 67:1113–1117

Anscher MS, Prosnitz LR (1991) Multivariate analysis of factors predicting local relapse after radical prostatectomy – possible indications for postoperative radiotherapy. Int J Radiat Oncol Biol Phys 21:941

Banker FL (1988) The preservation of potency after external beam irradiation for prostate cancer. Int J Radiat Oncol Biol Phys 15:219–220

Berthelsen JC, Skakkebaek NE (1983) Gonadal function in men with testis cancer. Fertil Steril 39:68

Bohle A, Balck F, von Wietersheim J, Jocham D (1996) The quality of life during intravesical bacillus Calmette-Guerin therapy. J Urol 155:1221–1226

Catalona WJ, Bigg SW (1990) Nerve-sparing radical prostatectomy: evaluation of results after 250 patients. J Urol 143:538

Doerr A, Skinner EC, Skinner DG (1993) Preservation of ejaculation through a modified retroperitoneal lymph node dissection in low stage testis cancer. J Urol 149: 1472–1474

Donohue J, Foster R (1990) Preservation of ejaculation with nerve-sparing retroperitoneal lymphadenectomy (NS RPLND). Proc Ann Meet Am Soc Clin Oncol 9:A507

Douchez J, Droz JP, Desclaux B, Allain Y, Fargeot P, Caty A, Charrot P (1993) Quality of life in long-term survivors of nonseminomatous germ cell testicular tumors. J Urol 149:498–501

Einhorn LA, Donohue JP (1977) Cis-diamminedichloroplatinum, vinblastine and bleomycin combination chemotherapy in disseminated testicular cancer. Ann Intern Med 87:293–298

Formenti SC, Lieskovsky G, Simoneau AR, Skinner D, Groshen S, Chen SC, Petrovich Z (1996) Impact of moderate dose of postoperative radiation on urinary continence and potency in patients with prostate cancer treated with nerve sparing prostatectomy. J Urol 155:616–619

Fossa SD, Reitan JB, Ous S, Kaalhus O (1987) Life with an ileal conduit in cystectomized bladder cancer patients; expectation and experience. Scan J Urol Nephrol 21:101

Freeman JA, Lieskovsky G, Cook DW, Petrovich Z, Chen SC, Groshen S, Skinner DG (1993) Radical retropubic prostatectomy and postoperative adjuvant radiation for pathological stage C (PCN0) prostate cancer from 1976 to 1989: intermediate findings. J Urol 149:1029

Gibbons RP, Cole BS, Richardson RG, et al. (1986) Adjuvant radiotherapy following radical prostatectomy: results and complications. J Urol 135:65

Gritz ER, Wellish DK, Wang HJ, Siau J, Landsverk JA, Cosgrove MD (1989) Long-term effects of testicular cancer on sexual functioning in married couples. Cancer 64: 1560–1567

Hammond GD (1986) The cure of childhood cancers. Cancer 58:408–413

Javadpour N (1980) Germ cell tumor of the testis. Cancer 30:242–255

Jones DR, Norman AR, Horwich A, Hendry WF (1993) Ejaculatory dysfunction after retroperitoneal lymphadenectomy. Eur Urol 23:169–171

Karling P, Hammar M, Varenhorst E (1994) Prevalence and duration of hot flushes after surgical or medical castration in men with prostatic carcinoma. J Urol 152:1170–1173

Kubo HD, Shipley WU (1982) Reduction of the scattered dose to the testicle outside the radiation treatment fields. Int J Radiat Oncol Biol Phys 8:1741–1745

Libman E, Fichten CS, Rothernberg P, et al. (1991) Prostatectomy and inguinal hernia repair: a comparison of the sexual consequences. J Sex Marital Ther 17:27–34

Marshall FF, Mostwin JL, Radebaugh LC, Walsh PC, Brendler CB (1991) Ileocolic neobladder post-cystectomy: continence and potency. J Urol 145:502–504

McNeal BJ, Weichselbaum T, Pauker SG (1978) Fallacy of the 5-year survival in lung cancer. N Engl J Med 299:1397–1401

McNeal BJ, Weichselbaum T, Pauker SG (1981) Speech and survival tradeoff between quality and quantity of life in laryngeal cancer. N Engl J Med 305:982–987

Myers RP, Fleming TR (1983) Course of localized adenocarcinoma of the prostate treated by radical prostatectomy. Prostate 4:461

Nijman JM, Schraffordt KH, Oldhoff J, Kremer J, Jager S (1987) Sexual function after bilateral retroperitoneal lymph node dissection for nonseminomatous testicular cancer. Arch Androl 18:255–267

Nijman JM, Jager S, Bower PW, Kremer J, Oldhoff J, Koops HS (1992) The treatment of ejaculation disorders after retroperitoneal lymph node dissection. Cancer 50:2967–2971

Nordstrom GM, Nyman CR (1992) Male and female sexual function and activity following ileal conduit urinary diversion. Br J Urol 70:33–39

Ofman US (1995) Preservation of function in genitourinary cancers. Psychosexual and psychosocial issues. Cancer Invest 13:125–131

Oishi K, Arai Y, Hashimura T, Takeuchi H, Yoshida O, Okada Y (1993) Quality of life of the patients with continent ileal reservoir. Hinyokika Kiyo 39:7–14

Olweny LM, Juttner CA, Rofe P, et al. (1993) Long term effects of cancer treatment and consequences of cure: cancer survivors enjoy quality of life similar to their neighbours. Eur J Cancer 29A6:826–830

Opjordsmoen S, Fossa SD (1994) Quality of life in patients treated for penile cancer. A follow-up study. Br J Urol 74:652–657

Perez CA, Eisbruch A (1993) Role of postradical prostatectomy irradiation in carcinoma of the prostate. Semin Radiat Oncol 3:198

Perez CA, Hanks GE, Leibel SA, Zietman AL, Fuks Z, Lee WR (1993) Localized carcinoma of the prostate (stages T1b, T1c, T2, and T3). Review of management with external beam radiation therapy. Cancer 72:3156–3173

Petrovich Z, Lieskovsky G, Langholz B, Luxton G, Jozsef G, Skinner DG (1991) Radiotherapy following radical prostatectomy in patients with adenocarcinoma of the prostate. Int J Radiat Oncol Biol Phys 21:949–954

Petrovich Z, Lieskovsky G, Freeman J, et al. (1995) Surgery with adjuvant irradiation in patients with pathological stage C adenocarcinoma of the prostate. Cancer 76: 1621–1628

Petrovich Z, Lieskovsky G, Langholz B, Baert L, Formenti S, Streeter O, Skinner DG (1998) Radical prostatectomy and postoperative irradiation in patients with pathological stage C (T3). Int J Radiat Oncol Biol Phys (in press)

Quinlan DM, Epstein JI, Carter BS, Walsh PC (1991) Sexual function following radical prostatectomy: influence of preservation of neurovascular bundles. J Urol 145:998

Rieker PP, Fitzerald EM, Kalish LA, Richie JP, Lederman GS, Edbril SD, Garnick MB (1989) Psychosocial factors, curative therapies and behavioral outcomes; a comparison of testis cancer survivors and a control group of healthy men. Cancer 64:2399–2407

Rieker PP, Fitzgerald EM, Kalish LA (1990) Adaptive behavioral responses to potential infertility among survivors of testis cancer. J Clin Oncol 8:347–355

Rosen MA, Goldstone L, Lapin S, Wheeler TG, Scardino PT (1992) Frequency and location of extracapsular extension and positive surgical margins in radical prostatectomy specimens. J Urol 148:331

Russeau L, Dupont A, Labrie F, Couture M (1988) Sexuality changes in prostate cancer patients receiving antihormonal therapy combining the antiandrogen flutamide with medical (LHRH agonist) or surgical castration. Arch Sex Behav 17:87–98

Schover LR (1987) Sexuality and fertility in urologic cancer patients. Cancer 60 (Suppl):553–558

Schover LR, Fife M (1985) Sexual counseling and radical pelvic or genital cancer surgery. J Psychosoc Oncol 3:21–41

Schover LR, Von Eschenbach AC (1985a) Sexual and marital relationships after treatment for nonseminomatous testicular cancer. Urology 25:251–255

Schover LR, Von Eschenbach AC (1985b) Sexual function and female radical cystectomy: a case series. J Urol 134:465–468

Schover LR, Evans R, Von Eschenbach AC (1986) Sexual rehabilitation and male radical cystectomy. J Urol 136:1015–1017

Schover LR, Von Eschenbach AC, Smith DB, Gonzalez J (1994) Sexual rehabilitation of urologic cancer patients. A practical approach. Cancer 34:66

Shevlin BE, Mittal BB, Brand WN, Shetty RN (1989) The role of adjuvant irradiation following primary prostatectomy, based on histopathologic extent of tumor. Int J Radiat Oncol Biol Phys 16:1425

Singer PA, Tasch ES, Stocking C, Rubin S, Siegler M, Weichselbaum R (1991) Sex or survival? Trade-offs between quality and quantity of life. J Clin Oncol 9:328–334

Smith DB, Babaian FJ (1989) Patient adjustment to an ileal conduit after radical cystectomy. J Enterostom Ther 16:244–246

Sogani PC, Whitmore WF (1988) Flutamide and other antiandrogens in the treatment of advanced prostatic carcinoma. Cancer Treat Res 39:131–145

Stein JP, Grossfeld GD, Freeman JA, et al. (1997) Orthotopic lower urinary tract reconstruction in women using the Kock ileal neobladder: updated experience in 34 patients (see comments). J Urol 158:400–405

Van Herrings C, De Schryver A, Verbeek E (1988) Sexual function disorders after local radiotherapy for carcinoma of the prostate. Radiother Oncol 13:47–52

Walsh PC (1988) Technique of radical retropubic prostatectomy with preservation of sexual function: an anatomic approach. In: Skinner DG, Lieskovsky G (eds) Diagnosis and management of genitourinary cancer. Saunders, Philadelphia, pp 753–778

Walsh PC, Mostwin JL (1984) Radical prostatectomy and cystoprostatectomy with preservation of potency. Results using a new nerve-sparing technique. Br J Urol 56:694–697

Whitmore WF Jr, Mackenzie AR (1959) Experiences with various operative procedures for the total excision of prostate cancer. Cancer 12:396

Witkin MH, Kaplan HS (1983) Sex therapy and penectomy. J Sex Marital Ther 8:209–221

Zinreich ES, Derogatis LR, Herpst J, Auvil G, Piantadosi S, Order SE (1990) Pretreatment evaluation of sexual function in patients with adenocarcinoma of the prostate. Int J Radiat Oncol Biol Phys 19:1001–1004

# 37 Racial Differences in the Incidence, Behavior, and Management of Tumors of the Genitourinary Tract

O.E. Streeter, Jr. and M. Roach III

CONTENTS



## 37.1
## Introduction

"Every aspect of American society has been affected by racial discrimination and segregation. Cancer has been no exception." These are the opening lines of the introduction to *Minorities and Cancer* (Organ 1989), a compilation of articles from the first Biennial Symposium on Minorities and Cancer held in Houston, Texas during the third week of April 1987, which by American Presidential Resolu-

O.E. Streeter, Jr., MD, Associate Professor of Clinical Radiation Oncology, University of Southern California School of Medicine; Chief, Radiation Oncology, USC/Norris Comprehensive Cancer Center, 1441 Eastlake Avenue, NOR 002, Los Angeles, CA 90033-0804, USA
M. Roach, III, MD, Associate Professor of Radiation Oncology, Medical Oncology, and Urology, University of California at San Francisco School of Medicine, Mt. Zion Cancer Center, 2356 Sutter Street, San Francisco, CA 94115, USA

tion is "National Minority Cancer Awareness Week." It is in this context that we will attempt to clarify the role of race in the behavior and management of prostate, bladder, renal, and testicular cancers, which account for the vast majority of genitourinary tumors.

## 37.1.1
## The Notion of Race, Behavior, and Disease

We start with the notion of "race," which comes from the Late Latin root *ratio* (Guralnik 1984), which provides a convenient, though crude way of organizing phenotypic features such as skin pigmentation, hair color, hair texture, lip shape, brow size, and the form of one's nasal bridge, to name a few characteristics. The inadequacy of this construct is based on the phenotypic traits selected; the racial groupings for one person or group can change based on that person or group performing the categorization. This was best exemplified by self-identification in the 1990 American census, when Americans claimed membership in nearly 300 races of ethnic groups and 600 American Indian tribes and 70 Hispanic categories (Begley 1995).

The question rarely asked by those who write about "racial differences" in cancer, is how did this process of classification by phenotypic features come about? It comes from polygenism, an idea about race that predates Darwin's theory of evolution, fully examined in *Race and Human Evolution*, by paleoanthropologists Wolpoff and Caspari (1997). Polygenists believe that races have different evolutionary origins and are different species (Wolpoff and Caspari 1997). This archetypal construct became popular in Europe before Columbus, and was based on the fact that during the time of European exploration, the people encountered along the way looked different. People were later ranked in the genus and species classification system of the Swedish taxonomist Carl Linneaus into four races: white (Europeans), red (Native Americans), dark (Asians) and black (Africans) (Begley 1995).

Disease was not prescribed at this time on racial terms, but behavior was by Linnaeus. This association between skin color and behavior gave subjugation of one race by another race a scientific underpinning. One's place of dwelling and environmental factors did not play a role in our understanding of cancer origins until a hundred years ago, when we started to connect parasites to "cancer houses" and cancer areas (PACE and SULLIVAN-FOWLER 1997).

## 37.1.2
### The Historical Development of Genetics and Disease

Prior to the parasitic model of cancer, the basic science of genetics was being formulated in the field of botany by Gregor Johann Mendel (1822–1884) in the 1860s with his pea plant studies and in entomology by the U.S. zoologist Thomas Hunt Morgan (1866–1945) and other investigators who studied the vinegar fly, *Drosophila melanogaster*, two models that have short generation time and a simple genomic structure (GELEHRTER and COLLINS 1990). These studies, however, still only dealt with phenotypic variants we now can trace to mutations in the nucleotide sequence of the genomic code.

The concept of molecular disease ironically was defined first with sickle cell anemia (mutant hemoglobin S), a condition first observed in West Africa and seen in a small portion of blacks living in the United States. This disease results in anemia and pain in the bones, abdomen, and retinal hemorrhages in its more severe form. Although many other hemoglobinopathies exist (BABIOR and STOSSEL 1984), sickle cell anemia became the prototype condition in our understanding of gene-protein synthesis. Linus Pauling viewed sickle cell anemia as a molecular variant in 1949 (PAULING et al. 1949), but it took another 7 years for Ingram to show that the dif-ference was due to the substitution of valine for glutamic acid as the sixth amino acid of the β chain of hemoglobin (INGRAM 1956). The hemoglobinopathies are not only seen in a subpopulation of West African descent; rather there are other hereditary hemoglobinopathies in Sicilians, Spanish, and Chinese ethnic groups, more genetic differences being exhibited within one ethnic group than between that group and another (BABIOR and STOSSEL 1984; LAU et al. 1997).

## 37.1.3
### The Role of Socioeconomic Status, Environment, and Disease

Some investigators believe that one or more of these phenomena result from biologic differences corresponding to the phenotypic features of "race." Unfortunately, "race" interacts with socioeconomic status (SES), and SES independently affects survival from cancer (AYANIAN and KOHLER 1993; ROACH and ALEXANDER 1995; ROACH et al. 1997). Such factors as poor health status, diet, life-style, and the quality, of health care received are difficult to quantify, making invoking "race" problematic, particularly when there is no clear-cut biologic definition of "what race really is."

The role of diet (GIOVANNUCCI et al. 1995), culture, and SES often do not fit into statistical analysis techniques. The issue of *"sustained intergenerational well-being"* is rarely explored, but it too is part of one's environment and affects one's response to health promotion, disease prevention, and sense of overall well-being (FOSTER et al. 1993; FOSTER 1997).

A direct challenge to the genetic concept of race was described in a study comparing birth weight among infants of U.S.-born blacks, African-born blacks, and U.S.-born whites. Infants of African-born blacks weighed more than infants of comparable black women born in the United States, but the same as infants of U.S.-born white women (DAVID and COLLINS 1997).

It is against this background that we examine differences in the occurrence of genitourinary cancer, understanding that we have yet to move beyond race in our classification of incidence and mortality. One of the most reliable databases which will be used for comparative incidences is from the International Agency for Research on Cancer (IARC) of the World Health Organization (PARKIN et al. 1992).

## 37.2
### Prostate Cancer

## 37.2.1
### Observations of Incidence and Mortality

Among men, the prostate is the leading cancer site, accounting for 26.5% of new cancer cases in males in the United States. The United States' National Cancer Institute's Surveillance, Epidemiology, and End Results (SEER) Program adjusted downward the estimated number of new cases of prostate cancer in the

United States to 209 000 in 1997, based on a 24% decline in incidence between 1992 and 1994 (PARKER et al. 1997; RIES et al. 1997), a direct outcome of increased screening for this disease in the U.S. population. The highest recorded incidence was in 1992, when the rate was 190.1/100 000 population, falling to 144/100 000 population in 1994 with no change in the mortality of 26/100 000 population (RIES et al. 1997).

African American men have been reported to have the highest incidence and mortality rates for prostate cancer in the world. It is noteworthy that Gambians from West Africa have the lowest rates, and blacks in Connecticut have lower rates than those who live in the state of Utah, which has very few blacks (Table 37.1). No definitive explanation currently exists to explain these observations, especially given that almost all the descendants of African Americans were forcibly brought to the United States from West Africa.

ROACH (1998) has recently reviewed the published literature on race and survival rates in patients with prostate cancer. He made the point that Scandinavian countries have among the highest incidence/ mortality rates in the world for prostate cancer (PARKER et al. 1997), while Africa has among the lowest mortality rates, casting doubts on the independent significance of race (SILVERBERG 1980; WALKER et al. 1993). He further argued that if "black genes" were critical, Africans should have the highest rates, while African Americans (in whom 30% of the gene pool is thought to be of European origin) should have an intermediate incidence of prostate cancer (CAVALLI-SFORZA 1991). He also noted the well-known fact that the incidence of prostate cancer increases among Asians following their migration to the United States. Since these large variations in the prostate cancer incidence/mortality rates extend across racial lines, "factors" other than "race" must dominate the impact of race on determining incidence and mortality. Roach argued that until these "factors" are identified and accounted for, we should not be confident in invoking "race" as the culprit.

Numerous studies demonstrate that blacks have a higher incidence of most common cancers for which established causes are well known (lung cancer, esophageal cancer, and carcinoma of the head and neck). They also note a lower survival for blacks for most common tumors for which early detection and treatment are thought to be valuable (e.g., breast cancer, colon cancer, uterine cancer, and cervical cancer). Since neither the increased incidence nor the differences in mortality rates between blacks and whites are unique to prostate cancer, it is unlikely

**Table 37.1.** Highest and lowest incidences of cancer of the prostate recorded worldwide (separated by the horizontal bar in the middle of the table). (ICD-9 185 ARC Registry) (modified from PARKIN et al. 1992)

| Geographic area | Cases | Rate/100 000 males |
|---|---|---|
| USA, Atlanta: blacks | 832 | 102 |
| USA, Bay Area: blacks | 944 | 95.6 |
| USA, Detroit: blacks | 2 210 | 94.2 |
| USA, Alameda: blacks | 497 | 93.5 |
| USA, Los Angeles: blacks | 1 734 | 82.7 |
| USA, Seattle | 7 712 | 82.4 |
| USA, Utah | 3 019 | 77.9 |
| USA, Connecticut: blacks | 296 | 65.0 |
| Bermuda: blacks | 45 | 64.0 |
| USA, Los Angeles: other whites | 9 414 | 51.9 |
| Sweden | 22 283 | 50.2 |
| USA, Connecticut: whites | 5 184 | 47.2 |
| USA, Los Angeles: Spanish surname, white | 1 069 | 38.4 |
| New Zealand: Maori | 97 | 37.3 |
| New Zealand: non-Maori | 3 492 | 35.4 |
| USA, Los Angeles: Japanese | 110 | 32.9 |
| USA: Puerto Ricans | 3 543 | 33.1 |
| USA, Los Angeles: Filipinos | 145 | 28.6 |
| Philippines, Manila | 572 | 16.9 |
| USA, Los Angeles: Chinese | 65 | 19.8 |
| Japan, Hiroshima City | 237 | 10 |
| Japan, Nagasaki City | 129 | 9.3 |
| USA, Los Angeles: Korean | 11 | 8.9 |
| Japan, Miyagi Prefecture | 518 | 7.8 |
| Mali, Bamako | 21 | 6.3 |
| Kuwait: Kuwaitis | 27 | 4.4 |
| India, Ahmedabad | 143 | 4.1 |
| Thailand, Chiang Mai | 59 | 4.0 |
| Thailand, Khon Kaen | 19 | 2.7 |
| India, Madras | 100 | 2.1 |
| Algeria, Serif | 21 | 2.0 |
| China, Shanghai | 323 | 1.7 |
| The Gambia | 6 | 1.2 |
| China, Tianjin | 84 | 1.2 |
| China, Qidong | 20 | 0.8 |

Reported from registries recognized by the International Association of Cancer Registries between 1983 and 1987, with an estimated median reporting year of 1985.

that there is some special "biologic relationship" between prostate cancer and race. Thus it is far more plausible that factors that contribute to the excess incidence and mortality rates for other cancer types also contribute to the risk of developing prostate cancer risk (VIJAYAKUMAR et al. 1996).

## 37.2.2
## Androgen Response and Genetic Polymorphism

The prostate gland is the only organ that actually increases in size with age in males who are not castrated before puberty or born phenotypically female, providing early evidence that biologically the prostate is an androgen-responsive organ. With the high incidence of prostate carcinoma in African American males, Ross et al. looked at a possible biological cause for this increase in a study showing that African American males have higher levels of 5α-reductase activity which leads to higher levels of dihydrotestosterone, which stimulates prostate epithelium division, compared with whites or Japanese men (Ross et al. 1992).

This has led to extensive research into the model of genetic susceptibility to cancer from exogenous and endogenous exposures for bladder, prostate, and breast cancer (Ross et al. 1997). It operates on the principle that potential genetic markers exist within and between ethnic groups that affect steroid hormone metabolism. Ross and his research colleagues at University of Southern California School of Medicine (USC) have proposed a polygenic model. The model states that there are functionally important genetic polymorphisms that encode enzymes involved in steroid hormone biosynthesis or meta-bolism which lead to the differences we see in susceptibility to breast and prostate cancer (Ross and Coetzee 1996). The word polymorphism is defined in the *The Dictionary of Cell Biology* as the existence in a population of two or more alleles of a gene, where the frequency of the rarer alleles is greater than can be explained by recurrent mutation alone (typically greater than 1%) (Lackie and Dow 1995).

The androgen receptor gene (AR) contains glutamine (CAG) and glycine (GGC) repeats that are each polymorphic in length (Hakimi et al. 1997). Investigators have examined prostate tissue in patients who were treated for clinically localized stage B (organ-confined) disease with radical retropubic prostatectomy. Pathologically patients had locally advanced tumors with high-grade disease. Both tumor DNA and nontumor DNA were examined for somatic mutations in the AR-CAG and GGC repeats. Hakimi et al. (1997) found that somatic mutations are rare, and the range of germ-line repeat lengths in men with prostate cancer was similar to the general white population controls. However, there was a subpopulation of men with clinical prostate cancer who had a higher frequency of AR alleles (10%) than the general population (1.6%). Among the prostate cancer patients who had an AR gene with 16 or 17 CAGs, 83% had lymph node-positive disease, suggesting that the short AR-CAG allele may be a risk factor for the development of lymph node-positive

prostate cancer, while short GGC repeats may be a risk factor for the development of clinical prostate cancer (Hakimi et al. 1997).

The largest examined CAG repeat length and the relationship of a higher risk of prostate cancer was in a review of the Physician's Health Study Database (Giovannucci et al. 1997). This was a nested case-control study of 587 newly diagnosed cases of prostate cancer detected between 1982 and 1995, and 588 controls without prostate cancer. Less than 5% of the population examined was black. In this population, shorter CAG repeat sequences were associated with a higher risk of total prostate cancer relative risk, extracapsular extension, node-positive disease, and more aggressive histology.

One study does have a multiethnic cohort (Irvine et al. 1995). In this group there were shorter alleles in blacks and longer alleles in Asian Americans relative to whites. However, the entire reported cohort is less than 200.

Though there are several studies that suggest that CAG repeats are associated with more aggressive disease and one suggesting that CAG repeats are shorter in blacks, larger studies need to be performed to bear this out. Whether or not short CAG repeats predict the biologic behavior of prostate cancer also is not known, and the frequency of short repeats is not known in the U.S. population as a whole.

### 37.2.3
### Race and Survival from Prostate Cancer

Because the major causes for prostate cancer remain elusive, it is difficult to exclude the possibility that exposure to some yet to be characterized factor(s) is responsible for the differences in incidence (Steele et al. 1971; Hsing et al. 1990; Reichman et al. 1990; Carter et al. 1993; Corder et al. 1993; Hsing and Comstock 1993; Lyn et al. 1993; Matzkin and Soloway 1993; Rotimi et al. 1993; Hiatt et al. 1994; Braun et al. 1995; Corder et al. 1995; Demark-Wahnefried et al. 1995; Monroe et al. 1995; Reichardt et al. 1995; Wu et al. 1995; Coughlin et al. 1996; Dale et al. 1996; Doll et al. 1996; Godley et al. 1996; Taylor et al. 1996; Ingles et al. 1997; Rodriguez et al. 1997). It is somewhat easier to address the issue of the excess mortality.

With earlier diagnosis in both whites and blacks, the relative 5-year survival rates have already shown a statistically significant increase from 68% from 1974–1976 to 89% for U.S. whites in the period 1986–1992, when prostate-specific antigen (PSA) testing became common. During the same periods, for blacks, the 5-year survival increased from 58% to 73%, reflecting an increased receptivity to screening by African American men (MYERS et al. 1994).

By adjusting for other well-known prognostic factors it is possible to estimate the independent contribution to outcome attributable to race. The critical question to be answered is: "Is race an independent prognostic factor for survival from prostate cancer?" Answering this question may shed light on other aspects of this complex problem. It is important to determine whether race has independent prognostic significance or whether it is simply associated with primary factors such as socioeconomic status or access to care. For example, during the time slavery was still legal in the United States, the slaves had a very high infant mortality (FRANKLIN and MOSS 1994). It was assumed by many historians at that time that the high mortality was characteristic of these people of African origin. We now know that the high mortality simply reflected the social circumstances into which the individuals were born. Poor prenatal and postnatal care and not race was the explanation for the excess mortality.

For the purposes of this discussion, the term "race" will be used to describe different populations in the United States characterized as "black" and "white" based on phenotypic characteristics. Although this would seem to be an unnecessary point of clarification, it is important to realize that in this country, individuals who are of mixed origin are generally classified as "black" even if one of their parents is half black and half white and the other parent is white. To address this issue it is also important to use the same convention to answer questions such as: "Does a specific type of medical intervention prolong survival?"

This type of question is best answered by conducting a prospective randomized trial. Therefore, whenever possible, we should emphasize data based on prospective randomized trials. Data based on retrospective subset analysis from single institutions adjusting for major prognostic factors are probably next most likely to be accurate. This conclusion is based on the belief that patients treated at single institutions are likely to have received a more uniform quality of treatment. Other types of retrospective studies which adjust for known prognostic factors are likely to provide the next most accurate form of data for addressing the problem of race and outcome. When evaluating the prognostic significance of race, we are not asking whether stage at presentation, quality of care, or access to care con-

tribute to mortality, but rather whether "race" is an independent prognostic factor.

To identify papers relevant to the topic of outcome following treatment for prostate cancer and race, Roach performed a literature search using "prostate cancer and race" as key words. He attempted to include all papers published in the last 15 years that assessed the independent significance of race for survival or disease-free survival among patients with prostate cancer. These papers were categorized as: (1) those based on prospective randomized trials, (2) single-institution studies, or (3) relatively "crude" population-based studies.

### 37.2.3.1
### Randomized Trials Looking at Race and Prostate Cancer

Table 37.2 summarizes major prospective randomized trials published to date reporting outcome by race. CRAWFORD et al. (1990) reported their results in patients with metastatic prostate cancer and found that although blacks tended to present with more advanced metastatic disease, when adjusted for the number of metastases and severity of disease, race was not an independent prognostic factor. In a retrospective analysis of 1200 men treated by three prospective randomized trials in the Radiation Therapy Oncology Group (RTOG), ROACH et al. (1992) reported that race did not appear to be a significant independent prognostic factor. Once again, blacks tended to present with more advanced disease as manifested by higher serum prostatic acid phosphatase. VOGELZANG et al. (1995) also noted no independent significance of race based on data from a prospective randomized trial. Among patients with hormone-refractory prostate cancer, treated in three randomized trials, blacks tended to do better than whites (SMITH et al. 1996). KENNEALEY et al. (1996) initially suggested that there were differences in outcome between blacks and whites in a 1995 abstract but, by the time of the poster presentation, they concluded that race was not a significant factor. Thus, although there are scattered reports suggesting that race is an independent factor in carcinoma of the prostate, in every major prospective randomized trial to date, race has been shown to have no independent prognostic significance.

**Table 37.2.** Randomized trials reporting outcomes following treatment for prostate cancer by race (adapted from ROACH 1998)

| Authors | Stages | Treatment | DFS/survival difference | Comparable care?[a] | Comments |
|---|---|---|---|---|---|
| CRAWFORD et al. (1990) | D2[b] | Leuprolide ±flutamide | NA/no | Yes | Race not significant when corrected for severity of extent of disease |
| KENNEALEY et al. (1996)[c] | D2 | LHRH drugs + bicalutamide or flutamide | NA/no (based on updated poster presentation) | Yes | Race not significant when corrected for severity of extent of disease |
| ROACH et al. (1992) | T1N0M0 through T4N2M0 | XRT | No/conflicting findings | Yes | Survival difference seen for 1 of 3 studies, probably due to differences in the extent of disease as suggested by higher acid phosphatase in blacks |
| SMITH et al. (1996)[c] | Refractory, metastatic | Systemic | No/no | Yes | Blacks tended to do better than whites |
| VOGELZANG et al. (1995) | D2[b] | Goserelin vs orchidectomy | NA/no | Yes | Race not significant when corrected for severity of extent of disease |

DFS, Disease-free survival; NA, not available; XRT, radiotherapy.
[a] Comparable care was assumed when care was delivered on a standardized protocol.
[b] A–D staging according to the American Urologic System.
[c] Abstracts only.

### 37.2.3.2
### *Nonrandomized Retrospective Single-Institution Studies Looking at Race and Prostate Cancer*

The major retrospective single-institution series reporting outcome by race are summarized in Table 37.3. In none of these 15 studies was race clearly demonstrated to independently impact survival. Of note, in one report it was concluded that race was an independent prognostic factor despite the fact that after adjustment for margin status the differences were no longer statistically significant (MOUL et al. 1996). PEREZ et al. (1989) found race to be significant in men with locally advanced disease but not in those with early disease. In the report by POWELL et al. (1995) it was concluded that young black men had a lower survival but older black men had a higher survival than whites. In the report by KIM et al. (1995), blacks were noted to have much higher serum PSA levels, with the mean and median being 31.7 and 15.8 vs 71.6 and 68.4, respectively, for whites and blacks (KIM et al. 1995). Furthermore, 40% of blacks had high-grade tumors compared to 26% of whites ($P < 0.001$). Since no adjustment was made for these pretreatment prognostic factors it is not surprising that blacks had a worse outcome.

In addition to the published papers, several abstracts based on patients who were thought to have received relatively uniform care have demonstrated that when adjusted for literacy or other prognostic factors, the survival of blacks was equal to or exceeded that of whites (HART et al. 1996; NAUTIYAL et al. 1996; WEINBERGER et al. 1996). At single institutions it is reasonable to assume that the quality of treatment was relatively uniform. Overall these studies suggest that race is probably not an independent prognostic factor.

### 37.2.3.3
### *Other Nonrandomized Retrospective Studies Looking at Race and Prostate Cancer*

Other major retrospective series reporting outcome by race are summarized in Table 37.4. Most of these studies suggest that there is a difference in outcome by race. However, in these studies is it likely that the initial workup, treatment, and evaluation were not uniform. In addition to a lack of uniformity of treatment, these studies are also characterized by "lumping" a wide range of disease stages into crude categories such as "local," "regional," and "distant." Because of these shortcomings the conclusions based on the studies summarized in Table 37.4 cannot be assumed to be as accurate as those based on the studies cited in Tables 37.2 and 37.3. Despite their

**Table 37.3.** Retrospective prostate cancer studies from single institutions: outcomes by race (adapted from ROACH 1998)

| Authors | Stages | Treatment | DFS/survival difference | Comparable care?[a] | Comments |
|---|---|---|---|---|---|
| AUSTIN et al. (1990) | T2–3 | XRT | NA/conflicting findings | No | Younger Blacks did worse but older blacks had a similar survival to that of older whites |
| AZIZ et al. (1988) | T2–T4N2M0 | XRT | NA/no | Yes | No survival difference if corrected for stage and grade |
| BAGSHAW (1990)[c] | T1–3 | XRT | NA/no | Yes | No difference in survival by race |
| DAYAL and CHIV (1982) | Local, regional, and distant | Non-standard | NA/conflicting findings | No | Race no longer significant after adjustment for socioeconomic status |
| EPSTEIN et al. (1986) | A1[b] | Surgery | NA/no | Yes | Early stages and small numbers from Johns Hopkins |
| FOWLER and TERRELL (1996) | A–D1[b] | Surgery | No/no | Yes | VA Hospital in Jackson Mississippi |
| HART et al. (1996)[d] | T1NxM0–T4NxM0 | XRT | No/no | Yes | Large contemporary series with PSA follow-up, from Wayne State University in Detroit |
| HUSSAIN et al. (1992) | A–D[b] | XRT | NA/yes | Yes | No difference when adjusted for smoking and grade |
| KIM et al. (1995) | A–D1[b] | XRT | Yes/yes | Yes | Blacks had more advanced disease; no adjustment was made for these differences |
| LAWTON et al. (1994) | A–D[b] | XRT | No/no | Yes | Blacks presented at an earlier age and later stage |
| LEVINE and WILCHINSKY (1979) | A–D[b] | NA | NA/no | Yes | Blacks presented at an earlier age and later stage |
| MOUL et al. (1996) | Clinical T1–2 | Surgery | Conflicting findings [d]/NA | Yes | No difference if adjusted for surgical margin status |
| NAUTIYAL et al. (1996) | T1–T3NxM0 | XRT | No/no | Yes | Large contemporary series with PSA follow-up, University of Chicago |
| PEREZ et al. (1989) | T1–T4NxM0 | XRT | Conflicting findings | Yes | Race not significant for stages T1Nx M0–T2NxM0 |
| POWELL et al. (1995) | Local, regional, and distant | NA | No/conflicting findings | Yes | SEER data, VA in Detroit area. No difference by race in men over the age of 70 or in men with metastatic disease |

DFS, Disease-free survival; NA, not available; XRT, radiotherapy; VA Veterans Administration.
[a] Comparable care is assumed when care was delivered at the same institution and with the same type of treatment (surgery or XRT).
[b] A–D staging according to the American Urologic System.
[c] Personal communication from Malcolm A. Bagshaw, Nov. 20, 1990.
[d] Abstract only.

limitations, even the studies cited in Table 37.4 raise serious doubts about the independent prognostic significance of race.

## 37.2.4
## Can Prostate Treatment Outcome Be Explained by Race?

The most likely explanation for the appearance of a difference in outcome for survival due to race is an epidemiologic phenomenon that Roach has called "extent of disease bias" (ROACH and ALEXANDER

**Table 37.4.** Other prostate cancer studies with outcomes reported by race (adapted from ROACH 1998)

| Authors | Stages | Treatment | DFS/survival difference | Comparable care?[a] | Comments |
|---|---|---|---|---|---|
| AUSTIN and CONVERY (1993) | T2–3 | XRT | NA/conflicting findings | No | Based on tumor registry data in Connecticut; younger blacks did worse but older blacks had a similar survival to that of older whites |
| METTLIN et al. (1994) | I–IV | Surgery, radiation, hormonal therapy | NA/yes | No | Survival differences not adjusted for differences in stage at diagnosis |
| MURPHY (1981) | A–D[b] | NA | NA/yes | No | American College of Surgeons data |
| NATARAJAN et al. (1989) | T1–4 | NA | Conflicting findings[c] | No | American College of Surgeons updated data |
| OPTENBERG et al. (1995) | A–D2[b] | Surgery, radiation, hormonal therapy | NA/no | No | Department of Defense Tumor Registry |
| PAGE and KUNTZ (1980) | Local, regional, and distant | Non-standard | NA/no | Yes and no | National VA data |
| PIENTA et al. (1995) | Local, regional, and distant | NA | NA/yes and no | No | SEER data, Detroit area; no difference by race in men over the age of 70 or in men with metastatic disease |

DFS, Disease-free survival; NA, not available; XRT, radiotherapy; VA, Veterans Administration.
[a] Care is assumed *not* to be comparable when it was *not* delivered at the same institution, with the same type of treatment or on a standardized protocol.
[b] A–D staging according to the American Urologic System.
[c] No difference in T1; <10% differences in T2 and T4.

1995). This bias results from the fact that when two different populations have different distributions of the severity of disease, comparison of the two populations without adequate adjustment for other factors such as the true extent of disease and treatment is likely to create the false impression of a difference due to the fact that a person belongs to that population. For example Surveillance Epidemiology and End Results (SEER) data, long considered "the gold standard" for reporting large population-based studies, lump cases of prostate cancer into "local," "regional," and "distant." Within the category of patients with local disease, there are patients who have a 10% risk of failure at 5 years and patients who have a 75% risk of failure at 5 years. These are not accounted for in the staging systems that are currently used. Numerous studies have demonstrated that African Americans tend to present with higher serum PSA levels and higher Gleason scores and that a higher percentage are likely to belong to the groups with the higher risk of failure, creating the false impression that difference in outcome is due to race.

## 37.3
## Bladder and Kidney Cancers

Bladder cancer tends to be common in societies with high rates of kidney cancer (PARKIN et al. 1992), suggesting common carcinogenic influences. The highest rates are in white males in the United States (23.9/100 000) and Canada, closely followed by the Nordic countries; blacks in the United States have less than half the incidence among U.S. whites (10.5/100 000), and the lowest rates are found in Algeria, Satif (2.2/100 000), and Gambia (1.8/100 000). In countries such as the United States where schistosomal infection is not an issue, bladder cancer is more common in whites than in blacks (2.3 : 1) (Table 37.5).

Table 37.5. Highest and lowest incidence rates of cancer of the bladder recorded worldwide (separated by the horizontal bar in the middle of the table). The case numbers and rates for women are given in parentheses. (Modified from PARKIN et al. 1992)

| Geographic area | Cases | Rate/100 000 males |
|---|---|---|
| USA, whites | 13 793 (4 745) | 23.9 (5.9) |
| Canada | 15 836 (5 430) | 21 (5.7) |
| Norway | 3 414 (1 138) | 19.7 (5.0) |
| Australia, Victoria | 2 437 | 19.5 |
| Sweden | 6 497 (2 195) | 16.9 (4.6) |
| Hong Kong | 2 019 (759) | 16.1 (4.6) |
| Australia, Tasmania | 203 (66) | 15.1 (3.7) |
| Switzerland, Geneva | 195 (77) | 15.8 (3.7) |
| Australia: Capital Territory | 54 (21) | 13 (3.5) |
| Switzerland, Basel | 211 (80) | 12.7 (3.1) |
| New Zealand: non-Maori | 1 192 (396) | 12.7 (3.2) |
| Mali, Bamako | 51 (19) | 12.4 (3.5) |
| USA, blacks | 585 (287) | 10.5 (3.8) |
| China, Shanghai | 1 283 (403) | 6.8 (1.8) |
| China, Tianjin | 517 (149) | 6.4 (1.8) |
| Philippines, Manila | 162 (65) | 4.0 (1.4) |
| New Zealand: Maori | 15 (16) | 4.5 (4.5) |
| Philippines, Rizal Province | 115 (46) | 3.7 (1.4) |
| China, Qidong City | 89 (39) | 3.8 (1.1) |
| Algeria, Setif | 24 (2) | 2.2 (0.2) |
| The Gambia | 13 (3) | 1.8 (0.7) |

Reported from registries recognized by the International Association of Cancer Registries between 1983 and 1987, with an estimated median reporting year of 1985.

## 37.3.1
## Bladder Cancer

### 37.3.1.1
### *Procarcinogens for Bladder Cancer*

The causality of bladder cancer appears to follow an environmental procarcinogen model (PERSAD et al. 1997). The most significant procarcinogen for transitional cell carcinomas is tobacco (ZHANG et al. 1994), followed by alcohol intake, although there is greater uncertainty regarding the role of the latter. A summary of selected comparisons of racial differences between blacks and whites is provided in Table 37.6.

Procarcinogens for squamous cell carcinoma are urinary stasis (EL-MASRI and FELLOWS 1981) and exposure of the uroepithelium to chronic infection (VIZCAINO et al. 1994; WARREN et al. 1995). The effect of the trematode worms *Schistosoma haematobium* and *S. mansoni* on the vesical plexus of the urinary bladder is well known. The worm is seen in East Africa and the Middle East, as well as in South Africa townships (GROENEVELD et al. 1996).

In developing countries, the effective management of squamous cell carcinoma of the bladder in the African patient will require eradication of schistosomiasis and early diagnosis when radical treatment may still cure (GROENEVELD et al. 1996).

Table 37.6. Selected series comparing blacks and whites with bladder cancer

| Authors | Type of study | Comments |
|---|---|---|
| AXTELL and MYERS (1978) | SEER data; 1966–73 study of many cancer sites | Greatest differences in survival, with 5-year survival nearly twice as high for whites |
| PAGE and KUNTZ (1980) | VA series study of numerous cancer sites | Blacks showed similar survival to whites for all sites except the bladder |
| HANKEY and MYERS (1987) | SEER data; 1977–80 study of bladder cancer | Much lower survival for blacks despite bladder cancer being less common |
| MAYER and McWHORTER (1989) | Comparison of treatment patterns in 20 764 whites and 882 blacks | Blacks more likely not to receive treatment after adjustment for age, stage at diagnosis, sex, and tumor histology |
| MALLIN et al. (1989) | Comparison of bladder cancers and occupations in blacks and whites in Illinois | Excess risk suggested for whites who were blue-collar workers, butchers, or workers in the electrical power industry, but possibly too few blacks were considered |
| HARRIS et al.(1990) | Case-controlled study; 1534 whites and 129 blacks and 4930 case controls | Steeper dose response to smoking cigarettes among whites than blacks getting bladder cancer |
| HOWARD et al. (1992) | NCI collaborative study comparing differences for bladder cancer as well as several cancer sites | Final results pending |

VA, Veterans Administration.

One of the problems is that schistosomes can live in the urinary bladder for up to 30 years, with a mean life span of 3–6 years, and can produce up to 300 eggs/day/female, which are deposited in the subepithelial tissues of the urinary bladder and ureters (WARREN et al. 1995). It is interesting that the rate of *p53* mutations in Egyptian (Nile delta) urothelial tumors was 39.4% (39/99) compared with 32.5% (118/363) in a cohort in Surrey, England; this difference was not statistically significant, but 5'-CpG-3' mutations were significantly (~3.5 times) more frequent in the Egyptian cancer cohort. By contrast, the G → T and G → C transitions had similar proportions in the English and the Egyptian cohort. These findings may indicate a role for an exogenous mutant, such as phenacetin, tobacco, or N-nitroso compounds. Also, early antibilharzial drugs used in the 1970s, which were known to be mitogenic, may have also played a significant role in 5'-CpG-3' mutations.

Occupational exposure to potential bladder carcinogens occurs in the following workers or industries: those who work with asbestos, auto mechanics, lorry servicing, carpentry, chemical industry, coal mining, construction industry, diesel exhaust (lorry drivers), train engineers, dyestuff manufacturing, fertilizer manufacturing, gardeners (exposed to weed killers and pesticides), glass processing industry, industrial cleaners, machinists, house painters, petroleum industry, photography (developer), printing industry, tobacco industry, rubber industry, and the smelting industry (PERSAD et al. 1997).

### 37.3.1.2
### *Race and Bladder Cancer Survival*

In the United States, surgery is used in the treatment of 90% of bladder cancer patients (American Cancer Society 1997). Despite the fact that blacks in the United States have a lower incidence of bladder cancer than whites, the relative 5-year survival rate from 1986 to 1992 was only 60%, compared to 82% for whites. However, there has been a statistically significant improvement for black survival since 1974–1976, when it was only 47%, reflecting an awareness of the symptoms and the opportunity for more curative treatment. This is also reflected in the improvement in survival from only 74% in 1974–1976 (ACS 1997).

Using SEER data including patients with a variety of cancer diagnoses, AXTELL and MYERS (1978) assessed differences in 5-year survival rates between blacks and whites. They concluded that the largest differences in survival for any cancer site was for bladder cancer, with blacks being nearly twice as likely to have died of tumor at 5 years. PAGE and KUNTZ (1980) similarly evaluated differences in black and white survival among American veterans treated in Veteran Administration Medical Centers. They noted similar survival rates in respect of all cancer sites except for bladder cancer, where they noted a higher risk of death among blacks. HANKEY and MYERS (1987) used more recent SEER data to make the point that blacks continued to have much lower survival rates from bladder cancer. They also noted that much of the difference could be explained by well-known prognostic factors. Hankey and Myers further suggested that "lead-time bias" or lack of diagnosis of benign lesions in blacks or other factors might explain the remaining differences. MAYER and McWHORTER (1989) made the important observation that after adjustment for age, stage, sex, and tumor histology, blacks were more likely not to receive treatment for bladder cancer. They concluded that this might explain a portion of the difference in survival. Hopefully an ongoing study being conducted by the National Cancer Institute will help answer the many questions raised by these data (HOWARD et al. 1992).

Several studies have suggested that there may be differences in the risk factors contributing to the development of bladder cancer by race. For example, MALLIN et al. (1989) studied occupations and cancer mortality in whites and blacks diagnosed in the State of Illinois between 1979 and 1984. They noted an excess risk among blue-collar workers, butchers, and electrical workers who were white but the number of blacks included was rather small. HARRIS et al. (1990) noted a steeper dose response for smoking and risk of acquiring bladder cancer in whites than in blacks, but again the sample size for blacks was rather small. These studies are compared in Table 37.6.

### 37.3.2
### Kidney Cancer

Renal cell carcinoma is more common in persons of European ancestry than in those of African or Asian descent (Table 37.7). It occurs most commonly as a sporadic form and rarely as a familial form. Smoking (DAYAL and KINMAN 1983) and renal dialysis (MATSON and COHEN 1990) have been associated with an increased incidence of this disease. In the United States, the probability of surviving after diag-

**Table 37.7.** Highest and lowest incidence rates of cancer of the kidney and renal pelvis recorded worldwide (separated by the horizontal bar in the middle of the table). The case numbers and rates for women are given in parentheses. (ICD-9 189 IARC Registry) (modified from PARKIN et al. 1992)

| Geographic area | Cases | Rate/100 000 males |
|---|---|---|
| USA, whites | 5629 (3331) | 10.3 (4.9) |
| Sweden | 3989 (2846) | 11.5 (6.6) |
| Switzerland, Geneva | 136 (77) | 11.1 (4.2) |
| USA, blacks | 495 (318) | 8.9 (4.4) |
| New Zealand: non-Maori | 672 (376) | 7.8 (3.8) |
| Hong Kong | 433 (311) | 3.3 (2.2) |
| Australia, Tasmania | 87 (57) | 6.8 (3.8) |
| New Zealand: Maori | 37 (15) | 8.5 (3.9) |
| Philippines, Rizal Province | 93 (64) | 2.4 (1.5) |
| Mali, Bamako | 15 (6) | 2.3 (1.3) |
| China, Tianjin | 189 (114) | 2.3 (1.4) |
| Philippines, Manila | 160 (119) | 3.3 (2.1) |
| China, Shanghai | 380 (261) | 2.0 (1.2) |
| China, Qidong City | 16 (12) | 0.7 (0.4) |
| The Gambia | 4 (4) | 0.3 (0.5) |
| Algeria, Setif Wilaya | 5 (12) | 0.2 (0.6) |

Reported from registries recognized by the International Association of Cancer Registries between 1983 and 1987, with an estimated median reporting year of 1985.

nosis of renal cancer has been improving since 1940 regardless of race, sex, and age at diagnosis (DAYAL and KINMAN 1983). In a study by BLOT and FRAUMENI (1979) there was clustering of renal cancer deaths in U.S. counties among white males and females in the upper north-central part of the country, with an increase in mortality with urbanization for males only. The major factor correlating with mortality was ethnicity, not race. Mortality was elevated in counties with high percentages of residents of German, Scandinavian, and especially Russian descent (BLOT and FRAUMENI 1979).

### 37.3.2.1
### Genetics of Kidney Cancer

Genetic association is clearly seen between von Hippel-Lindau disease, an autosomal dominant disease, and retinal angiomas, central nervous system hemangioblastomas, and renal cell carcinomas. Deletion is commonly seen in the short arm of chromosome 3 (3p) in renal cell carcinoma associated with von Hippel-Lindau disease. In the rare familial forms of renal cell carcinoma, translocations affecting chromosome 3p are uniformly present. Sporadic renal cell carcinoma of the nonpapillary type is also associated with 3p deletions (SCHMIDT et al. 1995).

### 37.3.2.2
### Survival of Kidney Cancer by Race

The only effective treatment in the management of renal cell carcinoma is nephrectomy or, in carefully selected patients, partial nephrectomy. Blacks in the United States have a slightly lower incidence of this disease than whites. The relative 5-year survival rates from 1986 to 1992 were 55% and 60% for blacks and whites, respectively (ACS 1997).

## 37.4
## Testicular Carcinoma

Testicular cancer is a rare cancer which accounts for only 1% of all cancers in men. Cryptorchidism and Klinefelter's syndrome are predisposing factors in the development of germ cell tumors arising from the testis and mediastinum, respectively (NICHOLS et al. 1987); otherwise there are no other known causative factors.

### 37.4.1
### Incidence of Testicular Carcinoma by Ethnicity

Worldwide, the incidence of testicular tumors is lower in Asians and blacks than in whites. The highest rates of incidence are in northern Europe, where they are about twice as high as in the United States, Canada, England, and Australia. The lowest rates are found in African Americans, Africans, and Chinese. In the United States, the incidence has increased about 2% per year since 1973; the largest increase has been in whites, and the rate in African Americans has remained flat. Denmark has the highest incidence of testicular cancer and Gambia has the lowest (Table 37.8).

### 37.4.2
### Racial Incidence and Treatment
### of Testicular Tumors

Because of the rarity of testicular tumors in blacks in the United States, there have been no large series looking at the care for this disease specifically in blacks. In the U.S. military the white/black incidence ratio was found to be 40:1 (DANIELS et al. 1981), whereas outside of the military it is 5:1 (Table 37.8). A retrospective review of 66 black patients treated at seven military medical centers compared these patients with the general testicular cancer

**Table 37.8.** Highest and lowest incidence rates of cancer of the testis, recorded worldwide (ICD-9 186 IARC Registry) (modified from PARKIN et al. 1992)

| Geographic area | Cases | Rate/100 000 males |
|---|---|---|
| Denmark | 1194 | 8.4 |
| Norway | 738 | 6.6 |
| Switzerland, Geneva | 66 | 6.2 |
| New Zealand: Maori | 47 | 6.0 |
| New Zealand: non-Maori | 426 | 5.3 |
| Australia, Tasmania | 61 | 5.0 |
| USA, whites | 2640 | 4.9 |
| Australia, Victoria | 483 | 4.2 |
| Sweden | 894 | 4.0 |
| England and Wales | 4851 | 3.7 |
| Japan, Hiroshima City | 33 | 1.2 |
| Hong Kong | 160 | 1.1 |
| Philippines, Manila | 65 | 0.9 |
| China, Shanghai | 148 | 0.8 |
| USA, blacks | 49 | 0.7 |
| Philippines, Rizal Province | 43 | 0.7 |
| Mali, Bamako | 4 | 0.5 |
| China, Tianjin | 45 | 0.5 |
| China, Qidong City | 13 | 0.4 |
| The Gambia | 2 | 0.2[†] |

Reported from registries recognized by the International Association of Cancer Registries between 1983 and 1987, with an estimated median reporting year of 1985.

population (MOUL et al. 1994). The distribution between seminoma and nonseminoma in the black patients was similar to that in the general population but there was a younger age at presentation; increased delay in diagnosis was found for blacks as compared with whites. Nevertheless, survival has improved for all races due to the wide use of cisplatin-based chemotherapy (BOSL and MOTZER 1997).

## 37.5
## Conclusions

The preponderance of evidence suggests that race is not an independent prognostic factor for survival in prostate cancer. Since most or all of the discrepancies in survival between blacks and whites can be explained on the basis of incidence and stage at diagnosis, resources allocated to research should focus on these areas. Although race does not appear to be an independent prognostic factor for survival from prostate cancer, poor initial workup, poor treatment, and restricted access to care are.

"Race-based" explanations for differences in survival should be viewed with skepticism for a number of reasons. First, as previously suggested, the term "race" does not refer to distinct biologic categories. Secondly, it is important to remember that one of the major tenets in medicine is not to assign multiple explanations or diagnoses if a single explanation (or set of explanations) will do. It seems untenable to assume that African American men die at a higher rate from laryngeal cancer for one biologic reason, from esophageal cancer for another biologic reason, from colon and rectal cancer for other biologic reasons and from bladder and prostate cancer for unique biologic reasons. For these and other cancer sites as well, differences in the extent of disease at the time of diagnosis, access to care, and the quality of care received can explain the discrepancies in survival.

## References

ACS (ed) (1997) Cancer facts and figures – 1997. Atlanta, American Cancer Society, Inc.

Austin JP, Convery K (1993) Age-race interaction in prostatic adenocarcinoma treated with external beam irradiation. Am J Clin Oncol 16:140–145

Austin JP, Aziz H, Potters L, et al. (1990) Diminished survival of young blacks with adenocarcinoma of the prostate. Am J Clin Oncol 13:465–469

Axtell LM, Myers MH (1978) Contrast in survival of black and white cancer patients, 1960–1973. J Natl Cancer Inst 60:1209–1215

Ayanian JZ, Kohler BA (1993) The relation between health insurance coverage and clinical outcomes among women with breast cancer. N Engl J Med 329:326–331

Aziz H, Rotman M, Thelmo W (1988) Radiation-treated carcinoma of the prostate. Am J Clin Oncol 11:166–171

Babior BM, Stossel TP (1984) Hematology: a pathophysiological approach. Churchill Livingstone, New York

Begley S (1995) Three is not enough. Newsweek 125:67–69

Blout WJ, Fraumeni JF Jr. (1979) Geographic patterns of renal cancer in the United States. J Natl Cancer Inst 63:363–366

Bosl GJ, Motzer RJ (1997) Testicular germ-cell cancer. A review article. N Engl J Med 337:242–253

Braun MM, Helzlsouer KJ, Hollis BW (1995) Prostate cancer and prediagnostic levels of serum vitamin D metabolites (Maryland, United States). Cancer Causes Control 6:235–239

Carter BS, Bova GS, Beaty TH, Steinberg GD, Childs B, Isaccs WB, Walsh PC (1993) Hereditary prostate cancer: epidemiologic and clinical features. J Urol 150:797–802

Cavalli-Sforza LL (1991) Genes, peoples and languages. Sci Am 11:104–110

Corder EH, Guess HA, Hulka BS, et al. (1993) Vitamin D and prostate cancer: a prediagnostic study with stored sera [see comments]. Cancer Epidemiol Biomarkers Prev 2:467–472

Corder EH, Friedman GD, Vogelman JH, Orentreich N (1995) Seasonal variation in vitamin D, vitamin D-binding protein, and dehydroepiandrosterone: risk of prostate cancer in black and white men. Cancer Epidemiol Biomarkers Prev 4:655–659

Coughlin SS, Neaton JD, Sengupta A (1996) Cigarette smoking as a predictor of death from prostate cancer in 348874 men screened for the Multiple Risk Factor Intervention Trial. Am J Epidemiol 143:1002–1006

Crawford ED, Blumenstein BA, Goodman PJ (1990) Leuprolide with and without flutamide in advanced prostate cancer. Cancer 66:1039–1044

Dale W, Vijayakumar S, Lawlor EF, Merrell K (1996) Prostate cancer, race, and socioeconomic status: inadequate adjustment for social factors in assessing racial differences. Prostate 29:271–281

Daniels JL, Stutzman RE, McLeod DG (1981) A comparison of testicular tumors in black and white patients. J Urol 125: 341–342

David RJ, Collins JW (1997) Differing birth weight among infants of U.S. born blacks, African-born blacks and U.S.-born whites. N Engl J Med 337:1209–1214

Dayal HH, Chiu C (1982) Factors associated with racial differences in survival for prostatic carcinoma. J Chron Dis 35: 553–560

Dayal H, Kinman J (1983) Epidemiology of kidney cancer. Semin Oncol 10:366–377

Demark-Wahnefried W, Strigo T, Catoe K, Conaway M, Brunetti M, Rimer BK, Robertson CN (1995) Knowledge, beliefs, and prior screening behavior among blacks and whites reporting for prostate cancer screening. Urology 46:346–351

Doll JA, Suarez BK, Donis-Keller H (1996) Association between prostate cancer in black Americans and an allele of the PADPRP pseudogene locus on chromosome 13 [letter]. Am J Hum Genet 58:425–428

El-Masri WS, Fellows G (1981) Bladder cancer after spinal cord injury. Incidence, presentation, histology and prognosis compared with bladder cancer in the non-paralyzed population. Paraplegia 19:265–270

Epstein JI, Paull G, Eggleston JC, Walsh PC (1986) Prognosis of untreated stage A1 prostatic carcinoma: a study of 94 cases with extended followup. J Urol 136:837–839

Foster HW Jr. (1997) The enigma of low birth weight and race. N Engl J Med 337:1232–1233

Foster HW Jr., Thomas DJ, Semenya KA (1993) Low birthweight in African Americans: does intergenerational well-being improve outcome? J Natl Med Assoc 85:516–520

Fowler JE Jr., Terrell F (1996) Survival in blacks and whites after treatment for localized prostate cancer. J Urol 156:133–136

Franklin JH, Moss AA (1994) From slavery to freedom. McGraw-Hill, New York

Gelehrter TD, Collins FS (1990) Principles of medical genetics. Williams and Wilkins, Baltimore

Giovannucci E, Ascherio A, Rimm EB, Stampfer MJ, Colditz GA, Willett WC (1995) Intake of carotenoids and retinol in relation to risk of prostate cancer. J Natl Cancer Inst 87:1767–1776

Giovannucci E, Stampfer MJ, Krithivas K, et al. (1997) The CAG repeat within the androgen receptor gene and its relationship to prostate cancer. Proc Natl Acad Sci USA 94:3320–3323

Godley PA, Campbell MK, Miller C, Gallagher P, Martinson FE, Mohler JL, Sandler RS (1996) Correlation between biomarkers of omega-3 fatty acid consumption and questionnaire data in African American and Caucasian United States males with and without prostatic carcinoma. Cancer Epidemiol Biomarkers Prev 5:115–119

Groeneveld AE, Marszalek W, Heyns CF (1996) Bladder cancer in various population groups in the greater Durban area of KwaZulu-Natal, South Africa. Br J Urol 78:205–208

Guralnik DB (ed) (1984) Webster's New World dictionary. New York, Simon and Schuster, New York

Hakimi JM, Schoenberg MP, Rondinelli RH, Piantadosi S, Barrack ER (1997) Androgen receptor variants with short glutamine or glycine repeats may identify unique subpopulations of men with prostate cancer. Clin Cancer Res 3:1599–1608

Hankey BF, Myers MH (1987) Black/white differences in bladder cancer patient survival. J Chron Dis 40:65–73

Harris RE, Chen-Backlund J-Y, Wynder EL (1990) Cancers of the urinary bladder in blacks and whites. A case-control study. Cancer 66:2673–2680

Hart KB, Porter AT, Reddy S, Pontes JE, Forman JD (1996) The relationship of race to the presentation and natural history of prostate cancer. Proc ASCO 15:247

Hiatt RA, Armstrong MA, Klatsky AL, Sidney S (1994) Alcohol consumption, smoking, and other risk factors and prostate cancer in a large health plan cohort in California. Cancer Causes Control 5:66–72

Howard J, Hankey BF, Greenber RS, Austin DF, Correa P, Chen VW, Durako S (1992) A collaborative study of differences in the survival rates of black patients and white patients with cancer. Cancer 69:2349–2360

Hsing AW, Comstock GW (1993) Serological precursors of cancer: serum hormones and risk of subsequent prostate cancer. Cancer Epidemiol Biomarkers Prev 2:27–32

Hsing AW, McLaughlin JK, et al. (1990) Diet, tobacco use, and fatal prostate cancer: results from the Lutheran Brotherhood cohort study. Cancer Res 50:6836–6840

Hussain F, Aziz H, Macchia R, Avitable M, Rotman M (1992) High grade adenocarcinoma of prostate in smokers of ethnic minority groups and Caribbean Island Immigrants. Int J Radiat Oncol Biol Phys 24:451–461

Ingles SA, Haile RW, et al. (1997) Strength of linkage disequilibrium between two vitamin D receptor markers in five ethnic groups: implications for association studies. Cancer Epidemiol Biomarkers Prev 6:93–98

Ingram VM (1956) A specific chemical difference between the globins of normal human and sickle cell anemia hemoglobin. Nature 178:792–794

Irvine RA, Yu MC, Ross RK, Coetzee GA (1995) The CAG and GGC microsatellites of the androgen receptor gene are in linkage disequilibrium in men with prostate cancer. Cancer Res 55:1937–1940

Kennealey GT, Vogelzang NJ, Soloway MS, et al. (1996) Analysis of time to treatment failure by extent of disease and race in a randomized, multicenter trial comparing Casodex (bicalutamide) (C) with Eulexin (flutamide) (E), each combined with luteinizing hormone releasing hormone. Proc ASCO 15:251

Kim JA, Kuban DA, El-Mahdi EM, Schellhammer PF (1995) Carcinoma of the prostate: race as a prognostic indicator in definitive radiation therapy. Radiology 194:545–549

Lackie JM, Dow JAT (eds) (1995) The dictionary of cell biology. Academic Press, San Diego

Lau Y-L, Chan L-C, Chan Y-Y, Ha S-Y, Yeung C-Y, Waye JS, Chui DHK (1997) Prevalence and genotypes of alpha and β-thalassemia carriers in Hong Kong – implications for population screening. N Engl J Med 336: 1298–1301

Lawton CA, Cantrell JE, Derus SW, Murray KJ, Byhardt RW, Wilson JF (1994) Prostate cancer: are racial differences in clinical stage and survival explained by differences in symptoms? Radiology 192:37–40

Levine RL, Wilchinsky M (1979) Adenocarcinoma of the prostate: a comparison of the disease in blacks versus whites. J Urol 121:761–762

Lyn D, Cherney BW, Lalande M, et al. (1993) A duplicated region is responsible for the poly(ADP-ribose) polymerase polymorphism, on chromosome 13, associated with a predisposition to cancer. Am J Hum Genet 52:124–134

Mallin K, Rubin M, Joo E (1989) Occupational cancer mortality in Illinois white and black males, 1979–1984, for seven cancer sites. Am J Ind Med 699–717

Matson MA, Cohen EP (1990) Acquired cystic kidney disease: occurrence, prevalence, and renal cancers. Medicine 69: 217–226

Matzkin H, Soloway MS (1993) Cigarette smoking: a review of possible associations with benign prostatic hyperplasia and prostate cancer. Prostate 22:277–290

Mayer WJ, McWhorter WP (1989) Black/white differences in non-treatment of bladder cancer patients and implications for survival. Am J Public Health 79:772–775

Mettlin C, Murphy GP, Menck H (1994) Trends in treatment of localized prostate cancer by radical prostatectomy: observations from the Commission on Cancer National Cancer Database, 1985–1990. Urology 43:488–492

Monroe KR, Yu MC, Kolonel LN, Coetzee GA, Wilkens LR, Ross RK, Henderson BE (1995) Evidence of an X-linked or recessive genetic component to prostate cancer risk [see comments]. Nat Med 1:827–829

Moul JW, Schanne FJ, Thompson IM, et al. (1994) Testicular cancer in blacks. A multicenter experience. Cancer 73: 388–393

Moul JW, Connelly RR, Harris JA, Mooheyhan RE, Srivastava SK, McLeod DG (1995) Prostate specific antigen (PSA) values at initial prostate cancer diagnosis are higher in African-American men: multivariable analysis of 541 patients. Proceedings of the American Urological Association 153:417A

Moul JW, Douglas TH, McCarthy WF, WcLeod DG (1996) Black race is an adverse prognostic factor for prostate cancer recurrence following radical prostatectomy in an equal access health care setting [see comments]. J Urol 155:1667–1673

Murphy GP (1981) Prostate cancer today. Urology 17:1–3

Myers RE, Wolf TA, Balsheim AW, Ross EA, Chodak GW (1994) Receptivity of African American men to prostate cancer screening. Urology 43:480–487

Natarajan N, Murphy GP, Mettlin C (1989) Prostate cancer in blacks: an update from the American College of Surgeons' Patterns of Care Studies. J Surg Oncol 40:232–236

Nautiyal J, Vaida F, Awan A, Weichselbaum, Vijayakumar S (1996) The impact of race on biochemical outcome in patients receiving irradiation for prostate cancer. Int J Radiat Biol Phys 36(Suppl):305

Nichols CR, Heerema NA, Palmer C, Loehrer PJ, Williams SD, Einhorn LH (1987) Klinefelter's syndrome associated with mediastinal germ cell neoplasms. J Clin Oncol 5: 1290–1294

Optenberg SA, Thompson IM, Friedrichs P, Wojcik B, Stein CR, Kramer B (1995) Race, treatment, and long-term survival from prostate cancer in an equal-access medical care delivery system. JAMA 274:1599–1605

Organ C Jr. (1989) Introduction. In: Jones LL (ed) Minorities and cancer. Springer, New York Berlin Heidelberg

Pace BP, Sullivan-Fowler M (1997) "Cancer houses" and cancer areas: JAMA 100 years ago, January 30, 1987. JAMA 277:1420

Page WF, Kuntz AJ (1980) Racial and socioeconomic factors in cancer survival. Cancer 45:1029–1040

Parker SL, Tong T, Bolden S, Wingo PA (1997) Cancer statistics, 1997. CA Cancer J Clin 47:5–27

Parkin DM, Muir CS, Whelan SL, Gao YT, Ferlay J, Powell J (eds) (1992) Cancer incidence in five continents. International Agency for Research on Cancer, Lyon

Pauling L, Itano HA, Singer SJ, Wells IC (1949) Sickle cell anemia: a molecular disease. Science 110:543–548

Perez CA, Garcia D, Simpson JR, Zivnuska F, Lockett MA (1989) Factors influencing outcome of definitive radiotherapy for localized carcinoma of the prostate. Radiother Oncol 16:1–21

Persad R, Fleming C, Chern HD, et al. (1997) Environmental procarcinogen hypothesis of bladder cancer in humans: dapsone hydroxylation as a susceptibility risk factor for aggressive bladder cancer. Urol Oncol 3:18–26

Pienta KJ, Demers R, Hoff M, Kau TY, Montie JE, Severson RK (1995) Effect of age and race on the survival of men with prostate cancer in the Metropolitan Detroit tricounty area, 1973 to 1987. Urology 45:93–101; discussion 101–102

Powell I, Gelfand D, Heilbrun L, Parzuchowski J, Franklin A (1995) Results of early detection of prostate cancer in 1100 African American men. Deed program update. Proceedings of the American Urological Association 153:417A

Reichardt JK, Makridakis N, Henderson BE, Yu MC, Pike MC, Ross RK (1995) Genetic variability of the human SRD5A2 gene: implications for prostate cancer risk. Cancer Res 55: 3973–3975

Reichman ME, Hayes RB, Ziegler RG, Schatzkin A, Taylor PR, Kahle LL, Fraumeni JF Jr. (1990) Serum vitamin A and subsequent development of prostate cancer in the First National Health and Nutrition Examination Survey Epidemiologic Follow-up Study. Cancer Res 50: 2311–2315

Ries LAG, Kosary CL, Hankey BF, Miller BA, Harras A, Edwards BK (eds) (1997) SEER cancer statistics review, 1973–1994. National Cancer Institute, Bethesda

Roach M III (1998) Is race an independent prognostic factor for survival from prostate cancer? J Natl Med Assoc (in press)

Roach M III, Alexander M (1995) The prognostic significance of race and survival from breast cancer: a model for assessing the reliability of reported survival differences. J Natl Med Assoc 87:214–219

Roach M III, Krall J, Keller JW, et al. (1992) The prognostic significance of race and survival from prostate cancer based on patients irradiated on Radiation Therapy Oncology Group Protocols (1976–1985). Int J Radiat Oncol Biol Phys 24:441–449

Roach M, Lu J, et al. (1997) Long-term survival in 1500 men treated for prostate cancer with radiotherapy alone (XRT): based on Radiation Therapy Oncology Group (RTOG) protocols 7706, 7506, 8531, and 8610. American Urological Association (Abstract submitted). JAMA (Pending Submission)

Rodriguez C, Tatham LM, Thun MJ, Calle EE, Health CW Jr. (1997) Smoking and fatal prostate cancer in a large cohort of adult men. Am J Epidemiol 145:466–475

Ross RK, Coetzee GA (1996) The epidemiology and etiology of prostate cancer. In: Petrovich Z, Baert L, Brady LW (eds) Carcinoma of the prostate. Innovations in management. Springer, Berlin Heidelberg New York, pp 1–11

Ross RK, Bernstein L, Lobo RA (1992) 5-Alpha-reductase activity and risk of prostate cancer among Japanese and US white and black males. Lancet 339:887–889

Ross RK, Feigelson HS, Yu MC, Coetzee GA, Reichardt JKV, Henderson BE (1997) Genetic susceptibility to cancer from exogenous and endogenous exposures. In: Fortner JG, Sharp PA (eds) Accomplishments in cancer research 1996. Lippincott-Raven, Philadelphia, pp 208–220

Rotimi C, Austin H, Delzell E, Day C, Macaluso M, Honda Y (1993) Retrospective follow-up study of foundry and engine plant workers. Am J Ind Med 24:485–498

Schmidt L, Li F, Brown RS (1995) Mechanism of tumorigenesis of renal carcinomas associated with the constitutional chromosome 3;8 translocation. Cancer J Sci Am 1:191–195

Silverberg E (1980) Cancer statistics. CA Cancer J Clin 30:23–38

Smith DC, Trump DL, Vogelzang NJ, Redman BG, Flaherty LE, Pienta KJ (1996) The effect of African American race on response and survival in phase II trials of patients with hormone-refractory prostate cancer. Proc ASCO 15(Suppl):242

Steele R, Lees REM, Kraus AS, Rao C (1971) Sexual factors in the epidemiology of cancer of the prostate. J Chron Dis 24:29–37

Taylor JA, Hirvonen A, Watson M, Pittman G, Mohler JL, Bell DA (1996) Association of prostate cancer with vitamin D receptor gene polymorphism. Cancer Res 56:4108–4110

Vijayakumar S, Weichselbaum R, Vaida F, Hellman S (1996) Prostate-specific antigen levels in African-Americans correlate with insurance status as an indicator of socioeconomic status. Cancer J Sci Am 2:225–233

Vizcaino AP, Parkin DM, Boffetta P, Skinnerq MEG (1994) Bladder cancer: epidemiology and risk factors in Bulawayo, Zimbabwe. Cancer Causes Control 5:517–522

Vogelzang NJ, Chodak GW, Soloway MS, et al. (1995) Goserelin versus orchiectomy in the treatment of advanced prostate cancer: final results of a randomized trial. Zoladex Prostate Study Group. Urology 46:220–226

Walker AR, Walker BF, Segal I (1993) Cancer patterns in three African populations compared with the United States black population. Eur J Cancer Prev 2:313–320

Warren W, Biggs PJ, El-Baz M, Ghoneim MA, Stratton MR, Venitt S (1995) Mutations in the $p53$ gene in schistosomal bladder cancer: a study of 92 tumours from Egyptian patients and a comparison between mutational spectra from schistosomal and non-schistosomal urothelial tumours. Carcinogenesis 16:1181–1189

Weinberger M, Williams B, Davis T, Mata JA, Eastham J, Venable DD, Sartor O (1996) Low literacy scores predict advanced stage prostate cancer presentation in African-American men. Am Urol Assoc 155:606A

Wolpoff M, Caspari R (1997) Race and human evolution. Simon and Schuster, New York

Wu AH, Whittemore AS, Kolonel LN, et al. (1995) Serum androgens and sex hormone-binding globulins in relation to lifestyle factors in older African-American, white, and Asian men in the United States and Canada. Cancer Epidemiol Biomarkers Prev 4:735–741

Zhang ZF, Sarkis AS, Cordon CC, et al. (1994) Tobacco smoking, occupation, and p53 nuclear overexpression in early stage bladder cancer. Cancer Epidemiol Biomarkers Prev 3:19–24

# 38 Risk of Second Malignancies Following Treatment for Genitourinary Tumors

S.C. FORMENTI and F.A. CORSO

CONTENTS



## 38.1 Introduction

The advances in the diagnosis and therapy of genitourinary cancers during the last two decades have significantly improved the prognosis and prolonged the survival of genitourinary cancer patients. The therapeutic success has been accompanied by concerns for long-term side-effects of treatments, including therapy-related second malignancies (BOYER and RAGHAVAN 1992). Due to their low curability, most second cancers significantly compromise the prognosis of these patients, often nullifying the success of curing the primary cancer.

Several studies have focused on the role of radiotherapy and/or chemotherapy in inducing second tumors after therapy for primary genitourinary cancer. Most secondary malignancies occurring after a primary treatment for genitourinary tumors arise among patients originally affected by germ cell tumors of the testis and Wilms' tumors. Most of these patients, in fact, can be cured of their primary


S.C. FORMENTI, MD, Associate Professor, Department of Radiation Oncology, University of Southern California School of Medicine, 1441 Eastlake Avenue, Los Angeles, CA 90033, USA
F.A. CORSO, MD, Department of Radiation Oncology, University of Southern California School of Medicine, 1441 Eastlake Avenue, Los Angeles, CA 90033-0804, USA


tumor but at the cost of a high probability of exposure to late effects of treatment. Data about treatment-related hazard are fundamental both to fully inform the patient at the time of the treatment decision and to promote research in modifying/adjusting the therapy without compromising cure rates.

The interpretation of the existing literature on this subject is made complex by methodological differences among studies that range from analysis of tumor registries to description of specific subsets of patients such as recipients of chemotherapy only. In addition, most studies focus on second neoplasms excluding synchronous or preceding tumors. Moreover, a large range of relative risks (RR) of developing secondary malignancies are reported, reflecting insufficient length of follow-up in some reports or the heterogeneity of treatment and outcome among the patients studied. For instance, among germ cell tumors infradiaphragmatic radiotherapy has been the conventional treatment of early-stage seminoma for decades, resulting in large cohorts of survivors at risk for second malignancies. Consequently, available studies on second malignancies after radiotherapy tend to have a longer median follow-up that allows the detection of long-term increase in the relative risk. This is in contrast to studies on nonseminoma survivors, in whom high cure rates with platinum-based regimens were established only 20 years ago, resulting in limited data on long-term risk of secondary malignancies. To address this problem, BOKEMEYER and SCHMOLL (1993) have suggested calculating the incidence of second tumors per year of follow-up, which corrects for the different length of observation among studies. They suggested that reports on secondary malignancies should describe the incidence of these tumors during 5-year intervals. This would provide data for risk estimates at specific time points.

In summary, the evidence to support links between the primary treatment and secondary malignancies is still evolving. Studies of long-term survivors of childhood cancers have taught us how to best interpret the nature of these second cancers.

In fact, overall, pediatric malignancies are more successfully treated than adult tumors. As a result, a large population of childhood cancer survivors has emerged. During the course of analyzing the long-term outcome of these survivors, including the risk of second cancers, the Late Effects Study Group (LESG) identified the association of certain combinations of tumors with underlying genetic syndromes (MEADOWS et al. 1977). Recent research in the field of molecular epidemiology research has provided us with the biological basis for understanding some of these syndromes.

## 38.2
## Genetic Predisposition to Second Cancerogenesis in Germ Cell Tumors

It is of importance to address the issue of whether or not patients affected by a specific cancer possess a genetic predisposition that may put them at an increased risk for additional malignancies, irrespective of therapy. For instance, MALKIN et al. (1992) have described a familial syndrome that manifests as breast cancers, sarcomas, and other neoplasms (brain tumors, leukemias, and adrenocortical carcinomas) in patients with germ line mutations of the p53 gene. Similarly, families affected by Li-Fraumeni syndrome characteristically include a patient who had a sarcoma diagnosed at a pediatric age and two close relatives with cancers diagnosed before the age of 45 (LI et al. 1988; FRIEND et al. 1986; DRAPER et al.1986; WIGGS et al. 1988). Furthermore, germ line mutations of the tumor suppresser gene p53 have been reported to predispose children who are carriers of this defect to an increased risk of second malignant neoplasms, even in the absence of a Li-Fraumeni setting. MALKIN et al. (1992) analyzed genomic DNA from the blood of 59 children and young adults with a second primary tumor. These investigators were able to demonstrate in 4/59 (6.8%) patients the presence of p53 gene mutations and found that five close relatives of three of the four patients were carriers of p53 mutations. These findings suggested the inherited nature of the disorder (MALKIN et al. 1992).

A genetic predisposition to multiple neoplasms in the same individual can be associated with inherited DNA repair deficits. In such a setting the addition of radiation therapy dramatically increases the risk of developing secondary malignancy. For example, patients with the hereditary form of retinoblastoma have an increased risk of a second tumor, frequently

osteosarcoma. The inclusion of radiation therapy in the management of retinoblastoma doubles the incidence of second tumors at 10 years (20% vs 10% among nonirradiated retinoblastoma patients). At 30 years the risk among irradiated versus nonirradiated patients is 90% versus 68%, respectively. Fibroblasts from patients affected by the inherited form of retinoblastoma are more radiosensitive and display impaired DNA repair: fibroblasts from their siblings display a similar defect (FRIEND et al. 1986; DRAPER et al. 1986; WIGGS et al. 1988; CAVENEE et al. 1983; YANDELL et al. 1989).

Consequently, while it is undeniable that patients with germ cell tumors have an increased incidence of a second neoplasm (see below), it is safe to assume that only part of the risk of second malignancy can be attributed to treatment. For instance, testicular cancer patients have a baseline higher relative risk of contralateral testicular cancer (DIECKMANN et al. 1986; VON DER MAASE et al. 1986; ANONYMOUS 1988). These second germ cell tumors probably develop from an in situ lesion in the contralateral testis. The treatment with platinum-based chemotherapy regimens is known to markedly reduce the risk of contralateral testicular cancer, possibly by eradicating microscopic, subclinical disease (VAN LEEUWEN et al. 1993a). Cryptorchidism is recognized as a major risk factor for testicular cancer. The underlying genetic defect, however, could explain why only a minority of individuals affected by cryptorchidism develop testicular cancer (CHILVERS and PIKE 1989). Forman et al. studied 42 families with two or more cases of testicular cancer reported to the UK Register for Familial Testicular Cancer. The authors found that the incidence of undescended testes in these familial cases was between 8% and 10%. As with other forms of cancer, familial cases were diagnosed at a younger age than nonfamilial cases. They also tended to be more frequently bilateral, with a prevalence of bilateral testicular cancer of 6% compared to 2.5% for nonselected cases. In these authors' estimate familial cases represented approximately 1.5% of all testicular cancers. Moreover, they estimated the relative risk for a brother of a testicular cancer patient to develop testicular cancer as 9.8, using actuarial methods in comparison with national registration rates (FORMAN et al. 1992). This risk is much higher than that of most other cancers, for which the risk is usually less than fourfold (EASTON and PETO 1990). FORMAN (1989) concluded that the described familial association supported the hypothesis of a genetic predisposition of tumor induction. Other indirect clinical evidence includes the following: (1) frequent association of testicular cancer with congenital disorder of sexual differentiation (SAVAGE and LOWE 1990); (2) the difference in the incidence of testicular cancer among races (FORMAN 1989); and (3) the fact that migration does not alter the incidence of this disease (MUIR et al. 1987). To our knowledge, no published report is available that compares the outcome of patients with the familial form tumors to that of nonselected testicular cancer patients.

In conclusion, only a minority of testicular cancer cases are familial. Further studies are needed to explain the genetic features of the familial forms. Whether the familial cases also have a predisposition to develop second malignancies remains unanswered.

Patients with testicular cancer have a higher risk for secondary malignancies than patients with other genitourinary tumors. DIECKMANN et al. (1994) reviewed the records of 584 consecutive patients with testicular germ cell tumors treated in Berlin from 1969 to 1992. A total of 23 patients (3.9%) were identified who, in addition to a primary testicular cancer, developed a nontesticular malignancy. In four (17%) of these 23 patients the nontesticular malignancy included: melanoma, colon carcinoma, bronchogenic carcinoma, and Hodgkin's disease which preceded the diagnosis of germ cell tumor. Three (13%) patients had a synchronous nontesticular tumor, including two patients with bladder cancer and one patient with a renal cell carcinoma. The remaining 16 patients had metachronous tumors outside of the testicle. The authors hypothesized in these patients a genetic predisposition for tumor development. To address the question of whether patients with testicular germ cell tumors have an increased risk of multiple neoplasms, the authors compared them with a population of patients with other urological cancer treated during the same period of time at the same institutions. A 3.3% prevalence of multiple neoplasms was identified among the latter group. In view of the fact that the median age of this group was 68 years compared with a median age of 42 years among the testicular cancer patients, the authors concluded that "patients with testicular cancers are indeed at a slightly increased risk of a second malignancy" (DIECKMANN et al. 1994). A similar conclusion has been reached by authors who used tumor registries to address this issue. KLEINERMAN et al. (1985) reported an analysis of the data of the Connecticut Cancer Registry for the period 1935–1982. They demonstrated a twofold increase for the relative risk of secondary solid tumors and a fivefold increase for the relative risk of leukemia in patients with testicular cancer who had not been treated with radiotherapy. VAN LEEUWEN et al. (1993a) estimated the risk of secondary tumors among 1909 patients with testicular cancer diagnosed in the Netherlands from 1971 to 1985. They detected a significantly increased risk of secondary malignancies in patients treated with radiotherapy or with a combination of radiotherapy and chemotherapy and increased relative risk of leukemia with either radiotherapy, chemotherapy or both. However, the patients who had undergone surgery as the only treatment suffered only an increased risk of developing contralateral testicular tumors (Table 38.1).

The best patient population to address the question of a possible genetic predisposition to secondary malignancies after germ cell tumors is emerging from data on patients diagnosed in the last 10–15 years. During that period, trials of "observation only" for selected patients with early disease were started. In two recent studies (BOKEMEYER and SCHMOLL 1993; VON DER MAASE et al. 1993) using either observation-only in stage I disease or surgery alone in germ cell tumor patients with retroperitoneal lymph node metastases, no increased risk for second tumors was detected. However, the reported 5-year median follow-up is a length of time insufficient to draw definite conclusions. It is anticipated that future reports from these series may finally settle this important issue.

**Table 38.1.** Relative risk of second solid tumors and leukemias in testicular cancer patients treated with radiotherapy, chemotherapy, a combination of both, or surgery only (VAN LEEUWEN et al. 1993a)

| | No. of patients | Relative risk | | | | Median follow-up (years) |
| --- | --- | --- | --- | --- | --- | --- |
| | | Stomach | All GI | Contralateral testis | Leukemia | |
| Radiotherapy | 1007 | 4.4 | 2.9 | 44.7 | 5.2 | 8.6 |
| Chemotherapy | 370 | 0 | 0 | 0 | 20.0 | 5.3 |
| Chemotherapy + radiotherapy | 286 | 8.3 | 5.5 | 0 | 2.9 | 3.4 |
| Surgery only | 207 | 0 | 1.1 | 100 | 0 | 6.0 |

Conversely, development of leukemia independently of therapy has been described in patients with primary mediastinal germ cell tumors (NICHOLS et al. 1990). In these cases an isochromosome 12p [i(12p)] that is a cytogenetic marker for testicular cancer has been identified in the leukemic cells. Patients with this genetic syndrome might therefore develop leukemia because of a common genetic abnormality shared by both germ cells and leukemia cells (NICHOLS et al. 1990; BOSL et al. 1989).

In summary, a baseline increased risk for contralateral testicular cancer exists among testicular cancer patients and it is more frequent among those affected by the familial type. An increased risk for synchronous other cancers of the genitourinary tract is also present. A genetic predisposition to develop leukemia has been reported among patients with primary mediastinal germ cell tumors. No clear genetic predisposition to develop other solid tumors has been proven among patients affected by genitourinary malignancies. More studies are necessary to elucidate a potential link between genetics and secondary malignancies among these patients.

## 38.3
## Role of Radiotherapy in Second Malignancies

Radiation therapy has been widely accepted as the standard treatment for early-stage germ cell tumors. However, its use and indications have changed throughout the last 10–20 years. Reduced radiation doses and smaller treatment fields are now used for the treatment of seminoma while radiation is rarely indicated for nonseminomatous testicular tumors and mediastinal germ cell tumors. Therefore, most of the studies regarding long-term sequelae of radiotherapy, and in particular second neoplasms, include patients diagnosed several decades ago when they were treated with higher doses and wider fields than are currently used. For instance some studies include patients diagnosed in the 1930s (KLEINERMAN et al. 1985), 1940s (MOELLER et al. 1993) and 1950s (HAY et al. 1984; HELLBARDT et al. 1990; FOSSA et al. 1989). In these series characterized by higher dose of radiation treatment, a cumulative incidence of second malignancies ranging from 7.9% to 11.6% was reported (KLEINERMAN et al. 1985; MOELLER et al. 1993; HAY et al. 1984; HELLBARDT et al. 1990; FOSSA et al. 1989). Noticeably, FOSSA et al. (1989) reported the highest cumulative incidence of second malignancies, 21.8%, among the subset of patients who, in addition to the standard abdominal radiotherapy, also received mediastinal radiotherapy (FOSSA et al. 1989).

More recent reports that examined patients treated in the 1970s and 1980s, when the indications, field sizes, and doses of radiotherapy were closer to the current practice, reported a much lower cumulative incidence of second malignancies. This incidence ranged from 2.7% to 3.6%, respectively (BOKEMEYER and SCHMOLL 1993; HANKS et al. 1992) (Table 38.2).

In addition to the use of different radiation doses and fields, the variable duration of follow-up makes it difficult to compare the published studies. It is probably for these reasons that the reputed relative risk (RR) of developing a second neoplasm falls within a wide range, with RR values ranging from 1.3 to 7.5. However, BOKEMEYER and SCHMOLL (1993) noticed that the particularly high relative risk (RR = 7.5) in their patient population was caused by the high frequency of second cancers developing in patients who were irradiated during earlier years for

**Table 38.2.** Radiotherapy for testicular cancer with cumulative incidence and relative risk of developing a second malignancy

| References | Period | No. of patients | No. of second tumors | Median follow-up (years) | Cumulative incidence (%) | Total relative risk |
|---|---|---|---|---|---|---|
| KLEINERMAN et al. (1985) | 1935–1982 | 844 | 67 | 9.3 | 7.9 | 2.0 |
| MOELLER et al. (1993) | 1943–1987 | 3256 | 337 | 11.6 | 10.3 | 1.5 |
| HAY et al. (1984) | 1950–1969 | 547 | 57 | 15.4 | 10.4 | 1.9 |
| | | | | >15 | | 2.9 |
| HELLBARDT et al. (1990) | 1951–1986 | 116 | 12 | 8.0 | 10.3 | 2.0 |
| FOSSA et al. (1989) | 1957–1977 | 394 | 46 | >10.0 | 11.6 | 1.3 |
| | | 64[a] | 14 | >10.0 | 21.8 | 4.1 |
| BOKEMEYER and SCHMOLL (1993) | 1970–1990 | 332 | 9 | 5.1 | 2.7 | 7.5 |
| HANKS et al. (1992) | 1973–1974 | 387 | 14 | 15.0 | 3.6 | 3.4 |

[a] Also received mediastinal radiotherapy.

nonseminomatous testicular cancer with a high dose of radiotherapy (>40 Gy). In this study, when the relative risk was calculated only for patients with seminoma and lower radiation doses, a relative risk of 2.3 was demonstrated. This relative risk is close to that reported in the other studies (BOKEMEYER and SCHMOLL 1993). Several authors have measured the relative risk of second tumors after adjustment based on radiation dose and the size of radiation fields. The large range of relative risk initially reported was then decreased to 1.5–2.9 (KLEINERMAN et al. 1985; MOELLER et al. 1993; HAY et al. 1984; HELLBARDT et al. 1990; STEINFELD and SHORE 1990; VAN LEEUWEN et al. 1993a).

The series reported by FOSSA et al. is particularly interesting. When the authors analyzed their data on patients treated with abdominal radiation therapy alone they found a relative risk of 1.3, which was not statistically significant when compared with that of nonirradiated patients. However, for patients who received both abdominal and mediastinal radiotherapy, a 4.1 relative risk was detected (FOSSA et al. 1989).

The issues of site and histology of second malignancies also deserve attention. In most reports at least 80% of second solid tumors are found inside the radiation field (KLEINERMAN et al. 1985; MOELLER et al. 1993; HELLBARDT et al. 1990; BOKEMEYER and SCHMOLL 1993; STEINFELD and SHORE 1990; VAN LEEUWEN et al. 1993a; JACOBSEN et al. 1993). Only two authors (HAY et al. 1984; HANKS et al. 1992) reported no difference in the frequency of second cancers within or outside the radiation fields.

Radiation-induced second malignancies typically include gastrointestinal tumors (stomach, colon, and pancreas), genitourinary cancers (bladder and kidney), and sarcomas. Increased incidence of lung cancer and skin cancers, including melanoma, have also been reported (FOSSA et al. 1989).

In germ cell tumor patients treated by abdominal radiotherapy alone, the relative risk of stomach cancer has been found to range from 1.1 to 4.4 (MOELLER et al. 1993; VAN LEEUWEN et al. 1993a). The excess risk of stomach cancer increases over time and is the greatest after 10 years (VAN LEEUWEN et al. 1993a). The risk is directly proportional to the radiation dose. Although the interpretation of data is hampered by the fact that the different histologies of testicular cancer were treated with different radiation doses, it is noticeable that patients with seminoma who received a 30 Gy radiation dose had an increase in the relative risk of stomach cancer of 3.2, whereas patients with nonseminomatous germ cell

tumors who received 40–50 Gy had a 26 times increased risk of stomach cancer (VAN LEEUWEN et al. 1993b).

Relative risk of bladder cancer has been estimated by different authors at 2.1 (MOELLER et al. 1993), 2.9 (HAY et al. 1984), and 6.9 (HELLBARDT et al. 1990). It is difficult to interpret such a variable range of relative risk. The use of different radiation doses and different fractionation schedules in the treatment is probably the determining factor to explain the different relative risk reported for second bladder cancer. In the series of Fossa's patients treated with mediastinal radiation, an 8.3 relative risk of stomach cancer, a 7.7 relative risk of lung cancer, and a 7.7 relative risk of melanoma were reported (FOSSA et al. 1989). Most lung cancers were diagnosed 10 years after radiation exposure. These findings are similar to those reported for Hodgkin's disease, where, as in germ cell tumors, large fields with considerable internal scattered radiation are employed (KALDOR et al. 1987). Regarding the increased incidence of melanomas reported by Fossa et al., since their diagnosis peaked between 1 and 4 years from the occurrence of testicular cancer, it is conceivable that it could just express increased detection due to the closer medical follow-up undergone by testicular cancer patients.

At least three studies have reported an excess in the risk of leukemia of 2.3, 2.6, and 5.2, respectively. These groups included patients treated with radiation for germ cell testicular cancer who did not receive chemotherapy. Acute myeloid, acute lymphatic, chronic myeloid, chronic lymphatic, and other unspecified types of leukemia were described (KLEINERMAN et al. 1985; MOELLER et al. 1993; VAN LEEUWEN et al. 1993a).

Numerous reports on second sarcomas have been published during the past 20 years (STEINFELD and SHORE 1990; STOCK et al. 1979; LYNCH and HERR 1981; SCHMIDT et al. 1988; GILKS et al. 1988; O'BRIEN et al. 1989; RAZ et al. 1989; YOSHITAKE et al. 1991; AMICHETTI and BOI 1993). The relative risk of developing sarcomas has been specifically addressed by JACOBSEN et al. (1993) in a study examining Danish seminoma patients treated by radiotherapy in the period between 1943 and 1987. A 4.7 relative risk of developing sarcomas was found in seminoma patients compared with a 1.3 relative risk in nonseminoma testicular cancer patients (JACOBSEN et al. 1993). This difference needs to be taken with caution, since in the late 1970s, before the introduction of platinum-based chemotherapy, most patients with nonseminomatous tumors died within 1 or 2 years from diagnosis. Therefore their lower risk of developing a second neoplasm could simply reflect their shorter survival. Noticeably, 80% of the sarcomas were within the radiotherapy field and the remaining 20% at the edge of the radiation field. The median time interval between radiotherapy and the occurrence of sarcomas was 12 years, but second sarcomas were also observed as early as 1 year and as late as 34 years after therapy. ROBINSON et al. (1988) studied the latency to develop second sarcoma after radiation for other malignancies. A longer latency was found after treatment with orthovoltage radiotherapy than after supervoltage radiotherapy.

Similarly, the Danish study found that the time interval from therapy to the development of second malignancy decreased from 21 years for secondary tumors that developed before the 1960s to approximately 11 years after supervoltage treatment was introduced. However, since both the radiation sources and the radiation dose and volume of interest changed over the years covered by this study, it is impossible to draw conclusions about a specific risk associated with any of these variables. While several reports of radiation-induced sarcomas among germ cell testicular cancer patients have described their association with radiation doses greater than 35 Gy (LYNCH and HERR 1981; SCHMIDT et al. 1988; GILKS et al. 1988; RAZ et al. 1989; YOSHITAKE et al. 1991; AMICHETTI and BOI 1993), second sarcomas can also occur after treatment with lower radiation doses (21–32 Gy) (STEINFELD and SHORE 1990; STOCK et al. 1979; O'BRIEN et al. 1989).

The relative risk of developing solid cancers increases with a longer duration of follow-up. HAY et al. (1984) studied 547 patients with testicular cancer, treated with radiotherapy. The total relative risk of their patients developing a second malignancy was 1.9 with a median follow-up of 15.4 years. However, when the authors calculated the total relative risk only for the patients in their study who had a longer follow-up (>15 years), the total RR of developing a second malignancy was 2.9 (HAY et al. 1984).

MOELLER et al. (1993) (Table 38.3) observed three patterns of increased relative risk for second malignancies over a period of time. Second tumors such as renal cell, bladder, and prostate carcinomas, melanoma, and skin and colon cancer displayed the highest risk of development after 20 years or more from the diagnosis of the primary tumor. The relative risk of other second tumors including those originating in the gastrointestinal tract, such as carcinoma of the rectum, stomach, or pancreas and lung cancer, peaked at 10–19 years after diagnosis of primary tumor. The relative risk of leukemia,

**Table 38.3.** Number of second malignancies (*n*) and relative risk (RR) by interval after testicular cancer treatment (MOELLER et al. 1993)

| Tumor sites | 0–9 years | | 10–19 years | | >20 years | |
|---|---|---|---|---|---|---|
| | *n* | RR | *n* | RR | *n* | RR |
| All sites | 146 | 1.5* | 146 | 1.7* | 176 | 1.6* |
| Leukemia | 13 | 4.6* | 3 | 1.3 | 2 | 0.8 |
| Rectum | 4 | 0.7 | 9 | *1.8* | 4 | 0.7 |
| Stomach | 10 | 1.6 | 16 | *3.2** | 8 | 1.5 |
| Pancreas | 3 | 1.0 | 9 | *3.1** | 9 | 2.6* |
| Lung | 12 | 0.7 | 24 | *1.4* | 16 | 0.7 |
| Kidney | 8 | 2.6* | 4 | 1.4* | 9 | *2.7** |
| Bladder | 11 | 1.6 | 14 | 2.0* | 22 | *2.5** |
| Prostate | 4 | 0.7 | 4 | 0.6 | 19 | *1.8** |
| Melanoma | 4 | 1.6 | 3 | 1.8 | 3 | *2.2* |
| Other skin ca. | 17 | 1.5 | 19 | 1.8* | 32 | *2.5** |
| Colon | 8 | 1.3 | 7 | 1.2 | 13 | *1.8* |

Italics are used for the numbers that express the highest relative risk for that tumor site.
* $P < 0.05$.

however, was more elevated within the first 9 years from the diagnosis of the primary cancer (MOELLER et al. 1993).

In view of the fact that some second malignancies can occur 20 years after treatment of the primary tumor, treating physicians should remain alert to this risk in the long-term follow-up of survivors of testicular cancer.

## 38.4
## Role of Chemotherapy in Second Malignancies

Only a few studies have analyzed the risk associated with chemotherapy alone in the development of second solid tumors after a primary genitourinary malignancy. Table 38.4 summarizes results of these studies. Probably the largest and most informative study is that reported by VAN LEEUWEN et al. (1993a), who described, among 1909 patients, 370 cases of testicular cancer treated by initial surgery followed by standard PVB chemotherapy regimen (cisplatin, vinblastin, and bleomycin) and observed for a median follow-up of 5.3 years. Within the period of observation, this subset of patients had a zero relative risk of developing second solid cancers but a 20 relative risk for developing leukemia. During the same period, patients who received radiotherapy only, had a relative risk of 1.8 for all second tumors, 4.4 for stomach cancer, and 5.2 for leukemia (Table 38.1, VAN LEEUWEN et al. 1993a). Therefore, based on the currently available data, with the limitation of

**Table 38.4.** Chemotherapy for testicular cancer and relative risk (RR) of developing solid second tumors and leukemia

| Reference | Period | No. of patients | Second tumors RR | Second leukemias RR | Median follow-up (years) |
|---|---|---|---|---|---|
| COLEMAN et al. (1987) | 1961–1980 | 2013 | 0.7 | 2.5 | 6.8 |
| VAN LEEUWEN et al. (1993a) | 1971–1985 | 370 | 0 | 20.0 | 5.3 |

the short follow-up, there is no clear evidence that PVB chemotherapy elevates the risk of second solid cancers in patients with malignant germ cell tumors. Similarly, COLEMAN et al. (1987) studied 2013 testicular cancer patients with a median follow-up of 6.8 years. The study patients were treated in the period ranging from 1961 to 1980. The authors found only 22 secondary solid tumors, i.e., no significantly elevated risk (RR = 0.7) for the development of second solid tumors. There was a higher, but still not statistically significant relative risk, for secondary leukemia (RR = 2.5).

Conversely, the association of chemotherapy with the risk of developing secondary leukemias is well known. Treatment-related risk of secondary leukemia generally emerges within the first 5 years after completion of therapy. Several reports of secondary leukemia after chemotherapy in testicular cancer patients have been published within the past 15 years (VAN LEEUWEN et al. 1993a; KERBRAT and LEPRISE 1985; REDMAN et al. 1984; VAN IMHOFF et al. 1986; DE VORE et al. 1989; PEDERSEN-BJERGAARD et al. 1991; BOKEMEYER et al. 1992; OLIVER et al. 1991; NICHOLS et al. 1993; BAJORIN et al. 1993). In these studies the chemotherapy regimens include the classic PVB regimens and etoposide-containing regimens. Only a few cases of PVB-induced leukemia have been reported (VAN LEEUWEN et al. 1993a; VAN IMHOFF et al. 1986; DE VORE et al. 1989), while several large studies have now documented the absence of leukemia risk post PVB (BOKEMEYER and SCHMOLL 1993; PEDERSEN-BJERGAARD et al. 1991; ROTH et al. 1988; OZOLS et al. 1988).

In contrast the risk associated with the use of etoposide is more consistent (BOKEMEYER and SCHMOLL 1993; PEDERSEN-BIERGAARD et al. 1991; NICHOLS et al. 1993; BAJORIN et al. 1993; BOSHOFF et al. 1994). Etoposide induces an acute nonlymphocytic leukemia that can be clinically and genetically differentiated from the classic leukemia associated with treatment utilizing alkylating agents. The secondary leukemias reported after the use of alkylating agents occur most frequently after an interval of 5–7 years and are preceded by a preleukemic myelodysplastic phase. There are also cytogenetic abnormalities of chromosomes 5 and 7 which

have been identified in these patients (LEBEAU et al. 1986). Conversely, the leukemias observed after treatment with etoposide tend to occur earlier after therapy. Patients do not have a preleukemic phase and show balanced chromosomal translocations involving a locus on the long arm of chromosome 11, at 11q23 (PEDERSEN-BJERGAARD and PHILIP 1991; WHITLOCK et al. 1991). Molecular investigations have shown that the oncogene ALL-1 is involved in the chromosomal translocation at the locus 11q23 (CIMINO et al. 1991).

The role of the total dose of administered etoposide in the development of secondary leukemia has received particular attention during the past 5 years. A summary of the results of some of the most significant studies on etoposide dose-effect is shown in Table 38.5. For instance, in the study by PEDERSEN-BJERGAARD et al. (1991) high doses of cisplatin, etoposide, and bleomycin were used. Five (6%) out of the 82 patients who received a cumulative dose of etoposide of $2\,g/m^2$ or more developed myeloid leukemia, whereas no leukemia occurred among 130 patients who had received lower doses of etoposide. The incidence of leukemia was 6% in patients receiving doses of etoposide above $2\,g/m^2$ and 0% in patients receiving lower drug doses. These data were confirmed by BOSHOFF et al. (1994), who observed a 0.6% incidence of secondary leukemia among patients receiving $<2\,g/m^2$ of etoposide compared with an 8% incidence in patients receiving $>2\,g/m^2$. Three other studies (BOKEMEYER and SCHMOLL 1993; NICHOLS et al. 1993; BAJORIN et al. 1993) that examined a total of 1102 patients receiving total etoposide doses $<2\,g/m^2$ reported only four (0.3%) cases of leukemia.

Data from the pediatric population suggest that the risk of etoposide-related leukemia may also depend on the schedule of administration (PUI et al. 1991; SUGITA et al. 1993). Children with primary lymphoproliferative diseases had a consistently higher cumulative risk of developing acute myeloid leukemia when etoposide was administered either weekly or twice a week in the management of their primary tumor (PUI et al. 1991; SUGITA et al. 1993). Even if a similar total cumulative dose was administered, the risk was very low when etoposide was

**Table 38.5.** Etoposide dose and incidence of second leukemias among testicular cancer patients

| Reference | No. of patients | Cumulative etoposide dose (mg/m$^2$) | No. of second leukemias (%) | Median follow-up (years) |
| --- | --- | --- | --- | --- |
| PEDERSEN-BJERGAARD et al. (1991) | 82 | >2000 | 5 (6) | 5.4 |
| | 130 | <2000 | 0 (0) | 5.4 |
| BOSHOFF et al. (1994) | 25 | >2000 | 2 (8) | >5.0 |
| | 636 | <2000 | 4 (0.6) | >5.0 |
| NICHOLS et al. (1993) | 538 | <2000 | 2 (0.37) | 4.9 |
| BAJORIN et al. (1993) | 343 | <2000 | 2 (0.6) | >5.0 |
| BOKEMEYER and SCHMOLL (1993) | 221 | <2000 | 0 (0) | 5.5 |

**Table 38.6.** Etoposide schedule, cumulative dose, and cumulative risk of developing acute myeloid leukemia (AML) in children treated for lymphoid malignancies

| Reference | No. of patients | Schedule | Cumulative etoposide dose (mg/m$^2$) | No. of second AMLs | Cumulative risk of AML (%) | Median follow-up (years) |
| --- | --- | --- | --- | --- | --- | --- |
| PUI et al. (1991) | 85 | Twice weekly | 9 240 | 6 | 12.3 | 6 |
| | 84 | Weekly | 19 200 | 7 | 12.4 | 6 |
| | 148 | Every other week | 19 200 | 2 | 1.6 | 6 |
| SUGITA et al. (1993) | 38 | Twice weekly | 5 600 | 5 | 18.4 | 4 |
| | 46 | Daily × 4 | 5 200–10 000 | 0 | 0 | 4 |

administered either every other week (PUI et al. 1991) or daily ×4 (SUGITA et al. 1993). Table 38.6 summarizes these data. It is conceivable that schedule-dependent effects may be also relevant in testicular cancer patients although no studies have, so far, specifically addressed this issue.

The leukemogenic effect of etoposide could also be potentiated by the association with cisplatin (PEDERSEN-BJERGAARD et al. 1992; TAN et al. 1987) and the higher risk observed by PEDERSEN-BJERGAARD et al. (1991) could be attributed to the combination of a dose-effect and a synergistic effect.

In summary, based on the currently available data, it can be concluded that the risk of etoposide-induced leukemia is proportional to the dose administered, the use of weekly schedules, and concurrent cisplatin treatment.

## 38.5
## Role of the Combination of Radiotherapy and Chemotherapy in Second Malignancies

The combination of chemotherapy and radiation dramatically increases the risk of secondary leukemias and solid tumors in patients with Hodgkin's disease (COLEMAN et al. 1982). In genitourinary tumors, the impact of combining radiotherapy and chemotherapy has been investigated only by a few studies (MOELLER et al. 1993; VAN LEEUWEN et al. 1993a).

MOELLER et al. (1993) examined 6180 patients with testicular cancer with a median follow-up of 9.5 years. This study included patients who underwent either radiotherapy alone from 1943 to 1970 or a combination of radiotherapy and chemotherapy from 1970 to 1987. The increased incidence of solid tumors reached a maximum after 15–20 years following radiotherapy, therefore including the patients with a longer follow-up who underwent radiotherapy alone. The duration of follow-up for the patients treated with chemotherapy as well was shorter and therefore the marked increase in secondary solid tumors observed in this study was probably independent of the use of chemotherapy and mainly related to radiotherapy.

VAN LEEUWEN et al. (1993a) analyzed 1909 patients. The authors demonstrated that among 286 patients who received a combination of radiotherapy and chemotherapy, a relative risk of 5.5 for all secondary gastrointestinal tumors and of 8.3 for stomach cancer was observed. Such a risk was significantly higher than the risk for chemotherapy or radiotherapy alone (all gastrointestinal tumors RR of 0 and 2.9 respectively and stomach cancer RR of 0 and 4.4, respectively). These data supported a possible synergistic effect between the two modalities in the genesis of second solid tumors (Table 38.1, Van Leeuwen et al. 1993a).

A study examining chromosomal aberrations in peripheral blood lymphocytes of testicular cancer patients treated with chemotherapy and/or radiotherapy found the highest frequency of circulating aberrant cells in the subset of patients treated with second-line combined therapy, again suggesting a synergistic effect of chemotherapy and radiotherapy in increasing the risk of developing secondary malignancies (Gundy et al. 1992). It is apparent that further studies are needed to clarify this highly relevant issue.

## 38.6
## Second Malignancies Among Wilms' Tumor Survivors

A genetic predisposition to neoplasm susceptibility and/or a predisposition to a decreased genetic suppression of such neoplasms could be responsible for the development of some or most second malignant neoplasms among children. It has been shown that children who develop second neoplasms tend to have survived heritable tumors, such as retinoblastoma and Wilms' tumors, as initial cancers (Tucker et al. 1984). Especially since the use of chemotherapy and radiation therapy has significantly improved the long-term survival of Wilms' tumor patients (Green et al. 1991), an increased risk of second malignant neoplasms has emerged (Hawkins et al. 1987; Hartley et al. 1994).

In a study undertaken to document the incidence and characteristics of secondary malignancies, the records of 5278 Wilms' tumor patients accrued by the National Wilms' Tumor Study (NWTS) were reviewed. With a mean follow-up of 7.5 years, 43 secondary tumors were detected, including: 13 sarcomas, 13 carcinomas, nine leukemias, four lymphomas, three brain tumors, and one retinoblastoma. Three tertiary malignancies in three patients were also observed. In addition to the Wilms' tumor, one patient developed a basal cell carcinoma and a breast tumor, both found within the radiation field. Another patient was found to have a secondary malignant fibrous histiocytoma and a tertiary hepatocellular carcinoma diagnosed at autopsy. The third patient was diagnosed with a tumor of the cerebellum associated with acute myelogenous leukemia and a Wilms' tumor as well. The incidence of second malignancies rose with the increase in the dose of abdominal irradiation, the use of doxorubi-

cin, retreatment of relapse, and, as expected, the duration of follow-up (Breslow et al. 1995).

The standardized incidence ratio was estimated to increase by 43% for each 10 Gy of abdominal radiation in the absence of doxorubicin and to increase by 78% for each 10 Gy when radiation and doxorubicin were combined. Specifically, eight (3%) second malignant neoplasms were observed among 234 patients who received both doxorubicin and more than 35 Gy of abdominal radiation, whereas only 0.22% patients were expected. The risk of developing leukemia was 0.4% by the 8th year, after which no further cases occurred. Conversely, the risk of developing a solid tumor continued to increase with the increase in the duration of follow-up (Beir 1979). Retreatment at relapse increased the rate of second malignancies by a factor of 4.3 (Breslow et al. 1995). A recent study of risk factors for any second malignant neoplasm in childhood cancer patients demonstrated that the treatment with doxorubicin was the most significant factor identified using proportional hazards modeling (Green et al. 1994). Attempts have been made to clarify the role of doxorubicin in the pathogenesis of second malignancies. Doxorubicin inhibits the activity of topoisomerase II in the same fashion as other leukemogens such as etoposide (Long and Stringfellow 1988; Tewey et al. 1984), already mentioned in the chemotherapy of germ cell tumors. It is important to note that the doxorubicin dose used in all the published reports has been $300 \, mg/m^2$, while current protocols use lower doses. The cancerogenic effects of lower doses of doxorubicin have yet to be established. It is most likely that, as with etoposide therapy, doxorubicin-induced cancerogenesis may be dose-dependent.

Until more data are available, a policy of patient information and discussion of the known risks at the time of treatment decision is strongly recommended. The use of regimens that reduce radiation and doxorubicin doses should be encouraged. Moreover, physicians treating genitourinary cancer patients need to maintain an alertness to detect at an early stage the most common second tumors (GI tumors and sarcomas), since early diagnosis may significantly impact on these patients' survival.

## 38.7
## Outcome After Second Malignancies

The previously quoted study from Dieckmann et al. (1994) is quite interesting because it reports on the treatment used in patient management and the

**Table 38.7.** Clinical characteristics and outcome of the patients who developed second malignancies (excluding second cancers affecting the GI tract) (DIECKMANN et al. 1994)

| Patient no. | Histology of primary cancer | Age | Treatment of primary TC | Type of second cancer | Interval from TC (years) | Treatment | Outcome |
|---|---|---|---|---|---|---|---|
| 1 | Seminoma | 33 | Surgery | Basaloma RT | 23 | Surgery | NED 3 yr |
| 2 | Nonseminoma | 30 | Surgery | CML | 12 | CT | Dead of disease |
| 3 | Seminoma | 55 | Surgery | Bronchogenic ca. | 9 | Conservative | Dead of disease |
| 4 | Seminoma | 34 | Surgery RT | Promyelocytic leukemia | 6 | CT | NED 2 yr |
| 5 | Seminoma | 43 | Surgery RT | Laryngeal ca. | 13 | Surgery | Lost |
| 6 | Seminoma | 40 | Surgery RT | Renal cell ca. | 6 | Surgery | NED 18 mo |
| 7 | Seminoma | 24 | Surgery RT | Basaloma | 13 | Surgery | NED 5 yr |
| 8 | Seminoma | 42 | Surgery RT | Bronchogenic ca. | 16 | Surgery | NED 6 mo |

TC, Testicular cancer; RT, radiotherapy; CT, chemotherapy; NED, no evidence of disease.

**Table 38.8.** Clinical characteristics and outcome of the patients who developed secondary gastrointestinal malignancies (DIECKMANN et al. 1994; VAN LEEUWEN et al. 1993a)

| Patient no. | Histology of primary cancer | Age | Treatment of primary TC | Type of second cancer | Interval from TC (years) | Outcome |
|---|---|---|---|---|---|---|
| 1 | Seminoma | 40 | surgery RT | Stomach ca. | 12 | Dead of disease |
| 2 | Seminoma | 67 | RT | Stomach ca. | 7 | Dead of disease |
| 3 | MTI,T | 24 | RT | Stomach ca. | 12 | Dead of disease |
| 4 | Seminoma | 47 | RT | Stomach ca. | 9 | NED 88 mo |
| 5 | Seminoma | 48 | RT | Stomach ca. | 16 | Dead of disease |
| 6 | MUT,E | 58 | RT | Stomach ca. | 14 | Dead of disease |
| 7 | MTU,E | 24 | RT + CT | Stomach ca. | 9 | Dead of disease |
| 8 | Sertoli cell | 49 | RT | Stomach ca. | 9 | Alive, 25 mo |
| 9 | MTI,T | 38 | RT | Stomach ca. | 16 | Dead of disease |
| 10 | Seminoma | 42 | RT | Stomach ca. | 20 | Dead of disease |
| 11 | MTI,T | 36 | RT | Stomach ca. | 9 | Dead of disease |
| 12 | Seminoma | 51 | RT | Stomach ca. | 17 | NED 21 mo |
| 13 | Seminoma | 61 | surgery RT | Colon ca. | 1 | Dead of disease |
| 14 | Nonseminoma | 34 | surgery RT | Esophageal ca. | 14 | Lost |
| 15 | Nonseminoma | 23 | surgery RT | Pancreatic ca. | 12 | NED 6 mo |

MTI, Malignant teratoma intermediate; T, teratocarcinoma; MTU, malignant teratoma undifferentiated; E, embryonal carcinoma.

outcome for secondary malignancies. Table 38.7 summarizes the clinical characteristics and outcome of the patients who developed secondary malignancies (excluding second cancers affecting the GI tract) in this series. The outcome of second malignancies in patients from this small series suggests that non-GI tract tumors after treatment for testicular cancer behave similarly to their primary counterpart. This is important information for both treating physicians and testicular cancer patients.

The data regarding outcome after gastrointestinal tract second malignancies appear to be different. Table 38.8 combines the information made available by DIECKMANN et al. (1994) on four gastrointestinal tract second malignancies from their study and the data from VAN LEEUWEN et al. (1993a) on 11 patients who developed stomach cancer after testicular cancer. At the time of the reports 10/15 (67%) patients had died of their second malignancies, one patient was alive with disease, one was lost to follow-up, and only three (20%) were alive with no evidence of recurrent tumor. All the gastrointestinal malignancies occurred in irradiated patients and the median interval from the primary cancer to the diagnosis of the second malignancy was 12 years (range 1–20 years). These data are consistent with the known pattern of radiation-induced carcinogenesis (SMITH and DOLL 1981; KATO and SCHULL 1982).

Few data are available regarding the outcome of postirradiation secondary sarcomas in patients with primary germ cell tumors. ROBINSON et al. (1988) reported on postirradiation sarcomas and found a worse prognosis associated with second sarcomas compared with their primary counterpart. Most of these tumors were diagnosed at an advanced stage, were high grade, and responded poorly to treatment. Median survival was 12 months, with only 11% of the patients alive at 5 years (ROBINSON et al. 1988). However, only a minority of the described patients had an initial genitourinary tumor and among these most were survivors of Wilms' tumors.

## 38.8
## Conclusions

Despite the complexity of the available data on second malignancies in patients with genitourinary cancers and in spite of the possible pitfalls associated with their interpretation, several conclusions can be drawn. First of all, patients surviving germ cell tumors and those surviving Wilms' tumors are known to be the main two groups at risk for second malignancies.

Radiotherapy increases the relative risk of developing a second neoplasm by a factor of 2–3. This is true even in patients treated with the currently available standard technology and the use of new treatment regimens. The risk of second malignancies, although lower than that reported in older series, is still there. The risk for developing certain subgroups of tumors, such as sarcomas or carcinomas of the gastrointestinal or genitourinary tract, seems to be clearly higher (relative risk ranging from 2.7 to 3.6). Most second tumors (>80%) develop within the radiation fields. Radiation dose, radiation fields, and possibly radiation type play a significant role in the genesis of a second neoplasm. The development of new radiation techniques, like conformal therapy, might further decrease the risk of radiation-induced cancerogenesis. In the meantime, since the benefits of radiation therapy in the treatment of early-stage seminoma of the testicle clearly outweigh the risk involved, its use should continue (VAN LEEUWEN et al. 1993a). A routine surveillance for second cancers during follow-up, associated with avoidance of unnecessary radiation exposure, should be the only precaution. Since second solid cancers might occur even up to 20 years from the radiation therapy administration, the patients should be informed about this long-term risk and monitored periodically with particular attention to signs and symptoms that are typically associated with the more likely second malignancies.

The role of chemotherapy in the development of second solid tumors is negligible, while it is clearly defined in the pathogenesis of secondary leukemias. However, even in this case, the advantages of chemotherapy are usually far superior to its leukemogenic risk. Etoposide has been determined to be a dangerous drug in terms of the risk of second tumors. The risk associated with its administration can be markedly reduced when lower doses in a monthly schedule are used. As clearly documented by VAN LEEUWEN et al. (1993a) and by BRESLOW et al. (1995), the combination of radiotherapy and doxorubicin carries a synergistic effect in second cancerogenesis, as shown in the treatment of primary Wilms' tumors. Unfortunately, their combination is often warranted by the recurrence of a tumor resistant to the first-line therapy. In such a setting taking the risk of secondary malignancies is most of the time an inevitable choice.

Finally, while a baseline genetic predisposition to multiple malignancies (other than contralateral testicular cancer) among testicular cancer patients has not been fully proven, a familial type of testicular cancer has been described. Further studies will address the issue of whether familial testicular cancer is associated with an increased risk of secondary malignancies in addition to the already described increased incidence of contralateral testicular tumors.

In fact, a better understanding of genetic cancer syndromes and their molecular biology could support the hypothesis that a genetic predisposition may play a role in the development of additional cancers in the same patient or may predispose to the development of second neoplasms after radiotherapy and/or chemotherapy. Inherited deficits in cell repair could indeed manifest both as a genetic predisposition to multiple malignancies and as a higher risk of second tumors after mutagenic treatment.

## References

Amichetti M, Boi A (1993) Postirradiation sarcoma in a patient treated for testicular seminoma. Oncology 50: 264–266

Anonymous (1988) Cyclophosphamide and tamoxifen as adjuvant therapies in the management of breast cancer. CRC Adjuvant Breast Trial Working Party. Br J Cancer 57: 604–607

Bajorin DF, Motzer RJ, Rodriguez E, et al. (1993) Acute nonlymphocytic leukemia in germ cell tumor patients treated with etoposide-containing chemotherapy. J Natl Cancer Inst 85:60–62

Beir V (1979) Biological effects of ionizing radiation. United States Department of Health, Education and Welfare Public Health Services, National Institutes of Health, Bethesda, Md.

Bokemeyer C, Schmoll HJ (1993) Second neoplasms following treatment of malignant germ cell tumors. J Clin Oncol 11:1703–1709

Bokemeyer C, Freund M, Schmoll HJ, et al. (1992) Second lymphoblastic leukemia following treatment of a malignant germ cell tumour. Ann Oncol 3:772

Boshoff CH, Begent RHJ, Oliver RTD, et al. (1994) Second tumours following etoposide containing therapy for germ cell cancer (abstract). Proc Am Soc Clin Oncol 13:245

Bosl GJ, Dmitrovsky E, Reuter V, et al. (1989) Isochromosome of chromosome 12: clinically useful marker for male germ cell tumors. J Natl Cancer Inst 81:1874–1878

Boyer M, Raghavan D (1992) Toxicity of treatment of germ cell tumors. Semin Oncol 19:128–142

Breslow NE, Takashima JR, Whitton JA, Mokness J, D'Angio GJ, Green DM (1995) Second malignant neoplasms following treatment for Wilms'tumor: a report from the National Wilms' Tumor Study Group. J Clin Oncol 13:1851–1859

Cavenee WK, Dryja TP, Phillips RA, et al. (1983) Expression of recessive alleles by chromosomal mechanisms in retinoblastoma. Nature 305:779–784

Chilvers CED, Pike MC (1989) Epidemiology of undescended testis. In: Oliver RTD, Blandy JP, Hope-Stone HF (eds) Urological and genital cancer. Blackwell Scientific, Oxford, pp 306–321

Cimino G, Moir DT, Canaani O, et al. (1991) Cloning of ALL-1, the locus involved in leukemias with the t(4;11) q(21;23), t(9;11) (p22;q23), and t(11;19) (q23;p13) chromosome translocations. Cancer Res 51:6712–6714

Coleman C, Kaplan H, Cox R, et al. (1982) Leukemias, non-Hodgkin's lymphomas and solid tumours in patients treated for Hodgkin's disease. Cancer Surv 1: 734–744

Coleman MP, Bell CMJ, Fraser P (1987) Second primary malignancy after Hodgkin's disease, ovarian cancer and cancer of the testis: a population-based cohort study. Br J Cancer 56:349–355

De Vore R, Whitlock J, Hainsworth JD, et al. (1989) Therapy related acute nonlymphocytic leukemia with monocytic features and rearrangement of chromosome 11q. Ann Intern Med 110:740–742

Dieckmann KP, Boeckmann W, Brosig W, et al. (1986) Bilateral testicular germ cell tumors. Report of 9 cases and review of the literature. Cancer 57:1254–1258

Dieckmann KP, Wegner HEH, Krain J (1994) Multiple primary neoplasms in patients with testicular germ cell tumor. Oncology 51:450–458

Draper GJ, Sanders BM, Kingston JE (1986) Second primary neoplasms in patients with retinoblastoma. Br J Cancer 53:661–671

Easton D, Peto J (1990) The contribution of inherited predisposition to cancer incidence. Cancer Surv 9:395

Forman D (1989) Epidemiology of testis cancer. In: Oliver RTD, Blandy JP, Hope-Stone HF (eds). Urological and genital cancer. Blackwell Scientific, Oxford, pp 289–305

Forman D, Olover RTD, Brett AR, et al. (1992) Familial testicular cancer: a report of the UK family register, estimation of risk and an HLA Class 1 sib-pair analysis. Br J Cancer 65:255–262

Fossa SD, Aass N, Kaalhus O (1989) Radiotherapy for testicular seminoma stage I: treatment results and long-term post-irradiation morbidity in 365 patients. Int J Radiat Oncol Biol Phys 16:383–388

Friend SH, Bernards R, Rogelj S, et al. (1986) A human DNA segment with properties of the gene that predisposes to retinoblastoma and osteosarcoma. Nature 323:643–646

Gilks B, Hegedus C, Freeman H, et al. (1988) Malignant peritoneal mesothelioma after remote abdominal radiation. Cancer 61:2019–2021

Green DM, Finklestein JZ, Breslow NE, et al. (1991) Remaining problems in the treatment of patients with Wilms' tumor. Pediatr Clin North Am 38:475–488

Green DM, Zevon MA, Reese PA, et al. (1994) Second malignant tumors following treatment during childhood and adolescence for cancer. Med Pediatr Oncol 22:1–10

Gundy S, Baki M, Bodrogi I (1992) Spontaneous and cytostatic therapy induced chromosome aberrations in testicular cancer patients. Orv Hetil 133:3141–3146

Hanks GE, Peters T, Owen J (1992) Seminoma of the testis: long term beneficial and deleterious results of radiation. Int J Radiat Oncol Biol Phys 24:913–919

Hartley AL, Birch JM, Blair V, et al. (1994) Second neoplasm in a population-based series of patients diagnosed in renal tumours in childhood. Med Pediatr Oncol 22: 318–324

Hawkins MM, Draper GJ, Kingston JE (1987) Incidence of second primary tumours among childhood cancer survivors. Br J Cancer 56:339–347

Hay JH, Duncan W, Kerr GR (1984) Subsequent malignancies in patients irradiated for testicular tumours. Br J Radiol 57:597–602

Hellbardt A, Mirimanoff RO, Obradovic M, et al. (1990) The risk of second cancer (sc) in patients treated for testicular seminoma. Int J Radiat Oncol Biol Phys 18:1327–1331

Jacobsen GK, Mellemgaard A, Engelholm SA, et al. (1993) Increased incidence of sarcoma in patients treated for testicular seminoma. Eur J Cancer 29:664–668

Kaldor JM, Day NE, Band P, et al. (1987) Second malignancies following testicular cancer, ovarian cancer and Hodgkin's disease: an international collaborative study among cancer registries. Int J Cancer 39:571–585

Kato H, Schull WJ (1982) Studies of the mortality of the A-bomb survivors. 7. Mortality, 1950–1978. Part 1. Cancer mortality. Radiat Res 90:395–432

Kerbrat P, LePrise PY (1985) Acute leukemia following testicular carcinoma. J Clin Oncol 3:1287

Kleinerman RA, Lieberman JV, Li FP (1985) Second cancer following cancer of the male genital system in Connecticut, 1935–82. NCI Monogr 68:139–147

LeBeau MM, Albain KS, Larson RA, et al. (1986) Clinical and cytogenetic correlations in 63 patients with therapy-related myelodysplastic syndromes and acute nonlymphocytic leukemia: further evidence for characteristic abnormalities of chromosomes no. 5 and 7. J Clin Oncol 4:325–345

Li FP , Fraumeni JF Jr, Mulvihill JJ, et al. (1988) A cancer family syndrome. JAMA 48:5358–5362

Long BH, Stringfellow DA (1988) Inhibitors of topoisomerase II: structure-activity relationships and mechanisms of action of podophyllin congeners. Adv Enzyme Regul 27:223–256

Lynch DF, Herr HW (1981) Radiation-induced sarcoma following radiotherapy for testicular tumor. J Urol 126: 845–846

Malkin D, Jolly KW, Barbier N, et al. (1992) Germ line mutations of the p 53 tumor-suppressor gene in children and young adults with second malignant neoplasms. N Engl J Med 326:1309–1315

Meadows AT, D'Angio GJ, Mike V, et al. (1977) Patterns of second malignant neoplasms in children. Cancer 40: 1903–1911

Moeller H, Mellemgaard A, Jacobsen GK, et al. (1993) Incidence of second primary cancer following testicular cancer. Eur J Cancer 29:672–676

Muir C, Wterhouse J, Mack T, et al. (1987) Cancer incidence in five continents, vol 5. International Agency of Research on Cancer, Lyon

Nichols CR, Roth BJ, Heerema N, et al. (1990) Hematologic neoplasia associated with primary mediastinal germ cell tumours. N Engl J Med 322:1425–1429

Nichols CR, Breeden ES, Loehrer PJ, et al. (1993) Second leukemia associated with conventional dose of etoposide: review of serial germ cell tumor protocols. J Natl Cancer Inst 85:36–40

O'Brien WM, Abbondanzo SL, Chun BK, et al. (1989) Neurogenic fibrosarcoma following radiation therapy for seminoma. Urology 33:420–423

Oliver RT, Ong JYH, Raja MA, et al. (1991) Second preleukemia and etoposide. Lancet 338:359–363

Ozols RF, Ihde DC, Linehan WM, Jacob J, Ostchega Y, Young RC (1988) A randomized trial of standard chemotherapy vs high dose chemotherapy regimen in the treatment of poor prognosis nonseminomatous germ-cell tumors. J Clin Oncol 6:1031–1040

Pedersen-Bjergaard JP, Philip P (1991) Balanced translocations involving chromosome bands 11q23 and 21q22 are highly characteristic of myelodysplasia and leukemia following therapy with cytostatic agents targeting at DNA-topoisomerase II. Blood 78:1147–1148

Pedersen-Bjergaard J, Daugaard G, Hansen SW, et al. (1991) Increased risk of myelodysplasia and leukemia after etoposide, cisplatin and bleomycin for germ cell tumors. Lancet 338:359–363

Pedersen-Bjergaard J, Sigsgaard TC, Nielsen D, et al. (1992) Acute monocytic or myelomonocytic leukemia with balanced chromosome translocations to band 11q23 after therapy with 4-epi-doxorubicin and cisplatin or cyclophosphamide for breast cancer. J Clin Oncol 10:1444–1451

Pui C-H, Ribeiro R, Hancock M, et al. (1991) Acute myeloid leukemia in children treated with epipodophyllotoxins for acute lymphoblastic leukemia. N Engl J Med 325: 1682–1687

Raz HR, Maurer R, von Hochstetter A, et al. (1989) Angiosarkomnach Teratokarzinom: "Mutation", sukzessives Malignom oder Bestrahlung. Helv Chir Acta 56: 355–357

Redman JR, Vugrin D, Arlin ZA, et al. (1984) Leukemia following treatment of germ cell tumours in men. J Clin Oncol 2:1080–1087

Robinson E, Neugut AI, Wylie P (1988) Clinical aspects of postirradiation sarcomas. J Natl Cancer Inst 80: 233–240

Roth BJ, Greist A, Kubilis PS, Williams SD, Einhorn LH (1988) Cisplatin-based combination chemotherapy for disseminated germ cell tumors: long-term follow-up. J Clin Oncol 6:1239–1247

Savage MO, Lowe DG (1990) Gonadal neoplasia and abnormal sexual differentiation. Clin Endocrinol 32:519–533

Schmidt A, Kob D, Kosmehl H (1988) Zur Kenntnis strahlenbedingter Sarkome. Mitteilung über 2 Beobachtungen. Zentrabl Allg Pathol 134:41–45

Smith PG, Doll R (1981) Mortality among patients with ankylosing spondylitis after single treatment course with X-rays. Br Med J 284:449–460

Steinfeld AD, Shore RE (1990) Second malignancies following radiotherapy for testicular seminoma. Clin Oncol R Coll Radiol 2:273–276

Stock RJ, Fu YS, Carter JR (1979) Malignant peritoneal mesothelioma following radiotherapy for seminoma of the testis. Cancer 44:914–919

Sugita K, Furukawa T, Tsuchida M, et al. (1993) High frequency of etoposide (VP-16)-related second leukemia in children with non-Hodgkin's lymphoma. Am J Pediatr Hematol Oncol 15:99–104

Tan KB, Mattern MR, Boyce RA, Schein PS (1987) Elevated DNA topoisomerase II activity in nitrogen mustard-resistant human cells. Proc Natl Acad Sci USA 84: 7668–7671

Tewey KM, Chen GL, Nelson EM, et al. (1984) Adriamycin-induced DNA damage mediated by mammalian DNA topoisomerase II. Science 226:446–468

Tucker MA, Meadows AT, Boice JD Jr, Hoover RN, Fraumeni JF (1984) Cancer risk following treatment of childhood cancer In: Boice JD, Fraumeni JF Jr (eds) Radiation cancerogenesis: epidemiology and biological significance. Raven Press, New York, pp 211–224

van Imhoff GW, Sleijfer DT, Breuning MH, et al. (1986) Acute nonlymphocytic leukemia 5 years after treatment with cisplatin, vinblastine and bleomycin for disseminated testicular cancer. Cancer 57:984–987

van Leeuwen FE, Stiggelbout AM, van der Belt-Dusebout AW, et al. (1993a) Second cancer risk following testicular cancer: a follow-up study of 1909 patients. J Clin Oncol 11: 415–424

van Leeuwen FE, Stiggelbout AM, van der Belt-Dusebout AW, et al. (1993b) Second tumors after radiation treatment of testicular germ cell tumors (correspondence). J Clin Oncol 11:2286–2287

von der Maase H, Rorth M, Walbom-Jorgensen S, et al. (1986) Carcinoma in situ of contralateral testis in patients with testicular germ cell cancer: a study of 27 cases in 500 patients. Br Med J 293:1398–1401

von der Maase H, Specht L, Jacobsen GK, et al. (1993) Surveillance following orchiectomy for stage I seminoma of the testis. Eur J Cancer 29:1931–1934

Whitlock JA, Greer JP, Lukas JN (1991) Epipodophyllotoxin-related leukemia. Identification of a new subset of second leukemia. Cancer 68:600–604

Wiggs J, Nordenskjold M, Yandell D, et al. (1988) Prediction of the risk of hereditary retinoblastoma, using DNA polymorphism within the retinoblastoma gene. N Engl J Med 318:151–157

Yandell DW, Campbell TA, Dayton SH, et al. (1989) Oncogenic point mutations in the human retinoblastoma gene: their application to genetic counseling. N Engl J Med 321:1689–1695

Yoshitake T, Takahama T, Suzuki T, et al. (1991) Osteosarcoma developing after radiation and chemotherapy for primary mediastinal seminoma. Nippon Kyobu Geka Gakkai Zasshi 39:424–429

# Subject Index

# List of Contributors

Joost A. L. L. Baert, MD
Pediatric Urologist
Beatrix Children's Hospital
University Hospital Groningen
Postbus 3001
9700 RB Groningen
The Netherlands

Luc V. Baert, MD, PhD
Professor and Chairman, Department of Urology
University Hospitals Gasthuisberg
Catholic University of Leuven
Herestraat 49
B-3000 Leuven
Belgium

Michael Bamberg, MD
Professor, Department of Radiotherapy
Eberhard-Karls-Universität
Hoppe-Seyler-Strasse 3
D-72076 Tübingen
Germany

Arie Belldegrun, MD
Professor of Urology
Chief, Division of Urologic Oncology
Department of Urology
UCLA School of Medicine
10945 LeConte Avenue
Suite 2333
Los Angeles, CA 90095
USA

Guy A. Bogaert, MD
Professor of Pediatric Urology
Department of Urology
University Hospitals Gasthuisberg
Catholic University of Leuven
Herestraat 49
B-3000 Leuven
Belgium

Roger Bouillon, MD, PhD
Professor and Chairman
Laboratory and Clinic of Experimental Medicine
and Endocrinology
University Hospitals Gasthuisberg
Catholic University of Leuven
Herestraat 49
B-3000 Leuven
Belgium

Luther W. Brady, MD
Hylda Cohn/American Cancer Society
Professor of Clinical Oncology, and
Professor, Department of Radiation Oncology
Allegheny University of the Health Sciences
Allegheny University Hospitals, Hahnemann
230 North Broad Street, Mail Stop 200
Philadelphia, PA 19102-1192
USA

Charles Catton, MD, FRCPC
Department of Radiation Oncology
The Princess Margaret Hospital
610 University Avenue, Room 4-728
Toronto, ON M5G 2M9
Canada

J. Classen, MD
Department of Radiotherapy
Eberhard-Karls-Universität
Hoppe-Seyler-Strasse 3
D-72076 Tübingen
Germany

Francesca A. Corso, MD
Department of Radiation Oncology
University of Southern California
School of Medicine
1441469 Eastlake Ave.
Los Angeles, CA 90033-0804
USA

Paola Dal Cin, PhD
Center for Human Genetics
University Hospitals Gasthuisberg
Catholic University of Leuven
Herestraat 49
B-3000 Leuven
Belgium

Dirk J.M.K. De Ridder, MD
Consultant Urologist
Department of Urology and Fertility Center Leuven
University Hospitals Gasthuisberg
Catholic University of Leuven
Herestraat 49
B-3000 Leuven
Belgium

Herlinde Dumez, MD
Resident, Department of Oncology
University Hospitals Gasthuisberg
Catholic University of Leuven
Herestraat 49
B-3000 Leuven
Belgium

MICHAEL DZEDA, MD
Department of Radiation Oncology
Allegheny University of the Health Sciences
Allegheny University Hospitals, Hahnemann
230 North Broad Street, Mail Stop 200
Philadelphia, PA 19102-1192
USA

ROBERT A. FIGLIN, MD
Professor of Medicine
Division of Hematology/Oncology
Department of Medicine
UCLA School of Medicine
10945 LeConte Avenue
Suite 2333
Los Angeles, CA 90095
USA

ARSENIO J. FIGUEROA, MD
Chief Resident
Department of Urology
University of Southern California
Norris Comprehensive Cancer Center, MS # 74
1441 Eastlake Avenue, Suite 7414
Los Angeles, CA 90033
USA

SILVIA C. FORMENTI, MD
Associate Professor
Department of Radiation, Oncology, and Medicine
University of Southern California
School of Medicine
1441 Eastlake Ave.
Los Angeles, CA 90033-0804
USA

BRIAN E. HENDERSON, MD
Department of Preventive Medicine and
Norris Comprehensive Cancer Center
1441 Eastlake Avenue
Los Angeles, CA 90033-0800
USA

SIMON HORENBLAS, MD, PhD
Head, Department of Urology
Netherlands Cancer Institute
Antoni van Leeuwenhoek Hospital
Plesmanlaan 121
1066 CX Amsterdam
The Netherlands

GABOR JOZSEF, PhD
Department of Radiation Oncology
University of Southern California
School of Medicine
Kenneth Norris Jr. Cancer Hospital
and Research Institute
1441 Eastlake Avenue
P.O. 33804
Los Angeles, CA 90033-0804
USA

BARRY A. KOGAN, MD
Professor and Chief
Division of Urology, K209/A-108
The Albany Medical College
47 New Scotland Avenue
Albany, NY 12208-3479
USA

JOHN E. LAHANIATIS, MD
Department of Radiation Oncology
Allegheny University of the Health Sciences
Allegheny University Hospitals, Hahnemann
230 North Broad Street, Mail Stop 200
Philadelphia, PA 19102-1192
USA

ROBERT LAVEY, MD
Department of Radiation Oncology
Children's Hospital Los Angeles
4650 Sunset Blvd.
Los Angeles, CA 90027
USA

BRIAN K. LEE, MD
Department of Radiation Oncology
Allegheny University of the Health Sciences
Allegheny University Hospitals, Hahnemann
230 North Broad Street, Mail Stop 200
Philadelphia, PA 19102-1192
USA

BIZHAN MICAILY, MD
Department of Radiation Oncology
Allegheny University of the Health Sciences
Allegheny University Hospitals, Hahnemann
230 North Broad Street, Mail Stop 200
Philadelphia, PA 19102-1192
USA

JEFF M. MICHALSKI, MD
Department of Radiology
Mallinckrodt Institute of Radiology
Washington University School of Medicine
St. Louis, MO 63110
USA

ANNE MOHRBACHER, MD
Department of Hematology
USC School of Medicine
1441 Eastlake Ave.
Los Angeles CA 90033
USA

PETER W. NICHOLS, MD
Professor of Pathology
Director of Laboratories
Kenneth Norris Jr. Cancer Hospital
and Research Institute
USC School of Medicine
1441 Eastlake Ave
Los Angeles CA 90033
USA

RIEN J.M. NIJMAN, MD, PhD
Head, Department of Pediatric Urology
Sophia Children's Hospital
University Hospital Rotterdam
Postbus 2060
3000 CB Rotterdam
The Netherlands

RAYMOND H. OYEN, MD, PhD
Adjunct Clinic Head
Department of Radiology
University Hospitals Gasthuisberg
Catholic University of Leuven
Herestraat 49
B-3000 Leuven
Belgium

Howard Ozer, MD
Chief, Hematology/Oncology
Department of Medicine
Cancer Center Director
Allegheny University Hospitals, Hahnemann
Broad & Vine Sts., Mail Stop 487
Philadelphia, PA 19102-1192
USA

A. Pawinski, MD
Department of Oncology
University Hospitals Gasthuisberg
Catholic University of Leuven
Herestraat 49
B-3000 Leuven
Belgium

C. Leigh Pearce, MPH
Department of Preventive Medicine
Norris Comprehensive Cancer Center
1441 Eastlake Avenue
Los Angeles, CA 90033-0800
USA

Zbigniew Petrovich, MD, FACR
Professor of Radiation Oncology and Urology
Chairman, Department of Radiation Oncology
University of Southern California
School of Medicine
Kenneth Norris Jr. Cancer Hospital
and Research Institute
1441 Eastlake Avenue
Room 34, P.O. 33804
Los Angeles, CA 90033-0804
USA

Henricus Raat, MD
Department of Radiology
University Hospitals Gasthuisberg
Catholic University of Leuven
Herestraat 49
B-3000 Leuven
Belgium

Mack Roach, III, MD
Associate Professor of Radiation Oncology,
Medical Oncology and Urology
University of California at San Francisco School of Medicine
Mt. Zion Cancer Center
2356 Sutter Street
San Francisco, CA 94115
USA

Tania Roskams, MD, PhD
Professor, Department of Pathology
University Hospitals (K.U. Leuven)
Minderbroederstraat 12
B-3000 Leuven
Belgium

Ronald K. Ross, MD
Department of Preventive Medicine
University of Southern California
Norris Comprehensive Cancer Center
1441 Eastlake Avenue
Los Angeles, CA 90033-0800
USA

Carol E. Salem, MD
Urologic Oncology Fellow
University of Southern California
School of Medicine
Department of Urology
1441 Eastlake Ave, Suite 7414, MS-74
Los Angeles, CA 90033
USA

Donald G. Skinner, MD
Professor and Chairman
University of Southern California
School of Medicine
Department of Urology
1441 Eastlake Ave, Suite 7414, MS-74
Los Angeles, CA 90033
USA

Eila C. Skinner, MD
Assistant Professor of Clinical Urology
Department of Urology
University of Southern California
Norris Comprehensive Cancer Center, MS # 74
1441 Eastlake Ave, Suite 7414
Los Angeles, CA 90033
USA

John P. Stein, MD
Assistant Professor of Urology
University of Southern California
School of Medicine
Department of Urology
1441 Eastlake Ave, Suite 7414, MS-74
Los Angeles, CA 90033
USA

Luc Stockx, MD
Department of Radiology
University Hospitals Gasthuisberg
Catholic University of Leuven
Herestraat 49
B-3000 Leuven
Belgium

Oscar E. Streeter, Jr., MD
Associate Professor of Clinical Radiation Oncology
University of Southern California
School of Medicine
Chief, Radiation Oncology
Norris Comprehensive Cancer Center
1441 Eastlake Avenue, NOR 002
Los Angeles CA 90033-0804
USA

Steven J. Tucker, MD
Fellow, Hematology/Oncology
Division of Hematology/Oncology
Department of Medicine
UCLA School of Medicine
10945 LeConte Avenue
Suite 2333
Los Angeles, CA 90095
USA

Boudewijn Van Damme, MD, PhD
Professor and Chairman
Department of Pathology
University Hospitals (K.U. Leuven)
Minderbroederstraat 12
B-3000 Leuven
Belgium

H. Van Den Berghe, PhD
Professor and Chairman
Center for Human Genetics
University Hospitals Gasthuisberg
Catholic University of Leuven
Herestraat 49
B-3000 Leuven
Belgium

A. Van den Bruel, MD
Laboratory and Clinic of Experimental Medicine
and Endocrinology
University Hospitals Gasthuisberg
Catholic University of Leuven
Herestraat 49
B-3000 Leuven
Belgium

Allan Van Oosterom, MD, PhD
Professor and Chairman
Department of Oncology
University Hospitals Gasthuisberg
Catholic University of Leuven
Herestraat 49
B-3000 Leuven
Belgium

Hein P. Van Poppel, MD, PhD
Professor of Oncologic Urology
Department of Urology
University Hospitals Gasthuisberg
Catholic University of Leuven
Herestraat 49
B-3000 Leuven
Belgium

Luc Vanuytsel, MD, PhD
Department of Oncology
Section of Radiotherapy
University Hospitals Gasthuisberg
Catholic University of Leuven
Herestraat 49
B-3000 Leuven
Belgium

Berit M. Verbist, MD
Department of Radiology
University Hospitals Gasthuisberg
Catholic University of Leuven
Herestraat 49
B-3000 Leuven
Belgium

Geert A. Verswijvel, MD
Department of Radiology
University Hospitals Gasthuisberg
Catholic University of Leuven
Herestraat 49
B-3000 Leuven
Belgium

W. Wynendaele, MD
Department of Oncology
University Hospitals Gasthuisberg
Catholic University of Leuven
Herestraat 49
B-3000 Leuven
Belgium

Cheng Yu, PhD
Assistant Professor of Radiation Oncology
Department of Radiation Oncology
University of Southern California
School of Medicine
Kenneth Norris Jr. Cancer Hospital
and Research Institute
1441 Eastlake Avenue
P.O. Box 33804
Los Angeles, CA 90033-0804
USA

Mimi C. Yu, PhD
Professor of Preventive Medicine
Department of Preventive Medicine
University of Southern California
Norris Comprehensive Cancer Center
1441 Eastlake Avenue
Los Angeles, CA 90033-0800
USA

Jian-Min Yuan, MD, PhD
Department of Preventive Medicine
University of Southern California
Norris Comprehensive Cancer Center
1441 Eastlake Avenue
Los Angeles, CA 90033-0800
USA

Chi-Shing Zee, MD
Department of Radiology
University of Southern California
School of Medicine
Kenneth Norris Jr. Cancer Hospital
and Research Institute
1441 Eastlake Avenue
P.O. 33804
Los Angeles, CA 90033-0804
USA

# MEDICAL RADIOLOGY
## Diagnostic Imaging and Radiation Oncology

*Titles in the series already published*

DATE DUE